CARDIAC RHYTHM DISORDERS

A Nursing Process Approach

CARDIAC RHYTHM DISORDERS

A Nursing Process Approach

PATRICIA LOUNSBURY, BSN, MEd, RN, CCRN
Clinical Nursing Specialist II
Coordinator of the Cardiovascular Rehabilitation Center
University of Iowa Hospitals and Clinics
Iowa City, Iowa

SUSAN J. FRYE, MSN, JD, RN
Health and Nursing Consultant
Attorney—Health and Environmental Law
Iowa City, Iowa

Second Edition

with 422 illustrations

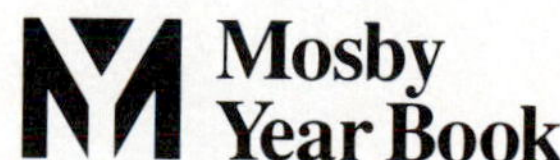

St. Louis Baltimore Boston Chicago London Philadelphia Sydney Toronto

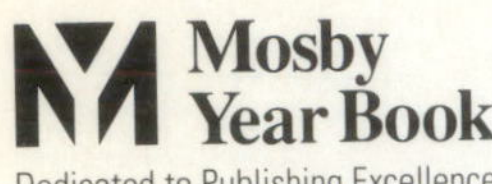

Dedicated to Publishing Excellence

Editor: Terry Van Schaik
Developmental Editor: Jeanne Rowland
Project Manager: Carol Sullivan Wiseman
Production Editor: Diana Lyn Laulainen
Designer: Julie Taugner
Cover Illustrator: Jean Calder

SECOND EDITION

Printed in the United States of America

Mosby–Year Book, Inc.
11830 Westline Industrial Drive
St. Louis, Missouri 63146

Library of Congress Cataloging in Publication Data
Lounsbury, Patricia S. Frye
Cardiac rhythm disorders : a nursing process approach / Patricia Lounsbury, Susan J. Frye.
p. cm.
Frye's name appears first on the earlier edition.
Includes bibliographical references and index.
ISBN 0-8016-6576-0 : $29.00
1. Arrhythmia—Nursing. 2. Electrocardiography. I. Frye, Susan J. II. Title.
[DNLM: 1. Arrhythmia—nursing. 2. Electrocardiography—nursing. WY i52.5 L889c]
RC685.A65L59 1992
616.1'28'0024613—dc20
DNLM/DLC
for Library of Congress

91-46329
CIP

92 93 94 95 96 CL/MV 9 8 7 6 5 4 3 2 1

Contributors

MICHAEL G. KIENZLE, MD

Associate Professor of Medicine,
Department of Internal Medicine,
Assistant Director, Division of Cardiovascular Diseases
Director, Clinical Cardiac Electrophysiology
University of Iowa Clinics and Hospitals
Iowa City, Iowa

MARY JO YTZEN, RN, CCRN

Critical Care and Cardiac Rehabilitation
Iowa Lutheran Hospital
Des Moines, Iowa

Dedicated to
William H. Lounsbury, Sr.
Mark C. Mathis II

Preface

Electrocardiography has, for the past several years, been a rather stable subject. Books on arrhythmias did not change much from edition to edition and treatments for arrhythmias remained relatively stable as well. In the last few years, however, electrocardiography and arrhythmia interpretation have enjoyed robust study and offer a rapidly changing discipline based on electrophysiology studies. Electrophysiology studies take much of the guesswork out of arrhythmia interpretation, and it is now time to educate new students of arrhythmias in the fundamental principles electrophysiology offers. Additionally, Holter monitoring is providing new definitions of "normal."

Cardiac Rhythm Disorders: A Nursing Process Approach grew out of a persistent need for a textbook on arrhythmias that *(1)* was based on electrophysiologic facts, *(2)* was written for the adult student using adult education principles, *(3)* was easy to understand, *(4)* was not directed solely to coronary care unit nurses, *(5)* included enough arrhythmias and 12-lead electrocardiogram analyses to allow independent and autonomous study, and *(6)* paved the way for further study in arrhythmias by providing a sturdy educational foundation in electrocardiography.

We have found, as countless others have, that teaching a course in arrhythmias requires formulating numerous study guides and photocopying countless arrhythmias to supplement the texts being used. Thus many instructors opt not to use a text at all because so many are found to be incomplete, inappropriate for their audience, and/or not factual. *Cardiac Rhythm Disorders: A Nursing Process Approach* is a reader-friendly work that can be used for an individualized learning project or as a text for a course in a classroom situation at the baccalaureate, graduate, or clinical level. Since it has many electrocardiographic illustrations, the instructor need not search for additional examples. The book is organized in such a way that the learner may progress through it without being impeded by unfamiliar terms.

Cardiac Rhythm Disorders: A Nursing Process Approach presents each arrhythmia in the nursing process format. Chapter 4 explains application of the nursing process and nursing diagnoses appropriate for arrhythmias. Such consistency in approach lends security to the new learner and fosters the development of the nursing process as a problem-solving method.

The second edition of *Cardiac Rhythm Disorders* is substantially expanded and revised. Thirteen chapters replace the former eight chapters. The bibliographies are significantly updated and enlarged.

We updated the book primarily in the areas of pharmacologic and nonpharmacologic antiarrhythmic therapy. Advances in cardiac monitoring are included with discussions of signal-averaged electrocardiography and heart rate variability. We added a new chapter on differential diagnosis of wide QRS complexes. The subjects of supraventricular and ventricular arrhythmias and nursing diagnosis of cardiac rhythm disorders are substantially revised. New information is included in the area of management of cardiac rhythm disorders in infants, children, and adolescents.

Because the book is intended for a variety of settings, it is not a critical care unit arrhythmia book. Although it contains information about arrhythmias associated with myocardial infarction, it transcends all age and diagnostic groups. It includes cardioactive drugs and nursing implications, cardiac pacing, and techniques of cardioversion and defibrillation.

We have found, through many years of teaching this subject, that numerous fallacies about arrhythmias are perpetuated like rumors, not based in fact. A factual volume such as this, and a bibliography of research-based articles helps alleviate this problem. This book is intended to be the foundation for a course in arrhythmias for a broad range of practitioners—from the telemetry nurse to the paramedic to the critical care units. We hope that it will instill an appreciation of the vast amount of knowledge required to be proficient at arrhythmia interpretation and will help the learner realize that much remains to be learned.

P.F.L.
S.J.F.

Acknowledgments

Most of the electrocardiograms found in this text are from the authors' collection through many years of experience. We thank the following for adding to this collection:

- Michael Kienzle, MD
- The critical care and emergency department staffs at Iowa Lutheran Hospital, Des Moines, Iowa
- Monica Sassmann, RN, Iowa Methodist Medical Center, Blank Children's Hospital, Des Moines, Iowa
- Maureen Buonanno, RN, Philadelphia, Pennsylvania
- Kathy Cantonwine, RN
- The many patients who provided us with unique arrhythmias and allowed us to learn from them so we might teach others.
- Electrocardiology Laboratory, University of Iowa Hospitals and Clinics, Iowa City, Iowa

Contents

Detailed Contents

PART THREE INTERVENTIONS

CARDIAC RHYTHM DISORDERS

A Nursing Process Approach

PART ONE

KNOWLEDGE BASE

CHAPTER ONE

Selected Topics in Cardiac Anatomy, Physiology, and Electrophysiology

▶ GOAL

You will have a basic understanding of relevant cardiac anatomy, physiology, and electrophysiology, allowing you to apply concepts to the clinical situation.

▶ OBJECTIVES

After studying this chapter, you should be able to:

1. Recall the sequence of circulation through the heart.
2. Compare the thickness of the left ventricle with that of the right, and explain the difference.
3. List the three layers of the heart's wall, explaining where each is in relation to structures such as the sinoatrial node and the coronary arteries.
4. Describe and relate each of the following coronary arteries to the area of myocardium it supplies: left main, left anterior descending, left circumflex, right, and posterior descending.
5. List structures of the conduction system supplied by each of the coronary arteries listed previously. Anticipate kinds of conduction disturbances that may accompany occlusion of these coronary arteries.
6. Explain the sequence of normal cardiac activation and the resultant wave forms produced on the ECG.
7. Recall the cardiovascular effects of increased vagal activity and compare these effects with those of increased sympathetic activity.
8. Recall two techniques by which vagal tone and sympathetic tone may be clinically increased.
9. Define the electrophysiologic terms *depolarization, repolarization, threshold potential, refractory period,* and *conduction.*
10. Explain the cardiac action potential and correlate it with ventricular depolarization on the ECG.
11. Compare and contrast fast and slow response tissues.
12. Differentiate between abnormal impulse formation and propagation as two mechanisms for arrhythmia genesis.
13. Classify the antiarrhythmic drugs and offer two examples for each category. Explain how each class works, relating to the action potential when appropriate.

An electrocardiogram (ECG) is the representation on the body surface of the summated electrical activity of the heart. Even though an ECG is an electrical event, its appearance depends highly on anatomic factors such as the relationship of the coronary arteries to the myocardium they supply, especially when the coronary arteries are diseased. The appearance of an ECG is also determined by the sequence of activation of the cardiac chambers, and this in turn is determined by the anatomy and electrophysiologic features of the cardiac conduction system. Finally, the mechanisms of cardiac arrhythmias, as well as responses to antiarrhythmic drugs manifested on the surface ECG, can be understood, in part, from the electrophysiology of single cardiac cells and specialized cardiac tissues. A detailed discussion of these topics would require many volumes. The purpose of this chapter is to relate cardiac anatomy and electrophysiology to the generation of an ECG. It is hoped that this will enhance your understanding of the chapters that follow.

GROSS CARDIAC ANATOMY

The heart is a muscular organ consisting of four chambers and four valves, connected by large vessels to the pulmonary and systemic circulations. The heart is enclosed within a fibrous sac called the *pericardium.* The position of the heart in the chest influences the electrocardiographic pattern. It is located in the thoracic cavity, between the lungs and in front of the thoracic aorta and esophagus. The heart rests on the diaphragm, giving rise to the term *dia-*

phragmatic surface of the heart, referring to the portion of the ventricle resting there. The heart is arranged obliquely in the chest such that the long axis (top to bottom) of the heart points down, forward, and to the left. Because of normal rotation of the heart, the right atrium and ventricle are arranged in front of the left atrium and ventricle and are closer to the anterior chest wall. Alterations in cardiac position because of congenital or normal variants or specific disease may have a marked effect on an ECG, which is primarily related to the electrical axis, or the main direction of depolarization, noted on the limb leads. In some cases the precordial leads may also be altered (e.g., in dextrocardia or right-sided heart). (Leads are discussed in detail in Chapter 3.)

The atria (right and left) serve primarily to collect blood returning from the systemic and pulmonary veins and channel its movement to the ventricles (Fig. 1-1). These atria are thin-walled and consist of two layers arranged at roughly right angles. Atrial contraction, which occurs just before ventricular contraction, serves to boost filling of the ventricle and cardiac output. The depolarization of the atrium, which starts the contraction process, gives rise to the P wave on an ECG (Fig. 1-2). The P wave is made up of the depolarization of both the right and left atria, with

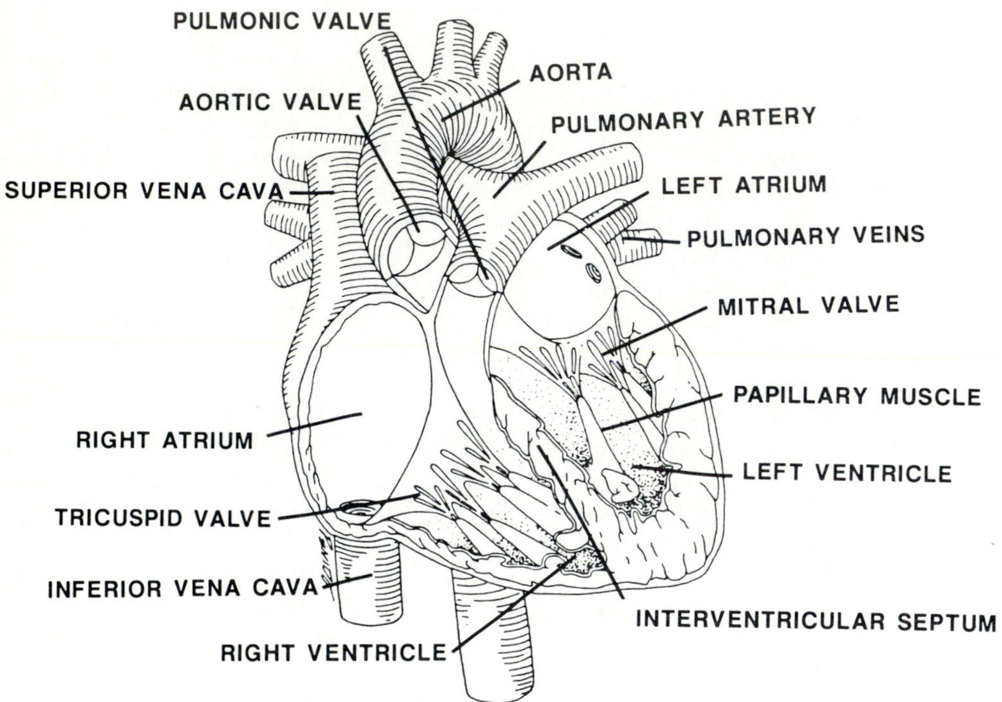

FIGURE 1-1 Schematic drawing of an open heart, revealing the relationship of atria, ventricles, and valves. The anterior walls of the atria and ventricles have been removed to reveal the intracardiac structures.

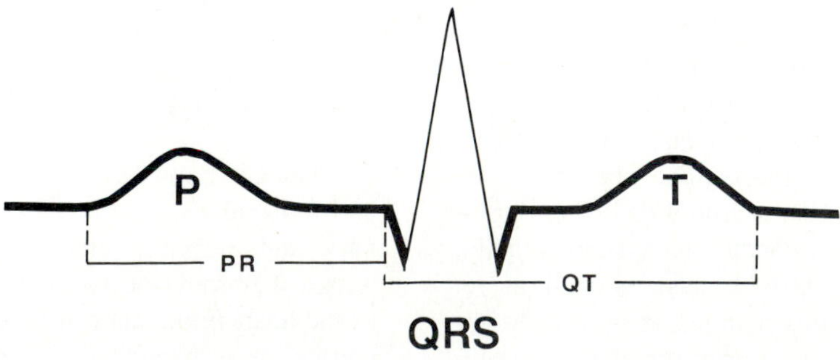

FIGURE 1-2 Components of a surface ECG. These represent atrial depolarization (P wave), ventricular activation (QRS), AV conduction (PR interval), and ventricular recovery (QT interval).

the right atrium inscribed first and the left atrium coinciding with the last portion of the P wave.

The ventricles are the main pumping chambers of the heart (see Fig. 1-1). Their purpose is to pump blood into the pulmonary and systemic circulations. The right and left ventricles are markedly different in regard to size and shape. The left ventricle is a thick-walled, cone-shaped chamber that pumps oxygenated blood to the rest of the body. Because of the need to pump against a high pressure the left ventricle is considerably thicker and heavier than the right ventricle, which pumps unoxygenated blood against a lower pressure into the pulmonary circulation. The right ventricle is a broad, thin-walled structure and looks crescent-shaped when cut in cross-section, compared with the thick circular left ventricle.

The ventricles are made up of a number of layers of muscle arranged at angles to one another. This arrangement results in the characteristic contraction pattern of the heart, in which blood is "wrung out" in a twisting motion that shortens both the transverse and apex-to-base dimensions of the heart. The ventricular wall has three layers, each roughly consisting of one third of the thickness of the wall. The inner, or endocardial, layer is in contact with chamber blood. The outer third is the epicardial layer, which is in contact with the large coronary arteries and pericardium. Between these two layers is the myocardium, or midmyocardial layer.

The electrical event of depolarization that initiates contraction (systole) of the ventricular myocardium makes up the QRS complex on a surface ECG (Fig. 1-2). Because of the difference in size between the right and left ventricles, the left ventricle makes the greatest contribution to the size and shape of the QRS complex. Processes that increase ventricular mass (right or left), like hypertrophy resulting from hypertension, may increase the height (amplitude) of the QRS in leads that record activity from the involved ventricle. Other ECG changes that accompany an increase in ventricular mass include widening of the QRS because of an increase in the time of activation of the ventricles and a shift in QRS axis toward the hypertrophied ventricle. In contrast, loss of ventricular myocardium, (e.g., after a myocardial infarction) reduces the amplitude of the QRS in the leads representing that area. A QRS axis shift away from the area of lost myocardium might also be seen.

Repolarization, or electrical recovery, of the ventricles produces a T wave on an ECG. The space between the end of the QRS complex to the T wave is the ST segment. Repolarization corresponds with diastole or ventricular filling.

Before considering the anatomy of the coronary arteries, let us follow the route of blood through the heart (see Fig. 1-1). Unoxygenated blood returning from the lower extremities and internal viscera is carried in the inferior vena cava. Blood from the head and upper extremities returns via the superior vena cava. These two vessels empty into the right atrium, which is separated from the right ventricle by the tricuspid valve, a large multileafleted structure. After the blood empties into the right ventricle it is ejected through the three-leaflet pulmonic valve into the pulmonary artery. The blood traverses this low pressure system, is oxygenated, and returns to the heart by the pulmonary veins. The four pulmonary veins empty into the left atrium, which is separated from the left ventricle by the large bicuspid mitral valve. After being emptied into the left ventricle, blood is ejected through the three-leaflet aortic valve into the coronary arteries and the aorta and then to the rest of the body. The exchange of oxygen and nutrients and waste products occurs throughout the body in the tiny capillary vessels, and then the venous blood starts its trek back to the heart, completing the circuit.

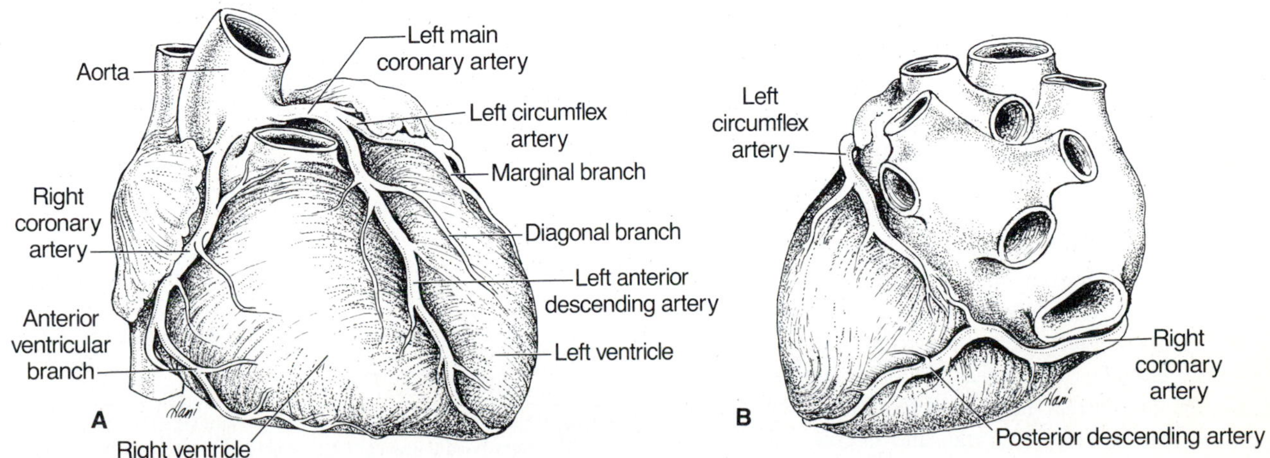

FIGURE 1-3 Schematic drawing of the coronary arteries. **A,** The branches of the coronaries viewed from the anterior aspect. **B,** The coronaries seen on the posterior aspect of the heart.

CORONARY ANATOMY

In the vast majority of patients the coronary arteries originate from the right and left sinuses of Valsalva, one of three dilatations above the aortic valve. At their origin they may be 1.5 to 5.5 mm in diameter. These vessels supply blood to the structures of the heart (Fig. 1-3).

Left Main Coronary Artery

The left main coronary artery arises as a main trunk from the center of the upper left coronary sinus of Valsalva. If oriented as the heart sits in the chest, this artery arises behind the pulmonary artery. It may be 1 mm to several centimeters long and divides into the left anterior descending and left circumflex coronary arteries. There may sometimes be an intermediate branch in addition to the two main divisions of the left main coronary artery.

Left Anterior Descending Coronary Artery

After branching from the left main coronary artery, the left anterior descending (LAD) coronary artery courses around from behind the pulmonary artery, proceeds in the anterior interventricular groove over the interventricular septum towards the apex, and often crawls around the apex onto the inferior wall. Its major branches are septal perforating arteries (averaging about 15) and free wall branches. The septal branches are generally not visible from the surface of the heart. The largest branch is often the first septal perforating branch. The LAD also gives off 2 to 6 diagonal branches that course at an angle away from the septum onto the free wall of the left ventricle. The septal perforating branches of the LAD supply the upper two thirds to three fourths of the septum (near the atria) and nearly all of the apical portions of the interventricular septum. The diagonal branches supply a variable amount of left ventricular free wall lateral to the septum. The LAD and its branches invariably supply approximately 50% of the left ventricular myocardium.

Left Circumflex Coronary Artery

After branching from the left main coronary artery the left circumflex coronary artery travels laterally and posteriorly under the left atrial appendage in the atrioventricular sulcus. As it proceeds in the atrioventricular (AV) groove it gives out 1 to 4 obtuse marginal branches that course over the lateral wall of the heart. In roughly 10% of patients the circumflex may continue posteriorly and run down the posterior interventricular groove, supplying the inferior wall of the heart. In 45% of patients the sinus node artery arises from the proximal left circumflex trunk. The circumflex may supply branches to provide blood for most of the left atrium. The circumflex provides blood flow for variable amounts of the anterior free wall and lateral wall and, as mentioned, may provide blood to the inferior wall as well. Overall, the circumflex provides blood for approximately 25% of the left ventricle.

Right Coronary Artery

The right coronary artery arises from the middle of the right coronary sinus of Valsalva, coursing anteriorly to the AV groove. It gives off few major branches before reaching the posterior interventricular groove. It provides branches to the sinus nodal (SA [sinoatrial] nodal artery) artery in 55% of patients and branches to the AV nodal artery in 90% of patients. After reaching the posterior interventricular groove, it supplies septal perforating vessels to the inferior one third of the septum posteriorly and very little to the septum near the apex.

The artery supplying the posterior descending branch has been called the *dominant coronary artery* (90% of the time right coronary artery, 10% of the time left circumflex). It is more correct to call the vessel supplying this branch the *dominant posterior artery*. In general the right coronary artery provides blood flow for approximately 25% of the left ventricle. However, there is a reciprocal anatomic relationship between the right and left circumflex coronary arteries. In other words, if the right coronary artery provides more blood flow to the left ventricle, the left circumflex provides less, and vice versa.

The right ventricle is supplied by branches from the left anterior descending artery, the right coronary artery, and occasionally the left circumflex coronary artery. Right

Table 1-1 Summary of Major Structures Supplied by Coronary Arteries*

Right coronary artery	Left coronary artery
Inferior wall LV (in 90%)	
SA node (in 55%)	Left anterior descending
AV node (in 90%)	Anterior wall LV
IV septum, a portion	IV septum, most of
RV	Apex
His bundle	His bundle
RBB (in some)	RBB, most of
Posterior inferior division LBB, a portion	Anterior superior division LBB
	Posterior inferior division LBB, a portion
	Circumflex
	Inferior wall LV (in 10%)
	Anterior, lateral walls LV
	SA node (in 45%)
	AV node (in 10%)
	Most of LA

*Key: IV = interventricular; LV = left ventricle; RV = right ventricle; RBB = right bundle branch; LBB = left bundle branch; LA = left atrium.

ventricular infarction may accompany the more common left ventricular infarction and may sometimes be an important part of the clinical picture. See Table 1-1 for a summary of the coronary arteries and structures they supply.

ECG PATTERNS OF ISCHEMIA AND INFARCTION

When the blood supply to myocardium is removed for several hours or more, irreversible ischemic damage occurs. This results in immediate loss of function of the ischemic myocardium and begins a process of cell death, cell removal, and eventual healing by replacement with fibrous scar tissue. This process is called *myocardial infarction*.

Acute Transmural Infarction

Immediately after the proximal occlusion of a large epicardial coronary artery, a variety of T-wave and ST-segment changes may be seen in the acute phase. Perhaps the earliest change to be seen is the appearance of tall, peaked T waves in leads representing the affected region. More commonly, however, elevation of the ST segment is seen (Fig. 1-4). ST-segment elevation may represent transient severe transmural ischemia as in coronary artery spasm and may resolve if coronary blood flow is restored.

Ischemia and Nontransmural Infarction

In situations where nontransmural infarction has occurred (of the subendocardial region) or where severe ischemia exists the most common ECG response is ST-segment depression, sometimes accompanied by T-wave inversion (Fig. 1-4). Again, these changes may be transient, and ST-segment depression may resolve if caused by reversible ischemia. It should be noted that there are a number of conditions unrelated to ischemia that may simulate ST-segment depression. The most common are the presence of left ventricular hypertrophy and the use of digoxin.

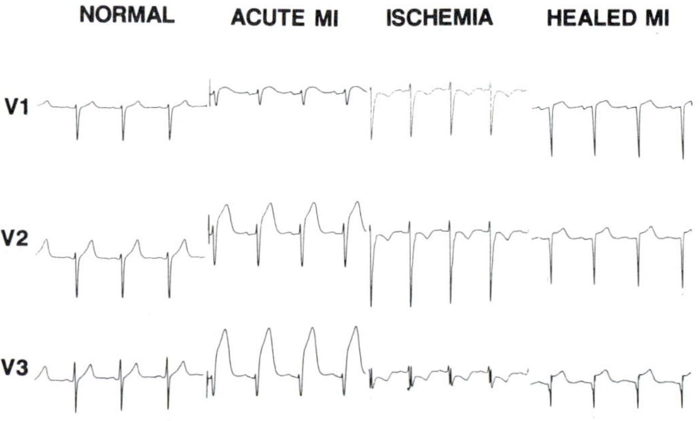

FIGURE 1-4 V_1 to V_3 QRS appearance in normal patient and patients with acute myocardial infarction (MI), ischemia, and healed MI. Note characteristic QRS and ST-segment appearance in V_1 to V_3, corresponding to the distribution of the left anterior descending coronary artery.

Chronic Infarction

The hallmark of chronic (healed) infarction is the presence of the q wave (see Fig. 1-4), an initial negative wave in the QRS complex. Small q waves may exist in normal patients in one or more leads as a manifestation of the axis, or direction of depolarization (e.g., lead III), or septal depolarization (i.e., leads I, aVL, and V_4 to V_6). In general, pathologic q waves are at least 0.04 seconds (i.e., one small box) or more wide and should constitute 25% or more of the QRS amplitude. Q waves of any size should be considered abnormal in precordial leads V_2 and V_3.

THE RELATIONSHIP OF THE LOCATION OF ISCHEMIA OR INFARCTION TO SURFACE ECG LEADS

Because of multilead ECG systems, processes involving different surfaces of the heart are reflected in different leads or groups of leads. Although this relationship may not be precise and is far from being totally sensitive or specific, an electrocardiogram correlates reasonably well with cardiac catheterization and autopsy data.

Anterior Wall

As previously mentioned, the anterior wall of the left ventricle is supplied for the most part by the LAD and left circumflex arteries.

Anteroseptal

As one can see from the previous discussion of coronary anatomy, processes involving the anteroseptal left ventricle (LV) are almost always due to involvement in the left anterior descending coronary artery. Changes are most often seen in precordial leads V_1 to V_4, although reciprocal (or opposite) ST-segment shifts may be seen in leads representative of uninvolved opposite or adjacent walls (e.g., leads II, III, and aVF).

Anterolateral

As discussed, the lateral wall of the heart is predominantly supplied by the circumflex coronary artery. Ischemia or infarction involving this region involves leads I and aVL and precordial leads V_4 to V_6 alone or in combination. There may also be accompanying ECG changes in the inferior leads. Occasionally large q waves are seen in the anterolateral leads in patients with hypertrophic cardiomyopathy without ischemia or infarction.

Inferior Wall

Processes involving the inferior wall generally represent disease in the right coronary artery and are generally reflected in leads II, III, and aVF, the *inferior leads*. The posterior wall (the portion of the inferior wall closest to the AV groove and mitral valve) and other portions of the inferior wall are relatively silent electrocardiographically compared with other regions of the heart. In posterior wall infarction the R wave is greater than the S wave in leads V_1 and V_2. Associated q waves are often seen in the inferior and/or lateral leads.

ANATOMY OF THE CONDUCTION SYSTEM

Sinus Node

The normal sinus impulse originates in the SA node. The SA node is an oval or crescent-shaped structure that is approximately 15 × 5 × 1.5 mm. It is located at the junction of the superior vena cava and the high lateral right atrium (Fig. 1-5). It is subepicardial in location and embedded in a matrix of elastic, collagen, and other supporting cells. SA nodal cells are small and are arranged in bundles.

The SA node is a richly innervated structure. Numerous anatomic studies have shown nerves in close contact with SA nodal cells. Histochemical studies have demonstrated high concentrations of catecholamines (norepinephrine) and strong anticholinesterase (breaks down acetylcholine) reactions in the SA nodal region, suggesting the presence of local sympathetic and parasympathetic influences.

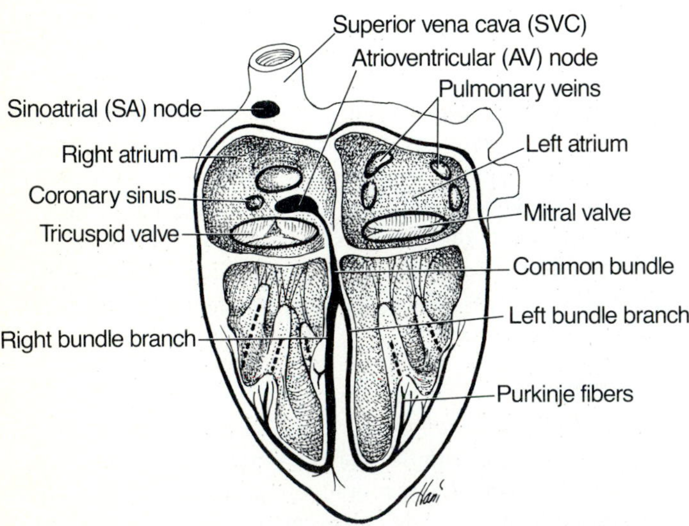

FIGURE 1-5 Schematic drawing of the conduction system. The components of the conduction system are shown with anterior atria and ventricles removed.

The SA node is supplied by its own blood vessel, the SA nodal artery, which runs right through the center of the nodal area. This vessel originates usually from the right coronary artery (55% to 65%), but 35% to 45% of the time the SA nodal artery arises from the proximal portion of the left circumflex coronary artery. The SA nodal artery is large relative to the size of the structure it supplies. This and other evidence suggest that a relationship exists between the SA nodal artery pulsations or flow and the electrical activity of the node.

Intraatrial Conduction

There has been a great deal of controversy regarding whether true specialized or preferential pathways of conduction exist in the atrium connecting the SA node to the AV node. A number of authors have described preferential pathways anatomically and electrophysiologically. The pathways primarily consist of the following three:

1. Anterior internodal tract—leaves the sinus node leftward and divides into branches to the left atrium and another across the intraatrial septum to the AV node.
2. Middle internodal tract—crosses the septum to the AV node.
3. Posterior internodal tract—crosses the crista terminalis portion of the right atrium to the right superior margin of the AV node.

The presence or absence of these specialized tracts remains unsettled. Not all investigations have demonstrated such tracts, and very few true conducting cells can be demonstrated in the proposed pathways. Most cells in the proposed pathways are normal working muscle. Moreover, these so-called pathways pass over wide muscle bands defined by normal anatomic obstacles such as the vena cava, rather than narrow cablelike structures. Some investigators maintain that the preferential nature of conduction is merely due to normal properties of atrial muscle rather than unique electrophysiologic properties of specialized conduction tissue.

Atrioventricular Node

The atrioventricular node is the control point for atrial impulses conducted to the ventricle. This important structure controls the ventricular response by slowing the impulses. This is especially important during very rapid atrial arrhythmias such as atrial fibrillation. The AV node serves to protect the ventricles from beating too fast.

The AV node is located between the opening of the coronary sinus and the posterior aspect of the membranous interventricular septum (Fig. 1-5). It is located beneath the right atrial endocardium above the insertion of the tricuspid valve.

Histologically the AV node is composed of several types of cells and fiber arrangements. The exact site of AV nodal delay is unclear.

Histologic studies suggest that the AV node is much less well innervated than the SA node, although studies of autonomic control have demonstrated that the AV node is under the influence of both sympathetic and parasympathetic limbs of the autonomic nervous system.

The blood supply to the AV node is the AV nodal artery, which is a branch of the posterior descending coronary artery (from right coronary artery 90%, left circumflex 10%). Other vessels also contribute to a plexus of vessels that renders the AV node fairly safe from persistent ischemic damage.

Common Bundle of His

The His bundle is in direct contact with the AV node and transmits impulses from the AV node to the remainder of the conduction system beyond. This tissue penetrates the central fibrous body of the heart and runs along the upper margin of the muscular interventricular septum (Fig. 1-5). In addition, as it penetrates the central fibrous body, it lies in close proximity to the aortic and mitral valve rings. At the top of the muscular septum, it gives off the left bundle branch as a broad ribbon and subsequently moves rightward to become the right bundle branch.

Histologically it is like a large telephone cable that is subdivided into smaller individual cables by collagen dividers.

The His bundle receives a dual blood supply from the AV nodal artery and the first septal branch of the LAD, as well as from smaller and less constant branches of other origins.

Right Bundle Branch

Of the two bundle branches the right bundle branch maintains a more discrete cablelike structure. It is classically divided into the following three portions:

1. The first portion runs in the subendocardium on the right surface of the interventricular septum (missing in 20% of patients).
2. The second part enters the myocardium in the middle third of the interventricular septum.
3. The third portion runs in the subendocardium down to the base of the anterior papillary muscle. This third portion is the first part of the right bundle branch to have a functional contact with the myocardium.

The blood supply to the proximal right bundle branch is either the AV nodal artery along with the first septal perforating branch of the LAD or one of these two arteries alone. If only one of the arteries supplies the right bundle, it usually is the first septal perforator. The more distal portions of the right bundle branch are supplied by anterior septal perforating arteries.

Left Bundle Branch

The exact configuration of the left bundle is uncertain. The left bundle as a bifascicular structure has been a popular concept, but more recent studies have shown the left bundle to be slightly more complex in configuration. The proximal portion of the left bundles starts between the noncoronary and the right coronary cusps of the aorta and may extend both anteriorly and inferiorly from there. Thereafter it divides into fascicles; most commonly the following 2 large main radiations are seen:

1. Anterior radiation—This fascicle runs to the anterior papillary muscle. It is often referred to as the *anterior superior division,* of the left bundle branch.
2. Posterior radiation—This fascicle usually appears as a continuation of the main left bundle branch and goes posteriorly to the base of the posterior papillary muscle. It is also known as the *posterior inferior division* of the left bundle branch.

Many variations are seen in the distribution of the remaining conducting tissue to the septal endocardium. In 60% a central radiation arises from the point of division or from the anterior or posterior radiation and continues to the midseptum. In 15% of hearts examined the septal endocardium receives conducting tissue from the posterior ramifications, and in 25% the septum is supplied by a complicated network contributed to by both the anterior and posterior fascicles. Electrophysiologic activation data support such a trifascicular concept of the left bundle branch.

The blood supply to the anterior and midseptal portions is provided by anterior septal branches from the left anterior descending artery. In 50% the AV nodal artery also supplies the proximal portions of these left bundle fascicles. The proximal portions of the posterior ramifications are supplied by the AV nodal artery or a combination of AV nodal and septal perforating branches. More distally, the left bundle branch receives a dual blood supply from both anterior and posterior perforating septal branches.

Cardiac Activation Sequence

Activation during sinus rhythm begins at the site of the SA node (Fig. 1-6). The depolarization of the SA node cannot be seen on a standard ECG. The activation of the right atrium corresponds to the initial portion of the P wave. Subsequent spread to the left atrium contributes the last part of the P wave. During the PR interval on an ECG, the

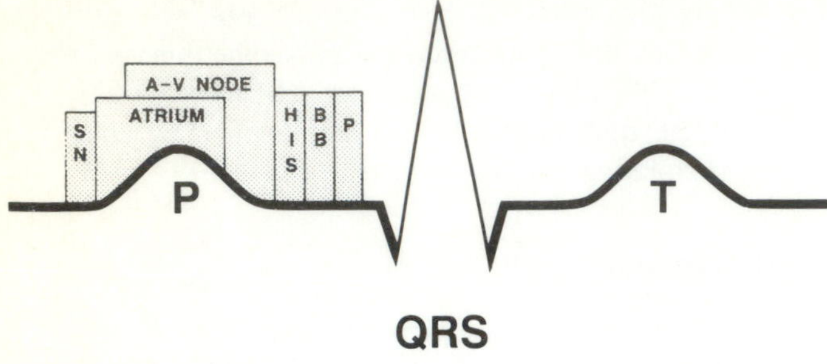

FIGURE 1-6 Schematic drawing of cardiac activation related to the surface ECG. The timing of activation of the components of the conduction system is superimposed on the surface ECG. SN = Sinus node; His = common bundle of His; BB = bundle branches; P = Purkinje network.

period from the beginning of the P wave to the beginning of the QRS complex, the AV node, His bundle, and bundle branches are activated. Therefore a prolonged PR interval can be caused by slowed conduction through the atrium, AV node, His-Purkinje system, or any combination of these.

Studies of the activation sequence of the human ventricles are relatively limited. These studies have consisted of epicardial activation mapping during open chest surgery, catheter mapping during electrophysiologic studies, and study of total cardiac activation in hearts removed at the time of death. These studies have shown that at least two separate sites of earliest endocardial activation can be detected during activation of the left ventricle. These sites include the midinferior septum and the anterior wall in the area of the insertion of the anterior papillary muscle. Studies in the isolated human heart have suggested a third endocardial breakthrough point at the inferior paraseptal region. After the initial activation the spreading wavefronts coalesce rapidly and converge at the apex. The last portion of the endocardial surface of the LV to be activated is the posterobasal region near the mitral valve. The first endocardial activation of the right ventricle starts near the insertion of the anterior papillary muscle 5 to 10 msec after the onset of left ventricular septal activation. Activation ends at the outflow tract of the RV.

Activation of the epicardium (which largely determines the appearance of the QRS on an ECG) largely follows the sequence on the endocardium. The earliest epicardial point of activation or breakthrough is most commonly in the anterior RV near the insertion of the anterior right ventricular papillary muscle with smooth excitation over both ventricles and with activation occurring last over the posterobasal portion of the heart.

For purposes of explaining the appearance of the QRS complex on an ECG the sequence of activation roughly proceeds in the following order: septum—posterior to anterior and left to right; ventricles—roughly simultaneous with most of the QRS morphology dominated by the larger left ventricle.

AUTONOMIC INFLUENCES

People are subjected to many types of of stress in the course of daily life. Among these are environmental (e.g., temperature, altitude, oxygen) and psychologic (e.g., anger, fear, pain) stresses and those related to exercise or illness. Cardiovascular function is an important component of the response to stress. The form that the cardiovascular response takes is generally related to alterations in: (1) the heart rate; (2) the vigor of cardiac contraction, or contractility; and (3) the tone of vascular resistance vessels. These three elements are measured clinically as heart rate, cardiac output, and blood pressure. The type and extent of cardiovascular response to stress are determined largely by the autonomic nervous system.

The autonomic nervous system is divided into the parasympathetic and the sympathetic systems. Many of the cardiovascular effects of these two systems are opposite in direction. These two limbs may have a balanced effect in certain circumstances, whereas at other times one system may predominate in its actions. The overall effect of interactions between sympathetic and parasympathetic nervous systems is intended to maintain cardiovascular homeostasis.

Parasympathetic System

The fibers of the parasympathetic system arise in centers in the neural medulla of the brain. These fibers give rise to right and left vagal nerves. After passing through the neck, in close association with the common carotid arteries, they traverse the mediastinum and synapse with postganglionic cells located within the heart. These are concentrated primarily near the SA and AV nodal tissues, where vagal nerve influence is most pronounced. The acetylcholine released from these nerve terminals is rapidly inactivated by cholinesterase, an enzyme in high concentration in SA and AV node tissue. Therefore the effects of vagal discharge may be brief at sites of vagal innervation. In the SA node, increased vagal activity slows, and vagal withdrawal speeds heart rate. The vagal, or parasympathetic, influence dominates the sympathetic contribution to heart rate. For example, at the beginning of exercise, the increase in heart rate is mediated almost entirely by withdrawal of vagal tone. Simultaneous stimulation of parasympathetic and sympathetic systems experimentally results in clear predominance of vagal effect. Other experimental studies in animals have suggested that the right vagus nerve exerts more influence than the left vagus in the SA node, whereas the left vagus has more effect in the AV node.

Resting AV nodal conduction is determined by a more balanced influence of parasympathetic and sympathetic systems. However, an increase in parasympathetic or vagal tone brings about slowing of AV nodal conduction and an increase in refractoriness, or electrical recovery. This may result in varying levels of heart block, usually with a Wenckebach pattern of conduction. Because of the parasympathetic predominance in some resting, healthy people (especially young and athletic individuals) or during sleep, asymptomatic periods of a Wenckebach type of AV block need not be interpreted as abnormal. More intense vagal effects, however, may result in symptomatic bradycardia because of sinus slowing or transient heart block.

The effects of the parasympathetic nervous system on His-Purkinje conduction tissue and ventricular muscle are less well worked out. It is safe to say that, in general, vagal stimulation prolongs refractoriness in His-Purkinje tissue and ventricular muscle, although these effects are small compared with those in sinus and AV nodes. Other parasympathetic effects include a decrease in contractility and peripheral vasodilation. Clinically, parasympathetic activation results in bradycardia, decreased cardiac output, and a decline in blood pressure.

Sympathetic System

The cardiac sympathetic fibers arise in the upper thoracic and lower cervical spinal cord and enter a chain of autonomic ganglia near the vertebral column. There they synapse with neurons that become part of a complex of sympathetic and parasympathetic nerves of the heart. These fibers run along the great vessels to the base of the heart and are distributed to various chambers along the epicardial cardiac surface. From the epicardium, they penetrate the myocardium to supply underlying cardiac structures.

There is regional variability in the distribution of sympathetic fibers in experimental animals and probably in man. Fibers arising in the right sympathetic chain, traveling via the right stellate ganglion, may be more densely distributed to the right atrium and sinus node, whereas the left stellate has more prominent distribution to ventricular myocardium. Stimulation of right sympathetic fibers increases heart rate predominantly, whereas left sympathetic stimulation may markedly enhance ventricular contractility. In addition, stimulation of the left stellate ganglion or blockade of the right stellate ganglion may induce QT-interval (from the beginning of the QRS complex to the end of the T wave) prolongation and a variety of ventricular arrhythmias. Imbalance between right and left sympathetic activity has been implicated in the long QT-interval syndrome in patients, a condition associated with syncope and sudden death resulting from ventricular tachyarrhythmias.

Activation of the sympathetic nervous system results in a number of cardiac effects. Heart rate is increased, and AV nodal function is enhanced. The heart rate at which block in the AV node occurs increases with increasing sympathetic stimulation, and a 1:1 ratio of AV conduction is usually maintained all the way to maximum heart rate. Sympathetic stimulation may shorten His-Purkinje and ventricular muscle refractoriness and improve conduction under certain circumstances in these tissues. Ventricular contractility and peripheral resistance are increased by sympathetic influence. Therefore the clinical hallmarks of sympathetic discharge are tachycardia, hypertension, and increased cardiac output.

The sympathetic and parasympathetic nervous systems play a prominent role in reflex hemodynamic alterations. Cardiovascular reflex adjustments occur in response to a detected stimulus. These stimuli vary considerably and include the stresses listed at the beginning of this section. One of the most important and potent stimuli to reflex autonomic adjustment is blood pressure. Sensors of arterial and intracardiac pressure are present in the heart, pulmonary vasculature, aorta, and carotid sinus. A decline in blood pressure results in reflex inhibition of parasympathetic influence and activation of the sympathetic nervous system. This results in an increase in heart rate, increased cardiac contractility and output, and increase in peripheral vascular resistance, intended to reverse the detected decline in perfusing pressure.

In contrast an increase in blood pressure inhibits sympathetic activity and increases parasympathetic influence, resulting in a decline in heart rate, contractility, and peripheral resistance.

Another reflex action that commonly can be seen on an ECG is the phasic slowing and speeding of heart rate with respiration, called *sinus arrhythmia* (Fig. 1-7). This ECG

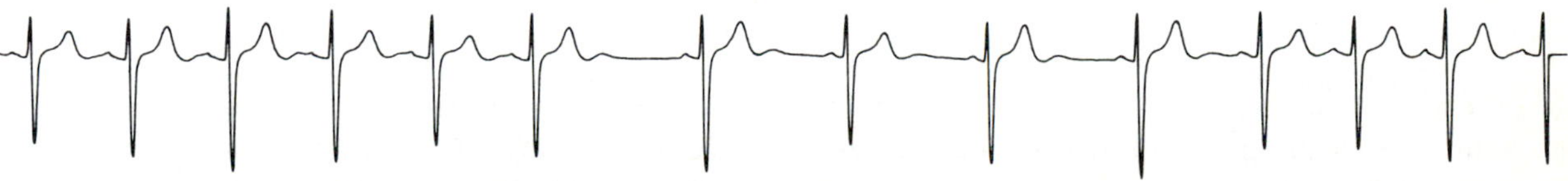

FIGURE 1-7 ECG showing sinus arrhythmia. The phasic speeding and slowing of heart rate correspond with respiration in this example from an 18-year-old patient with asthma.

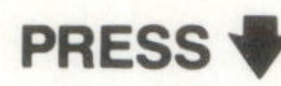

RELEASE

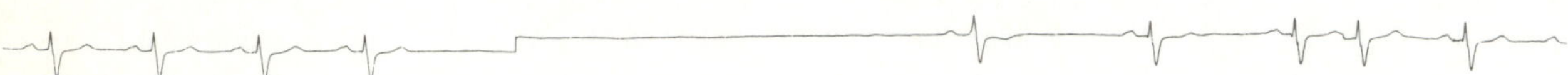

RIGHT CAROTID SINUS MASSAGE

FIGURE 1-8 ECG showing asystole resulting from carotid sinus massage in a patient with suspected carotid sinus hypersensitivity. Pressure on the right carotid resulted in asystole and reproduction of symptoms.

finding is probably due to more than one reflex stimulated by changes in intracardiac volume brought about by respiration. This arrhythmia is discussed in Chapter 4.

Occasionally it is helpful to produce increases in sympathetic or parasympathetic tone for diagnostic or therapeutic purposes. Sympathetic tone is increased most commonly with exercise or occasionally by immersion of the hand in ice water (cold pressor test). Increases in parasympathetic tone are produced by carotid sinus massage, which stimulates the sensors located there, simulating hypertension (Fig. 1-8). The Valsalva maneuver (voluntary increase in intraabdominal and intrathoracic pressure against a closed glottis —"bearing down") also produces increases in vagal tone. Finally, production of hypertension with a pressor agent like Neo-Synephrine results in reflex parasympathetic activation. The increase in vagal tone is often useful to terminate supraventricular tachycardia by producing block in the AV node.

Electrophysiologic Definitions

Depolarization—Movement of transmembrane potential in a positive direction.
Repolarization—Movement of transmembrane potential in a negative direction.
Threshold potential—Transmembrane potential at which an action potential is initiated.
Refractoriness—Inability of a cell or tissue to generate a normal response to stimulation.
Conduction—Movement or propagation of electrical impulse from cell to cell through tissue.

BASIC ELECTROPHYSIOLOGY

As previously mentioned, an ECG is the summation of electrical activity of individual cardiac cells. The electrical activity of single cardiac cells can be studied using extremely fine glass electrodes carefully inserted through the cell membrane. These electrodes measure the differences in electrical potential between the inside and the outside of the cell (transmembrane potential difference). Many of the concepts relating to the interpretation of an ECG can be seen in studies of single cardiac cells. Definitions of frequently used electrophysiology terms are listed in the box on this page.

Cardiac Action Potential

Classically the cyclic changes in membrane potential difference have been divided arbitrarily into a number of phases. This arbitrary division allows discussion of depolarization, repolarization, and ionic movement in a more precise manner (Fig. 1-9).

Resting Potential

In the absence of spontaneous pacemaker activity, most cardiac cells remain at a constant level of potential difference. In most instances, this potential difference is 80 to 90 mV with the inside of the cell negative relative to the outside. This transmembrane potential difference of the undisturbed cardiac cell is referred to as the *resting potential*.

Phase 0

During this phase of the action potential the potential difference rapidly changes from −80 to 90 to a +10 to 30 mV. This is the phase of rapid depolarization of the cardiac action potential. If one were measuring a potential difference in a ventricular muscle cell, phase 0 would correspond to the QRS complex on the surface ECG.

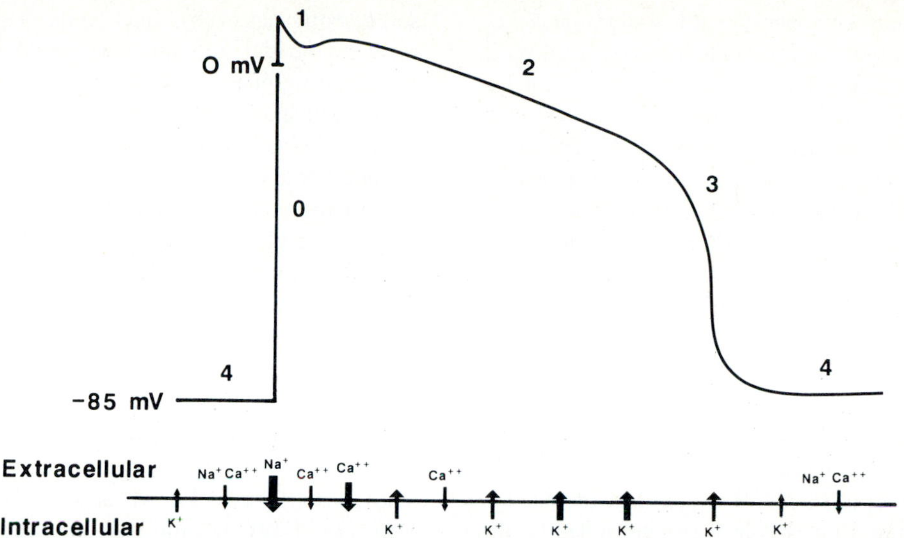

FIGURE 1-9 Schematic drawing of ionic movement during cardiac action potential. The components of the cardiac action potential and their relationship to the major ionic movements are shown.

Phase 1

A brief period of rapid repolarization (return toward negative potential) occurs during phase 1.

Phase 2

This phase is called the *plateau phase* or *slow repolarization phase* of the action potential.

Phase 3

Repolarization becomes more rapid during phase 3. The end of phase 3 corresponds with the end of the T wave on an ECG.

Phase 4

Phase 4 is the period of electrical diastole and may consist of a constant membrane potential (resting potential) or a period of constantly changing membrane potential in cells with automaticity.

Ionic Basis for the Cardiac Action Potential

The resting transmembrane potential difference is determined principally by the concentration gradient of potassium, which is the principal intracellular ion (150 mmolar inside versus 4 mmolar outside the cell). Constant movement of potassium from inside to outside the cell down the electrochemical gradient maintains the inside of the cell negative relative to the outside, hence the resting potential of −80 to −90 mV in most cardiac cells (see Fig. 1-9).

Phase 0 depends on rapid changes in permeability of the cardiac membrane to sodium ions and the rapid inward movement down the electrochemical gradient for sodium (150 mmolar outside versus 10 mmolar inside the cell). Changes in permeability are thought to be due to the opening and closing of specialized activation and inactivation "gates" or particles. The status of these gates depends on membrane potential, therefore the rapidity of phase 0 is markedly influenced by the level of resting potential. More sodium gates are available for more rapid depolarization when depolarization starts from a more negative level. The rapid inward current also activates a slower and longer lasting inward movement of calcium that contributes little, if any, to phase 0.

Phase 1, seen primarily in Purkinje and ventricular muscle fibers, is a brief and rapid period of repolarization (more negative potential) due to a transient surge of outward current, probably mediated by potassium.

During phases 2 and 3 the rate of repolarization is the result of the balance between continued slow inward currents of calcium and sodium, and outward currents of potassium, as well as inward current of chloride and the activity of the sodium-potassium exchange pump (which likely generates a net outward movement of sodium).

During phase 4 in working atrial and ventricular cells, resting membrane potential is maintained constant during diastole until an impulse arrives to cause depolarization. However, in other cells, such as some atrial and Purkinje cells, a gradual slow depolarization occurs until a specific membrane voltage or threshold potential occurs and this triggers a full action potential. Such cells are said to have automaticity. This gradual depolarization during phase 4 (phase 4 automaticity) is due to gradually decreasing movement of potassium ions from inside to outside the cell, whereas a small constant inward sodium leak remains, resulting in a net positive or depolarizing current. An alternative explanation has been suggested—namely, that a gradually increasing inward sodium leak occurs during a constant level of potassium movement. Nonetheless, either of these explanations would result in a net inward positive or depolarizing current, resulting in spontaneous and automatic depolarization. In other tissues with automaticity, such as the SA node, calcium is probably more important in the generation of pacemaker activity.

Functional Significance of Features of Depolarization and Repolarization

Cells or tissues in which depolarization (phase 0) is determined by the activation of sodium channels are known as *fast response tissues* (Fig. 1-10). The speed of conduction or propagation through tissues is in part determined by the rapidity of phase 0. Therefore, tissues possessing fast response characteristics, such as atrium, Purkinje, and myocardium, are capable of rapid conduction. Factors that reduce the movement of sodium by changing resting potential or changing sodium channel number or function (ischemia or drugs for example) may markedly reduce conduction and may be important in cardiac arrhythmias.

Tissues that normally do not possess sodium-dependent fast response properties are known as *slow response tissues* (Fig. 1-11). In these tissues, depolarization is mediated by the slow inward current of calcium (and probably some sodium as well). Such cells possess a less negative resting potential and once activated have a much more slowly rising phase 0. These tissues are not capable of the rapid conduction seen in fast response (sodium-dependent) tissues. Examples of predominantly slow response tissue include SA and AV nodes.

Fast response fibers that have been rapidly depolarized (experimentally or through disease) lose their rapid inward sodium current, leaving a predominance of calcium-mediated properties and may resemble a slow response tissue.

The duration of the periods of repolarization (phases 2 and 3) is a major determinant of the refractoriness of cardiac tissue. Tissues (or cells) that are refractory are unable to generate a normal response. In the early phase of repolarization, no stimulus, no matter how strong, can generate a response. This is known as the *absolute refractory period* (Fig. 1-12). Stimuli progressively later in the repolarization phase may result in progressively more normal responses, but any stimulus occurring before full recovery (during the relative refractory period) will result in an action potential with a reduced rate of rise of phase 0 and therefore decreased conduction in tissue. This is the electrophysiologic basis for some types of aberration (so-called phase 3 block).

In normal fast response fibers, full excitability (responsiveness to stimulation) returns with return to resting potential, whereas in diseased fast response and slow response tissues, full excitability may be delayed beyond

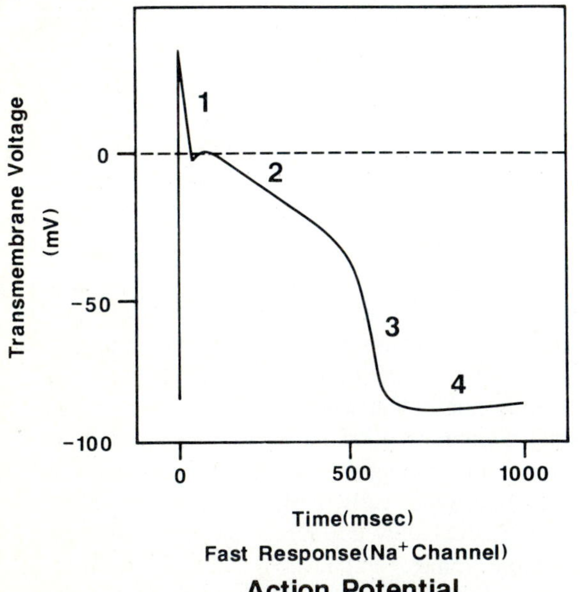

FIGURE 1-10 Schematic drawing of action potential from fast response tissue. The more negative resting potential and the rapid rise of phase 0 are characteristics of activation that is sodium-channel mediated.

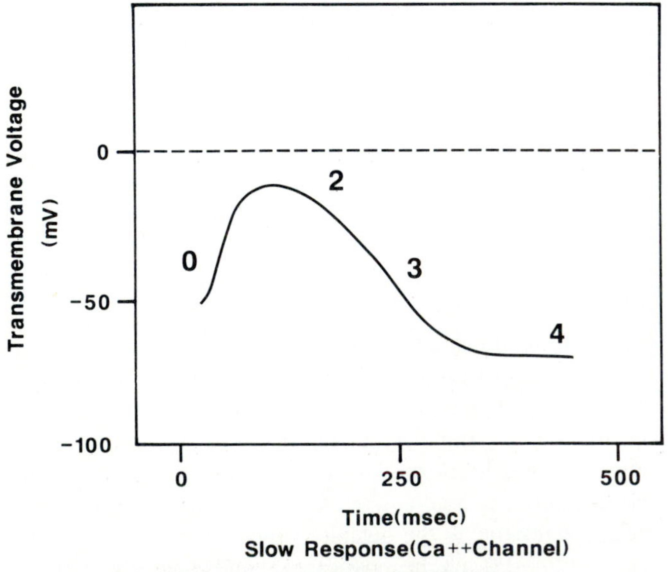

FIGURE 1-11 Schematic drawing of action potential from slow response tissue. This has a less negative resting potential compared with a fast response tissue and a slower rate of rise of phase 0.

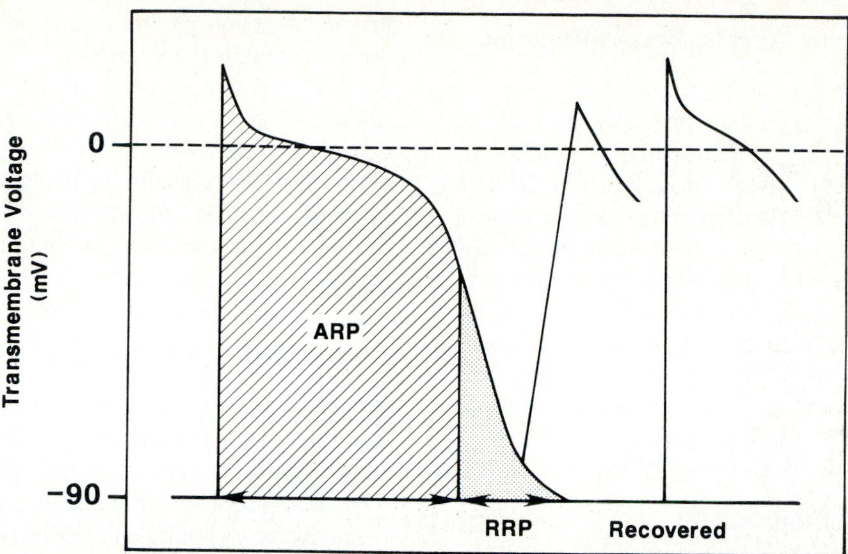

FIGURE 1-12 Schematic drawing of refractory periods of action potential. ARP = Absolute refractory period. RRP = Relative refractory period. An action potential occurring during the RRP has a slower phase 0 and slower conduction velocity. After recovery, phase 0 and conduction velocity are restored to normal.

recovery of resting potential. As can be seen from this discussion, slow response tissues are more likely to possess slowed conduction and increased likelihood for block. Such properties represent normal function in the AV and SA nodes but in theory could contribute to arrhythmia genesis under other circumstances.

EFFECTS OF ANTIARRHYTHMIC DRUGS ON ELECTROPHYSIOLOGIC CHARACTERISTICS

Antiarrhythmic drugs have been routinely classified by their effect on the action potential (Table 1-2). Such a classification is at best artificial and may bear little relationship to the antiarrhythmic effects seen in man.

Class I Antiarrhythmic Agents

Class I has been subdivided into classes IA, IB, and IC. Class IA drugs depress normal phase 4 automaticity of the action potential, reduce phase 0 at high dose and/or in diseased tissue, and may increase the period of refractoriness greater than increases in action potential duration. As one might expect, patients treated with drugs of this class show QRS widening and QT prolongation on the surface ECG. Class IB drugs, such as lidocaine and phenytoin, depress phase 4 of the action potential but have little effect on phase 0 except in ischemic and other abnormal tissues. These drugs may shorten the action potential duration and hasten repolarization. Drugs of this class have little or no effect on QRS width, but there may be some shortening of the QT interval. Drugs in the IC class slow the rate of rise of phase 0 but unlike IA drugs do this without appreciable effect on action potential duration (or recovery). Clinically, these drugs slow intracardiac conduction. On the surface ECG, this might result in PR prolongation and significant QRS widening without a great deal of QT prolongation.

Table 1-2 Antiarrhythmic Drug Classification

CLASS	Drugs	Effect on action potential
IA	Procainamide, Quinidine, Disopyramide, and Moricizine	Depressed depolarization
IB	Lidocaine, Tocainide, Mexiletine, and Phenytoin	Depressed depolarization
IC	Encainide, Flecainide, and Propafenone	Depressed depolarization
II	Propranolol, Metoprolol, Esmolol, and others	Beta-adrenergic blockade
III	Bretylium, Amiodarone, Sotalol, N-acetyl, and Procainamide	Prolonged repolarization
IV	Verapamil, Diltiazem, Nifedipine, and others	Calcium channel blockade

Class II Antiarrythmic Agents: Beta-Adrenergic Blockers

The effects of beta blockers are primarily a result of competitive inhibition of beta-receptors in the heart. Quinidine-like membrane effects may be seen at high doses of some beta blockers but are rarely seen in clinical doses used. Beta blockers reduce phase 4 automaticity by antagonizing the effects of catecholamines on this phase of the cardiac cycle. Electrocardiographically this would be expected to result in a reduction in resting heart rate and to blunt the increase in heart rate that is often seen with exercise, emotional upset, or the administration of beta-agonist (stimulating) drugs such as isoproterenol.

Class III Antiarrhythmic Agents

Class III drugs exert their antiarrhythmic effect by increasing total action potential duration, by slowing phase 0 and prolonging recovery of excitability. Individual drugs of this class may have indirect effects on catecholamine release or blockade and therefore may effect phase 4 automaticity. Common surface ECG features of drug action are QRS widening and QT prolongation.

Class IV Antiarrhythmic Agents: Calcium-Channel Blockers

Calcium-channel blockers act by blocking the transmembrane influx of calcium through the slow calcium channel. These drugs may have an effect on phase 4 depolarization of the action potential, particularly in the sinus node, which can be seen clinically as sinus slowing. The remainder of the action potential is largely unaffected by these drugs, except for acceleration of phase 2 of the action potential. Of note, recently it has been shown that some calcium blockers may also possess effects much like those of beta blockers. As one might expect, these drugs have been found most useful in the treatment of arrhythmias involving cardiac tissue that is predominantly slow response in nature, such as the sinus node and the AV node.

Unclassified Antiarrhythmic Agents

Adenosine is an antiarrhythmic agent that does not fit into the current classification scheme. Adenosine is an endogenously occurring substance involved in a wide variety of regulatory processes throughout the body, including the regulation of systemic and coronary vascular tone and fat and carbohydrate metabolism. It exerts electrophysiologic effects on calcium slow channel conductance and potassium conductance and is antiadrenergic in some tissues. Direct effects are mediated by interaction with a specific extracellular adenosine receptor. The most prominent effects are on sinus automaticity and atrioventricular conduction, depressing both. The drug is used principally to terminate supraventricular tachycardias that use the AV node as part of the reentrant circuit.

MECHANISMS OF ARRHYTHMIAS

In recent years, cardiac arrhythmias have been divided into those resulting from abnormal impulse formation and those arising because of abnormal impulse propagation. We discuss each of these individually.

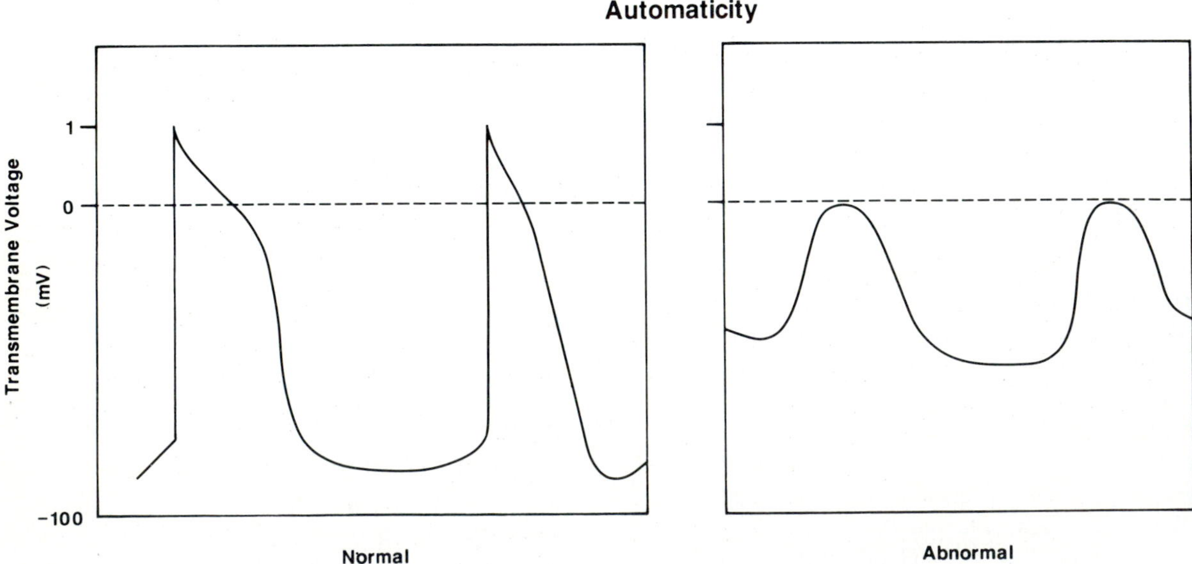

FIGURE 1-13 Schematic drawing of normal and abnormal automaticity. Differences in resting potential and action potential shape are apparent.

Abnormalities of Impulse Formation

Cells with normal automaticity characteristically have a resting potential less negative than cells that do not possess automaticity (Fig. 1-13). The automaticity of normal cells can be enhanced by substances such as catecholamines, but all normally automatic fibers can be suppressed by stimulation at a faster rate than the spontaneous rate of firing of the automatic fiber. After termination of this overdrive pacing, normally automatic fibers gradually recommence automatic firing after a brief pause. In contrast, cells made less negative experimentally or by disease may possess abnormal automaticity and produce automatic responses at a much faster rate than might otherwise be seen in that type of fiber (Fig. 1-13). This response is seen when the membrane potential is reduced towards −50 mV and may be the cause of arrhythmias seen in some damaged cardiac tissue. Overdrive pacing of tissues with abnormal automaticity does not display overdrive suppression, as seen in normally automatic tissue. As a matter of fact, actual acceleration of the abnormal automatic rate may be seen.

Another mechanism of abnormal impulse formation is triggered activity (Fig. 1-14). Triggered activity depends on the presence of delayed after-depolarizations. Delayed after-depolarizations are transient slow depolarizations that occur at the end of the action potential and depend on the action potential for their occurrence. They may increase in size with increasing rate of depolarization or with premature depolarizations. If these delayed after-depolarizations become large enough they may reach threshold and result

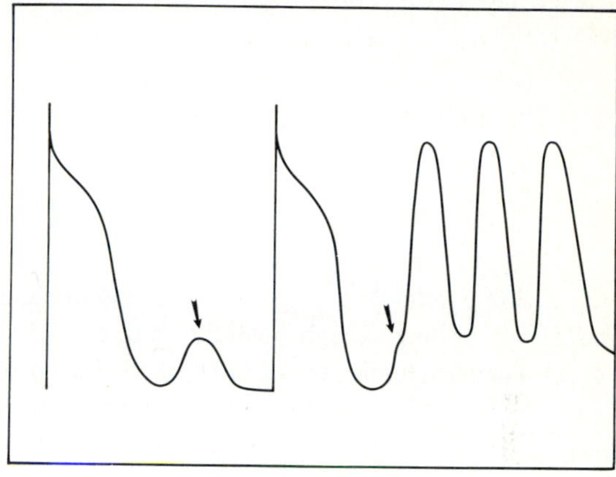

Triggered Activity

FIGURE 1-14 Schematic drawing of triggered activity. Delayed after-depolarizations *(arrows)* increase in size until triggered activity occurs.

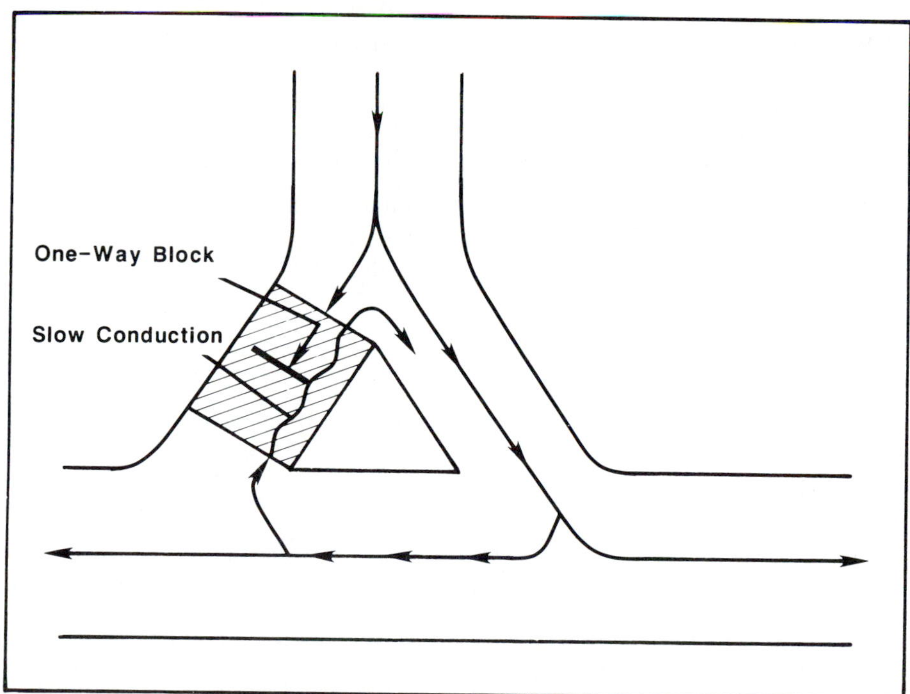

Reentry

FIGURE 1-15 Schematic drawing of reentrant activity. This represents a reentrant circuit in which an impulse blocks, takes a second pathway, and enters an area of slow conduction. When the wavefront of activation returns to the original area of block, the tissue has recovered and a reentrant beat occurs. If this continued, a tachycardia would occur.

Table 1-3 Possible Mechanisms of Clinical Arrhythmias

Automaticity	Triggering	Reentry
Escape beats—all types	Digitalis intoxication	AV nodal reentry
Ectopic atrial rhythms	?Multifocal atrial tachycardia	SA nodal reentry
Automatic atrial tachycardia	?Torsades de pointes	Reciprocating supraventricular tachycardia using bypass (Wolff-Parkinson-White syndrome)
Nonparoxysmal AV junctional tachycardia	?Ventricular tachycardia	Intraatrial reentry
Accelerated idioventricular rhythm		Atrial flutter and fibrillation
Parasystole		Ventricular tachycardia and fibrillation

in a full action potential, giving rise to an additional after-depolarization, another action potential, and so on, resulting in sustained rhythmic activity. Delayed after-depolarizations have been described in abnormal diseased ventricular myocardium and digitalis intoxication. The ionic basis of these depolarizations probably involves calcium and sodium currents. The involvement of calcium currents is supported by the observation that Ca^{++} channel-blocking drugs, like verapamil, may abolish delayed after-depolarization and triggered rhythms in experimental studies.

Abnormalities of Impulse Propagation

Abnormalities of impulse propagation may result in reentrant excitation. Reentry is the likely mechanism for most important arrhythmias in humans. Although the elements of the reentrant circuit may change, depending on the arrhythmia in question, the main ingredients in reentrant activity are the presence of block and slowed conduction. Reentry may occur when an impulse encounters an area of unidirectional block and must take an alternate pathway that conducts slowly. By the time the impulse returns to the original area of block the tissue has recovered and can again be excited—hence reentry (Fig. 1-15). The impulse enters the blocked areas, allowing it to activate the same tissue again, and the cycle is perpetuated. Block and slow conduction may be due to normal functional characteristics of tissue, such as in the AV node, or relatively fixed anatomic abnormalities, such as in scarred and disrupted myocardium of healed myocardial infarction. Examples of clinical arrhythmias that possibly fit into each of these categories are shown in Table 1-3.

SUGGESTED READINGS

Gross Cardiac Anatomy

Hollinshead WH. *Textbook of Anatomy*. 4th ed. New York: Harper and Row, 1985, Chapter 19, pp 522-541.

Coronary Anatomy

Baim DS, Grossman W. Coronary angiography. *In* Grossman W (ed). *Cardiac Catheterization and Angiography*. 3rd ed. Philadelphia: Lea and Febiger, 1986, Chapter 13, pp 173-199.

Levin DC, Gardiner GA. Coronary Arteriography. *In* Braunwald E (ed). *Heart Disease: A Textbook of Cardiovascular Medicine*. 3rd ed. Philadelphia: WB Saunders, 1988, Chap 10, pp 272-293.

Hollinshead WH. *Textbook of Anatomy*. 4th ed. New York: Harper and Row, 1985, Chapter 19, pp 530-532.

Electrocardiographic Patterns of Ischemia and Infarction

Fisch C. Electrocardiography and vectorcardiography. *In* Braunwald E (ed). *Heart Disease: A Textbook of Cardiovascular Medicine*. 3rd ed. Philadelphia: WB Saunders, 1988, Chapter 7, pp 180-222.

Anatomy of the Conduction System

Anderson RH, Ho SY, Becker AE. Gross anatomy and microscopy of the conducting system. *In* Mandel WJ (ed). *Cardiac Arrhythmias: Their Mechanisms, Diagnosis, and Management*. Philadelphia: JB Lippincott, 1987, Chapter 2, pp 13-52.

Autonomic Influences

Berne RM, Levy MN. Regulation of the heartbeat. *In* Berne RM, Levy MN (eds). *Physiology*. 2nd ed. St. Louis: The CV Mosby Co, 1988, Chapter 29, pp 451-471.

Mark AL, Mancia G. Cardiopulmonary baroreflexes in humans. *In Handbook of Physiology—The Cardiovascular System III*. Rockville, MD: American Physiological Association, 1980, Chapter 21, pp 795-813.

Basic Electrophysiology

Gadsby DC, Wit AL. Normal and abnormal electrical activity in cardiac cells. *In* Mandel WJ (ed). *Cardiac Arrhythmias: Their Mechanisms, Diagnosis, and Management*. 2nd ed. Philadelphia: JB Lippincott, 1987, Chapter 3, pp 53-80.

Hoffman BF. Mechanisms of antiarrhythmic action. *In* Zipes DP, Jalife J (eds.) *Cardiac Electrophysiology and Arrhythmias*. Orlando: Grune and Stratton, 1985, Chapter 22, pp 193-197.

Karagueuzian HS, Singh BN, Mandel WJ: Antiarrhythmic drugs: Mode of action, pharmacokinetic properties, and clinical applications. *In* Mandel WJ (ed). *Cardiac Arrhythmias: Their Mechanisms, Diagnosis, and Management*. 2nd ed. Philadelphia: JB Lippincott, 1987, Chapter 29, pp 697-737.

CHAPTER TWO

Cardiac Monitors and their Functions

▶ GOAL

You will be able to select and prepare a patient for cardiac monitoring and produce electrocardiographic data suitable for interpretation.

▶ OBJECTIVES

After reading this chapter, you should be able to:

1. Identify five major indications for monitoring in acute and ambulatory settings.
2. Describe the three types of monitoring systems and their energy sources.
3. Describe the capability features common to all hard wire monitors.
4. Identify the components of a telemetry monitoring system.
5. Determine what type of information enters a Holter diary and instruct the patient regarding entries and the description of symptoms.
6. Demonstrate the proper method of electrode application.
7. Recognize common sources of artifact, distinguish artifact from a cardiac rhythm, and identify ways to prevent or eliminate it.
8. Define signal-averaged electrocardiography and describe why it is used.

The electrical activity of the heart is monitored in several ways and in different settings. Monitoring is a standard feature of patient management in critical care units, the operating room, recovery room, and emergency department. Once confined to intensive care areas and diagnostic laboratories, monitoring is now performed in subacute or step down units, medical-surgical areas, and on an outpatient basis. Indications are for diagnostic and surveillance purposes and for evaluation of therapy.

TYPES OF MONITORING SYSTEMS

Monitoring is performed continuously through bedside electrical hard wire systems (for patients on bed rest), or via telemetry, in which radiofrequency signals transmit the electrical impulses (for the ambulatory patient). Both of these systems send information to centralized monitor stations in a hospital unit. Ambulatory electrocardiography, or Holter monitoring, is designed for intermittent, short-term use in the ambulatory setting. The Holter monitor is battery powered and stores heart activity on tape instead of displaying it on a screen. Emergency monitoring can be accomplished with the application of defibrillation paddles to the chest. Advancement in technology has led to increasingly lightweight, portable monitoring units, specialized pacemaker monitors, and models designed specifically for laboratories and operating suites. Combined defibrillator-monitor units have reached a level of sophistication in which 12-lead electrocardiography can be performed immediately after defibrillation.

Continuous Hard Wire Monitors

The term *hard wire* is used because the patient, generally on bed rest, is connected to a bedside monitor via a cable, and electrodes are attached to the skin to receive the current produced by the depolarization and repolarization of the heart. The currents are then transmitted through a cable to the monitor, magnified more than 1000 times, and displayed on the screen as wave forms. A monitor in the nurse's station records and displays the same activity as the bedside unit. Monitoring began in the early 1960s for patients with myocardial infarctions. It is now used for purposes of diagnosis, surveillance, and evaluation of therapy. The primary indications are summarized in the box on p. 20.

Indications for Bedside Monitoring

Emergency and life-threatening conditions
Acute myocardial infarction
Arrhythmia identification and evaluation
Chest pain
Evaluation of heart block and bundle branch block
Evaluation of ectopy
Detection and evaluation of changes in electrical axis (e.g., chamber hypertrophy)
Perioperative
Evaluation of pacemaker function
Evaluation of the effect of cardiac disease on heart function (e.g., pericarditis, mitral valve prolapse, valvular disease, cardiomyopathy, congestive heart failure)
Evaluation of the effect of noncardiac disease or injury on heart function (e.g., acute burn, hepatic failure, major trauma, chronic obstructive pulmonary disease)
Evaluation of response to drug therapy (e.g., antiarrhythmics or beta blockers)
Surveillance of heart rate

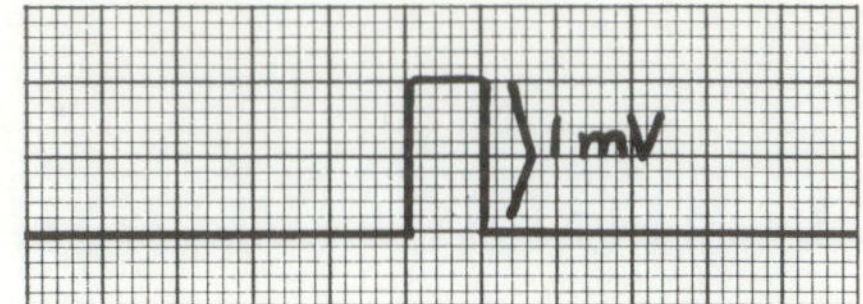

FIGURE 2-1 When 1 mV records 1-cm amplitude, the ECG is calibrated to standard size 1.

A wide variety of bedside monitors is on the market, but virtually all of them share the following standard features:

Power switch: turns machine on and off.

Oscilloscope: displays the moving electrocardiogram (ECG) wave forms on a CRT/VDT (cathode ray tube/video display terminal) screen. This may have one channel (which shows one ECG lead) or multiple channels to display simultaneous ECG leads or intracardiac pressure wave forms (pulmonary arterial pressure or systemic arterial pressure recordings). The nonfade screen has replaced the "bouncing ball" electron beam display in most modern clinical systems.

Brightness control: adjusts the brightness of the images on the oscilloscope.

Rate indicator: displays a digital heart rate number in beats per minute. Rate meters, as opposed to the digital number display, are still available and are quite accurate.

If the monitor is multichanneled, a digital number indicator corresponds with each channel on the oscilloscope. For example, a systemic arterial pressure wave form will show a digital number such as 110/60 mm Hg.

Alarm system: activates sound and light alarms if established limits are exceeded. High and low heart rates are dialed in, usually 10 to 20 beats above and below the patient rate. Alarm limits require adjustments according to the patient's changing status.

Alarm reset: resets the internal alarm after it has been activated.

Cable connector: connects the cable plug to the monitor. The patient's lead wires are connected to the other end of the cable. Both cable ends must be securely attached for proper transmission of impulses. Cable ends should never become wet.

Lead selector: allows the desired lead to be dialed in; 3-lead selectors offer leads I, II, or III; 5-lead selector systems permit monitoring of all 12 leads.

Position control: moves the tracing to the top, center, or bottom of the screen.

Gain control: adjusts the monitor's sensing of the QRS amplitude. Changes in amplitude (higher or lower) will be evident both on the screen and paper printout. Some monitors have a separate size button, which changes QRS amplitude on the screen and paper but does not affect the internal sensitivity function. If this is adjusted too high, the machine may register other wave forms as QRS complexes and exhibit erroneously high heart rates on the rate indicator.

1 mV/cal: allows the monitor to be calibrated. If the machine is accurately calibrated by adjusting the gain control, depressing the 1 mV/cal button will produce a 1 cm amplitude "square" wave form on the printout paper (or a height of 2 large boxes). This is standard size 1 (Fig. 2-1).

Sweep: refers to the speed at which the image is displayed on an oscilloscope. When the image is displayed on ECG paper, it is referred to as the *paper speed:* 25 mm/sec is standard speed; 50, 75, and 100 mm/sec are used for diagnostic purposes (e.g., QRS morphology) and make the complexes appear wider.

Printout/recorder: automatically prints the wave form on paper if the alarm sounds or on demand if the button is depressed.

QRS light: blinks with each QRS complex.

QRS volume: beeps with each QRS complex. The volume is adjustable.

Run/hold/record switch: allows the wave form to run continuously across the screen or be held or "frozen" and recorded for interpretation. Memory loops retain up to 60 seconds and return trace to screen.

Monitor/standby: allows temporary deactivation of alarms, for example, when the patient is being manipulated or electrodes are changed. Switch is generally placed on monitor mode. Changing it to standby is for deactivation.

Synchronizer outlet: allows for insertion of a cable that is connected to a defibrillator, if the patient requires cardioversion. This outlet may be in the front or back of the monitor.

Monitor/diagnostic: adjusts filtering. When the switch is turned to monitor, a filter is activated. Diagnostic indicates less filtering and is used for wave form diagnostic purposes.

Hard wire bedside monitoring systems use electricity as their energy source. Modern, functioning units are sufficiently grounded so that bathing, moist dressings, and routine patient care do not present electrical hazards to the patient, provided the equipment is properly installed and maintained. Fig. 2-2 illustrates features commonly found in monitors.

Information recorded at each bedside monitor is simultaneously recorded at the central monitoring station. This monitoring bank features multiple oscilloscopes, recorders, alarms, and arrhythmia detectors. It allows one person to observe and monitor the activity of a large number of patients (Fig. 2-3). Traditionally nurses have monitored at

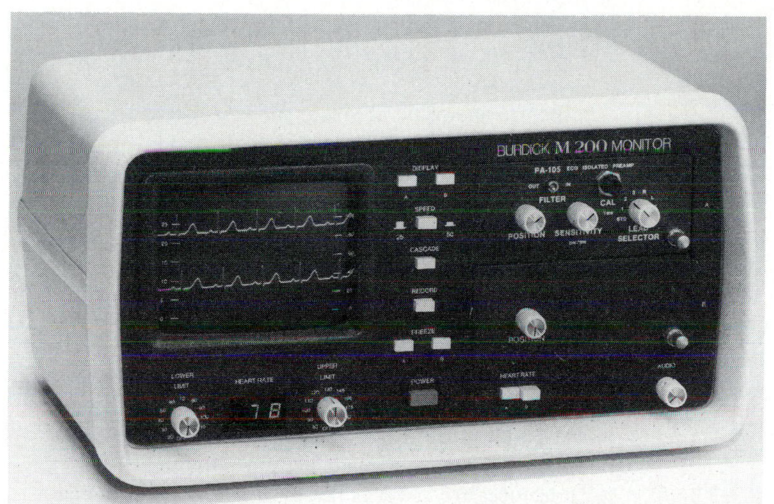

FIGURE 2-2 Basic monitoring system showing standard features. Courtesy of Burdick Division, Kone Instrument, Inc.

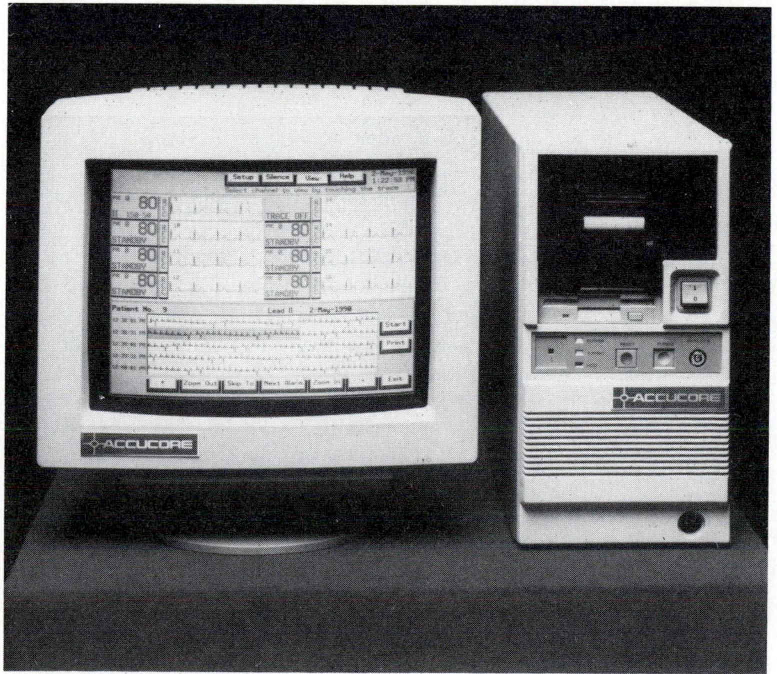

FIGURE 2-3 Contemporary monitoring system showing standard features. Courtesy of Accucore.

the central station. In recent years, some institutions have employed monitor technicians who are specially trained in arrhythmia identification. They provide continuous observation and free the nurses to leave the station to give patient care.

Many critical care units and telemetry services use computer microprocessor techniques for sophisticated monitoring of large patient groups. Computerized arrhythmia systems provide periodic and demand ECG monitoring, continuous scanning of ECG rhythms and patterns, a system of audio and visual alarms, and the capability to process trends in heart rate and rhythm. Some systems offer a preliminary arrhythmia interpretation. These are just some of the standard features (see box on this page and Fig. 2-4).

Telemetry

Telemetry monitoring was developed to permit continuous ECG surveillance without attaching the patient to a bedside monitor by lead wires. It is used primarily for arrhythmia analysis and to identify trends in heart rate and arrhythmia patterns. Telemetry offers convenience and practicality for convalescing and ambulatory patients.

The telemetry system has four components: the transmitter, the antennas, a receiver that monitors signals from the antenna network, and the monitoring recording devices (Fig. 2-5). The system uses 2 or 3 electrodes attached to the patient and connected to a battery-operated transmitter box that is placed in a pouch and tied to the patient's body. The actual energy source for transmission of the ECG tracing is radiofrequency waves, which are received in the central monitoring station.

Many centralized units have the capability for both bedside and telemetry monitoring. This is an attractive feature because it allows conversion from one type of monitoring to another. For example, patients may be monitored in one unit although they are actually housed and cared for in another. However, under these circumstances the care giver and the person responsible for monitoring must know where their responsibilities lie. Recently more versatile telemetry systems have been developed that also offer transmission of ECG, electromyelographic (EMG), and electroencephalographic (EEG) signals.

Ambulatory Electrocardiography

Holter Monitoring

Physicist Norman J. Holter developed the ambulatory monitor in the 1950s, after decades of research in radio telemetry and radio electrocardiography.[2] Clinical application of the Holter monitor was reported in 1954.[3] Holter is the common name for short-term (usually 24 hours) ambulatory/outpatient monitoring. Holters are useful in diagnosing patient complaints of skipped beats, extra beats, palpi-

Capabilities of Contemporary Monitoring Systems

- Systems compatible, microprocessor based, and software driven
- Multiple parameters detected, processed, and recorded:
  - ECGs
  - Central and systemic hemodynamic pressures
  - Body temperatures
  - Cardiac output
  - Peripheral pulses
- Rhythm analysis and trending:
  - Electrocardiographic event and rhythm detection
  - Simultaneous display, recording, and analysis of multiple leads
  - Storage and recall of single and cumulative events
  - Projection of trends and physiologic profiles
  - Scanning for analysis and summary of: ectopic beats, tachycardias, bradycardias, morphologies, and ST-segment changes
- Display of information:
  - Digital transmission of: data, colored graphics, and histograms (bar graphs showing frequency of events)
  - Printing of wave forms
  - Visual comparison of current parameters with previously recorded ones
  - Algorithms for feature extraction and template correlation (the monitor reproduces patterns and shapes of electrical events for purposes of analysis and comparison)
  - Preliminary arrhythmia interpretation
- Improvements in artifact suppression with early detection of improperly applied electrodes to minimize false alarms[1]
- Improvements in audible/visual graded alarms and alarm resetting
- Increased sophistication of hold/freeze, recall, and delay:
  - Retrieval of information several hours after real time occurrence
  - Cascading capabilities (enhanced storage and display that enable visualization of 15 to 20 seconds of elapsed data)
- Options for the display and positioning of wave forms on the oscilloscope
- Models designed for the special needs of anesthesia and surgical areas:
  - Improved visibility of parameters
  - Suppression of electrosurgical unit interference
- Detection and display of artificial pacemaker activity and parameters

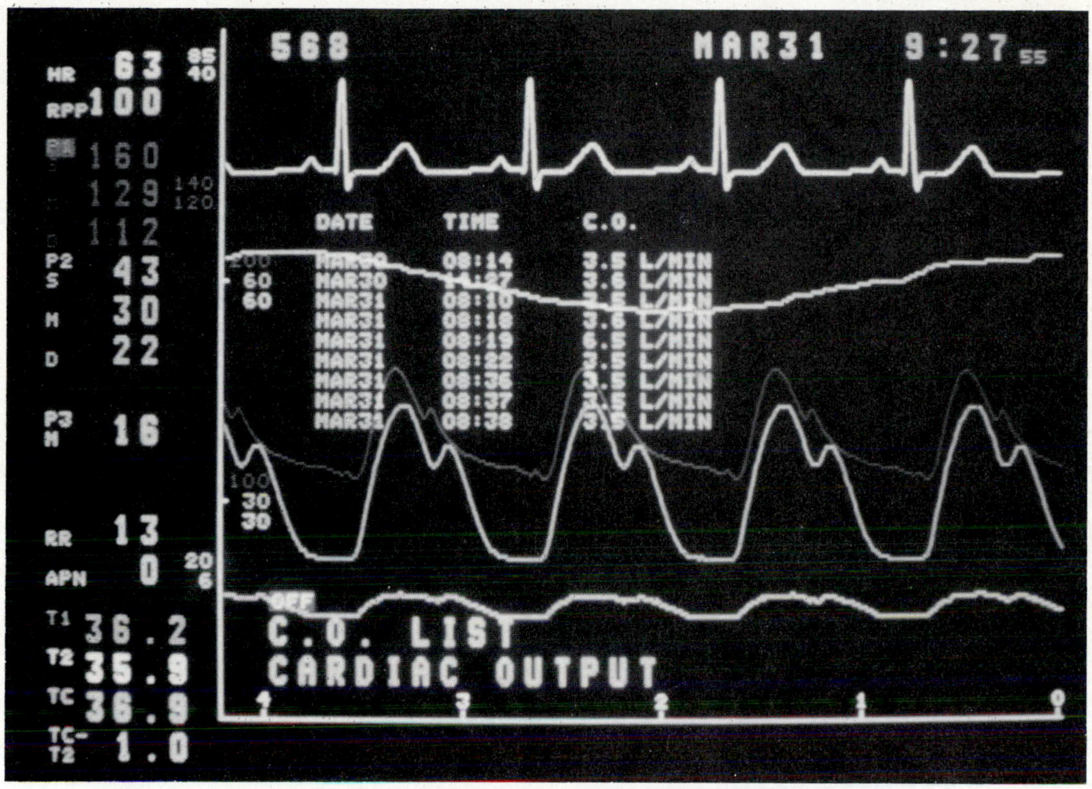

FIGURE 2-4 Single-patient monitor displaying multiple hemodynamic parameters (heart rate, various hemodynamic pressures, body temperatures, and trend of cardiac output measurements), date, and time. Courtesy of Burdick Division, Kone Instrument, Inc.

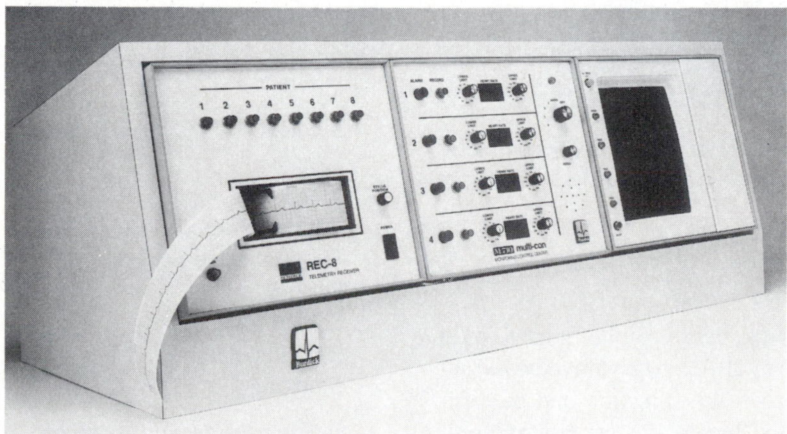

FIGURE 2-5 This photograph illustrates the basic design of a telemetry receiver. Courtesy of the Burdick Division, Kone Instruments, Inc.

Indications for Holter Monitoring

Diagnosis of arrhythmias
Diagnosis of ischemia[4,5]
Stress testing (treadmill)
Evaluation of malignant ventricular ectopy[6]
Evaluation of symptoms such as dizziness, dyspnea, chest pain, palpitations, syncope, fatigue, light-headedness
Evaluation of the efficacy of antiarrhythmic drug therapy
Ongoing evaluation of patients with structural and congestive heart disease
Identification of patients at risk for sudden cardiac death (SCD)[4]

Features of Holter Monitoring

Multiple, programmable formats
Multiple lead analysis
Morphology classification of components of the ECG: QRS complex, T wave, ST segment
Heart-rate analysis
Summary of tachycardias and bradycardias
Summary of ectopic events
Analysis of ST-segment elevation and depression (used to evaluate the occurrence of ischemia)

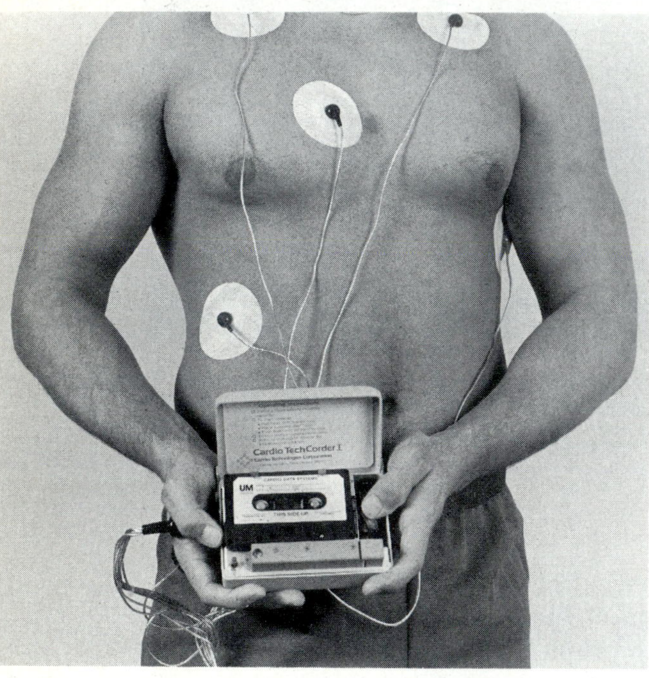

FIGURE 2-6 Patient shown with Holter-lead electrodes in place, holding the receiver/recorder. Photo by Judy Taylor, courtesy of United Medical Corporation.

tations, and other symptoms that may be related to a rhythm disturbance. They are also used postmyocardial infarction and to evaluate pacemaker function and the efficacy of antiarrhythmic drugs. Indications for Holter monitoring are listed in the box at the top of the column.

The design of the Holter monitor has been streamlined considerably in the last three decades. Operating with a single channel (records one lead), dual channels (records two leads simultaneously), or multiple channels, the unit is battery operated and worn on a belt (Fig. 2-6). Each heart beat is recorded on magnetic tape; the 24-hour tape of heart activity is later analyzed and summarized in a written report. Features of Holter monitoring are summarized in the box above.

For successful Holter monitoring with meaningful reports, patient care and education are important. Chest electrodes must be securely adhered for a complete recording. This is best accomplished by taping the electrodes to the patient's skin. Instruct the patient not to loosen the electrodes or shower during the monitoring interval. Stretchable net shirts are sometimes used to secure electrodes and lead cables for the prevention of artifact. Selection of Holter lead sites is discussed in Chapter 3.

Inpatients and outpatients are instructed to keep a diary during the 24-hour period, recording the times of activities and any associated symptoms. Physical activities are indicated by a patient-activated event marker found on the receiver. Most Holter companies provide a diary booklet. Instruct the patient to record in the diary the following activities or events:

Medications (especially antiarrhythmics)
Exercise
Meals
Urination/defecation
Bedtime/sleep period
Driving
Sexual intercourse
Emotional stress
Smoking

Instruct the patient to record any symptoms during the period, including fatigue, light-headedness, dizziness, chest pain, or palpitations. Make certain that the patient's medications and medical diagnosis are recorded in the diary. It is just as important to correlate symptoms that occur during an arrhythmia as it is to record symptoms in the absence of arrhythmias.

Symptom-Activated, Transtelephonic Event Recorders

A portable, symptom-activated, transtelephonic event recorder is sometimes used in place of Holter monitoring to evaluate infrequent, episodic symptoms that may be due to an arrhythmia. The device is kept at home with the patient for several weeks and used only when symptoms such as palpitations or light-headedness occur. When an event arises, the patient places the receiver over the chest and records the heart rhythm for approximately 30 seconds. The recording is then transmitted via telephone by the patient to the physician, who determines whether an arrhythmia has caused the symptom. Another transtelephonic method involves the use of electrodes placed in the axilla. Some devices have memory capabilities enabling the patient to record and transmit the recording at a later time.

Another recent development is the ECG memory loop recorder, which remembers and documents the ECG preceding the symptom, as well as during and subsequent to the symptomatic period.

Cardiac loop electrocardiographic recording is an important diagnostic test in patients with syncope unexplained by Holter monitoring.[7] This symptom-activated, transtelephonic recording device, unlike the portable recorder described previously, is worn continuously by the patient for weeks or months at a time. Its memory loop stores the preceding 1 to 4 minutes of cardiac rhythm when activated by a symptomatic patient. The patient then places a component of the recording system on the telephone and the recording is transmitted telephonically to a receiving station where a nurse or physician can conduct the initial interpretation of the rhythm.

MONITORING THE PATIENT

Electrodes and Leads

Monitoring is sophisticated and far more versatile and reliable than ever before. New features have simplified the process and it is now common for nurses to monitor from a choice of several lead systems. Whatever lead is studied, however, the underlying principles of obtaining and securing an accurate lead are the same. The electrode-lead system must be comfortable to the patient, provide maximum information, and be free of electrical artifact and interference. The electrode sites chosen should also allow maximum access to the chest for physical examination (auscultation), frequent 12-lead ECGs, cardioversion or defibrillation (room for correct application of paddles), and external cardiac massage. Electrodes are patches applied to the skin, generally the trunk, which pick up the small currents produced by electrical depolarization and repolarization of the heart. Skin electrodes can be positioned on the trunk or extremities in a number of patterns or locations to establish various lead systems. Two to five electrodes are used. Some useful principles in applying electrodes and reducing artifact are discussed before the description of lead systems.

Remember that for heart surgery and special diagnostic procedures, electrodes can be intracardiac or positioned as catheters on the epicardial or endocardial surfaces of the heart. The electrograms or wave forms produced are clear and detailed. Skin electrodes translate the same current but through the bone, muscle, and fluid of the body cavity. That is why the skin electrogram of bedside monitoring or ECGs looks different from the wave forms of intracardiac electrograms that are recorded during cardiac surgery or catheterization.

Normally, the impulses generated within the heart spread from the high right atrium to the left ventricle, having depolarized all chambers during the process. Because of its greater mass, the left ventricle generates more electrical activity. Because there are more cells to depolarize in the left ventricle, and because the impulses normally originate in the SA node, the predominant direction of depolarization is right to left and top to bottom (Fig. 2-7). The sum total of several, individual wavefronts of activation is the *mean vector force*. The same pattern of depolarization occurs repeatedly in the patient's heart (i.e., the overall direction does not change). Some individuals, because of anatomy, disease, or change in heart size or function, do not exhibit this pattern of normal depolarization. This is known as *axis deviation* and is discussed in Chapter 3.

Because the direction of depolarization is a constant, electrode position is a variable that causes the electrogram of one lead to look different from the others. If the impulse flows toward the positive electrode of a bipolar lead (one positive and one negative) or a unipolar electrode, the galvanometer or recording device records a positive or up-

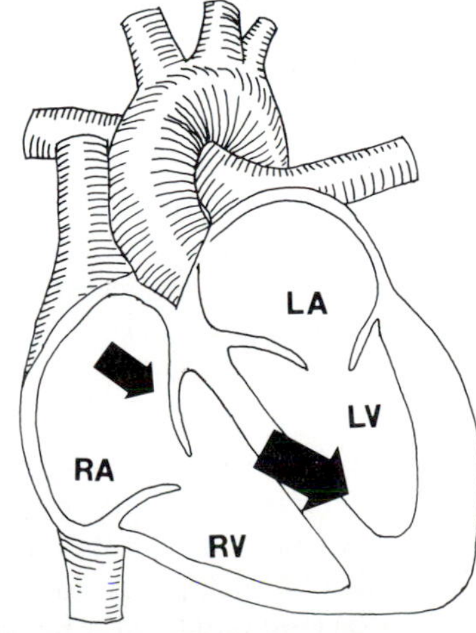

FIGURE 2-7 Schematic drawing illustrating the direction of depolarization for cardiac impulses originating in SA node and the comparatively thick aspect of the left ventricle (LV). LA = left atrium, RA = right atrium, RV = right ventricle.

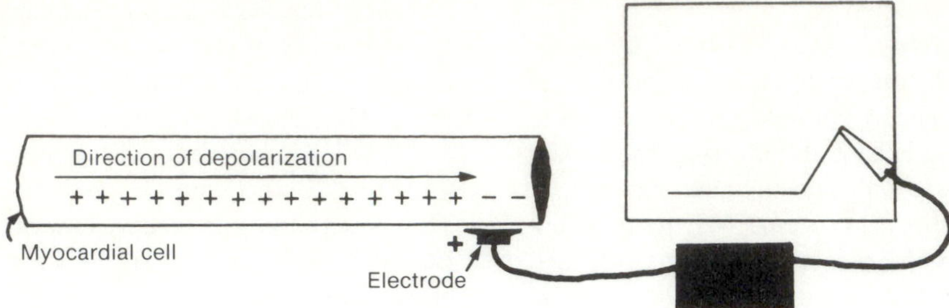

FIGURE 2-8 Schematic drawing illustrating wave of depolarization. When direction of depolarization is toward the positive electrode, a positive deflection is written on the ECG. For the purpose of simplicity, a negative electrode is not illustrated.

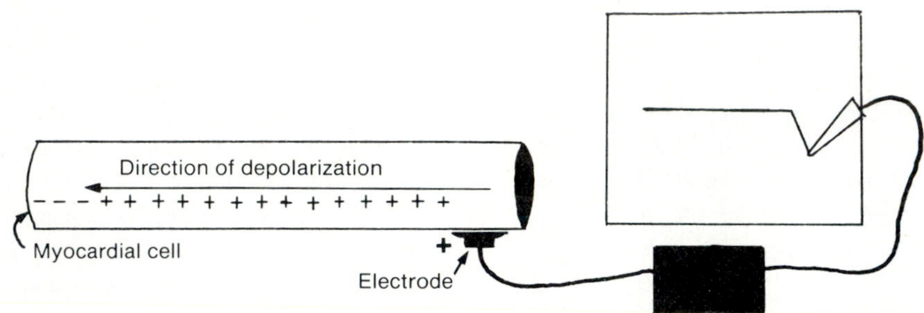

FIGURE 2-9 Schematic drawing illustrating wave of depolarization. When direction of depolarization is away from the positive electrode, a negative deflection is written on the ECG. For the purpose of simplicity, a negative electrode is not illustrated.

ward deflection. If the impulse flows either away from a positive electrode or toward a negative electrode (the negative pole of a bipolar lead), a negative or downward deflection is recorded (Figs. 2-8 and 2-9). The deflection increases or decreases until maximum depolarization occurs. It then peaks and recedes.

Proper electrode application is one important step in cardiac monitoring. Unless there is excellent electrode-to-skin contact, electrical resistance will distort the wave forms (electrogram) and cause artifact to appear. Hair, skin residues, sweat, body oils, and air spaces impede electrical flow and may interfere with transmission of the impulses.

There are three types of electrodes used for surface (skin) electrocardiography: the metal disk (metal plate, silver plate), the metal suction cup, and the disposable disk (floating disk). The metal plates and suction cups are placed on the chest and extremities for 12-lead ECGs and are not designed for monitoring. The self-adhering, pregelled disposable disk electrode is used for continuous hard wire, telemetry, and Holter monitoring and for signal-averaged electrocardiography. It consists of an adhesive paper, cloth, karaya, or foam synthetic ring with a conductive gel center. The conductive gel is usually of silver/silver chloride composition and saturates the sponge center. Needle electrodes are outmoded and are rarely seen. Fig. 2-10 illustrates a cross section of a disposable disk electrode.

Temporary monitoring can be achieved through the disk plates of defibrillator paddles. When placed on the chest, the paddles provide a crude but legible electrogram that is necessary in emergencies.

Electrode sites should be clean, dry, and provide a smooth and flat surface. Proper skin preparation is essential because it is a factor in preventing inaccurate readings. The following are guidelines for secure electrode application:

1. Shave hairy areas approximately 4 inches in diameter.
2. Rub briskly with a dry gauze pad to remove skin oil, cells, and residue. In general, it is best to avoid the excessive use of alcohol and solvents, since they become trapped and cause irritation and loss of adhe-

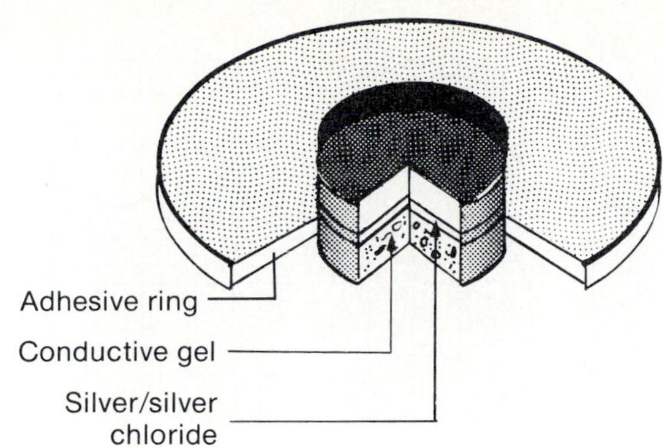

FIGURE 2-10 Cross section of disk electrode. The adhesive ring minimizes motion artifact. The gel sponge center conducts the skin surface voltage change.

sion. Alcohol may be necessary if the skin is greasy, but it must be allowed to dry. Avoid the use of acetone for cleansing and tincture of benzoin for adhesiveness. These agents are frequently irritating to the skin and may cause problems. If one must be used, place it on the perimeter of the area and not the center.

3. Electrodes should be kept at room temperature. Open the electrode package only when ready to use to prevent evaporation of the electrolyte gel. Remove the paper backing from the adhesive surface, tack one edge to skin, pull gently against it, and tack the other side. Then smooth the electrode with your finger in a circular motion. This helps to fix the gel and prevent motion artifact.
4. Attach lead wires to the electrodes and secure the cable to the patient's gown. Make sure the cable is fastened snugly into the monitor. In the case of telemetry the cable fits into the transmitter box. The box fits into a pouch and the patient wears it around his neck or waist. The Holter lead cable secures into the recorder and the device is worn belted around the waist. Because a Holter is a single 24-hour recording that is commonly used with outpatients, it is important additionally to secure the electrodes with tape or an elastic net vest.
5. Although mild abrasion of the skin is important for good electrode contact, never rub the skin until it is irritated or bleeding. Avoid using the sandpaper scratch pads found on many brands of electrodes; they are too abrasive. However, in some patients it may be necessary to mildly abrade the electrode contact sites with a small piece of ultra-fine sandpaper to reduce impedance further. Sometimes contact is difficult to maintain in profusely diaphoretic patients and in patients undergoing diagnostic testing in exercise laboratories and cardiac catheterization facilities. In these specialized settings, other methods for applying and securing electrodes will be found. There is a plethora of chemical abraders on the market. These products must be used carefully because they can be painful and cause bleeding or allergic reactions.
6. Specific locations for electrodes are discussed in Chapter 3. Regardless of the lead, an electrode should be placed approximately 8 inches from the heart, creating as large a triangle as possible.
7. Underlying bone is the most desirable location for an electrode. If this is impractical the electrode should be placed close to bone or over areas of soft tissue. Avoid muscle, skin folds, sharp bony protuberances and bony irregularities, and portions of the chest that move actively during breathing. These areas are more likely to produce artifact.
8. Electrodes should be changed every 2 to 3 days to maintain skin integrity. If the skin is irritated, do not reuse the site. Use the garment clip found on the cable to reduce lead wire strain.

Impedance of each electrode pair should be quantified with an appropriate testing device. Clochesy et al recently studied the effect of electrode site preparation techniques on reducing electrical potential (noise) in monitoring with skin electrodes. They concluded that offset potential, or artifact caused by the electrode-skin interface, can be significantly reduced by mild skin abrasion.[8]

Artifact

Artifact is incidental electrical activity and is caused by a flaw or problem in the monitoring process. There are multiple causes of artifact and practically all of them are avoidable. In troubleshooting this complication of monitoring, determine if the problem lies in the equipment or the patient. Whenever a bizarre rhythm appears or an alarm is triggered, always check the patient first. Is there a physiologic cause for the rhythm abnormality: cardiac arrest, respiratory distress, tremors, shivering, or movement? Check the electrodes to see that they are securely attached and are not over muscle or an actively moving part of the chest wall. Finally, check the lead wires and cable for disconnections and breaks. Make sure the cable end is inserted firmly into the monitor and not in close proximity to other electrical cords. Determine the appropriate lead, gain, and sensitivity on the monitor.

The following are common types of artifact with suggestions for preventing or correcting the problem:

- Movement artifact (Fig. 2-11) occurs when electrodes are placed over muscle mass and is easily prevented by choosing another site.

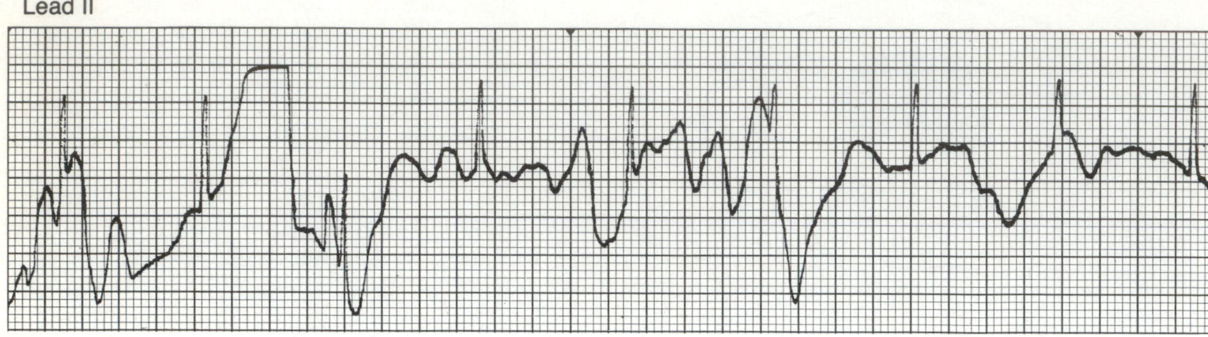

FIGURE 2-11 Artifact caused by patient movement. Most complexes are discernible. Artifact with this appearance resembles a serious rhythm disturbance and should be immediately evaluated.

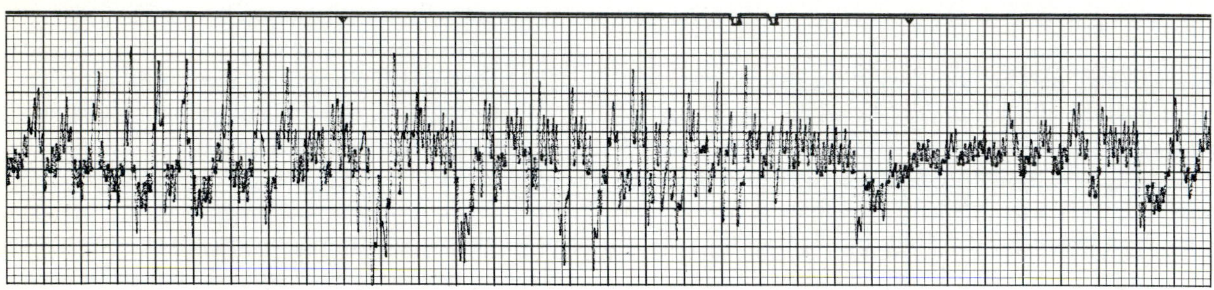

FIGURE 2-12 Tremor artifact. Unlike chaotic tracing or factitious artifact, tremor and muscle "noise" have more of a machine distortion appearance.

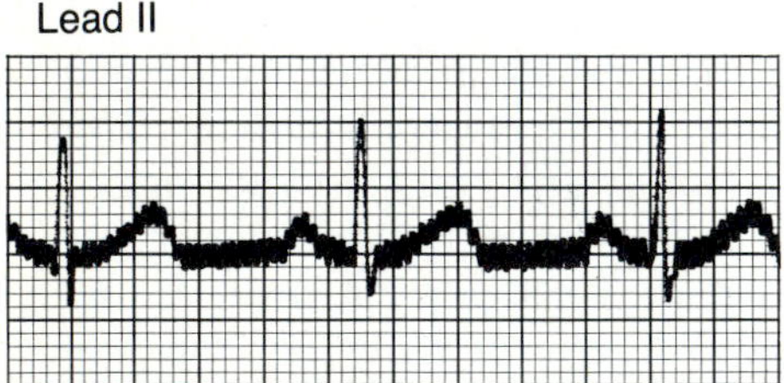

FIGURE 2-13 Example of 60-cycle interference. Note the baseline is widened by the regular, rapidly occurring spikes.

- Tremors (Fig. 2-12), tension, anxiety, seizures, or other "muscle noise" may cause an irregular, shaky baseline.
- Sixty-cycle (Fig. 2-13) or AC interference is a potentially hazardous artifact caused by extrinsic electrical sources. It produces a baseline widened and distorted by artifact spikes occurring 60 cycles/second. It has many sources: damaged lead wires, poor electrode contact, improper grounding, a cable that is in close proximity to the monitor's power cord, or current leakage from radios, electrical razors, fluorescent light fixtures, or defective equipment (e.g., ventilators, suction machines). Check the patient monitor series of connections for any breaks. Do not use a 5-electrode cable for a 3-lead system. If the electrodes, lead wires, cable connector, and cable are all securely connected and the cable is not close to the monitor cord, there is probably an extraneous source. The easiest and safest solution to this problem is to contact the hospital biomedical engineer.
- Chaotic tracing (Fig. 2-14) is what the name implies: a chaotic series of spikes and dips that obscure the underlying complexes. This is usually caused by poor electrode contact resulting from improper skin preparation, dried electrode gel, or loosening of the lead wires or cable.
- Wandering baseline (Fig. 2-15) is common and generally results from loose electrode-lead, wire-cable connections, damaged wires, loose or dry electrodes, excessive electrode gel, respiratory excursions, or movement of the cable with breathing. Checking the system for breaks and disconnections and reducing

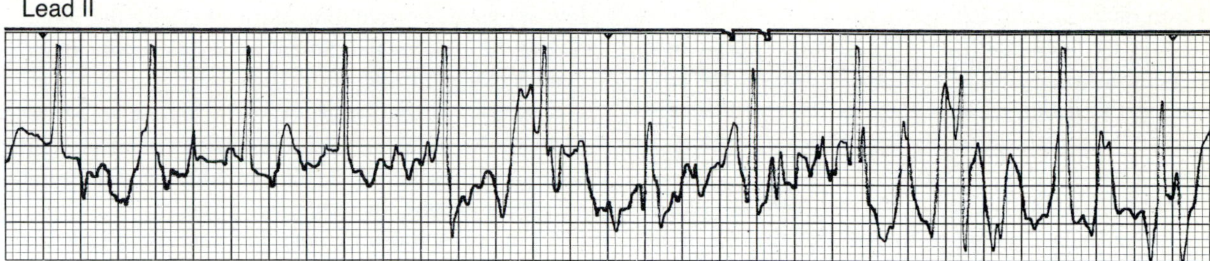

FIGURE 2-14 Chaotic tracing caused by poor electrode contact. Although very disorganized in appearance, chaotic tracing maintains most complexes and can mimic serious rhythm disturbances.

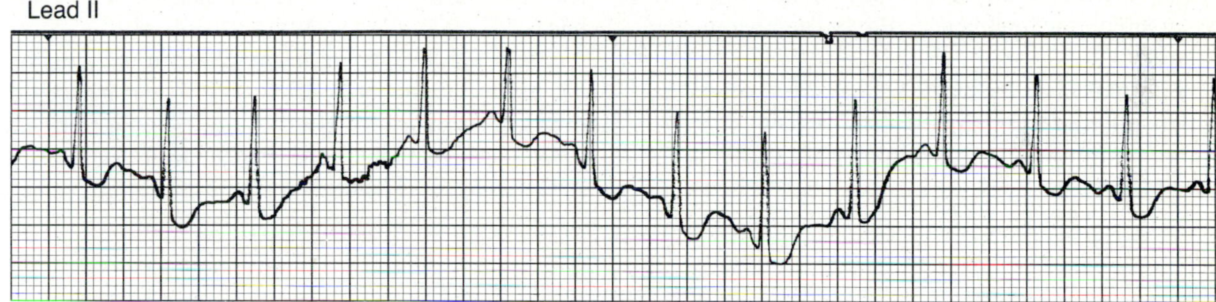

FIGURE 2-15 Exercise-induced sinus tachycardia (rate greater than 100 bpm) with wandering baseline. Diaphoresis frequently causes this wavering from the straight baseline.

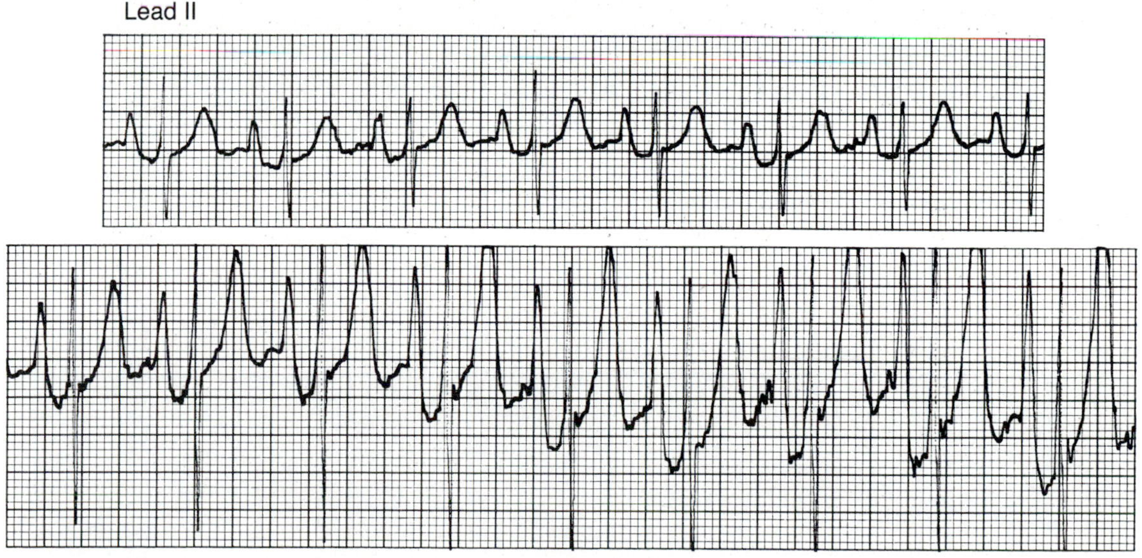

FIGURE 2-16 Falsely elevated heart rate. Initially, the monitor's rate meter read 94 bpm. Maximum amplitude adjustment resulted in P waves, T waves, and R waves all registering on the rate indicator, resulting in a false reading of 282 bpm at the end of the strip.

the tension on the electrodes, wires, and cable will prevent or eliminate this problem. It may be helpful to place the electrodes where respiratory excursions are minimal.

- A falsely elevated heart rate (Fig. 2-16) occurs when the monitor senses both the R and T waves, thereby doubling the patient's heart rate. To correct this, reduce the gain, reposition the electrodes, or select a different lead.
- A straight baseline (Fig. 2-17) or loss of signal always warrants examining the patient first. If it is not a patient emergency, the likely causes are a disconnection in the electrode-wire-connector-cable system, wrong setting on the lead selector, or insufficient gain. Continuity testers (circuit testers) are available for testing the integrity of lead wires. If the baseline persists after depressing the calibration (1 mV) button, the problem could be internal to the monitor.
- Weak batteries in a telemetry system will produce excessive artifact and small amplitude signals.
- Fig. 2-18 illustrates an example of artifact from factitious interference.

Alarms

The alarm system is the monitor's most critical safety feature. Nurses have many reasons for not using alarms and few are valid. Dismantling alarms because the sound is annoying or it keeps the patient awake is a potentially negligent nursing practice.

There are myriad causes of false alarms and a variety of methods for reducing their occurrence. It is important to reassure the patient that the sounding alarm is usually due to factors outside the actual heart rate.

Common sources of false low alarms include electrode disconnection, poor electrode contact, wrong lead, low QRS amplitude (because of a wrong lead, side lying position, obesity, thick chest wall), wide QRS complexes, insufficient gain, insufficient sensitivity, wandering baseline, damaged or disconnected lead wire, loose cable, and an alarm setting that is too close to the patient's intrinsic heart rate.

False high alarms are triggered when the monitor double counts (senses both the R and T) and may be due to high gain settings. AC electrical interference from infusion pumps and ventilators and artifact from movements and tremor may also contribute to this problem. The most

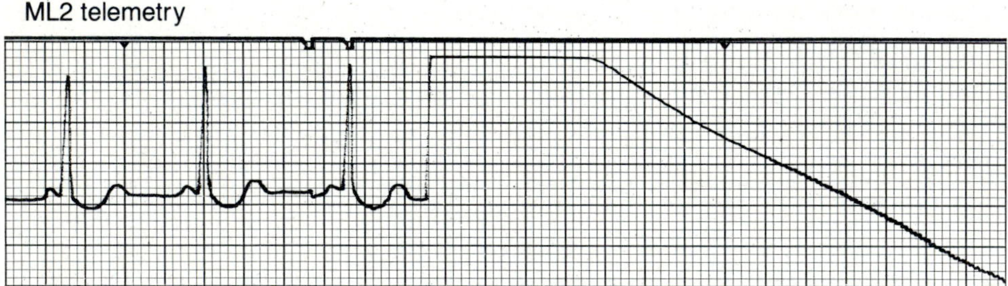

FIGURE 2-17 Loss of signal resulting from electrode detachment. This type of artifact also occurs when telemetry patients travel out of frequency range.

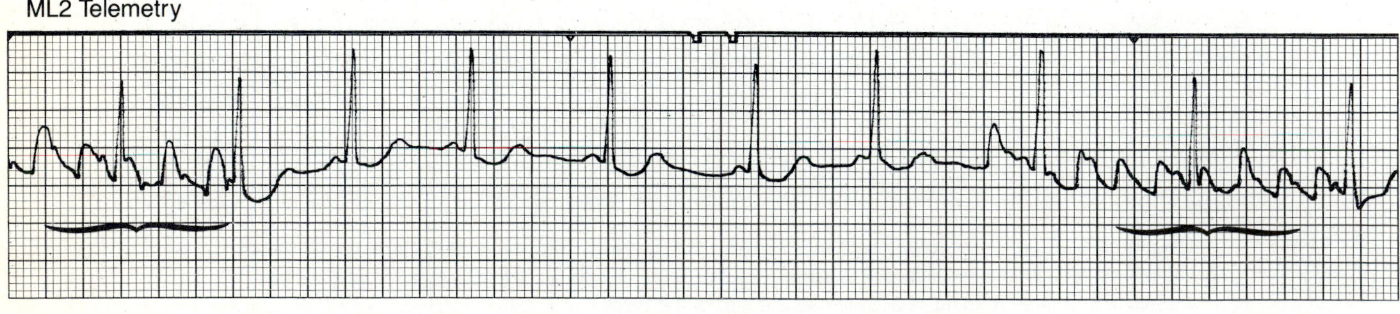

FIGURE 2-18 Normal sinus rhythm interrupted by factitious artifact, which resembles an arrhythmia. The artifact was produced by the patient tapping the positive electrode *(brackets)*.

common cause is an alarm setting that is too close to the patient's high rate.

Patient Education

It is important to educate patients on the purpose of monitoring. Often they are fearful of the procedure and misinterpret its intent. Some may need to be assured that the monitor is not a pacemaker, does not present an electrical shock hazard, and does not restrict movement a great deal. It is wise to show the patient how movement causes a false high rate reading and assure him or her that the nurses are able to differentiate this kind of artifact from rhythm disturbances.

ELECTROCARDIOGRAPHIC MONITORING STANDARDS

To cover the subjects of monitor instrumentation and performance, electrodes and lead systems, and personnel training, the reader is urged to review and adopt as needed the American Heart Association's "Instrumentation and Practice Standards for Electrocardiographic Monitoring."[9]

SIGNAL-AVERAGED ELECTROCARDIOGRAPHY

Signal-averaged or high-resolution electrocardiography is a noninvasive, computer-based diagnostic test used to predict or identify patients at high risk for sudden cardiac death from ventricular tachycardia.[10-12]It is also used to screen and evaluate patients with unexplained syncope after myocardial infarction[11,12] and postsubendocardial resection.[11]

Signal-averaged electrocardiography is used in conjunction with clinical electrophysiology and angiography, stress testing, echocardiography, and ambulatory electrocardiography. It may also be used to determine the need for invasive catheterization studies.

In recent years the use of the signal-averaging technique in the analysis of surface ECGs has revealed abnormal low-amplitude signals in the ECGs of patients with ventricular tachycardia.[11,13] These low-amplitude signals, or late potentials, occur in the terminal portion of the QRS complex and the beginning portion of the ST segment. Late potentials are believed to arise "in areas of abnormal myocardium exhibiting slow conduction (an essential requirement for reentrant ventricular tachycardia)."[13] The mechanism of reentry in tachyarrhythmias is discussed in Chapter 1 and subsequent chapters.

The value of the signal-averaged ECG lies in its ability to detect and display cardiac late potentials and to generate a noise-free recording through high-resolution electrocardiography. This signal enhancing capability is not achievable with conventional surface ECGs because noise from skeletal muscle, power lines, amplifiers, and electrodes cannot be sufficiently reduced. In signal-averaging, multiple signals are averaged to produce high-resolution, noise-free signals that can be amplified to detect and visualize the late potentials.

Depending on the system used, either the bipolar XYZ orthogonal (perpendicular to each other)[11,12] or the Frank XYZ[14] lead system is used. The electrodes must be securely attached and placed in areas where electrode artifact is minimized. There are myriad technologic differences among signal-averaged electrocardiographic systems, particularly filtering mechanisms, lead-electrode systems, and computer algorithms used to calculate the noise level and the result.

Signal-averaged electrocardiography is easily performed at the bedside and completed in less than 30 minutes. Ideally, the test is performed in an electronically isolated room. The patient should be told why the test is needed and the information it potentially yields. Instruct the patient to lie still (supine position), breathe normally, and remain quiet. It is important that the patient be relaxed during this procedure. To further minimize noise, unplug any unnecessary electrical equipment.

The reader is encouraged to review the American Heart Association's recently published standards concerning signal-averaged or high-resolution electrocardiography.[15]

REFERENCES

1. Weinfurt PT. Electrocardiographic monitoring: an overview. *J. Clin. Monit.*, Apr., 1990, 6(2): 132-8.
2. Holter NJ. New method for heart studies. *Science*, Oct. 20, 1961, 134(3486): 1214-20.
3. MacInnis HF. The clinical application of radio electrocardiography. *Can. Med. Assoc. J.*, 1954, 70: 574-6.
4. Antman EM. Clinical applications of Holter recording. *Consultant*, Mar. 30, 1985, 96-105.
5. DiMarco JP, Philbrick JT. Use of ambulatory electrocardiographic (Holter) monitoring. *Ann. Intern. Med.*, Jul. 1, 1990, 113(1): 53-68.
6. Horner SL. *Ambulatory Electrocardiography: Applications and Techniques*. Philadelphia: JB Lippincott, 1983.
7. Linzer M, Pritchett ELC, Pontinen M, McCarthy E, Divine GW. Incremental diagnostic yield of loop electrocardiographic recorders in unexplained syncope. *Am. J. Cardiol.*, Jul. 15, 1990, 66: 214-9.
8. Clochesy JM, Cifani L, Howe K. Electrode site preparation techniques: a follow-up study. *Heart & Lung*, 1991, 20(1): 27-30.
9. Instrumentation and practice standards for electrocardiographic monitoring in special care units: a report for health professionals by a task force of the Council on Clinical Cardiology, American Heart Association. Dallas: American Heart Association, 1989.
10. Moser DK, Wood MA, Stevenson WG. Noninvasive identification of patients at risk for ventricular tachycardia with the signal-averaged electrocardiogram. *Clin. Issues Crit. Care Nurs.*, May, 1990, 1(1): 79-86.
11. Lansdowne LM. Signal-averaged electrocardiograms. *Heart & Lung*, Jul., 1990, 19(4): 329-35.
12. Schlactman M, Green JS. Signal-averaged electrocardiography: a new technique for determining which patients may be at risk for sudden cardiac death. *Focus Crit. Care*, Jun., 1991, 18(4): 202-10.

13. McGuire M, Kucha D, Ganis J, Sammel N, Thorburn C. Natural history of late potentials in the first ten days after acute myocardial infarction and relation to early ventricular arrhythmias. *Am. J. Cardiol.*, Jun., 1, 1988, 61: 1187-90.
14. Frank E. An accurate clinically practical system for spatial vectorcardiography. *Circ.*, 1956, 13: 737.
15. Breithardt G, Cain ME, El-Sherif N, Flowers NC, Hombach V, Janse M, Simson MB, Steinbeck G. Standards for analysis of ventricular late potentials using high-resolution or signal-averaged electrocardiography. *Circ.*, Apr., 1991, 83(4): 1481-8.

SUGGESTED READINGS

Association for the advancement of medical instrumentation. American national standard for cardiac monitors, heart rate meters, and alarms (EC13-1983). Arlington: ANSI/AAMI, 1984; and Recommended practice for testing and reporting performance results of ventricular arrhythmia detection algorithms (ECAR/1986). Arlington: ANSI/AAMI, 1987.

Evaluation report: ECG monitors. *J. Med. Eng. Technol.*, Sept/Oct., 1983, 7(5): 234-6; Nov/Dec., 1983, 7(6): 288-91; Mar/Apr., 1984, 8(2): 66-70.

Ritz R. Clinical experience with computerized ICU-monitoring. *Resuscitation,* Mar., 1984, 11(3,4): 249-53.

Roberts WC, Silver MA. Norman Jefferis Holter and ambulatory ECG monitoring. *Am. J. Cardiol.*, Oct., 1983, 52(7): 903-6.

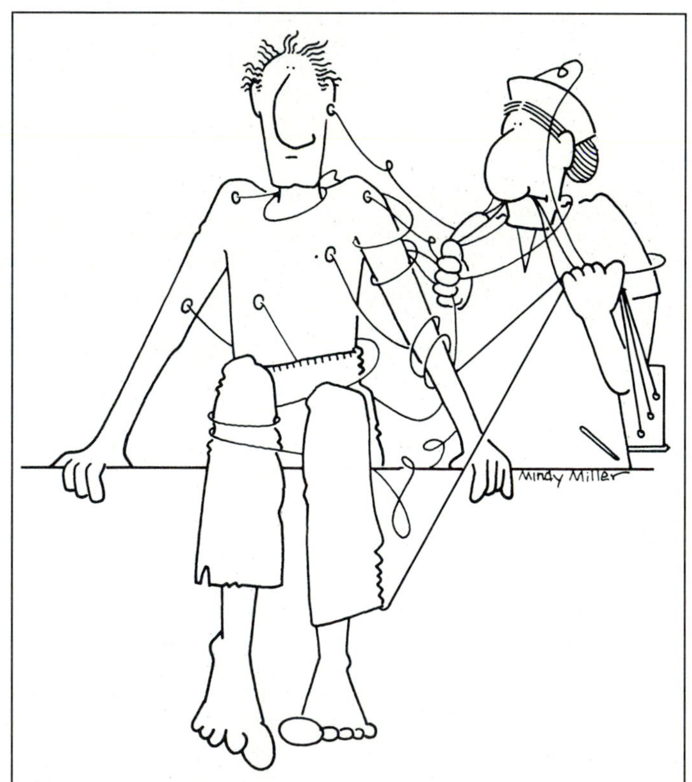

CHAPTER THREE

Monitoring the Patient

Identifying Electrocardiographic Complexes, Analyzing Rhythm, and Selecting a Lead

▶ GOAL

You will understand the leads of the 12-lead electrocardiogram (ECG) and use those most appropriate in assessing and evaluating your patients. You will recognize a "normal" ECG.

▶ OBJECTIVES

After studying this chapter and completing the self-assessment exercises, you will be able to:

1. Define time and voltage values on the ECG.
2. Calculate your patient's heart rate using three methods and state appropriate clinical situations for each method.
3. Recognize, describe, and define the components of the ECG.
4. Use descriptors in communicating the morphology of QRS complexes verbally and in documentation.
5. Recognize signs of myocardial injury and ischemia on the ECG, correlate these signs with the probable myocardial location of injury and ischemia, and discuss mechanical and physiologic variables that may distort ECG components.
6. List at least three causes of ST-segment elevation.
7. Correlate the duration of the QT interval with heart rate.
8. Analyze your patient's cardiac rhythm using a consistent format for interpretation.
9. Identify ECG criteria for normal sinus rhythm (NSR).
10. Describe and locate anatomic sites for the 12 leads and state which anatomic area of the heart each lead represents.
11. Explain how the QRS axis is determined using the hexaxial reference system. Draw the hexaxial reference system including correct location for the four quadrants of the frontal plane, degrees, leads, and positive and negative poles of each lead. State the general direction of the QRS with a normal axis in leads I and aVF.
12. Categorize the 12 leads into frontal and horizontal planes.
13. Demonstrate application of electrodes for the six precordial leads in proper anatomic locations.
14. Describe the "normal" appearance of the QRS complex in leads V_1 and V_6 using QRS descriptors.
15. Choose the appropriate lead for monitoring your patients based on appraisal of the clinical situation.

THE ELECTROCARDIOGRAPHIC COMPLEX ON PAPER

ECG paper is a special kind of graph paper that, when run through the recorder at standard speed, enables the interpreter to assign time and voltage values to the waves recorded. At the standard speed of 25 mm/sec, each small 1 mm square horizontally denotes 0.04 seconds (1 second divided by 25 mm/sec = 0.04 seconds). For visual convenience, every fifth line on the recording paper is darkened. The larger darkened square represents 0.20 seconds (Fig. 3-1). When a rhythm is described as *regular*, like deflections do not vary in distance from one another more than three small boxes (0.12 seconds) (Fig. 3-2).

Height is measured in millimeters and is called *voltage*. When calibrating the ECG machine, adjust the amplitude so that depressing the calibrate button writes a 1-cm de-

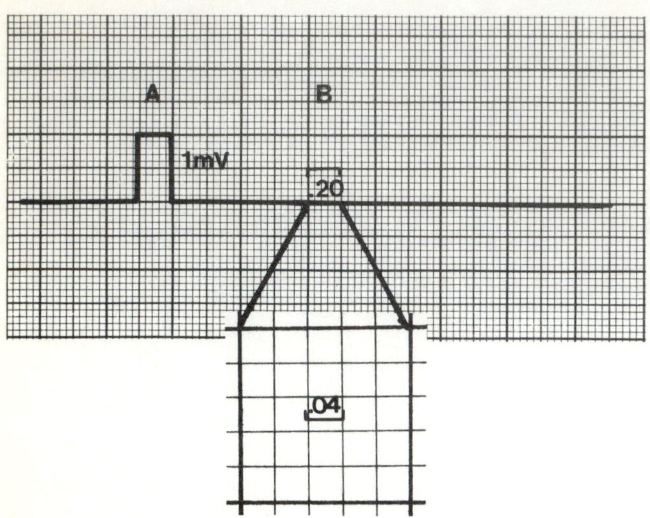

FIGURE 3-1 Time and voltage. Vertical lines measure voltage. When the ECG is calibrated to size 1, a 1-mV current writes a 1-cm deflection *(A)*. Horizontal lines represent time *(B)*. One small square (1 mm) is equal to 0.04 seconds. Five small squares are equal to 0.20 seconds.

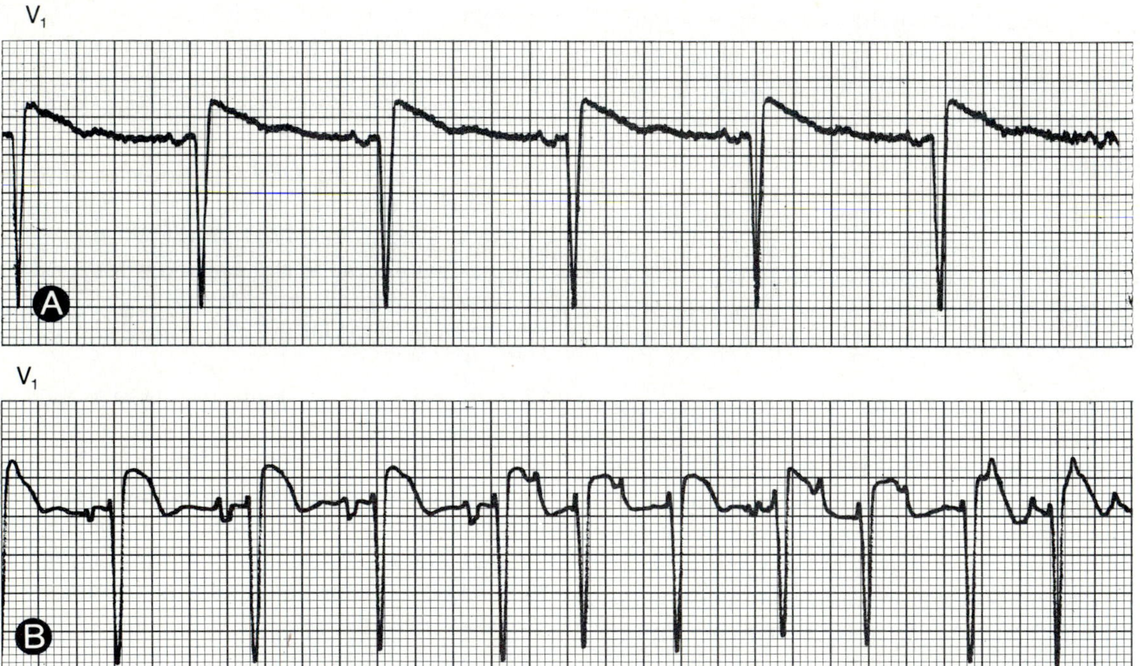

FIGURE 3-2 Regular and irregular rhythms. **A,** Regular rhythm. Like points on the ECG do not vary more than 0.12 seconds from one another. **B,** Irregular rhythm. Like points of the ECG vary more than 0.12 seconds from one another.

flection (two large squares vertically) on the ECG paper. The recording will then be standard size 1 (see Fig. 3-1).

Calculating Rate

As explained in the previous chapter, ECG monitors display heart rate (the number of QRS complexes per minute) on either a digital or analog display. Although the heart rate is usually an accurate display, it must not be relied on solely. Skills of rate determination must be developed that are accurate, yet faster than counting the heart rate for a full minute. At standard paper speed of 25 mm/sec, there are 1500 mm in 1 minute. The methods of determining rate from the ECG paper are based on this numerical value. Presented here are three popular methods for rate estimation.

The Box Method

Two requisite conditions for this method are a regular rhythm and a rate of roughly 120 beats per minute (bpm) or less. The slower the rate, the more accurate the estimation. Follow these steps to use the box method (Fig. 3-3):

1. Find a QRS complex that lands on a heavy line.
2. Place the following values on succeeding heavy lines: 300-150-100-75-60-50-43-37-35-30. If the next QRS complex falls on a heavy line, assign the appropriate rate value to it. If, however, the next QRS falls between two heavy lines, take the difference between the two values and divide by 5. Each small square is then worth that quotient. To use this method to its fullest advantage, it is necessary to memorize the sequence of numbers from 300 to at least 43. Based on this principle is Marriott's guide for rapid estimation (Fig. 3-4), which provides the precise heart rate value for each box. Memorization of the number sequence, however, is recommended for fastest calculation, since rulers can be misplaced.

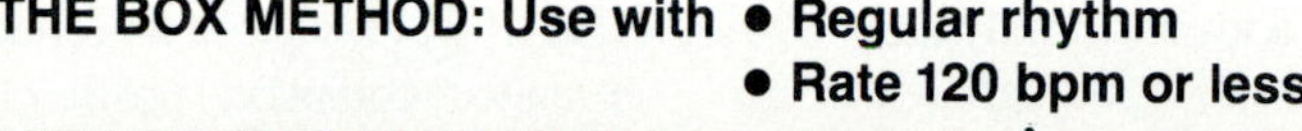

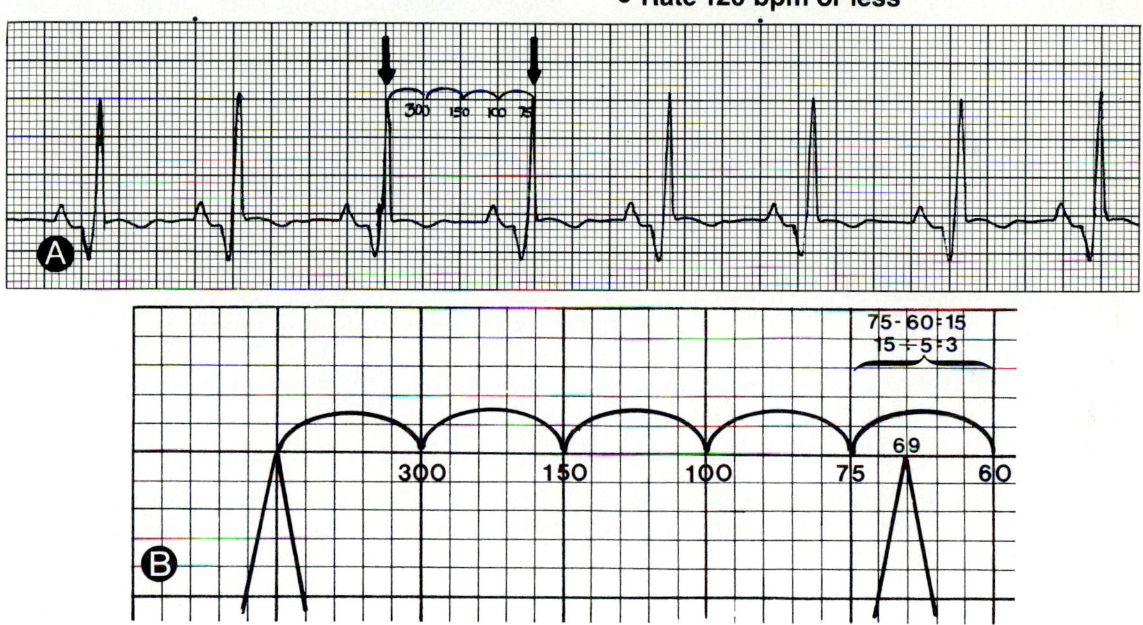

FIGURE 3-3 Calculating rate with the box method. **A,** In a regular rhythm, find a QRS that lands on a heavy line *(arrow)*. Ascribe values to succeeding heavy lines: 300-150-100-75-60 . . . The next QRS lands on a heavy line with the value 75. Thus the heart rate is 75 bpm. **B,** If the next QRS lands between two heavy lines, determine the difference in value between those two lines, divide that number by 5, ascribe the quotient to each small box.

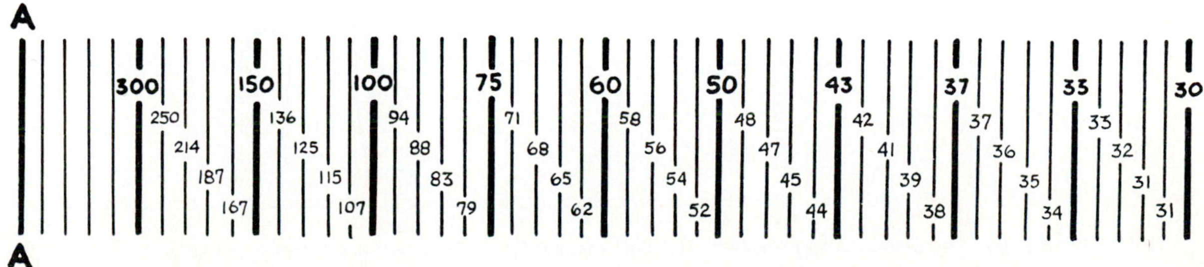

FIGURE 3-4 Marriott's rate ruler. From Marriott HJL. *Practical Electrocardiography.* 8th ed. Baltimore: Williams & Wilkins, 1988, p. 15.

The Division Method

Like the box method, the division method is used only with regular rhythms. This method can be used for high rates and is more accurate than the box method for rates above 120 bpm. The disadvantage in using this method is performing arithmetic functions under stressful conditions. (This method is the arithmetic basis for the box method. Again, Marriott's rate ruler provides the same values.) To use the division method, follow these steps:

1. Count the number of small boxes between two QRS complexes.
2. Divide 1500 by that number (Fig. 3-5).

The 6-Second Strip

For irregular rhythms and rates above approximately 120 bpm, the 6-second method is ideal. Although it can be used with any heart rate, it is more accurate with faster rates. To use the 6-second strip method follow these steps:

1. Count the number of complexes within a 6-second period.
2. Multiply that number by 10 (Fig. 3-6).

Components of the ECG

Before analyzing the cardiac rhythm, it is necessary to understand the components of the ECG. Although they have been mentioned briefly in preceding chapters, each is discussed in more detail.

P Wave

The P wave represents atrial depolarization. It is a gently rounded complex, positive in the inferior leads (those

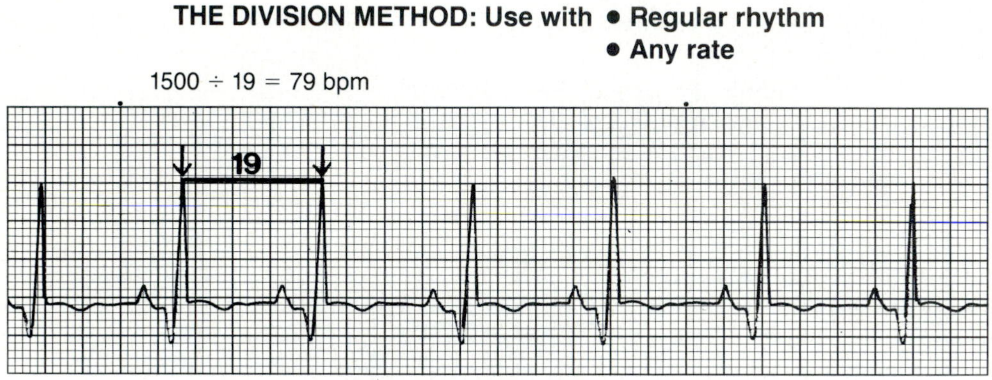

THE DIVISION METHOD: Use with • Regular rhythm
• Any rate

1500 ÷ 19 = 79 bpm

19

FIGURE 3-5 The division method. Determination of rate by this method involves counting the number of millimeters between two complexes of a regular rhythm. The quotient is the heart rate (HR) per minute: 1500/19 = 79 bpm.

THE 6-SEC STRIP: Use with • Irregular rhythm
• Any rate (the faster the rate, the more accurate the estimation)

11 complexes between two 3-sec markers: 11 × 10 = 110 bpm

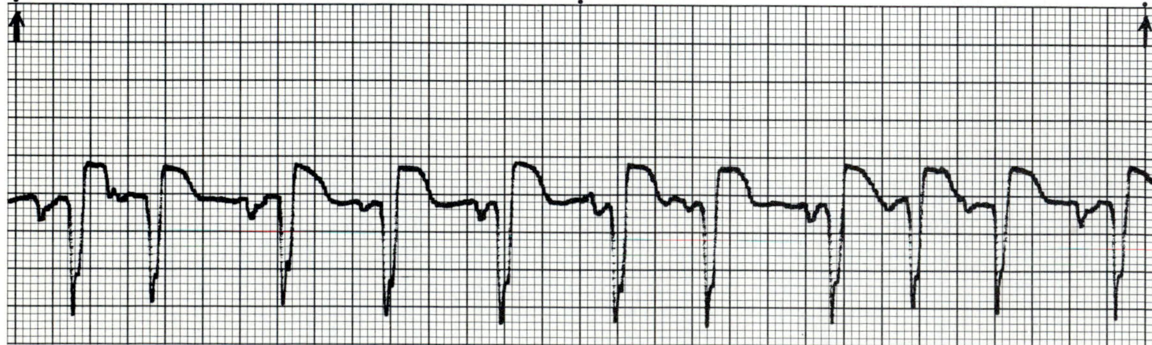

FIGURE 3-6 The 6-second strip method. The best method for rhythms that are irregular consists of locating a 6-second duration *(arrows)*. Distance between dots is 3 seconds, 15 large boxes. A 6-second distance is twice that. Count the number of complexes in 6 seconds and multiply by ten: 11 × 10 = 110 bpm.

leads that "look at" the inferior, or diaphragmatic, surface of the heart). Its duration should not exceed 0.10 seconds and its height should not exceed 2.5 mm[1] (Fig. 3-7). P waves measuring 0.11 seconds or longer and/or are irregular in shape indicate some defect in intraatrial conduction, which may be due to a variety of factors including atrial hypertrophy, fibrosis, and infarction. Hyperkalemia (elevated serum potassium), if severe enough, results in disappearance of the P wave.

PR Interval

The PR interval represents the time it takes the impulse to travel from the sinoatrial (SA) node to the ventricular Purkinje fibers. Measured from the beginning of the P wave to the beginning of the QRS complex, its normal value is between 0.12 and 0.20 seconds (Fig. 3-8). Normally there is an inverse relationship between heart rate and PR interval. That is, as the rate increases, the PR interval shortens. Age also affects the PR interval; children 1 year or younger average 0.11 seconds. Children usually reach 0.14 seconds by age 12 years, an average increase of 0.0025 seconds (2.5 msec) per year.[2]

PR intervals in excess of 0.20 seconds in the adult may be indicative of atrioventricular (AV) nodal conduction delay or block. Medications such as digitalis are known to cause lengthening of the PR interval. Refer to Chapter 11 for the specific effects other antiarrhythmic drugs have on the PR interval.

PR intervals measuring less than 0.12 seconds in the adult occur with what is known as *preexcitation arrhythmias*. Certain individuals have conductive fibers that bypass the AV node, allowing the impulse from the atria to enter the ventricles without having to go through the AV node. Examples of such arrhythmias include the Wolff-Parkinson-White (WPW) syndrome and the Lown-Ganong-Levine (LGL) syndrome.

QRS Complex

Representing ventricular depolarization, the QRS complex is measured from the beginning to the end of the waves that comprise it. Normal measures fall between 0.06 and 0.10 seconds (Fig. 3-9). Measurements of 0.12 seconds

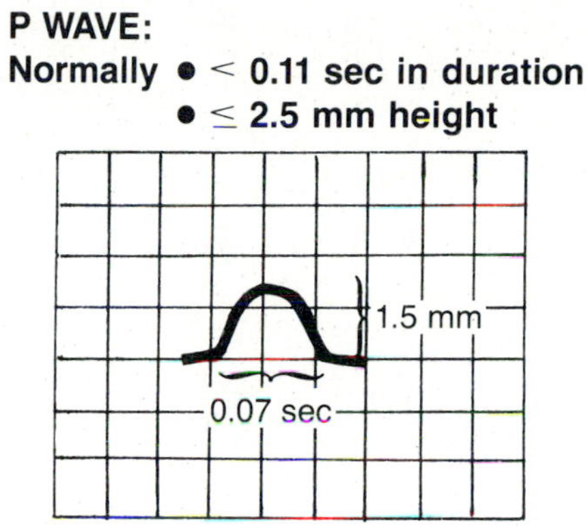

P WAVE:
Normally • < 0.11 sec in duration
• ≤ 2.5 mm height

1.5 mm
0.07 sec

FIGURE 3-7 Graphic representation of a normal P wave. This example is 0.07 seconds in duration and 1.5 mm in height.

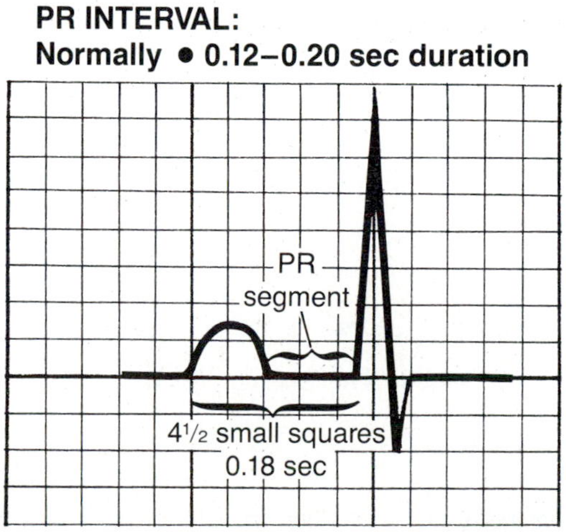

PR INTERVAL:
Normally • 0.12–0.20 sec duration

PR segment
4½ small squares
0.18 sec

FIGURE 3-8 Graphic representation of the PR interval. The PR interval is measured from the beginning of the P wave to the beginning of the QRS complex. In this example the PR interval is 0.18 seconds in duration. The space after the P wave to the beginning of the QRS complex is the PR segment.

QRS COMPLEX:
Normally • 0.06–0.10 sec in duration

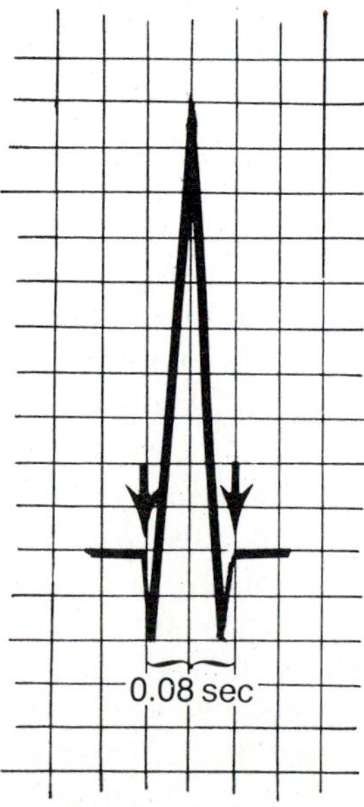

FIGURE 3-9 Graphic representation of QRS complex. QRS is measured from its beginning to its end *(arrows)*. In this example the QRS measures 0.08 seconds.

"I'm a QRS and I can look many different ways."
P!
T!
RS!
QR
rSR
qRS
Mindy Miller

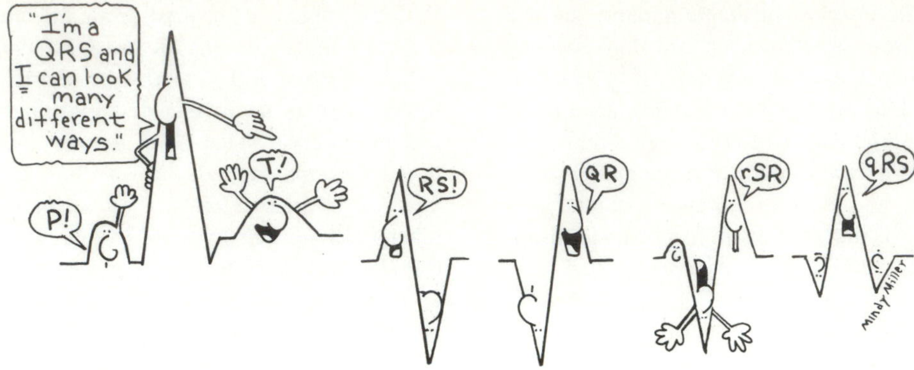

and above signify intraventricular conduction delays. Such delays are most often due to bundle branch blocks, but they may also be nonspecific delays as a result of metabolic disturbances (such as hyperkalemia), adverse drug effects (e.g., quinidine), or past myocardial infarction.[3] Values between 0.10 and 0.12 seconds may or may not be abnormal; these values are judged in light of the clinical situation. Hemiblocks (blocks involving a portion of the left bundle branch) may cause such a prolongation. (Hemiblocks and bundle branch blocks are discussed in Chapter 9).

When discussing the QRS complex displayed on the ECG, descriptors are used to enhance communication. Although we use the term *QRS*, a Q wave, an R wave, and an S wave may not all be present in the same complex. Indeed, all three are usually not displayed in the same complex.

A Q wave is the first negative deflection (below the isoelectric line). The R wave is the first positive deflection (above the isoelectric line). The S wave is the first negative deflection after the R wave. If there are two positive deflections in the same complex, the second is termed *R prime* (written R′). Likewise, if there are two negative complexes after an R wave, the second is written S′. Comparatively large waves are symbolized with a capital letter whereas relatively small waves are written with a lower case letter. Studying the diagram in Fig. 3-10 will help clarify these descriptors.

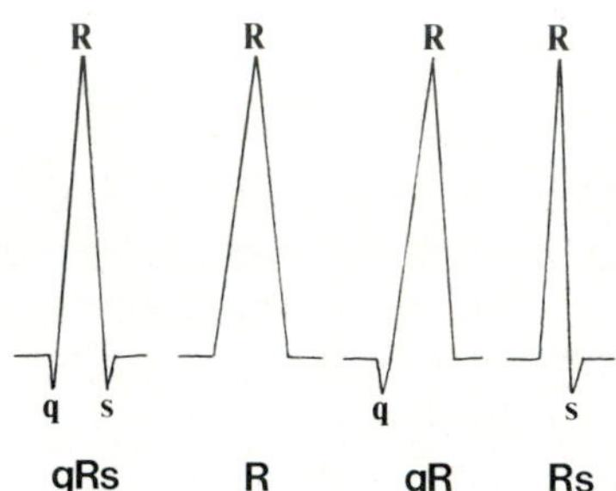

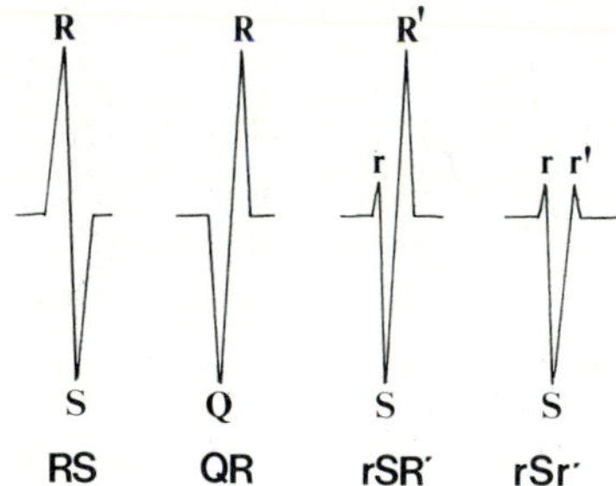

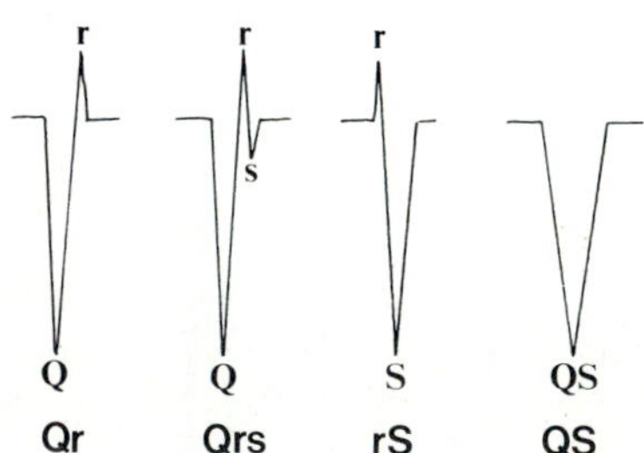

FIGURE 3-10 QRS descriptors.

ST Segment

The ST segment is located in the space from the end of the QRS complex to the beginning of the T wave. The point where the ST segment departs from the QRS is known as the *J point* or *J junction*. Normally the J point is isoelectric but may be elevated (above the baseline) or depressed (below the baseline) (Fig. 3-11). The ST segment gently slopes from the J point to the T wave. The midsection of the ST segment normally reaches the isoelectric line, but complete horizontality of it may indicate myocardial ischemia[4] (Fig. 3-12). On an ECG the isoelectric baseline is located in the interval between the end of the T or U wave (the TP interval) and the subsequent P wave and in the PR segment.

ST-segment elevation. Elevation of the ST segment (more than 1 mm above the baseline) (Fig. 3-12, *B*) is a significant finding. It may represent myocardial injury,

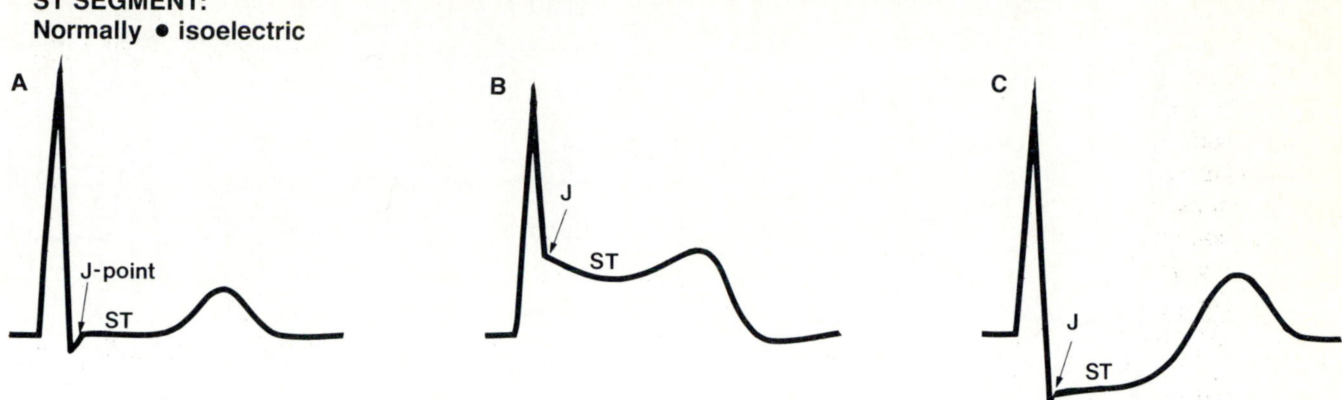

FIGURE 3-11 Graphic representation of the ST segment. The point where the ST segment departs from the QRS complex is known as the *J point (arrows).* The ST segment extends from the J point to the T wave. **A,** Isoelectric J point and ST segment. **B,** Elevated J point and ST segment. **C,** Depressed J point and ST segment.

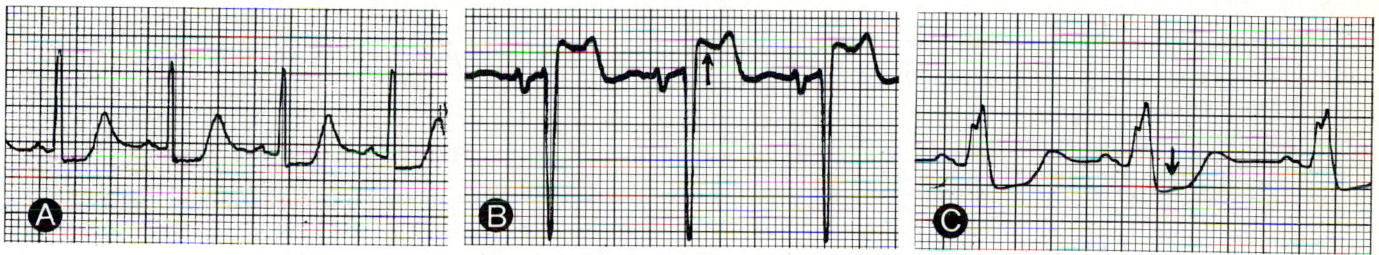

FIGURE 3-12 Variations of the ST segment. **A,** Horizontal ST segment that is also depressed 1 to 2 mm below baseline. **B,** Elevated ST segment. **C,** Depressed ST segment accompanying bundle branch block.

ventricular aneurysm, pericarditis, a normal variant, or accompany block of the left bundle branch.

Myocardial infarction (MI) produces myocardial injury and, in its early stages, ST-segment elevation is usually present. The ST-segment elevation appears in those leads that "look at" the particular surface of the heart that is injured (e.g., the inferior surface of the left ventricle or the anterolateral surface). Thus the more leads showing ST-segment displacement the more myocardium that may be in jeopardy.[5] ST-segment elevation is a rather transient sign, lasting hours to days. In some cases of angina (e.g., Prinzmetal's) the ST segments elevate during the ischemic episode and return to normal after the anginal episode subsides. Later in this chapter, you will learn which leads "look at" which portions of the myocardium.

Pericarditis and ventricular aneurysm are two other conditions producing ST-segment elevation. In contrast to myocardial infarction, pericarditis produces elevation in most or all of the leads. Ventricular aneurysm produces ST-segment elevation that is more persistent than that seen with myocardial infarction.

ST-segment elevation of up to 2 mm may, in some cases, be a normal variant.[4] Block of the left bundle branch produces deformation of the ST segment as a result of abnormal depolarization/repolarization process.

ST-segment depression. ST-segment depression more than 0.5 mm below baseline may reflect myocardial ischemia (Fig. 3-12, *A*). Progressive hypokalemia and bundle branch block (Fig. 3-12, *C*) also cause ST-segment depression.

Length of ST segment. The length of the ST segment may change in calcium imbalances. Low serum calcium tends to prolong the ST segment, whereas hypercalcemia results in shortening.[6]

T Wave

The T wave represents repolarization of the ventricles. It is rounded and slightly asymmetric with its upstroke longer than the downstroke (Fig. 3-13). T waves usually do not exceed 5 mm in height on the standard leads (leads I, II, III, aVR, aVL, and aVF) and 10 mm on precordial leads (V_1 to V_6).[4] T waves are best interpreted on a 12-lead

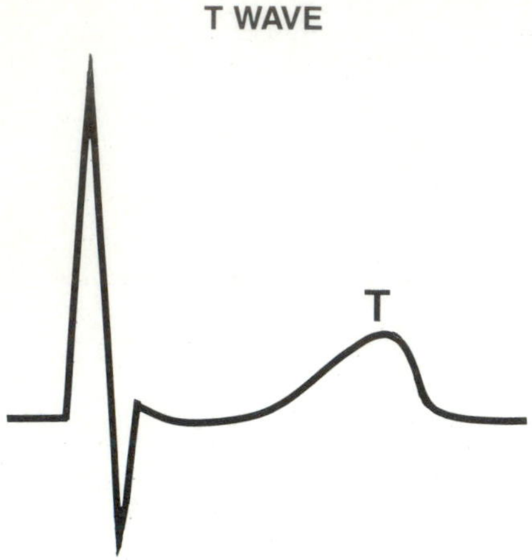

FIGURE 3-13 Graphic representation of T wave.

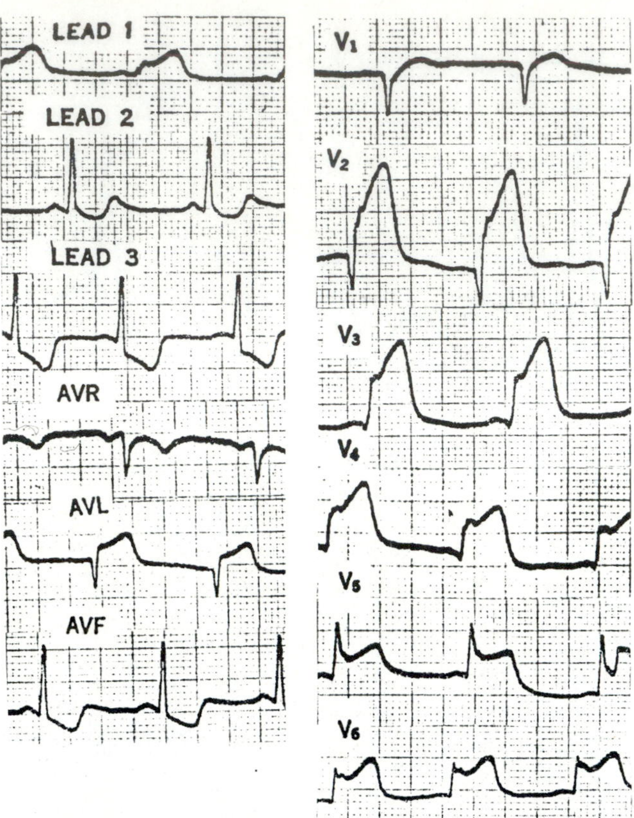

FIGURE 3-14 Tombstone T waves. In this ECG, tombstone T waves show on leads V_2, V_3, and V_4. Note that ST-segment elevation is not present in all leads. It appears only in those leads overlying the area of myocardial injury.

ECG because they are often distorted on bedside monitors or telemetry units because of electrode placement and amplitude adjustment.

Numerous chemical, pharmacologic, physiologic, and psychophysiologic processes can affect the appearance of the T wave. In the adult, T waves (like QRS complexes) are usually upright in leads I, II, and V_3 to V_6; inverted in aVR; and variable in leads III, aVL, aVF, V_1, and V_2.[4] Excessive height of the T wave can be the result of hyperkalemia, myocardial infarction or ischemia, or certain forms of ventricular overloading; it is seen in some psychotic patients and in patients who have had a cerebral vascular accident.[4] Very tall, symmetric T waves, dubbed *hyperacute T waves* by Schamroth,[7] occur in the early stages of acute myocardial infarction and represent acute transmural ischemia.[8] When accompanied by very high ST segments, the combination is sometimes referred to as *tombstone T waves* (Fig. 3-14).

When evaluating the height of T waves, it is important to consider relative changes.[8] For example, a change from an inverted to a flat T wave represents a relative increase in T amplitude.

Flat or inverted T waves may occur in the presence of hypokalemia, along with the appearance of a U wave (a result of prolonged repolarization), myocardial ischemia, as a normal variant,[5] or after a bout of tachycardia.[9] Fig. 3-15 illustrates three common T wave forms: upright, inverted, and flat (isoelectric).

The Ta wave. There is also a T wave for the P wave called the *Ta wave*. It is usually obscured by the QRS complex, though. It can be seen, however, in patients whose PR intervals are prolonged. Unlike the T wave of the QRS complex, the Ta wave is usually opposite in polarity to the P wave.

QT Interval

The QT interval represents the total time required for ventricular depolarization and repolarization (recovery). It is measured from the beginning of the QRS complex to the end of the T wave (Fig. 3-16) and is best done so in leads V_2 or V_3[10] (you will learn about leads later). The QT interval bears an inverse relationship to the heart rate; the faster the rate, the shorter the QT interval.[11] Since it varies with rate, its value must be adjusted, or corrected, for the heart rate before it can be compared with established normal values. When the QT interval has been corrected for heart rate, it is termed the *QTc*. Traditionally, the "normal" QTc did not exceed 0.44 seconds. However, recent studies[10,12] reveal that 6.5% to 18% of healthy persons exhibit QTc $\geq$ 0.44 seconds and that the upper limit of "normal" may well be 0.50 seconds.[12]

A formula commonly used for the purpose of calculating the QTc is Bazett's:

$$QTc = \frac{\text{QT interval (in seconds)}}{\sqrt{\text{R-R interval (in seconds)}}}$$

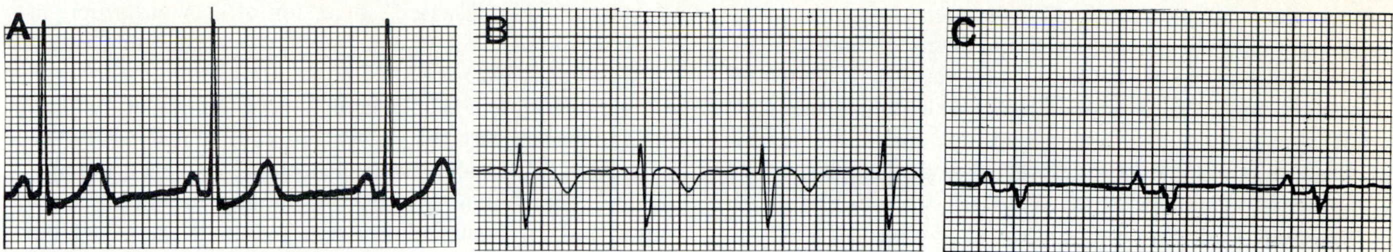

FIGURE 3-15 Three common T-wave forms. **A,** Upright. **B,** Inverted, **C,** Isoelectric (the T wave shows on another lead).

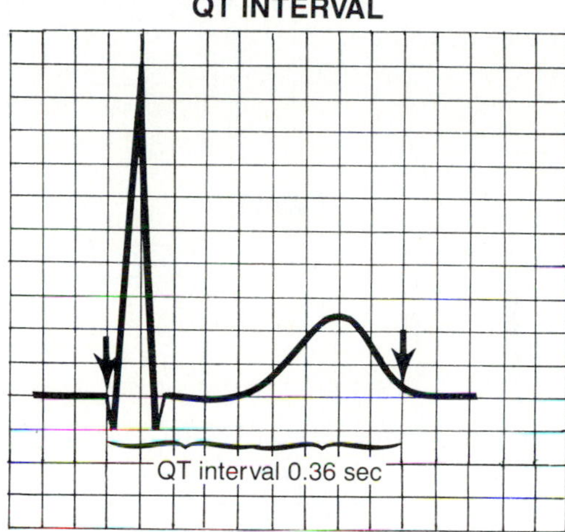

FIGURE 3-16 Graphic representation of QT interval. QT interval is measured from the beginning of the QRS complex to the end of the T wave *(arrows)*. In this example the QT measures 0.36 seconds.

Table 3-1 Approximate Normal Limits for QT Intervals in Seconds*

Heart rate/min	Men and children	Women
40	0.45-0.49	0.46-0.50
46	0.43-0.47	0.44-0.48
50	0.41-0.45	0.43-0.46
55	0.40-0.44	0.41-0.45
60	0.39-0.42	0.40-0.43
67	0.37-0.40	0.38-0.41
71	0.36-0.40	0.37-0.41
75	0.35-0.38	0.36-0.39
80	0.34-0.37	0.35-0.38
86	0.33-0.36	0.34-0.37
93	0.32-0.35	0.33-0.36
100	0.31-0.34	0.32-0.35
109	0.30-0.33	0.31-0.33
120	0.28-0.31	0.29-0.32
133	0.27-0.29	0.28-0.30
150	0.25-0.28	0.26-0.28
172	0.23-0.26	0.24-0.26

*Adapted from Ashman R, Hull E. *Essentials of Electrocardiography*. New York: Macmillan, 1945.

Nomograms and tables, such as the one in Table 3-1, are available for determination of normal length of the QT interval for various rates. There are two easy rules for determining the maximum QT interval for a particular rate. Although they are not as accurate as the tables, they are easy to remember:

1. As a general rule the QT interval should not exceed one half the previous R-R interval (the distance between two R waves). This rule can be applied for heart rates between 65 and 90 bpm.[4]
2. To determine what the QT interval should be for a particular rate, count the number of small squares between two R waves, add 18 and put a decimal point in front. For example, a heart rate of 75 bpm has 20 small squares between the two R waves. 20 + 18 = 38. Place a decimal point before the sum, and the maximum QT interval for a rate of 75 bpm is 0.38 seconds.

Besides varying with the heart rate, the QT interval varies with age and sex,[4] men and children displaying a slightly shorter QT interval than women. It also varies in any individual during a 24-hour period. One study demonstrated an average variability in the QTc of 0.076 seconds in healthy men.[13]

Abnormalities in the QT interval may be caused by drugs, hereditary factors, disease states, and electrolyte disturbances. Prolongation of the QT interval often accompanies the early stages of myocardial infarction.[14] It may occur in congestive heart failure,[4] organic heart disease, mitral valve prolapse, subarachnoid hemorrhage,[15] intracranial lesions,[16] or cerebrovascular accident,[17] or may be an effect of drugs such as quinidine[18] and other Class IA antiarrhythmics (see Chapter 11 for effects of various antiarrhythmic drugs on the QT interval), ketanserin, amiodarone, bepridil, sotalol, antidepressants, phenothiazines, erythromycin, antihistamines;[13] or electrolyte disturbances such as hypokalemia, hypocalcemia, or hypomagnesemia;[19] or sympathetic nervous system dysfunction.[20] Sudden death and syncopal episodes related to dangerous ventricular arrhythmias have been associated with idiopathic and acquired, prolonged QT-interval syndromes.[18-25] Hereditary QT-interval prolongation is related to sudden death in children and certain types of the syndrome are associated with deafness[23,25] and other ECG abnormalities.

Shortening of the QT interval is often evident in patients on digitalis,[19] patients with calcium excess, those with potassium intoxication,[4] and cardiac transplant patients.[26]

Although changes in the length of the QT interval are related to a variety of clinical situations, by itself, the QTc does not provide sufficient clinical or electrocardiographic information to definitively diagnose prolonged QT-interval syndrome[27] nor is it a good predictor of mortality and morbidity in healthy people.[28]

U Waves

U waves are small waves that, when present, follow the T wave and are usually in the same direction as the T wave[4] (Fig. 3-17). They are often most apparent in leads V_2 and V_3.[4,10] Conditions that may produce a U wave include hypokalemia,[6,29] digitalis administration,[29] myocardial infarction, and they are sometimes seen in people with no history of heart disease.[10] Inversion of previously upright U waves in response to exercise may be related to myocardial ischemic disease.[4]

Figs. 3-18 to 3-32 illustrate several normal and abnormal morphologies (wave-form shapes) to exemplify the preceding ECG components. Accompanying each example is an interpretation. You may not understand all the terms until you have studied this entire chapter (including the leads). Concentrate on identifying the wave forms, determine rate and rhythm, label the QRS complexes, and measure complexes and intervals. At the top of each strip, there is a recommended quick rate determination method.

Electrocardiographic features of common electrolyte disturbances are summarized in the box on p. 48. Figures 3-33 to 3-36 follow with electrocardiographic examples of electrolyte abnormalities.

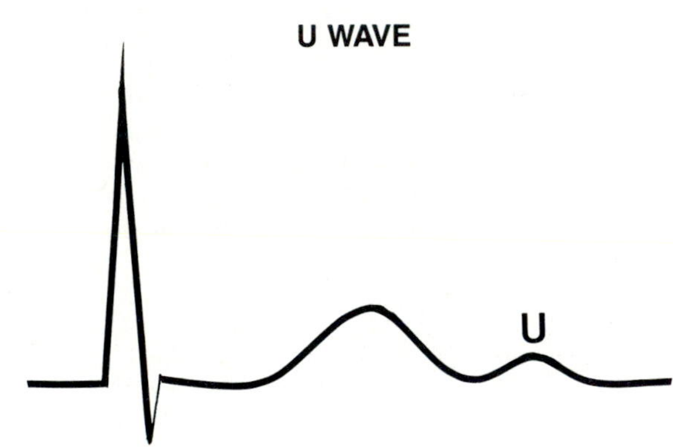

FIGURE 3-17 Graphic representation of U wave.

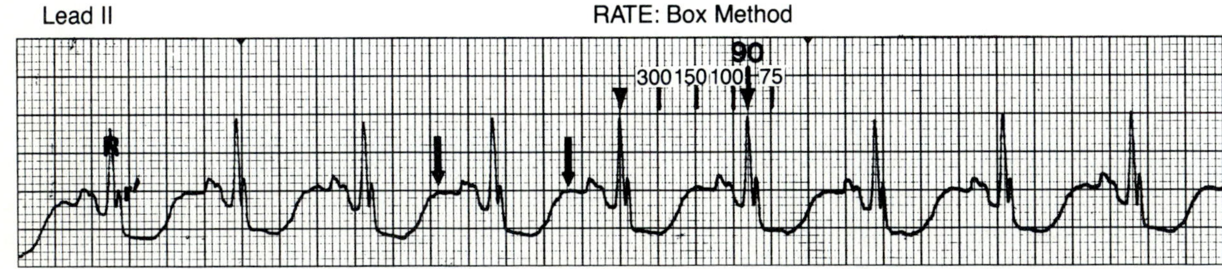

FIGURE 3-18 Sometimes particular components of the ECG are not readily identifiable on one or more of the leads. Such is the case with T waves in this example. The ends of the T waves are in the area marked with arrows. Visualization on other leads will assist in identifying such components. The isoelectric baseline in such an example is located in the PR segment.

Rate: 88 to 90 bpm
Rhythm: Regular
P waves: Notched, wide 0.11 to 0.12 seconds (intraatrial conduction delay). One precedes each QRS complex.
PR interval: 0.16 seconds
QRS complex: 0.10 seconds, Notched R wave; Depressed ST segments; QT interval 0.40 seconds, prolonged for this rate
Interpretation: Sinus rhythm, atrial conduction delay, prolonged QT interval

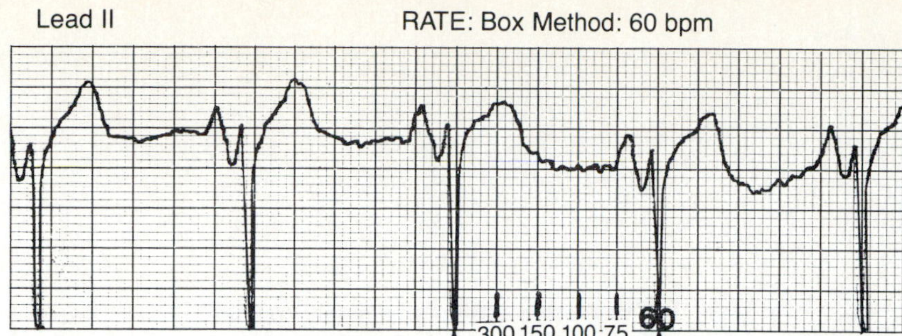

FIGURE 3-19

Rate: 60 bpm

Rhythm: Regular

P waves: Wide, 0.12 to 0.13 seconds. Tall (3 to 5 mm). One precedes each QRS complex.

PR interval: 0.16 to 0.18 seconds

QRS complex: 0.12 seconds (wide); Configuration is rS. ST segment elevated; QT interval 0.44 to 0.45 seconds, possible prolongation

Interpretation: Sinus rhythm, abnormal QRS axis; Intraatrial conduction delay, possible prolonged QT interval

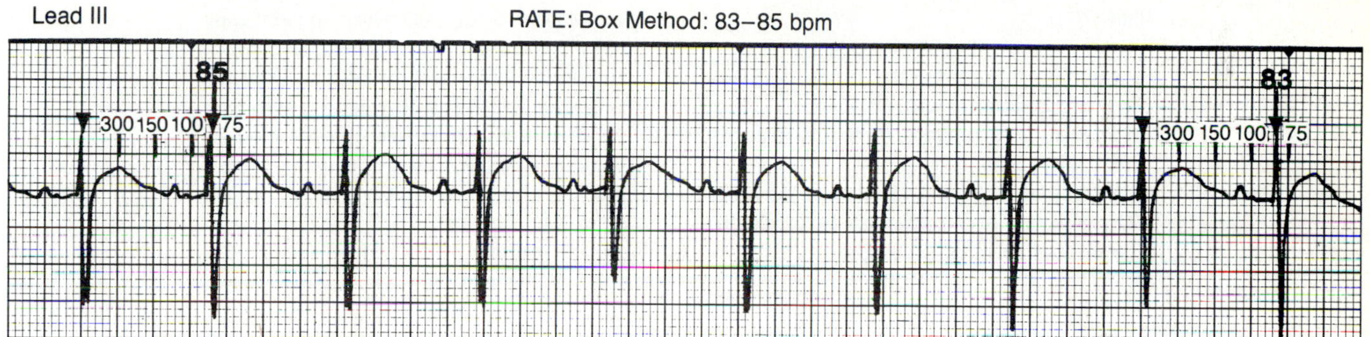

FIGURE 3-20

Rate: 83 to 85 bpm

Rhythm: Regular

P wave: 0.12 seconds (wide), notched, intraatrial conduction delay

PR interval: 0.20 to 0.22 seconds, prolonged

QRS complex: 0.08 to 0.10 seconds, rS configuration; QT interval 0.42 seconds, prolonged

Interpretation: Sinus rhythm, intraatrial conduction delay, PR and QT intervals prolonged

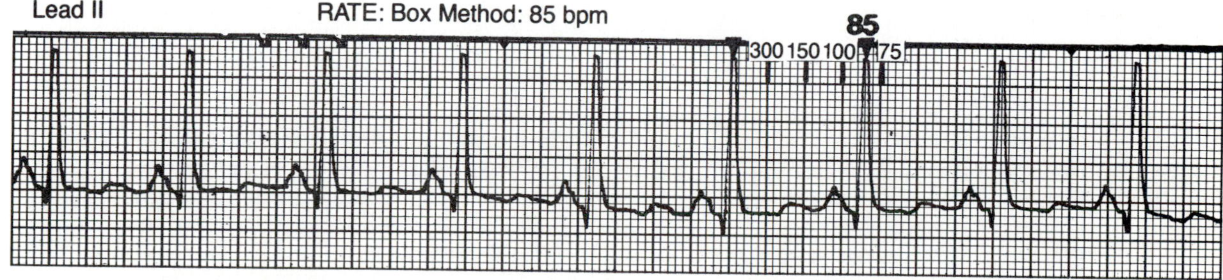

FIGURE 3-21

Rate: 83 to 85 bpm

Rhythm: Regular

P wave: 0.11 to 0.13 seconds (wide), 3 mm tall and notched, intraatrial conduction delay

PR interval: 0.16 seconds

QRS complex: 0.14 seconds, prolonged, intraventricular conduction delay, qR configuration, T waves flattened (normally upright in lead II); QT interval 0.47 to 0.48 seconds, prolonged (need to confirm measurement on a lead that shows T waves clearly)

Interpretation: Sinus rhythm, intraatrial and intraventricular conduction delays, T-wave flattening, QT-interval prolongation

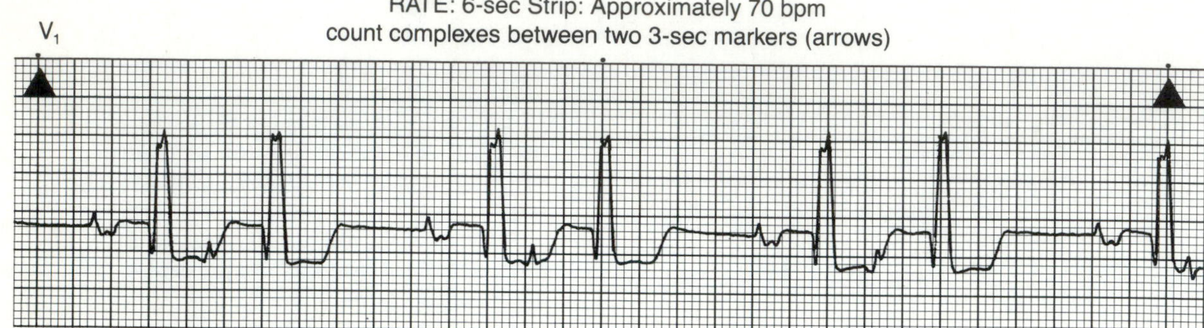

FIGURE 3-22 Irregular rhythm.

Rate: 70 bpm

Rhythm: Irregular (regular irregularity)

P wave: 0.14 seconds (too wide), diphasic, one precedes each QRS complex

PR interval: 0.30 seconds, up to 0.40 seconds with early beats

QRS complex: 0.12 to 0.13 seconds, too wide. Configuration is qR, abnormal for V_1; QT interval 0.44 seconds, prolonged

Interpretation: Sinus rhythm with frequent early beats, intraatrial and intraventricular conduction delays, prolonged PR interval. (You will later learn to call this arrhythmia first degree AV block with right bundle branch block, intraatrial conduction delay, bigeminal atrial premature beats conducted with PR interval up to 0.40 seconds.)

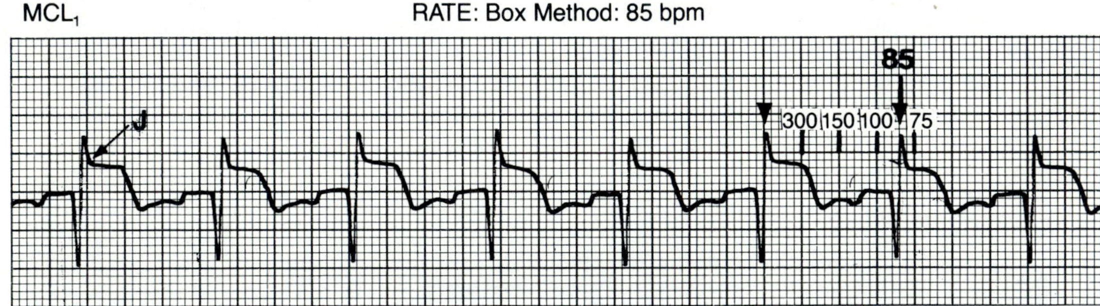

FIGURE 3-23

Rate: 83 to 85 bpm

Rhythm: Regular

P wave: Negative, acceptable for MCL_1, but more commonly is diphasic

PR interval: 0.24 seconds, prolonged

QRS complex: 0.09 to 0.10 seconds, QR configuration, initial r wave that is normally present in MCL_1 is absent, abnormal for lead MCL_1; ST-segment and J-point elevation. QT interval 0.36 seconds

Interpretation: Probable normal sinus rhythm (NSR), PR-interval prolongation, ST-segment and J-point elevation

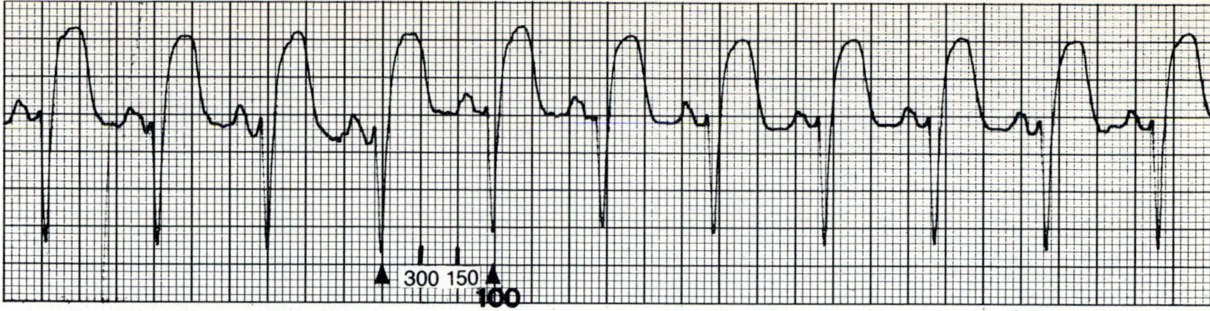

FIGURE 3-24

Rate: 100 to 102 bpm
Rhythm: Regular
P wave: 0.08 to 0.10 seconds
PR interval: 0.16 seconds
QRS complex: 0.10 seconds, rS configuration, ST-segment elevation; QT interval 0.32 to 0.36 seconds, prolonged for this rate
Interpretation: Sinus tachycardia (tachycardia because rate is above 100 bpm), intraatrial conduction delay, ST-segment elevation, QT-interval prolongation

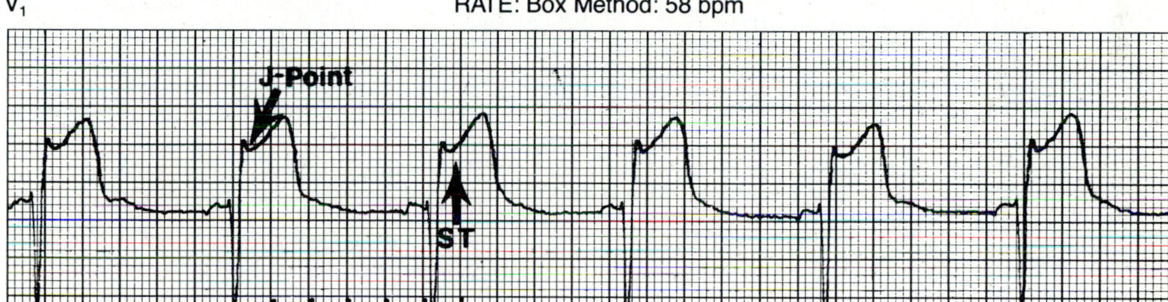

FIGURE 3-25

Rate: 58 bpm
Rhythm: Regular
P wave: Biphasic, negative-positive on lead V_1; suspect retrograde atrial depolarization, confirm on leads II, III, aVF (if P wave inverted, retrograde atrial depolarization is likely present)
PR interval: 0.12 to 0.14 seconds
QRS complex: 0.10 seconds, rSr′ configuration, abnormal for lead V_1; QT interval 0.40 seconds
Interpretation: Possible junctional rhythm with retrograde atrial depolarization and elevated ST segment

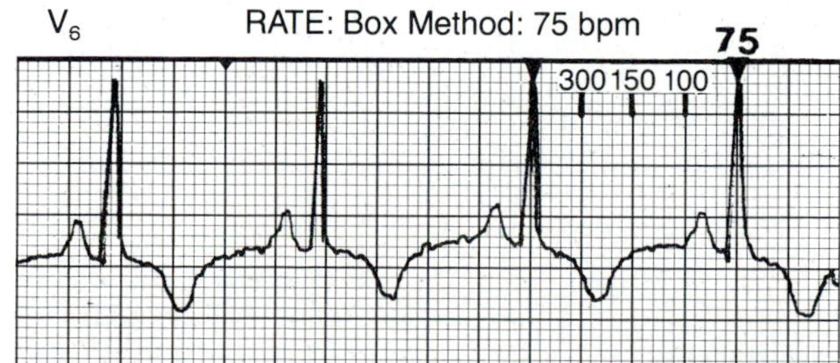

FIGURE 3-26 Normal upright QRS complexes of lead V_6 exhibiting inverted T waves.

Rate: 75 bpm
Rhythm: Regular
P wave: 0.12 seconds (wide), 3.5 mm tall, probable intraatrial conduction delay
PR Interval: 0.16 seconds
QRS complex: 0.09 seconds, R configuration, first and fourth are qR configuration, normal for V_6; T wave inverted; QT interval 0.40 seconds
Interpretation: Sinus rhythm with inverted T waves

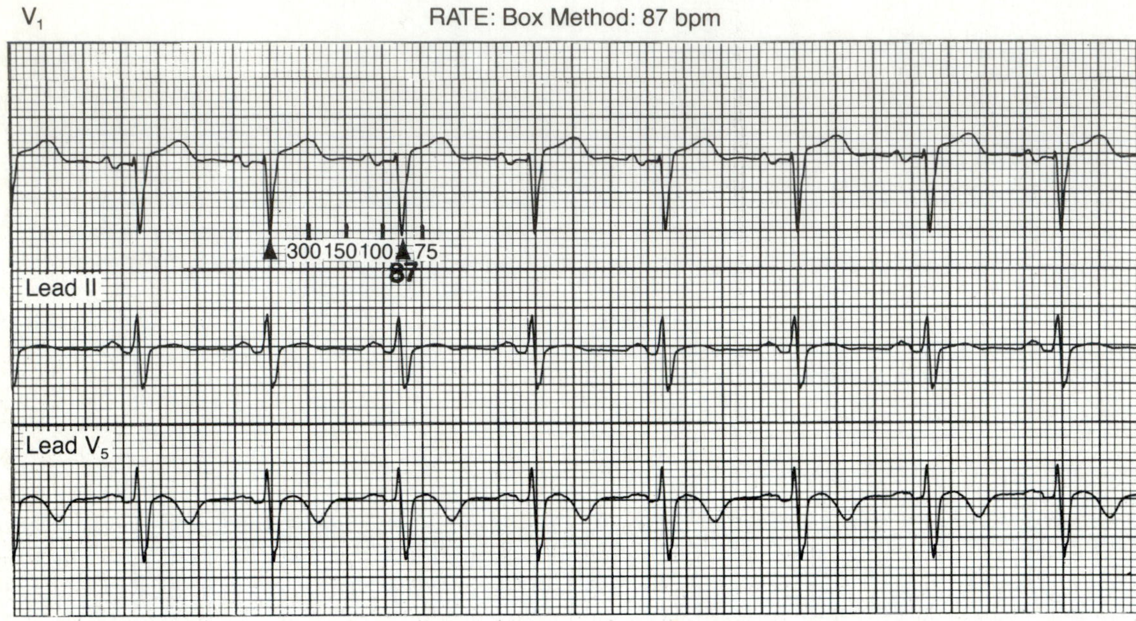

FIGURE 3-27 Simultaneous leads showing abnormal T waves. Inversion in one lead (third strip) is not evident in the first strip and questionable in the second. This illustrates the value of a 12-lead ECG for comparative evaluation.

Rate: 86 to 87 bpm
Rhythm: Regular
P wave: 0.12 seconds, prolonged, probable intraatrial conduction delay
PR Interval: 0.17 seconds
QRS complex: 0.10 seconds, normal rS configuration in V_1, but abnormal RS in lead II and rS in lead V_5; QT interval 0.39 to 0.40 seconds prolonged for this rate; inverted T wave in lead V_5
Interpretation: Sinus rhythm, intraatrial conduction delay, QT-interval prolongation, T-wave inversion in V_5

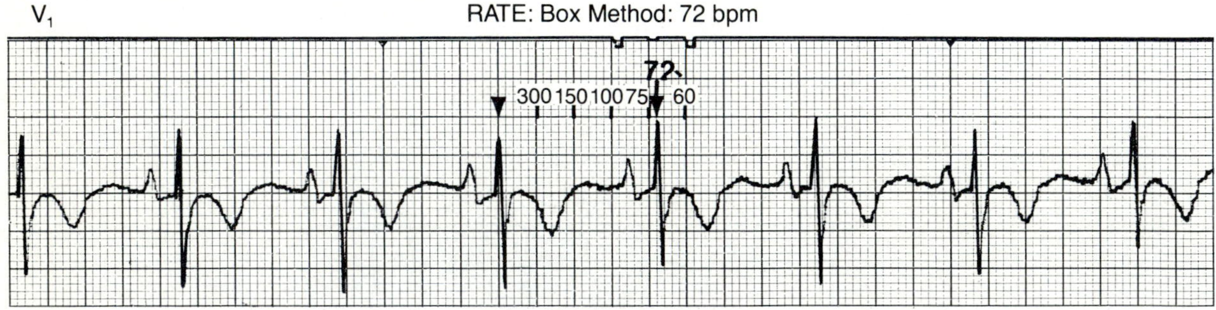

FIGURE 3-28

Rate: 72 bpm
Rhythm: Regular
P wave: 4 mm in height (too tall)
PR interval: 0.16 to 0.18 seconds
QRS complex: 0.11 seconds, RS configuration in V_1 may be abnormal; T-wave inversion; QT interval 0.39 to 0.40 seconds
Interpretation: NSR, T-wave inversion

Lead II

RATE: Box Method: 90 bpm

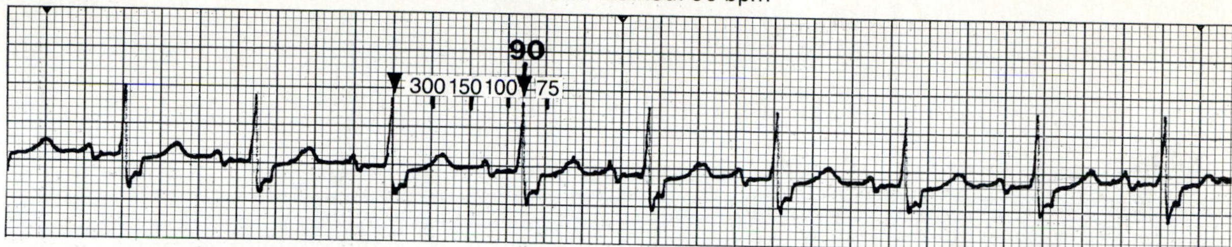

FIGURE 3-29

Rate: 87 to 90 bpm
Rhythm: Regular
P wave: Biphasic on lead II (normally round, upright)
PR interval: 0.20 seconds
QRS complex: 0.14 seconds, Rs configuration, intraventricular conduction delay; QT interval 0.37 seconds, prolonged for rate
Interpretation: NSR, intraventricular conduction delay, QT-interval prolongation

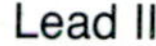
Lead II

RATE: Box Method: 72 bpm

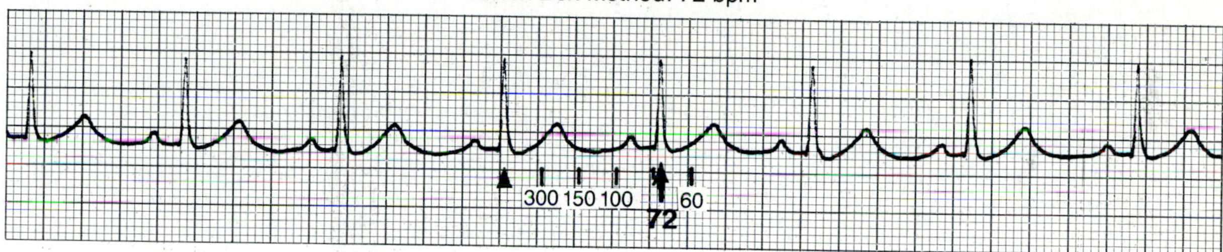

FIGURE 3-30

Rate: 72 bpm
Rhythm: Regular
P wave: Normal
PR interval: 0.16 to 0.18 seconds
QRS complex: 0.08 seconds, R configuration; QT interval 0.40 seconds. (Confirm on other leads. The terminal sloping may extend farther than is evident in this tracing.)
Interpretation: NSR

ML2 telemetry

RATE: Box Method: 43 bpm

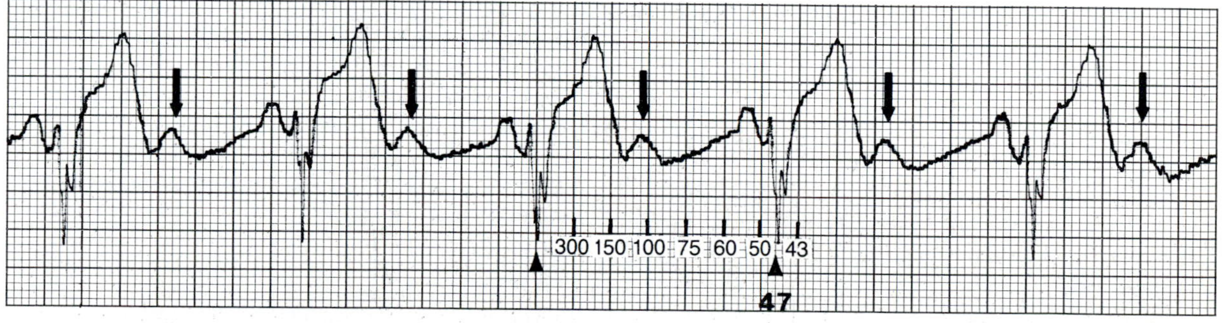

FIGURE 3-31 Pronounced U waves *(arrows)*.

Rate: 43 to 47 bpm
Rhythm: Regular
P wave: 0.11 to 0.12 seconds, wide , intraatrial conduction delay; 3.5 to 4 mm high (tall) (confirm on 12-lead ECG)
PR interval: 0.18 seconds
QRS complex: 0.12 to 0.15 seconds, prolonged, intraventricular conduction delay. Configuration is rS (with notched S wave) and predominantly negative. (Normally modified lead II of a telemetry system resembles lead II and the QRS is usually upright.) ST-segment elevation (may be secondary to bundle branch block). QT interval 0.52 seconds, prolonged; (Because heart rate is below 65 bpm, the "less than half R-R interval" rule does not apply. QT chart confirms prolongation.) U waves present
Interpretation: Sinus bradycardia (bradycardia because rate < 60 bpm), intraventricular and intraatrial conduction delays, prolonged QT interval, U waves

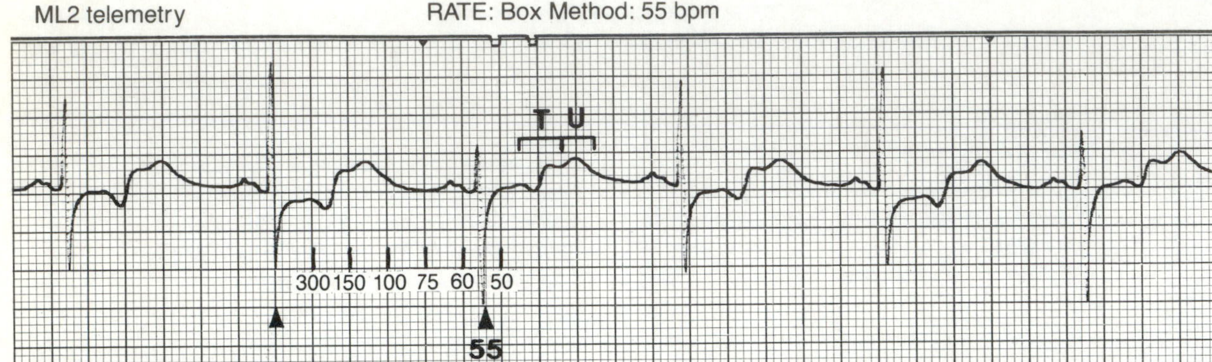

FIGURE 3-32 Sinus bradycardia with biphasic (bifid) T waves, U waves, variable QRS amplitude, and QT interval prolongation.

Rate: 55 bpm
Rhythm: Regular
P wave: 0.11 to 0.12 seconds, notched, intraatrial conduction delay
PR interval: 0.18 seconds
QRS complex: 0.11 seconds, RS configuration, variable QRS amplitude (cause unknown); Bifid T waves; QT interval 0.44 to 0.48 seconds, prolonged. Since heart rate <65 bpm, the "less than half R-R interval" does not apply.
Interpretation: Sinus bradycardia (bradycardia because rate < 60 bpm) with bifid T waves, QT-interval prolongation, variable QRS amplitude, and U waves

ECG Features of Electrolyte Disturbances[3,4,29-31]

Hypokalemia

Flat/inverted T wave
Depressed ST segment
Prominent U wave
Ventricular arrhythmias
Enhanced automaticity
Prolonged QT (QU) interval
Increased sensitivity to digitalis toxicity

Hyperkalemia

Diminished atrial activity
Disappearance of P wave
Widened QRS complex
Peaked T wave
Bradycardia
Ventricular arrhythmias
Asystole

As hyperkalemia progresses to a terminal condition, many of these features can be combined. The PR interval prolongs and eventually the P wave disappears and the QRS widens. This leads to what is known as a *sine wave* pattern, which eventually deteriorates into ventricular fibrillation.

Calcium changes are frequently extreme before producing electrocardiographic alterations.

Hypocalcemia

Long, flattened ST segment; prolonged ST segment
Prolonged QT interval

Hypercalcemia

Shortened ST segment
Shortened QT interval
Prolonged QRS complex
Prolonged PR interval

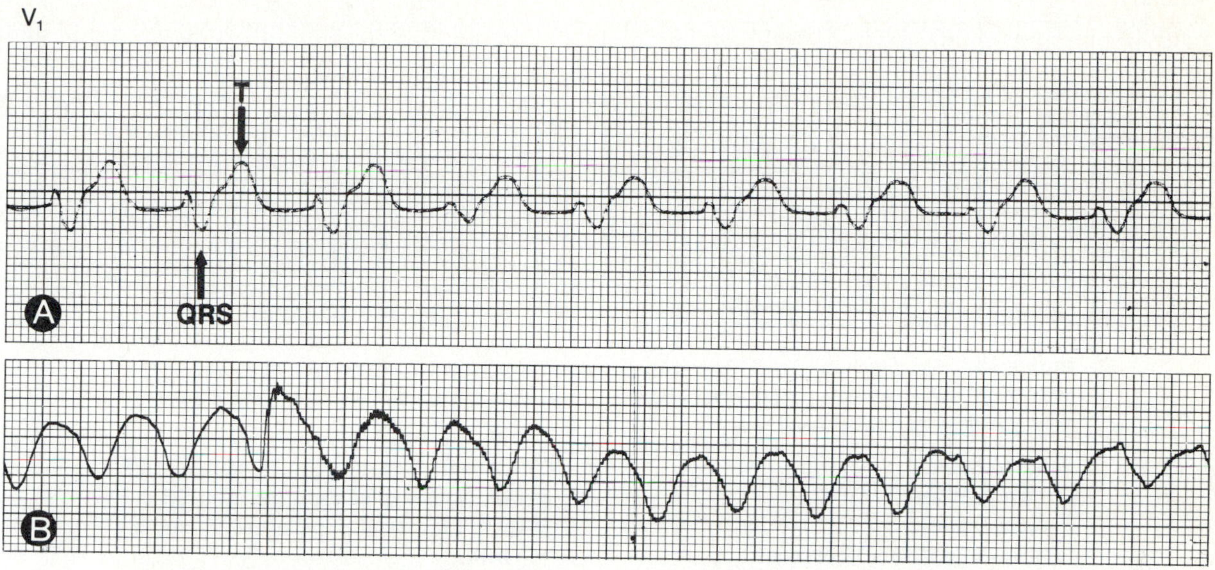

FIGURE 3-33 Hyperkalemia. **A,** Serum potassium 6.6 mEq. Note diminution of atrial activity, widened QRS complex, and merging P-QRS-T complex. Gradual widening of these complexes would produce the classic sine wave pattern of lethal hyperkalemia. **B,** Serum potassium 8.0 mEq. The patient was conscious at the time this tracing was taken.

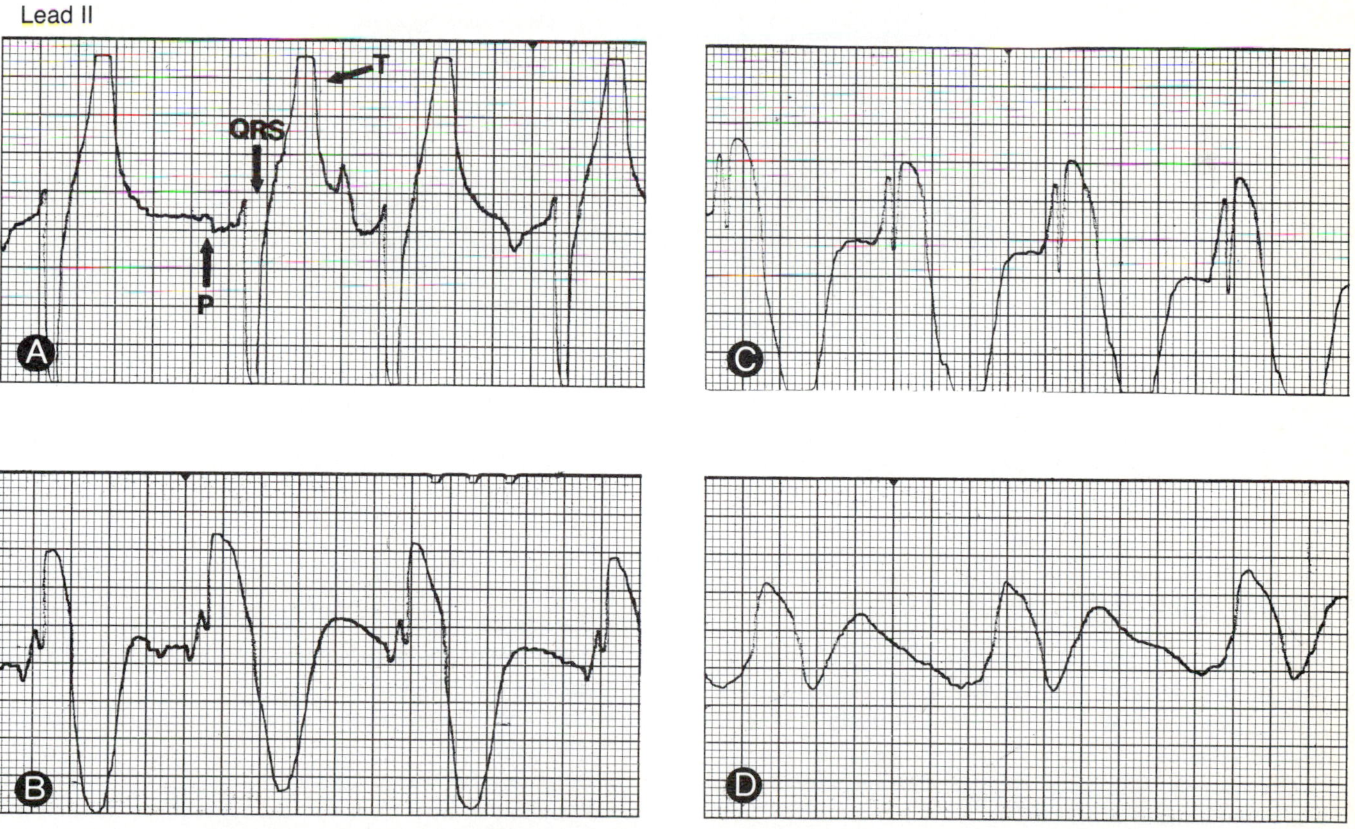

FIGURE 3-34 Terminal rhythm with hyperkalemia. A serum potassium drawn earlier was 6.6 mEq. **A** to **D** Note slowing of rate, loss of atrial activity, peaked T waves, progressive widening of the QRS complex to the terminal sine wave pattern.

Lead II

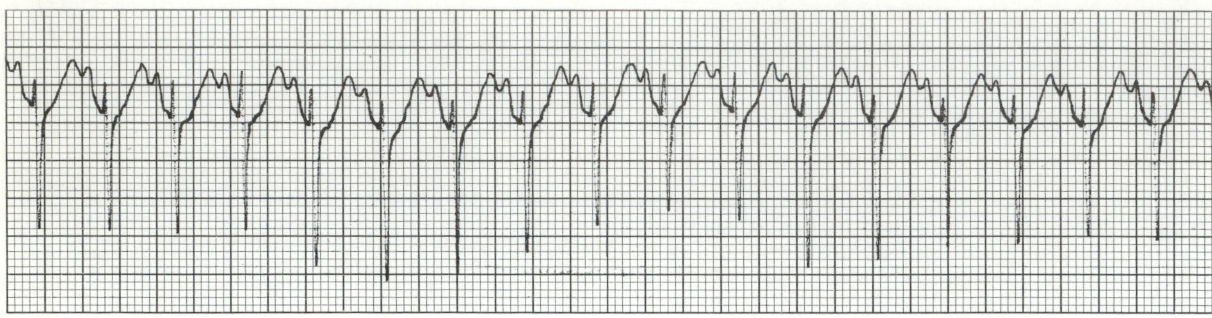

FIGURE 3-35 Sinus tachycardia, QT interval prolongation, hypokalemia present (serum potassium 3.1 mEq) in a 32-year-old male patient with diabetes mellitus. Hypokalemia can cause enhanced automaticity and prolonged QT interval.

Rate: 160 bpm
Rhythm: Regular
P wave: Normal
PR interval: 0.10 to 0.12 seconds
QRS complex: 0.08 seconds, rS configuration in lead II resulting from axis deviation. QT interval > 0.28 seconds, prolonged for rate of 160 bpm
Interpretation: Sinus tachycardia, QRS axis deviation, prolonged QT interval

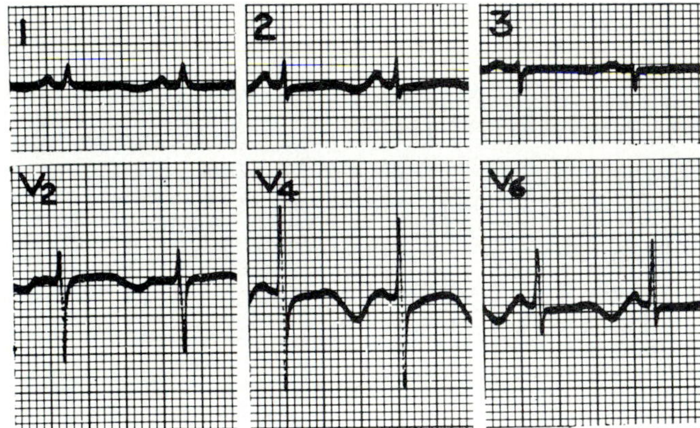

FIGURE 3-36 Hypocalcemia. Note prolonged ST segment and QT interval with late inversion of T waves. From a patient with serum calcium of 42 mg/100 ml. Reproduced with permission from Marriott HJL. *Practical Electrocardiography.* 8th ed. Baltimore: Williams & Wilkins, 1988, p. 528.

Rhythm Analysis

When examining a patient's rhythm strip, you should proceed in a consistently orderly fashion. If you analyze each rhythm in a systematic way, you are not likely to omit significant features.

Consider the following when approaching rhythm analysis (summarized in the box on p. 51):

- Determine the heart rate (rate of the QRS complexes), since this is the most important part of the ECG.
- Determine rhythm. Is the rhythm regular or irregular?
- P waves.
  - Does one P wave precede each QRS?
  - If the atrial rate is different from the ventricular rate, calculate both rates.
  - Does the P wave bear a constant relationship to the QRS complex?
  - Duration of P wave.
  - Morphology of P. Is the P wave upright in the inferior leads (leads II, III, aVF)?
- PR interval.
  - Duration.
  - Consistency.

Steps to Take for Rhythm Analysis

Rate
Rhythm
P waves
PR interval
QRS complex
QT interval

ECG Characteristics
Normal Sinus Rhythm

Rate: 60 to 100 bpm
Rhythm: Regular
P waves: Normal
PR interval: 0.12 to 0.20 seconds
QRS complex: 0.06 to 0.10 seconds

- QRS complex.
  - Duration.
  - Morphology.
- QT interval.
  - Duration.
  - Is it < one half the duration of the preceding R-R interval with rates between 65 and 90 bpm?

ECG Criteria for Normal Sinus Rhythm

Normal sinus rhythm (NSR) is defined as a rhythm originating in the SA node with the following characteristics (see the box at the top of the next column):

Rate:	60 to 100 bpm
Rhythm:	Regular (do not vary more than 0.12 seconds)
P wave:	Normal morphology
P/QRS ratio:	1:1 (one P wave precedes each QRS and bears a constant relationship to the QRS)
PR interval:	0.12 to 0.20 seconds
QRS complex:	0.06 to 0.10 seconds. The presence of an intraventricular conduction defect increases the duration of the QRS.

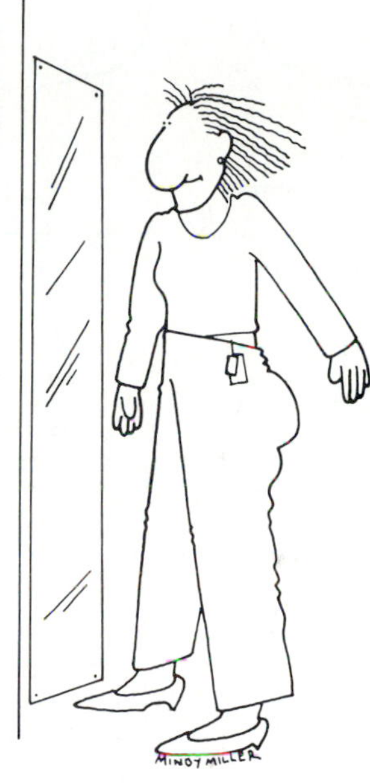

FIGURE 3-37 Only one view.

LEADS

We have examined the components of the ECG and the mechanics of monitoring (i.e., the series of components that comprise the patient-monitor circuit). The heart's electrical conduction system produces impulses that are sensed and transferred to a monitor via electrodes, lead wires, and cable. The current is then measured and amplified into a wave form that is displayed and printed by the monitor. Connecting the patient is only part of the process. Successful monitoring also necessitates a clear understanding of the definition and derivation of leads.

As was stated previously, electrodes, in combinations of two, three, four, or five, placed on different body sites offer visualization of the electrical activity of the heart from different angles and planes. Think of a lead as a particular "view" of the electrical activity of the heart. It is important to view this activity from several different vantage points. Consider the following analogy: when you shop for a pair of slacks, after trying them on, you look in the mirror. You use a three-way mirror if the store has it. If a three-way mirror is not available, you turn your body around to look at yourself from as many angles as possible. You do this because you realize that looking at yourself in those pants from only one angle may be very deceiving. The woman in Fig. 3-37 has no idea how she looks from the side and rear. Analyzing the heart's electrical activity is no different. It too requires examination from several angles.

Leads are used in continuous ECG monitoring and standard 12-lead ECGs. A lead is composed of negative and positive poles that, when connected to electrodes, sense the magnitude and direction of voltage. A vector is a symbol representing this force (Fig. 3-38). Leads enable visualization of the electrical activity of the heart on the **frontal plane** and the **horizontal plane** (Fig. 3-39).

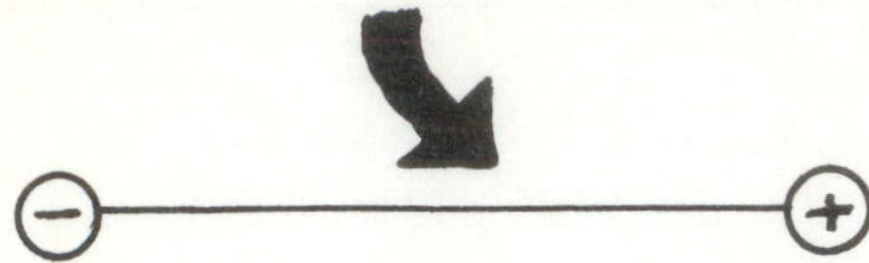

FIGURE 3-38 A lead is composed of a negative and a positive pole. A vector *(arrow)* symbolizes magnitude and direction of voltage.

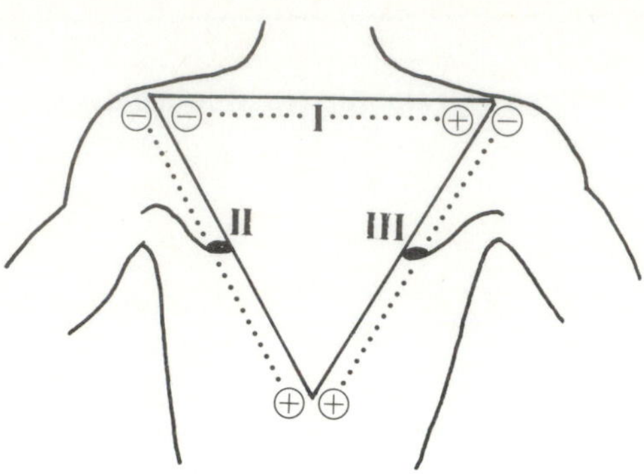

FIGURE 3-40 Einthoven triangle. Einthoven's equation states that a complex on lead II is equal to the sum of the same complex on leads I and III.

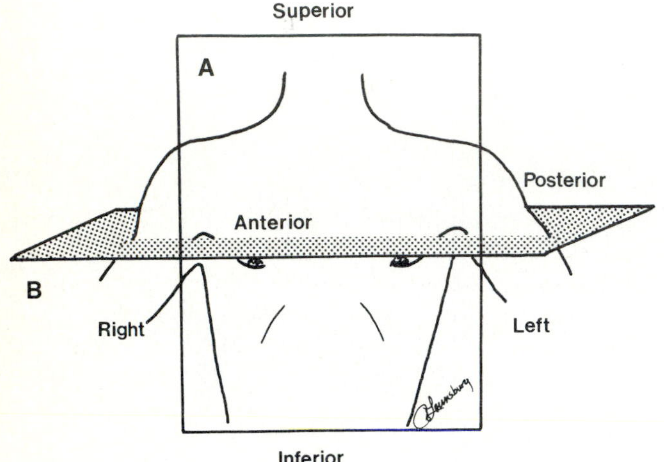

FIGURE 3-39 Frontal and horizontal planes. **A,** Frontal plane leads provide a view from the front of the body. Directions on this plane are right and left, superior and inferior. **B,** Horizontal plane leads view the heart as if the body were sliced in half. Directions on this plane are anterior and posterior and right and left.

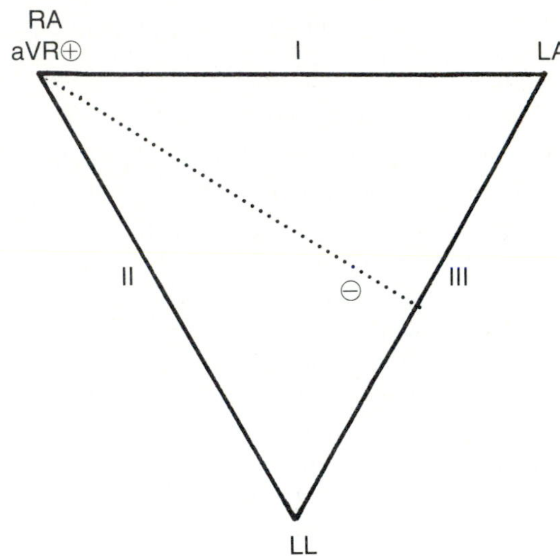

FIGURE 3-41 Lead aVR. This lead registers electrical variations at only one point, the right arm (RA) electrode. So the positive pole of this lead is the right arm. The negative pole is not on the body, but rather is a "null point" formed by and equidistant between, the other two points, the left leg (LL) and left arm (LA). Note the null point is directed toward the center of the triangle.

Leads of the Frontal Plane (the Limb Leads)

There are six leads on the frontal plane: three bipolar and three unipolar. The bipolar leads use a negative and positive electrode on the body's surface, whereas unipolar leads have only their positive pole on the body surface.

The Three Standard Bipolar Limb Leads

The standard bipolar limb leads are leads I, II, and III. All bedside monitors have the capability of monitoring these three leads, since only three skin electrodes are necessary. The three leads comprise Einthoven's triangle (Fig. 3-40). Lead I, with the negative electrode on the right arm and the positive one on the left arm, detects the current difference between these two electrodes. Likewise, lead II, with the negative electrode on the right arm and the positive one on the left leg, and lead III, with the negative electrode on the left arm and the positive one on the left leg, detect current differences between those respective sites.[32]

The Three Unipolar Limb Leads

The three unipolar limb leads are leads aVR, aVL, and aVF. The letter *a* stands for *augmented. V* is a traditional symbol for any exploratory unipolar lead. *R* denotes the right arm, *L* the left arm, and *F* is the symbol for the left leg or foot. Not all bedside units have the capability of monitoring the three augmented leads.

They may be considered unipolar, since they register the electric variations at only one point (right arm, left arm, or left foot) with respect to a null point. For example, in lead aVR, the electric potentials of the right arm are related to a null point, which is made by uniting the wires from the left arm and left leg[33] (Fig. 3-41). The other two leads, aVL and aVF, are similarly arranged (Fig. 3-42). Monitoring the augmented leads requires the connection of four skin electrodes and a monitor with a selector and the internal capability of augmenting the amplitude of the deflections.

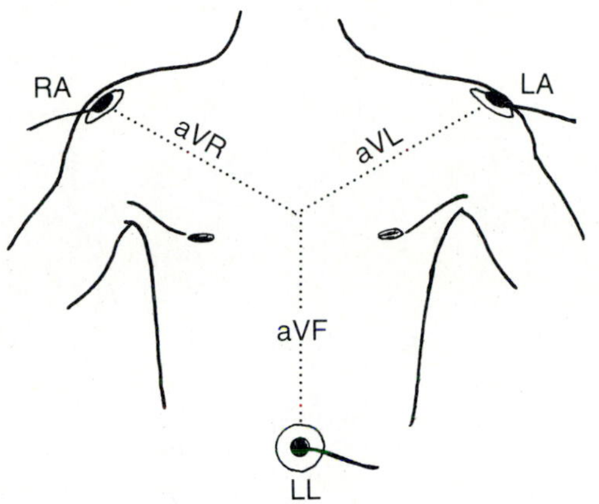

FIGURE 3-42 The unipolar limb leads aVR, aVL, aVF. RA = Right arm electrode. LA = Left arm electrode. LL = Left leg electrode.

The Appearance of the ECG on the Frontal Plane

As discussed previously, depolarization of the normal heart proceeds from superior to inferior and from right to left. Multiple, simultaneous wavefronts of activation converge in one dominant direction, the mean vector force (Fig. 3-43).

On lead I, with the positive electrode on the left arm and the negative electrode on the right arm, the mean vector force is directed more toward the positive than the negative electrode (Fig. 3-44, *A*). This results in a positive or upright P wave and QRS complex (Fig. 3-44, *B*).

On lead II, the positive electrode is on the left leg, and the negative electrode is on the right arm. The mean vector force again is directed toward the positive electrode, resulting in upright complexes (Fig. 3-45).

On lead III, the positive electrode is on the left leg and the negative one is on the left arm. The mean vector force is predominantly directed toward the positive pole (Fig. 3-46). What happens when the mean vector force is directed perpendicularly to the lead? In such situations, the QRS may be both above and below the baseline (isoelectric line) producing *biphasic* or *diphasic* complexes. When a complex is inscribed equally above and below the iso-

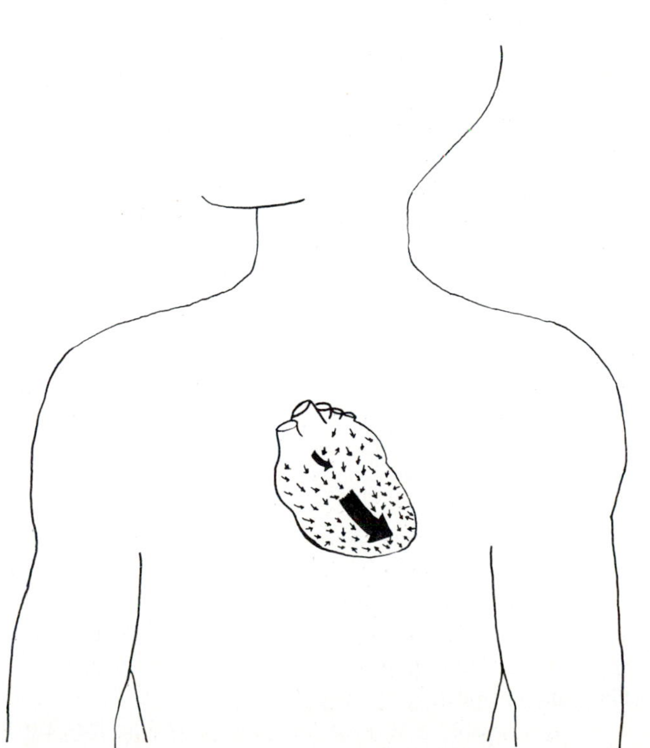

FIGURE 3-43 The mean vector force. Summation of multiple, simultaneous wavefronts creates the mean vector force.

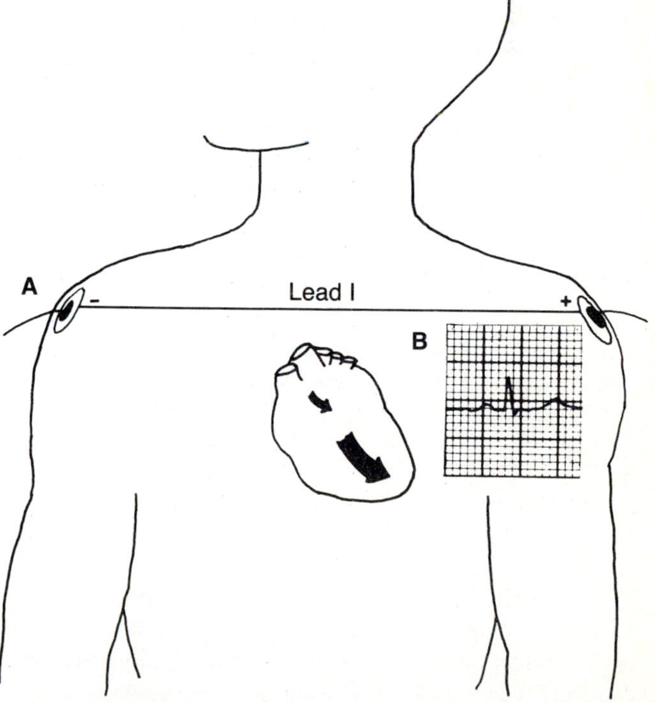

FIGURE 3-44 Lead I. With the negative electrode on the right arm *(A)* and the positive electrode on the left arm, the mean vector forces of the atria and ventricles are directed toward the positive electrode *(B)*, producing a positive P wave and QRS complex.

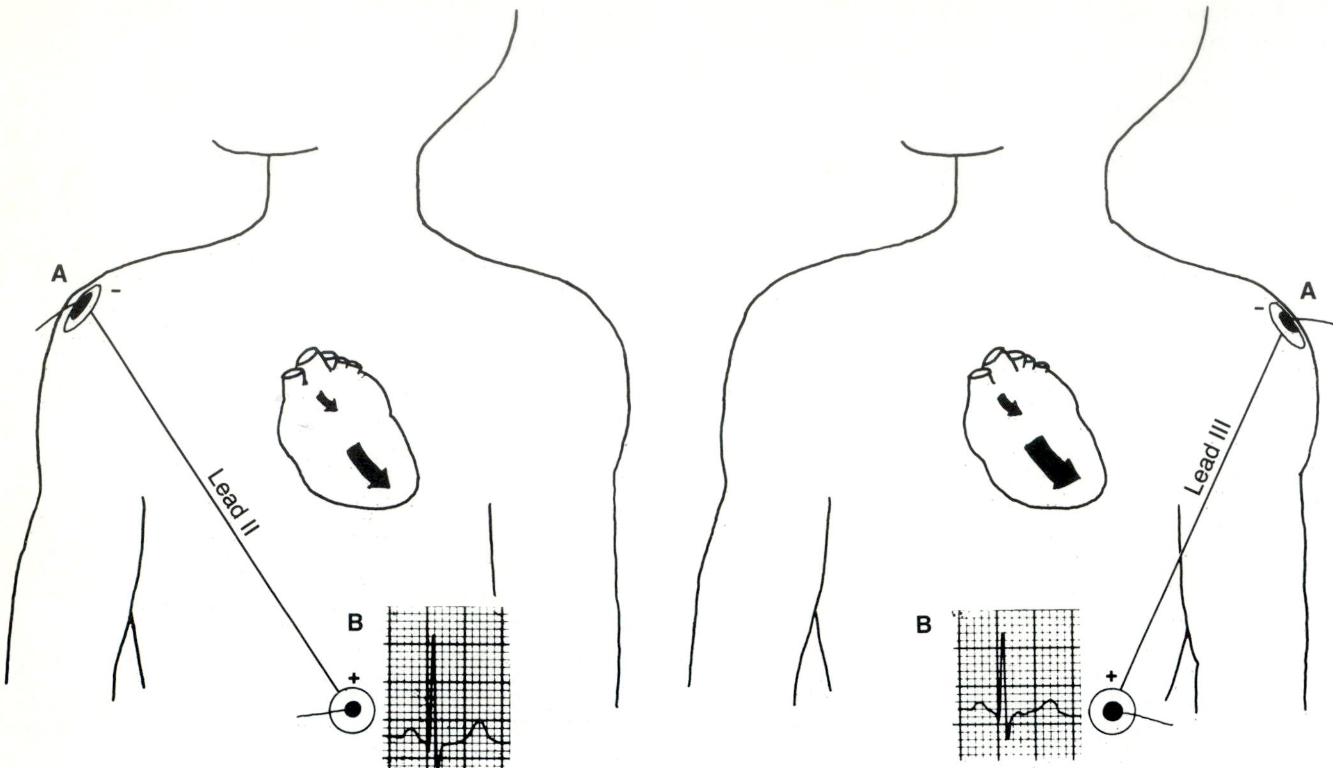

FIGURE 3-45 Lead II. The left leg electrode is positive, the right arm negative *(A)*. Mean vector forces are directed toward the positive electrode, resulting in a positive P wave and QRS complex *(B)*.

FIGURE 3-46 Lead III. The left leg electrode is positive, the left arm negative *(A)*. Mean vector forces are directed toward the positive electrode resulting in a positive P wave and QRS complex *(B)*.

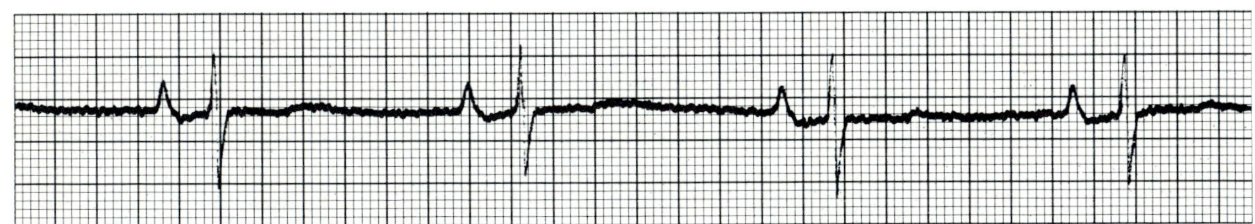

FIGURE 3-47 An equiphasic QRS complex. Note that the QRS complex is the same distance above and below the baseline.

electric line, regardless of amplitude, it is termed *equiphasic* (Fig. 3-47).

Lead aVR "looks" at the heart from the right shoulder. The mean vector force is normally directed away from this positive electrode, resulting in negative or downward deflecting P waves and QRS complexes (Fig. 3-48).

Lead aVL, with its unipolar positive electrode on the left shoulder, records the heart's activity with positive, negative, or diphasic complexes (Fig. 3-49).

Since the mean vector force is directed predominantly inferiorly, aVF records positive P waves and QRS complexes (Fig. 3-50).

Leads II, III, and aVF are often referred to as the *inferior leads,* since their positive electrodes are all located on the left leg. They view the heart from its inferior or diaphragmatic aspect.

Each of the lines formed from the preceding lead illustrations can be combined to intersect in the center (Fig. 3-51). If these intersecting lines are contained in a circle and assigned 360 degrees (Figs. 3-52 and 3-53), the mean

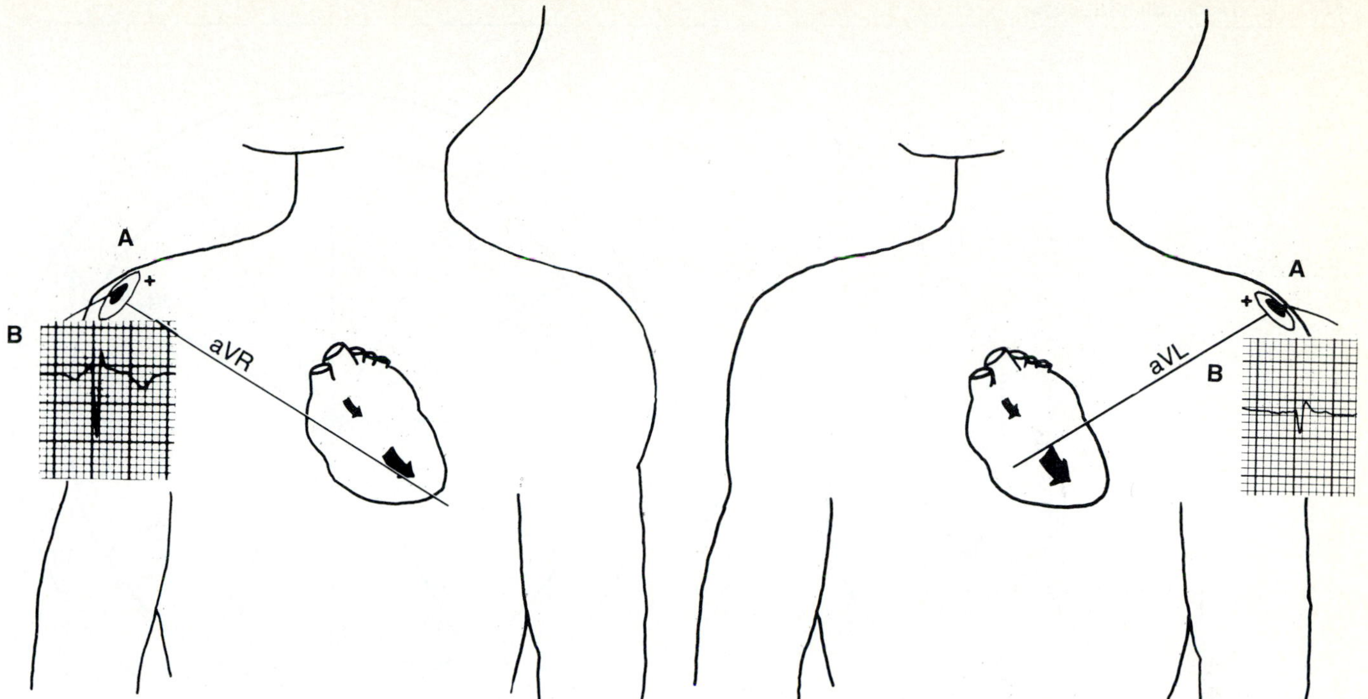

FIGURE 3-48 Lead aVR. With its positive pole on the right shoulder *(A),* mean vector forces are directed away from aVR, giving a negative P wave and QRS complex *(B).*

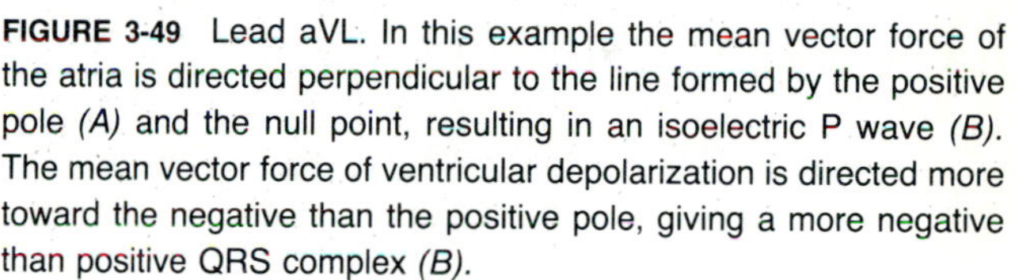

FIGURE 3-49 Lead aVL. In this example the mean vector force of the atria is directed perpendicular to the line formed by the positive pole *(A)* and the null point, resulting in an isoelectric P wave *(B).* The mean vector force of ventricular depolarization is directed more toward the negative than the positive pole, giving a more negative than positive QRS complex *(B).*

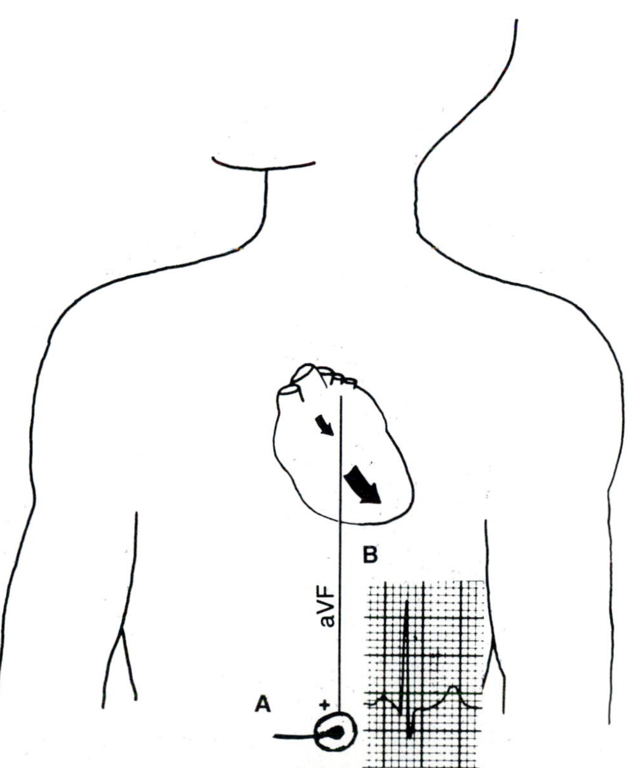

FIGURE 3-50 Lead aVF. With its positive electrode on the left leg *(A)* and negative pole directed straight up, mean vector forces of both the atria and ventricles are directed toward its positive pole, giving a positive P wave and QRS complex (*B*).

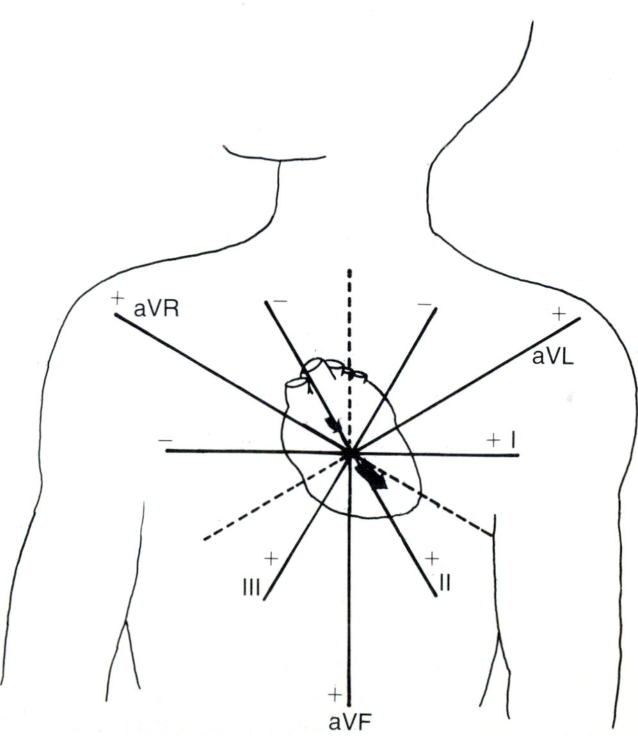

FIGURE 3-51 All leads of the frontal plane. When each lead line is placed to intersect in the center, all the leads of the frontal plane may be visualized simultaneously.

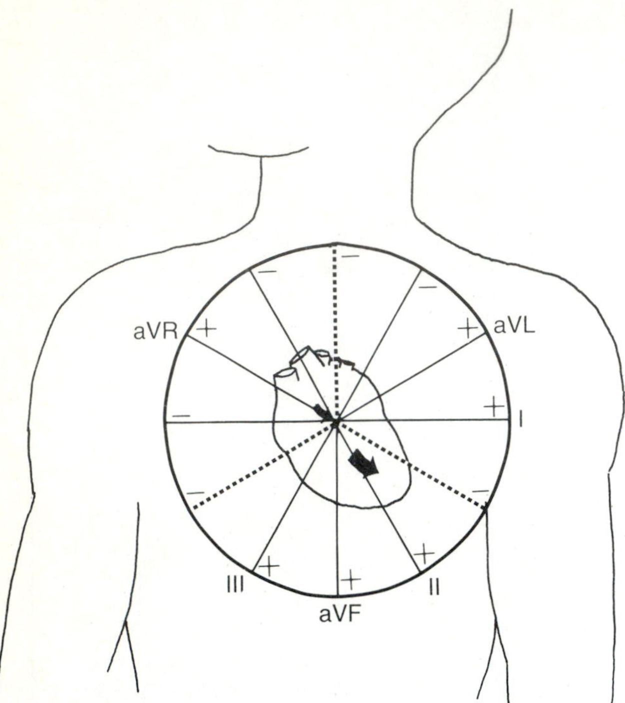

FIGURE 3-52 The leads of the frontal plane encircled.

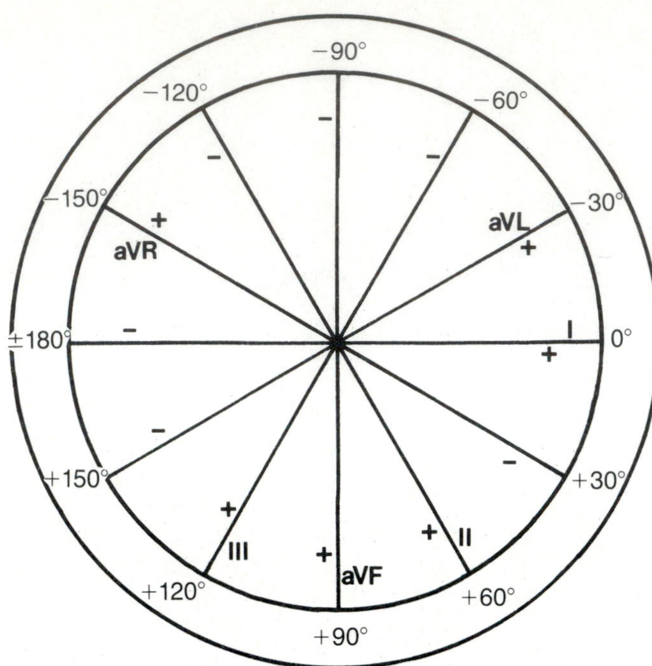

FIGURE 3-53 Degrees assigned to the leads of the frontal plane. Drawing a circle around the lead lines intersected in the center enables us to assign degrees to the leads. Leads are labeled on their positive poles.

Axis Determination

1. Check lead I.
   If positive, axis is left.
   If negative, axis is right.
   If isoelectric or equiphasic, axis is perpendicular to lead I, −90 or +90.
2. Check lead aVF.
   If positive, axis is inferior.
   If negative, axis is superior.
   If isoelectric or equiphasic, axis is perpendicular to lead aVF, 0 or +180.

vector force can be described in terms of degrees. This is known as the *hexaxial reference system*. The point to which the mean vector force is directed is called the *axis*. If we are discussing the mean vector force of the ventricles, we are referring to the QRS axis; likewise the mean vector forces of the P wave and T wave are referred to as the axes of the P wave and T wave, respectively. This discussion is limited to the *QRS axis*. Fig. 3-54 illustrates the quadrants for normal QRS axis and axis deviations and the box above illustrates a simple method for determining the axis quadrant.

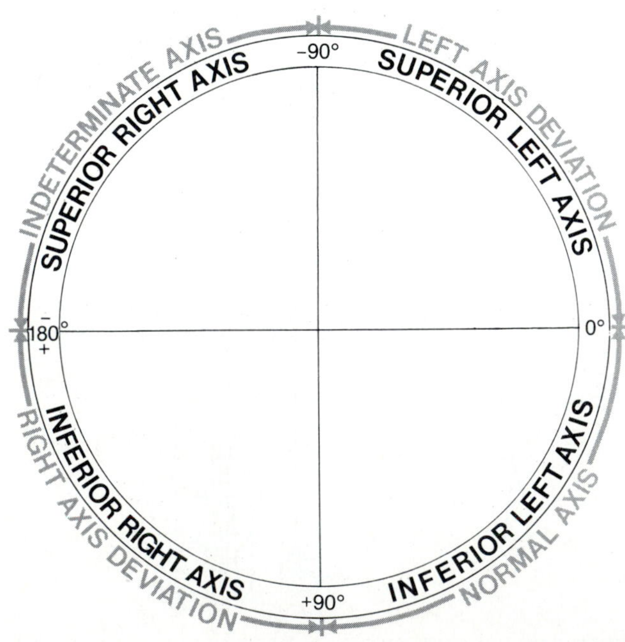

FIGURE 3-54 QRS axis quadrants. The terms on the outside of the circle—*normal axis, left axis deviation, right axis deviation,* and *indeterminate axis*—are common, traditional terms. Their synonymous terms, inside the circle, are gaining in popularity.

A few of the factors affecting axis include age, height, weight, and heart disease. A newborn baby has a QRS axis directed to the right, whereas elderly individuals often display axes to the left in the 0 to −30 degree range. Tall, thin people and those with chronic obstructive pulmonary disease (COPD) often have axes in the +90 degree range while short, obese, or those with protuberant abdomens may exhibit axes directed toward 0 degrees. Heart disease affecting conduction fibers may result in axes in the left axis deviation (LAD) or right axis deviation (RAD) quadrants. Figs. 3-55 to 3-58 illustrate normal and deviated QRS axes.

Test yourself by determining the QRS axes of the two ECGs in Figs. 3-59 and 3-60 using the quick method recommended (see the box on p. 56). You will find the answers in the lower right corner.

Leads of the Horizontal Plane (the Precordial Leads)

There are six leads on the horizontal plane and they are all unipolar, symbolized by the letter V. V_1 to V_6 are chest leads that, when placed in their specified locations, offer six close-up "views" (Figs. 3-61 and 3-62). On the horizontal plane, note how the electrodes "encircle" the heart (Fig. 3-63).

From V_1 to V_6 the QRS complex progresses from rS in V_1 to a qR in V_6 (Fig. 3-64). The change in the QRS com-

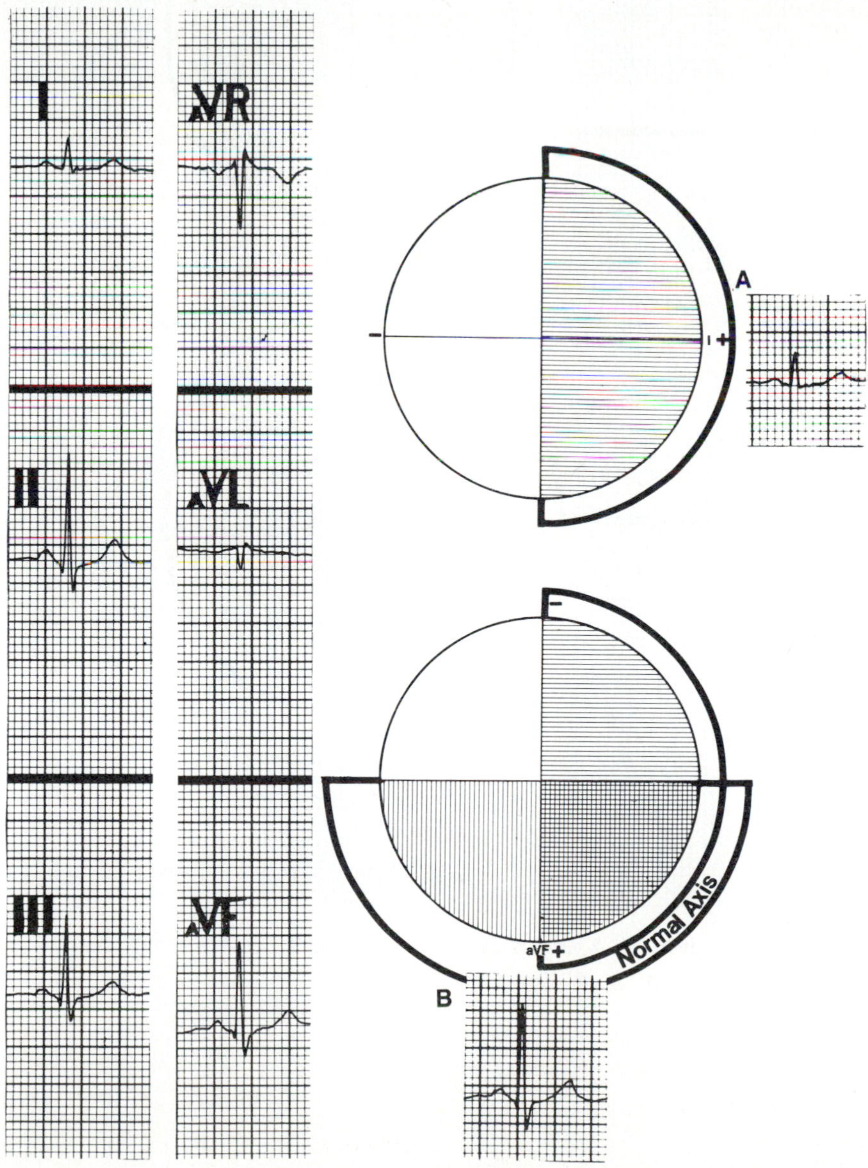

FIGURE 3-55 Normal QRS axis. **A,** Look at the QRS in lead I. It is positive, so the axis is left. **B,** The QRS in aVF is positive, so the axis is inferior.

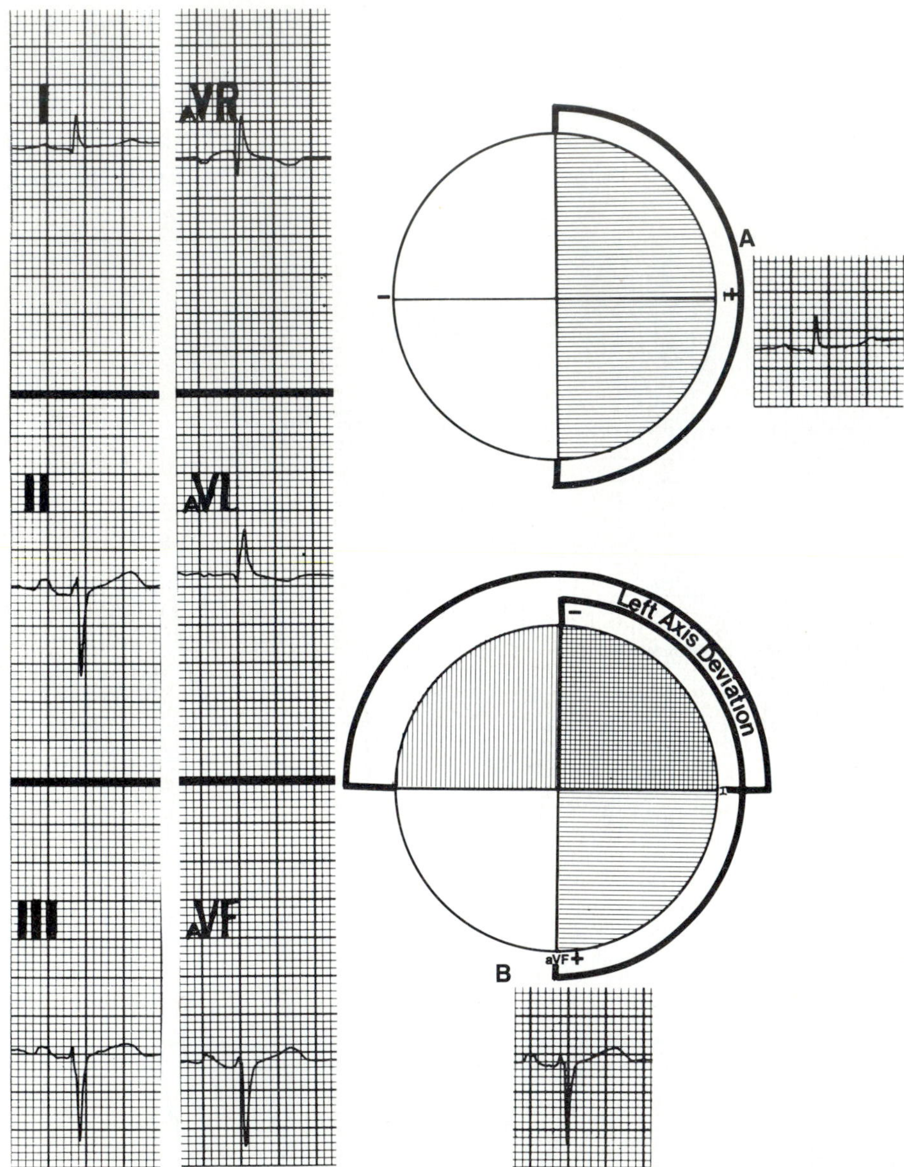

FIGURE 3-56 Left axis deviation. **A,** QRS is positive in lead I and **B**, negative in aVF, thus the axis is superior.

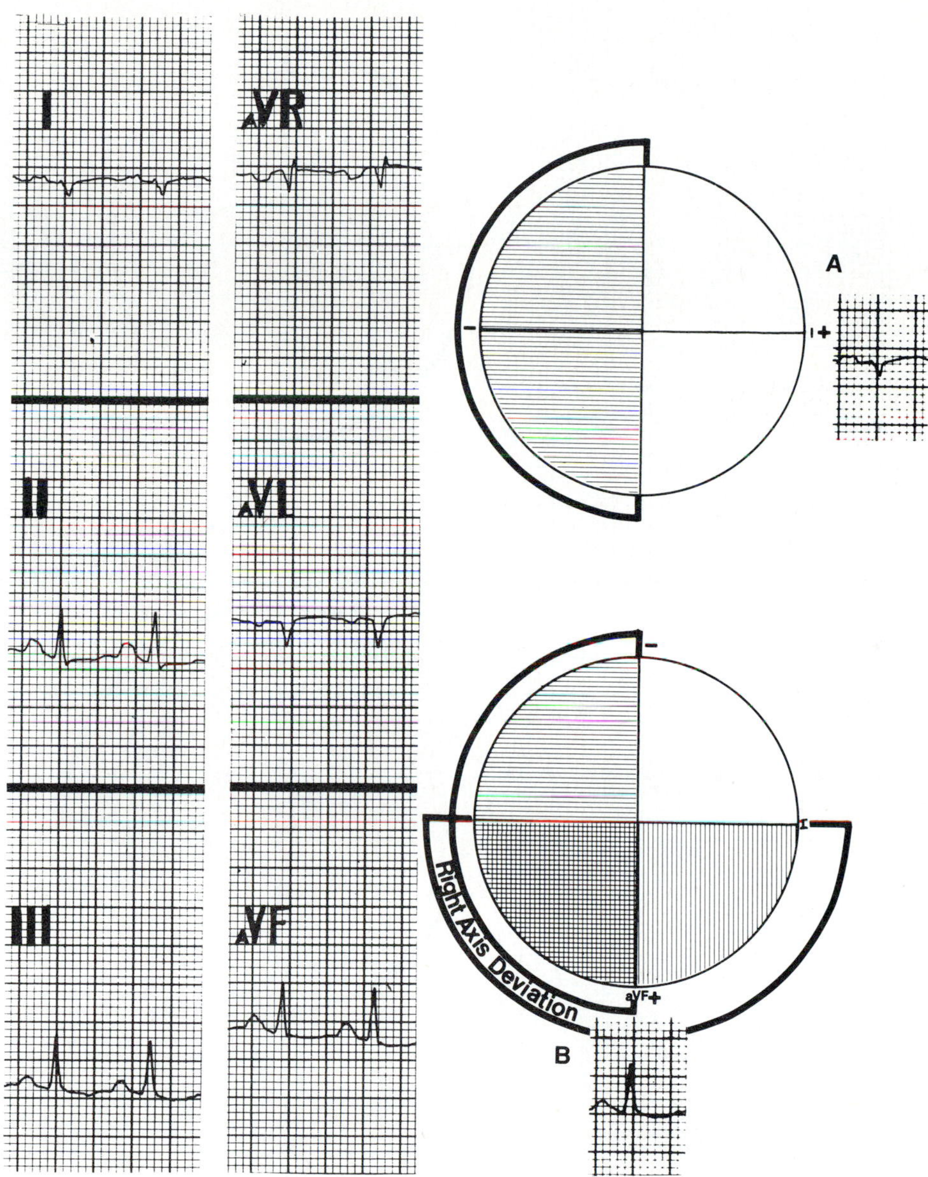

FIGURE 3-57 Right axis deviation. **A,** QRS is negative in lead I, so axis is right and **B**, positive in aVF, thus the axis is inferior.

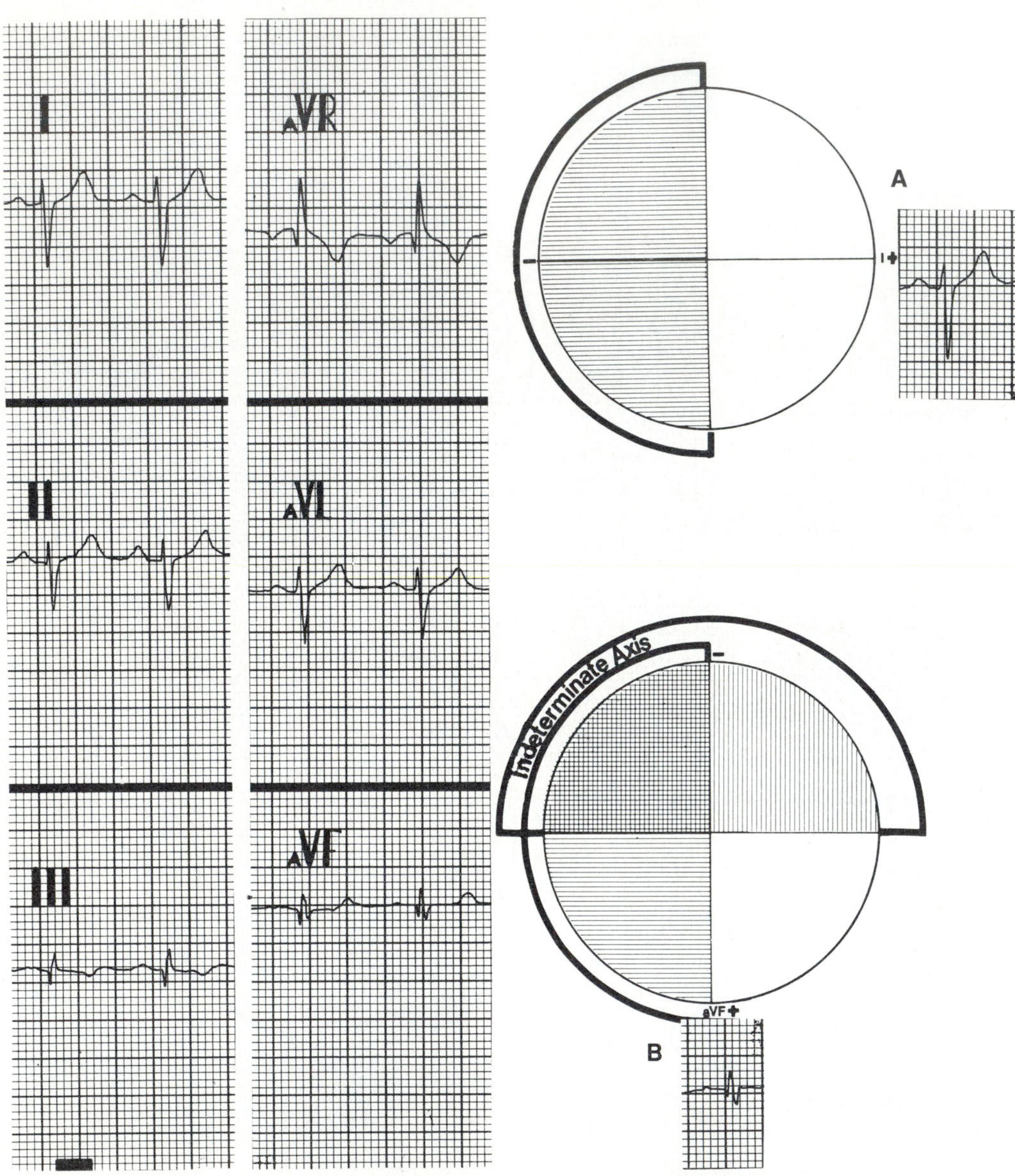

FIGURE 3-58 Indeterminate axis. **A,** QRS complex is negative in lead I, so axis is right, and **B**, equiphasic in aVF, so axis is perpendicular to aVF. Lead III is also equiphasic, therefore perpendicular to that lead line, causing the axis to fall in the −150 to −180-degree range.

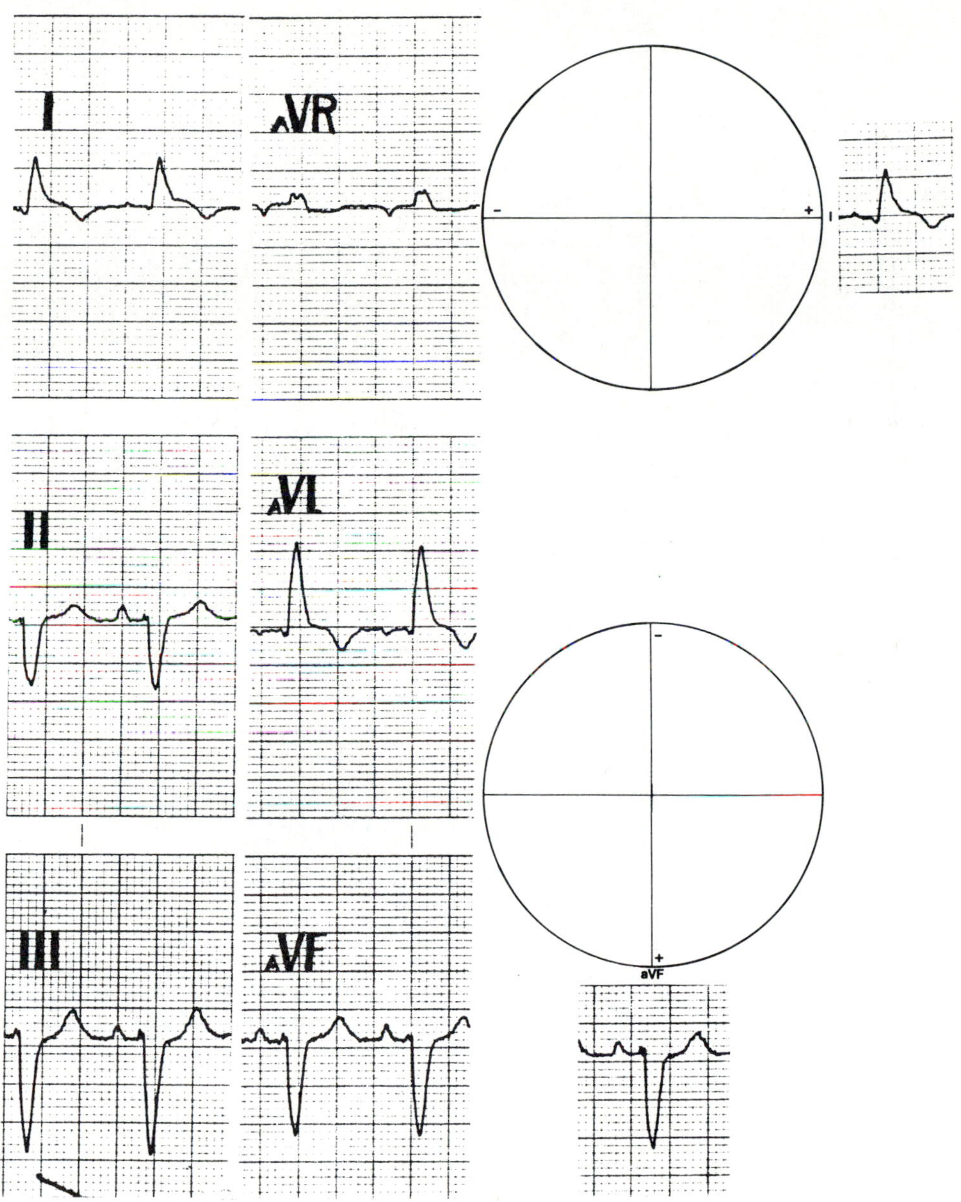

FIGURE 3-59 Test yourself.

Answer: Left axis deviation.

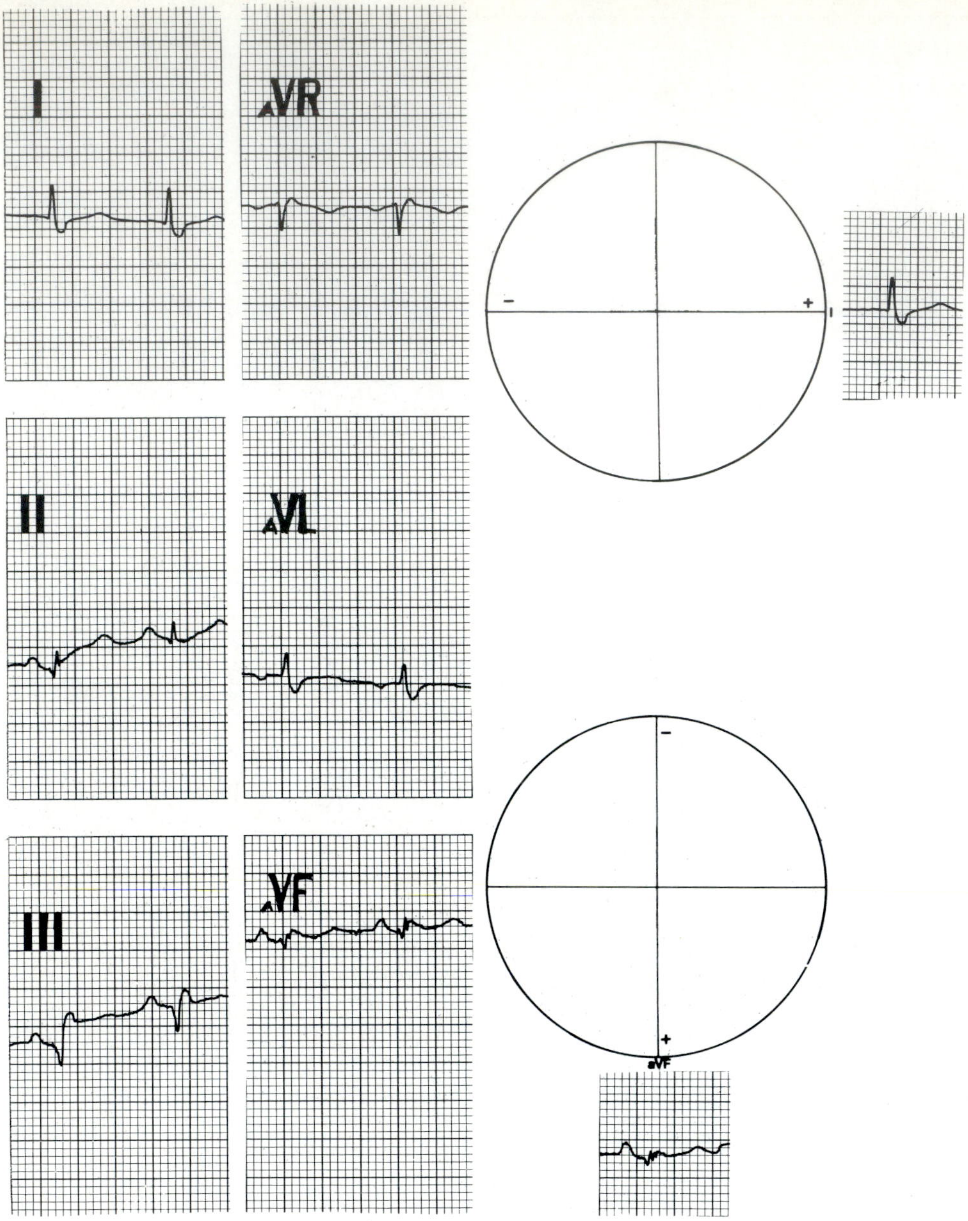

FIGURE 3-60 Test yourself.

Answer: QRS in aVF is equiphasic so axis is perpendicular to aVF. Since the QRS in lead I is positive, we know it is toward the positive pole of lead I. The axis is 0 degrees.

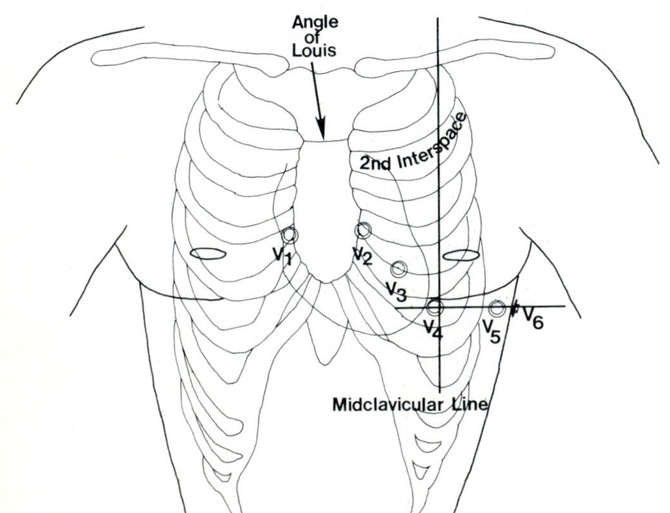

FIGURE 3-61 The leads of the horizontal plane.

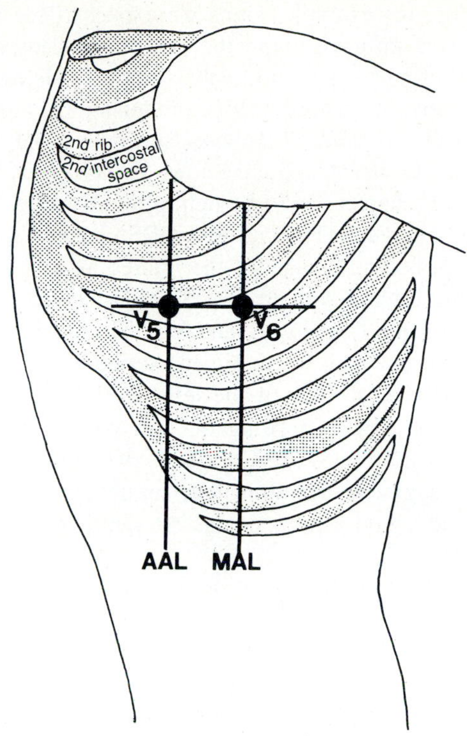

FIGURE 3-62 Leads V_5 and V_6. V_5 is on the same horizontal line as V_4, in the anterior axillary line (AAL). V_6 is also on the same horizontal line as V_4 but in the midaxillary line (MAL).

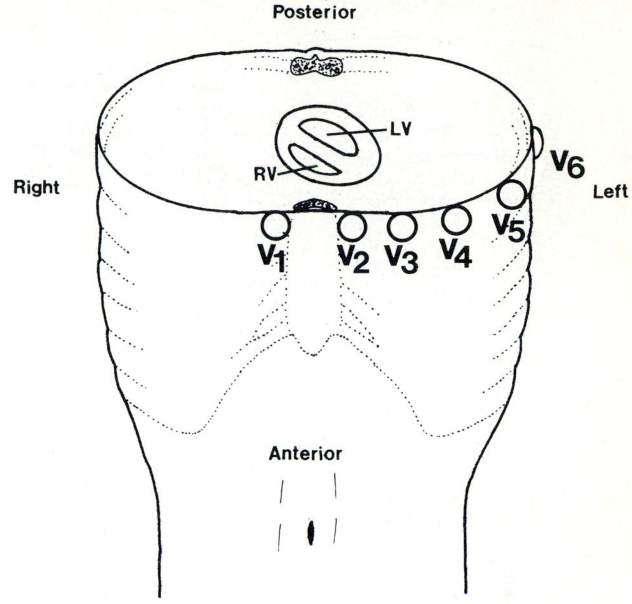

FIGURE 3-63 The precordial leads on the horizontal plane. LV = Left ventricle. RV = Right ventricle.

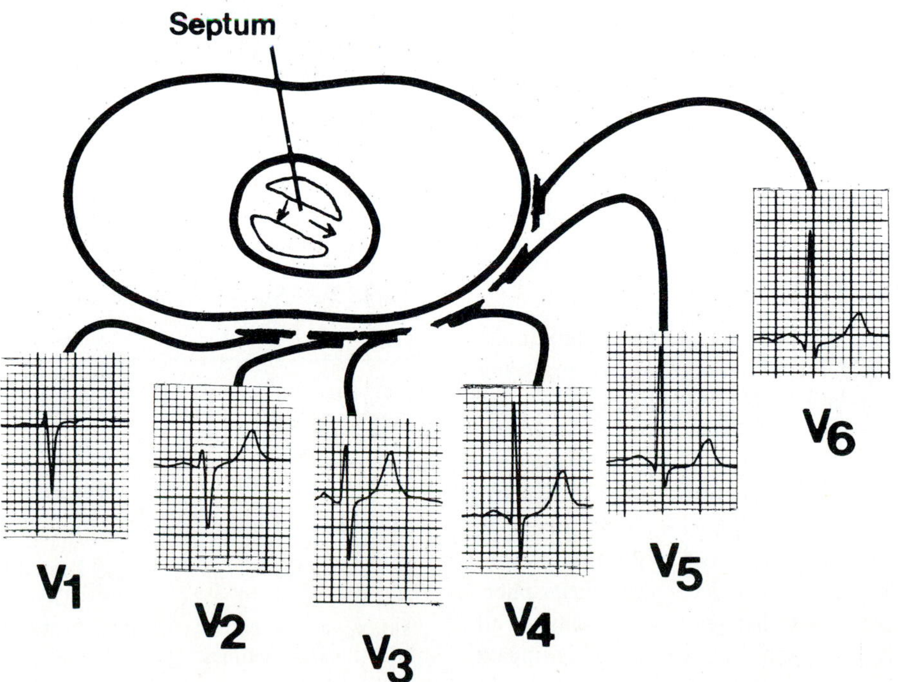

FIGURE 3-64 The precordial leads and their respective recordings. See text for discussion.

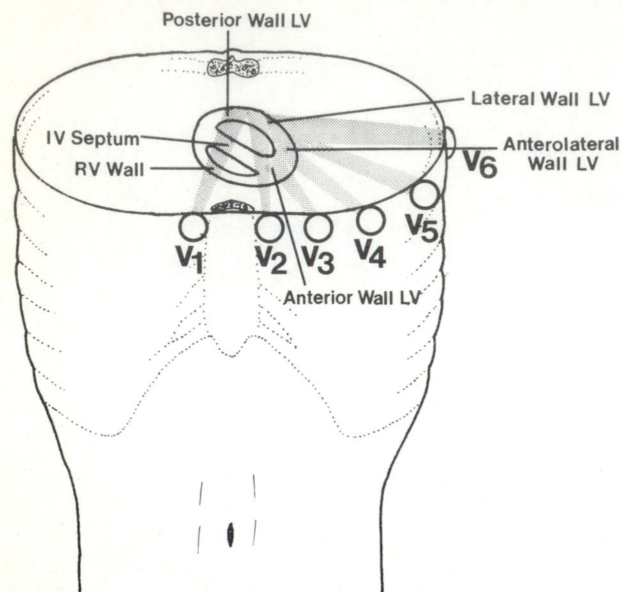

FIGURE 3-65 The precordial leads on the horizontal plane. The true posterior wall of the left ventricle is viewed indirectly by leads V_1 and V_2. IV = interventricular. LV = Left ventricle. RV = Right ventricle.

plex from predominantly negative to positive is known as *R-wave progression*. The initial r wave in V_1 and the initial q wave in V_6 result from septal depolarization that proceeds from left to right and from posterior to anterior.

Leads V_1, V_2, and sometimes V_3 reflect septal activity. Leads V_3 and V_4 record the activity of the anterior surface of the left ventricle. V_5 and V_6 (along with I and aVL) record activity from the lateral aspect of the left ventricle. Right ventricular abnormalities may be revealed in leads V_1 to V_3. Leads V_1 and V_2 also indirectly reflect activity from the true posterior surface (Fig. 3-65).

Location of Myocardial Infarction

It is now possible to understand how one can approximate the location of a myocardial infarction (MI) by analyzing all 12 leads of the standard ECG. The earliest ECG sign displayed during myocardial infarction is *ST-segment elevation,* signifying myocardial injury, in the leads that "look at" the injured area of the heart. High T waves, which are sometimes referred to as *hyperacute T waves,* in those same leads may also be apparent in the first hour(s) of the evolving infarction. *T-wave inversion* occurs later. The QRS complex also shows changes. It loses some or all of the height of its R wave and often develops significant *Q waves*, representing myocardial necrosis, over the area of transmural infarction. If a person has had a transmural anterior MI, for example, signs we expect to see include poor R wave progression in the precordial leads and replacement of r waves with Q waves in the leads overlying the infarction. Transmural MIs producing Q waves are known as *Q-wave MIs.* Likewise, subendocardial MIs do not produce Q waves and are known as *non-Q-wave MIs.* A review of Chapter 1 will be helpful at this time.

The ST-segment, T-wave, and QRS changes appear in the leads providing a view of the injured area. An MI involving the **lateral** wall of the left ventricle shows these changes in leads I, aVL, V_5 and V_6; the **anterior** wall of the left ventricle leads V_2 to V_4; the **septal** area, V_1 to V_3; and the **inferior** surface of the left ventricle, II, III, and aVF. Look at Figure 3-14 again. Can you determine the location of infarction? Leads I and aVL, and V_1 to V_6 show ST- segment elevation. The infarction involves the anterior and lateral aspects of the left ventricle, an **anterolateral** MI.

Although it sounds simple, unfortunately myocardial infarction does not always produce such clear electrocardiographic signs. A standard ECG reveals only *some* of the heart's activity. It is not unusual for a patient to have an MI with a normal ECG or an ECG with nonspecific abnormalities. It is therefore prudent to base the initial diagnosis of myocardial infarction on the patient's symptoms or history. If a patient presents with chest discomfort suggestive of myocardial ischemia, which is not relieved with nitroglycerin, the preliminary, presumptive diagnosis of myocardial infarction is made until more conclusive tests can be done.

The following pages (Figs. 3-66 to 3-77) and Table 3-2 summarize individual lead information of the leads presented thus far. Anatomic landmarks are given for bedside and telemetry ECG monitoring.

Table 3-2 Summary of Standard Leads

Lead	Also referred to as
I, II, III	Bipolar standard limbs leads
aVR, aVL, aVF	Unipolar augmented limb leads
I, II, III, aVR, aVL, aVF	Frontal plane limb leads
V_1-V_6	Unipolar precordial chest leads; Horizontal plane leads
V_2-V_4	Anterior chest leads
I, V_5, V_6, aVL	Lateral leads
V_1, V_2	"True" posterior leads
V_1, V_2, and sometimes V_3	Septal leads
V_1-V_4 and sometimes V_5	Anteroseptal leads
II, III, aVF	Inferior leads

Lead I

Lead I is also known by the following names:

Standard Lead I
Standard Limb Lead
Frontal Plane Lead
Monitoring Lead
Lateral Lead

Anatomic Landmarks

+ Left shoulder
− Right shoulder
G Right lower trunk (but may go anywhere) if a 4- or 5-lead cable is used. If a 3-lead cable with lead selector is used, the ground is usually placed on the lower left trunk.

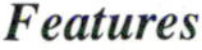

Features

- P, QRS usually positive.

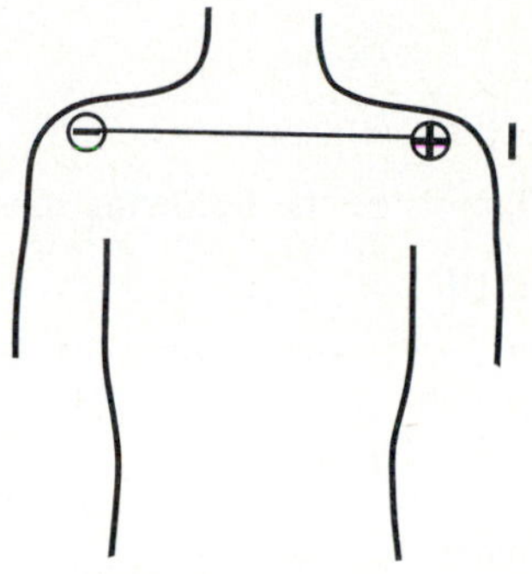

FIGURE 3-66 Lead I.

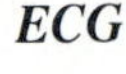

ECG

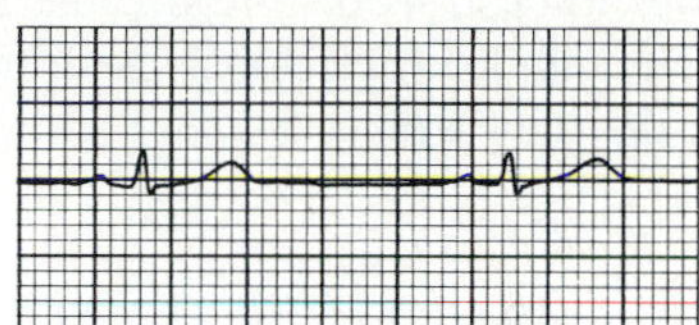

Lead II

Lead II is also known by the following names:

Standard Lead II
Standard Limb Lead
Frontal Plane Lead
Monitoring Lead
Inferior Lead

Anatomic Landmarks

+ Left lower trunk
− Right shoulder
G Right lower trunk, if using 4- or 5-lead cable. If 3-lead cable with lead selector is used, the ground is usually the left arm.

Features

- Popular lead for monitoring.
- Usually good P- and R-wave amplitude.
- Unable to differentiate right from left bundle branch block.
- Unable to differentiate ventricular ectopy from aberration. (This will be more meaningful in later chapters.)
- Good for detecting QRS axis shift.

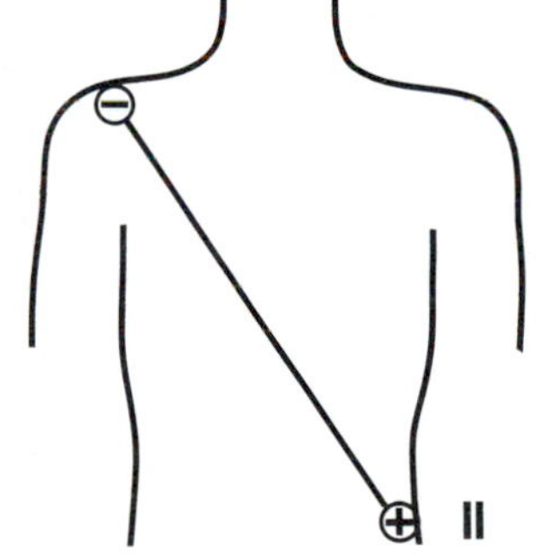

FIGURE 3-67 Lead II.

ECG

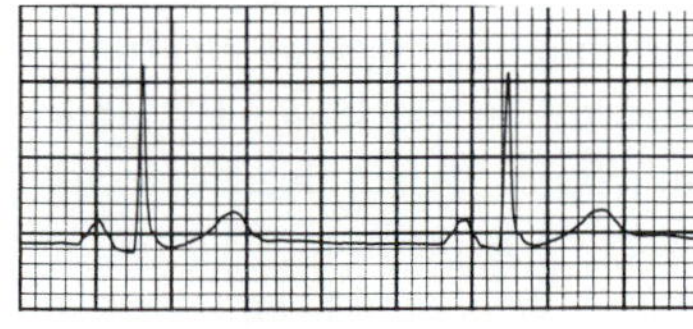

Lead III

Lead III is also known by the following names:

Standard Lead III
Standard Limb Lead
Frontal Plane Lead
Inferior Lead

Anatomic Landmarks

+ Left lower trunk
− Left shoulder
G Right lower trunk if 4- or 5-lead cable is used. If a 3-lead cable with lead selector is used, the ground is placed on the right arm.

Features

- Generally P, QRS positive but amplitude not as high as lead II.
- QRS may be diphasic.

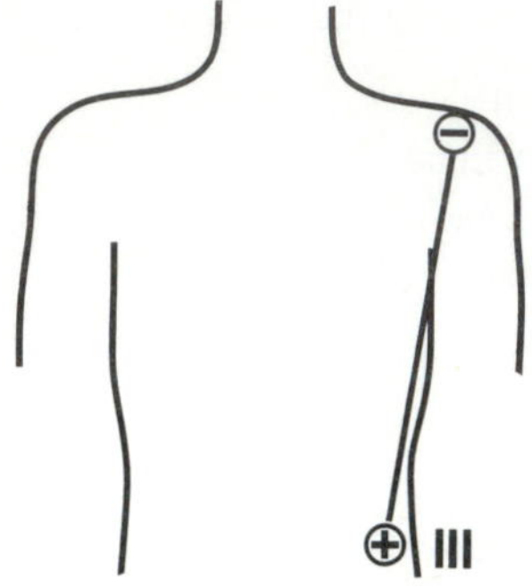

FIGURE 3-68 Lead III.

ECG

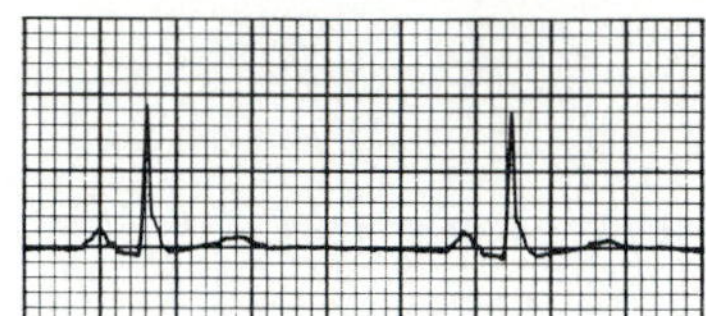

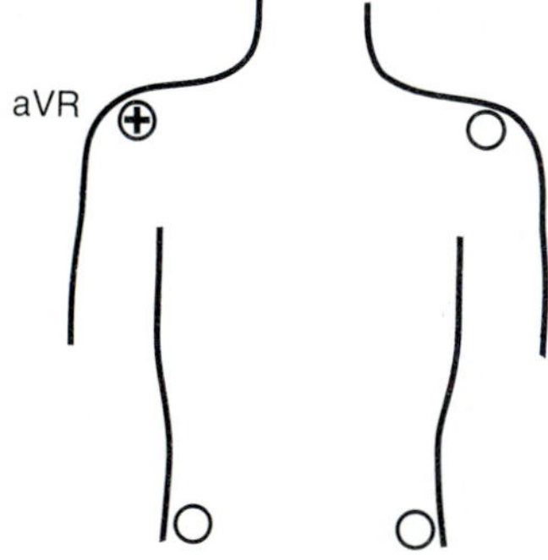

FIGURE 3-69 Lead aVR.

ECG

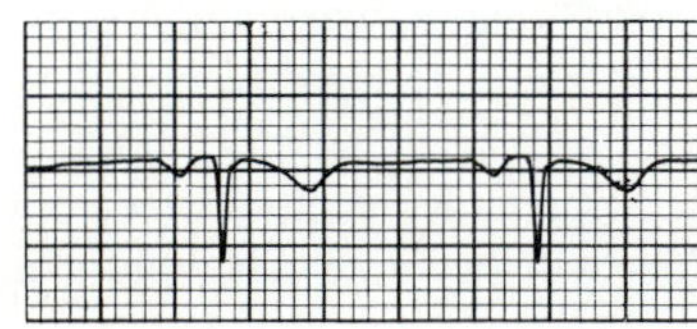

Lead aVR

Lead aVR is also known by the following names:

Augmented Limb Lead
Frontal Plane Unipolar Lead

Anatomic Landmarks

Four electrodes must be attached to body. The monitor must have aVR, aVL, and aVF capability. Place the RA electrode on right shoulder, the LA electrode on left shoulder, the LL electrode on the lower left abdomen, and the RL may go anywhere. When lead selector is turned to aVR the RA electrode is positive. The negative pole is not on the body surface; it is equidistant between LA and LL electrodes.

Features

- Negative P wave and negative QRS complex

Lead aVL

Lead aVL is also known by the following names:

Augmented Limb Lead
Frontal Plane Unipolar Lead
Lateral Lead

Anatomic Landmarks

Four electrodes must be attached to body. The monitor must have aVR, aVL and aVF capability. Place the RA electrode on right shoulder, the LA electrode on left shoulder, the LL electrode on the lower left abdomen, and the RL may go anywhere. When lead selector is turned to aVL, the LA electrode is positive. The negative pole is not on the body surface; it is equidistant between the RA and LL electrodes.

Features

- Flat, biphasic, or upright P wave.
- QRS complex can be upright, inverted, or biphasic.

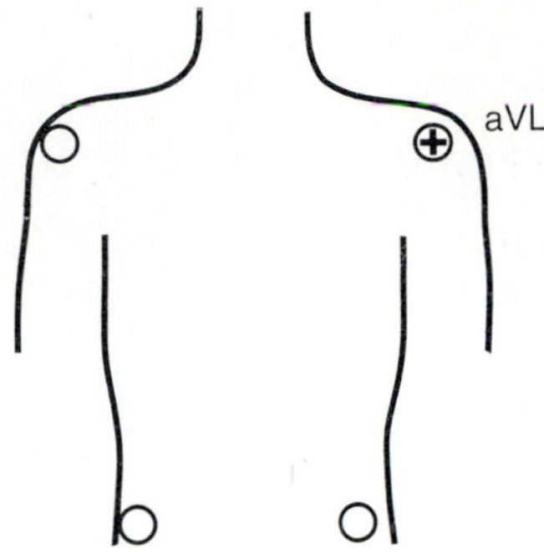

FIGURE 3-70 Lead aVL.

ECG

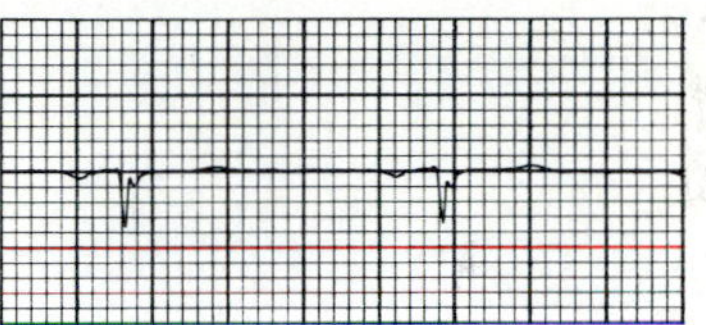

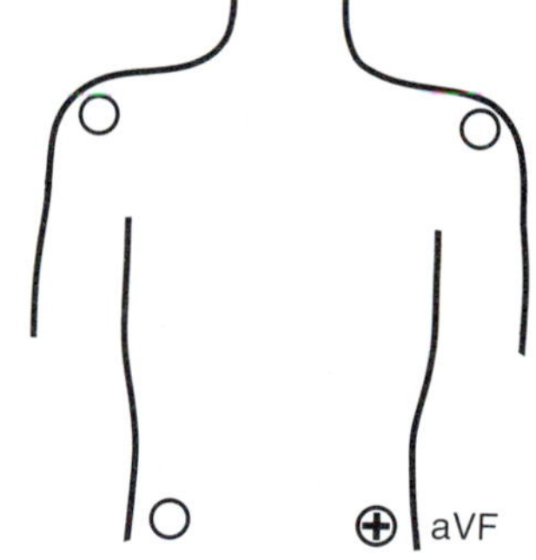

FIGURE 3-71 Lead aVF.

ECG

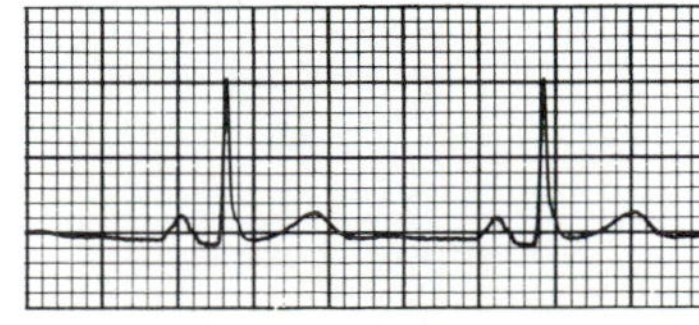

Lead aVF

Lead aVF is also known by the following names:

Augmented Limb Lead
Frontal Plane Unipolar Lead
Inferior Lead

Anatomic Landmarks

Four electrodes must be attached to body. The monitor must have aVR, aVL, and aVF capability. Place the RA electrode on right shoulder, the LA electrode on left shoulder, the LL electrode on the lower left abdomen, and the RL may go anywhere. When lead selector is turned to aVF, the LL electrode is positive. The negative pole is not on the body surface; it is equidistant between the RA and LA electrodes.

Features

- Upright P and QRS.
- Simultaneous monitoring of three leads often includes aVF.

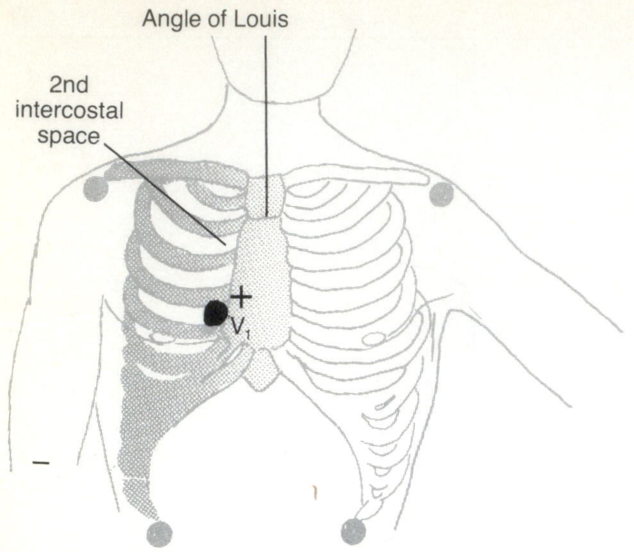

FIGURE 3-72 Lead V_1.

ECG

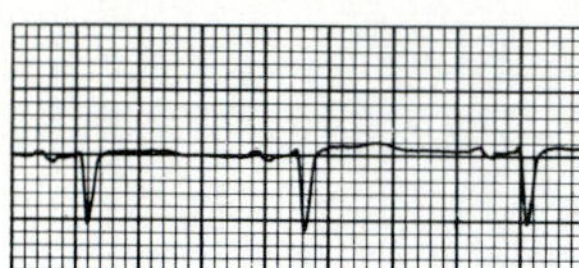

Lead V_1

Lead V_1 is also known by the following names:

Precordial, Horizontal, or Chest Lead
Anterior Lead
Septal Lead
True Posterior (Indirect) Lead

Anatomic Landmarks

To monitor any of the V leads, a 5-electrode system is required.

+ The V or C (chest) electrode is placed in the fourth intercostal space, right sternal border. Other electrodes placed as for augmented leads.

Features

- P wave may be positive or inverted, but is usually biphasic with positive deflection first. Retrograde atrial depolarization exhibits an initially negative biphasic P wave.
- P waves distinct. Excellent for analyzing atrial activity, including atrial flutter waves.
- QRS has initial r wave, deep S, resulting in a predominantly negative complex.
- Best lead for differentiating bundle branch blocks.
- Excellent lead for differentiating ventricular ectopy from aberration.
- Good lead for checking placement of right ventricular pacing catheter.
- Simultaneous recordings of three leads often include V_1.

Lead V_2

Lead V_2 is also known by the following names:

Precordial, Horizontal, or Chest Lead
Anterior Lead
Septal Lead
True Posterior (Indirect) Lead

Anatomic Landmarks

To monitor any of the V leads, a 5-electrode system is required.

+ The V or C (chest) electrode is place in the fourth intercostal space, left sternal border. Other electrodes placed as for augmented leads.

Features

- Not a common monitoring lead.
- Interferes with auscultation and external cardiac massage.
- P waves are upright or inverted.
- QRS has initial r wave, S wave is present but may not be as deep as in V_1. QRS is usually predominantly negative.
- Good for measuring QT interval.
- Good for identifying U wave, when present.

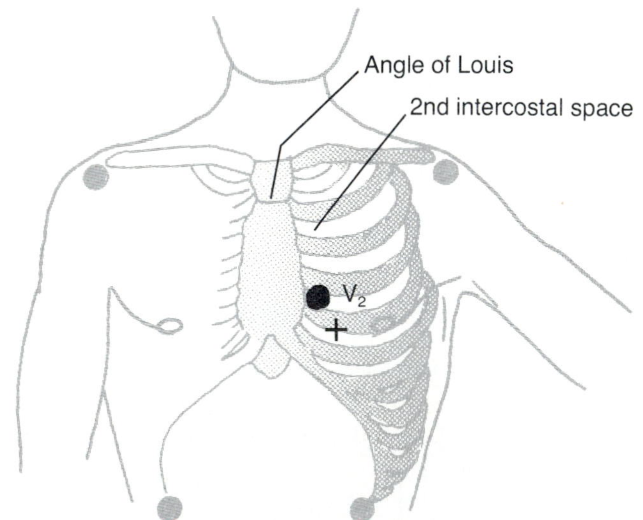

FIGURE 3-73 Lead V_2.

ECG

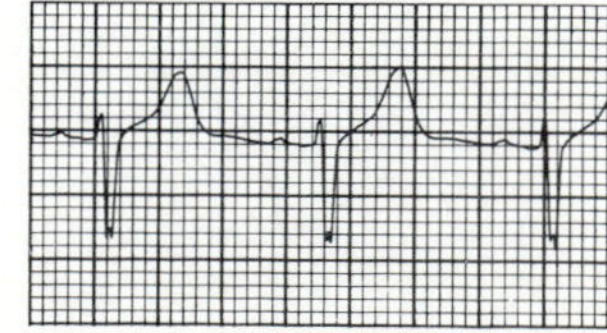

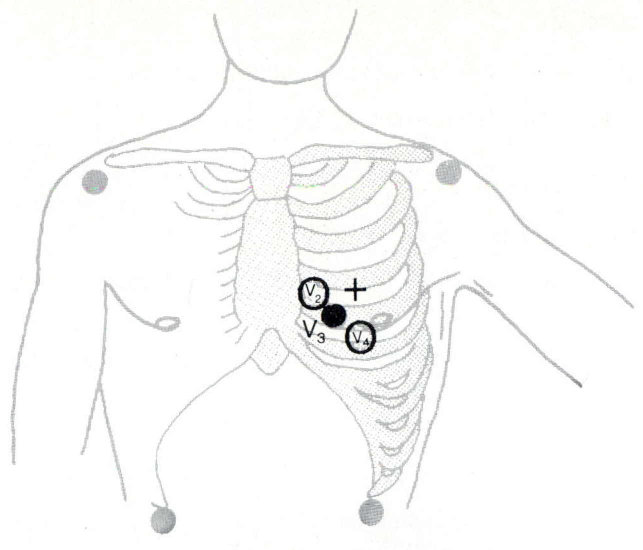

FIGURE 3-74 Lead V_3.

ECG

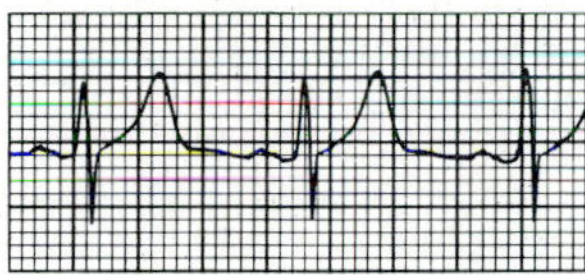

Lead V_3

Lead V_3 is also known by the following names:

Precordial, Horizontal, or Chest Lead
Anterior Lead
Septal Lead

Anatomic Landmarks

To monitor any of the V leads, a 5-electrode system is required.

+ The V or C (chest) electrode is placed equidistant between V_4 and V_2. (This means placing V_4 first.) Other electrodes placed as for augmented leads.

Features

- P wave usually upright.
- QRS may begin its transition in this lead and is often equiphasic.
- Useful for monitoring unstable angina patients.
- Good for measuring QT interval.
- Good for identifying U wave, when present.

Lead V_4

Lead V_4 is also known by the following names:

Precordial, Horizontal, or Chest Lead
Anterior Lead

Anatomic Landmarks

To monitor any of the V leads, a 5-electrode system is required.

+ The V or C (chest) electrode is placed in the fifth intercostal space, left midclavicular line (MCL). Other electrodes placed as for augmented leads.

Features

- P wave usually upright.
- QRS usually upright.
- Not a common monitoring lead for same reasons as V_2, V_3.

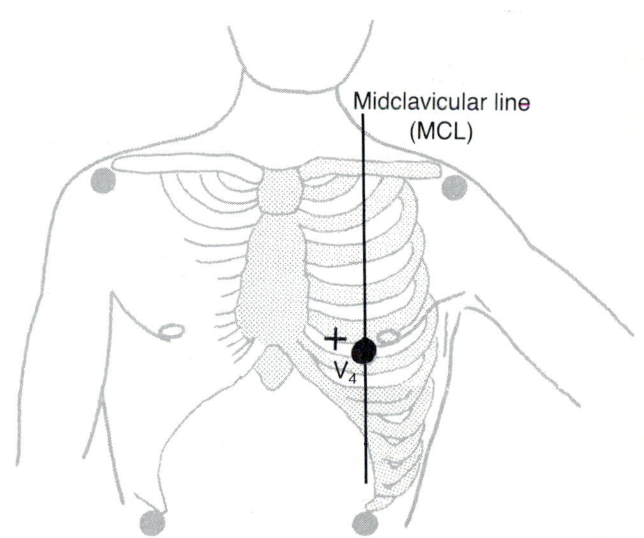

FIGURE 3-75 Lead V_4.

ECG

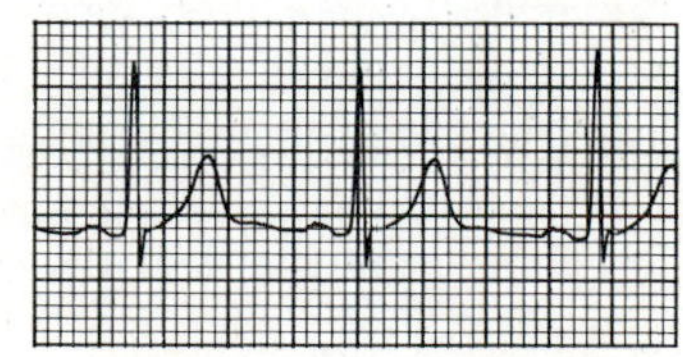

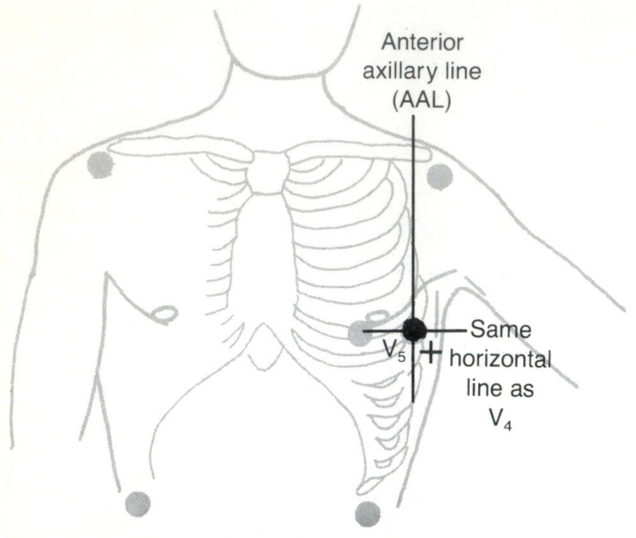

FIGURE 3-76 Lead V_5.

Lead V_5

Lead V_5 is also known by the following names:

Precordial, Horizontal, or Chest Lead
Anterior Lead
Lateral Lead

Anatomic Landmarks

To monitor any of the V leads, a 5-electrode system is required.

+ The V or C (chest) electrode is placed in the anterior axillary line (AAL), same horizontal line as V_4. Other electrodes placed as for augmented leads.

Features

- P wave usually upright.
- QRS at maximum positivity.
- Not a common monitoring lead for same reasons as V_2, V_3, V_4.
- Popular lead for monitoring exercising patients.
- Simultaneous recordings of three leads often includes V_5.

ECG

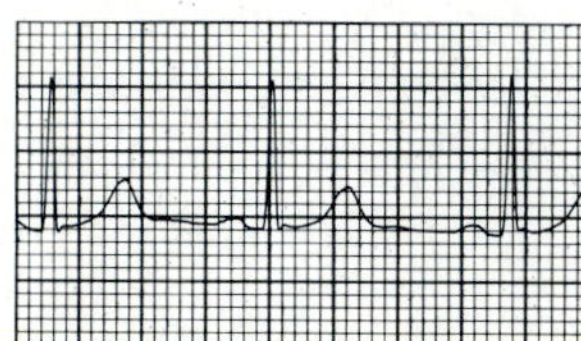

Lead V_6

Lead V_6 is also known by the following names:

Precordial, Horizontal, or Chest Lead
Lateral Lead

Anatomic Landmarks

To monitor any of the V leads, a 5-electrode system is required.

+ The V or C (chest) electrode is placed in the mid axillary line (MAL), same horizontal line as V_4. Other electrodes placed as for augmented leads.

Features

- P wave upright.
- QRS upright with an initial q wave resulting from septal depolarization.
- Common monitoring lead.
- Good for differentiating bundle branch blocks.
- Interferes with countershock.
- Good for differentiating ventricular ectopy from aberration.
- Good for observing right ventricular pacemaker complexes.

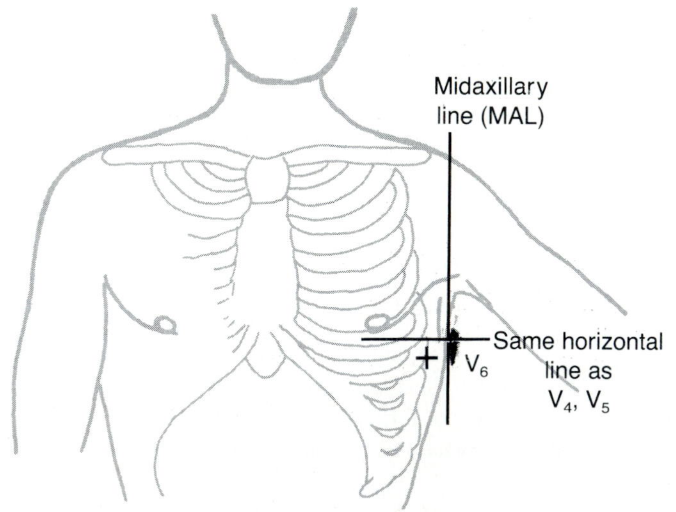

FIGURE 3-77 Lead V_6.

ECG

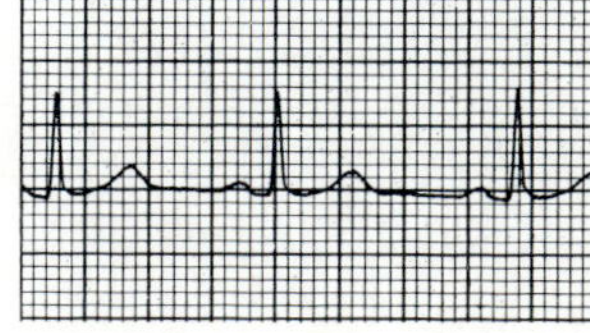

MCL_1 and MCL_6 Leads

The MCL leads introduced by Marriott[4] have evolved into popular choices for continuous monitoring leads using only three electrodes. The symbol *MCL* represents *m*odified—*c*hest (where the positive electrode of a three-lead system is placed)—L (for *l*eft arm, where the negative electrode is placed). These leads enable one to closely approximate the pattern of the V leads. Although all the V leads may be modified in such a fashion, V_1 and V_6 are the most common (Fig. 3-78). The electrocardiographic features and indications of MCL_1 and MCL_6 are the same as for V_1 and V_6 respectively.

If the monitor does not have a lead selector switch, it has been preset to monitor lead I or lead II. It is necessary to find what lead the monitor is preset for before placing the positive and negative electrodes. For example, if the monitor is preset on lead II (which many are), then the RA electrode is negative and the LL electrode is positive. Place the LL electrode (+) in either the V_1 or V_6 position and the RA electrode on the left clavicle. Remember if the monitor is a 5-electrode system there is no need to monitor the MCL leads because V_1 and V_6 are available. See the box below.

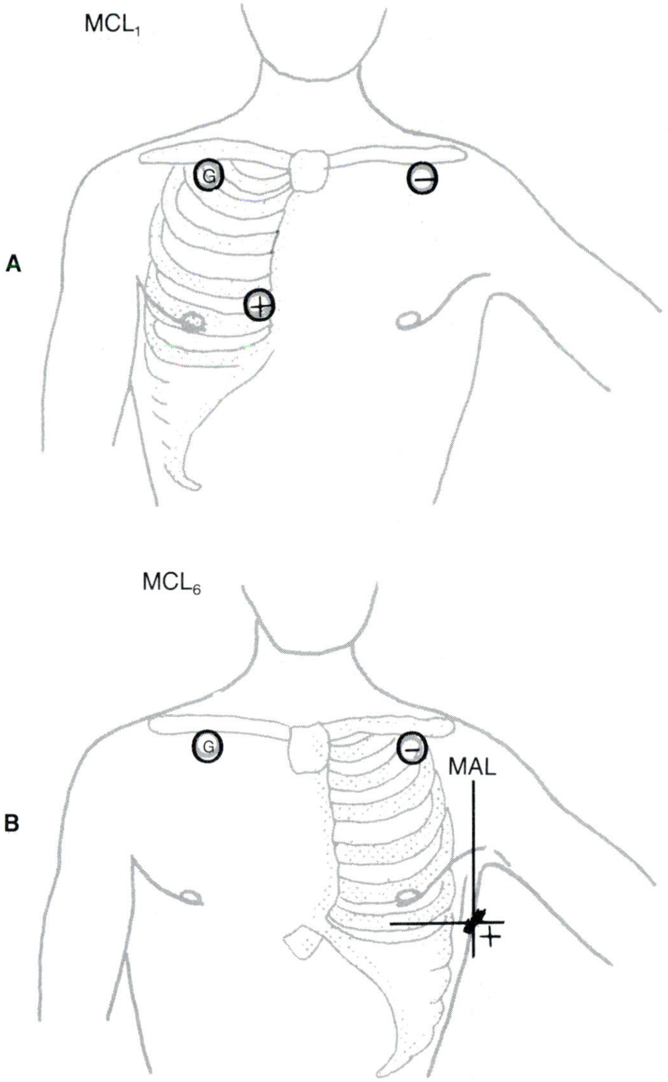

FIGURE 3-78 **A,** MCL_1 landmarks: + Fourth intercostal space, right sternal border (same as V_1)
– Left arm
G Anywhere
B, MCL_6 landmarks: + Mid-axillary line (MAL), same horizontal line as V_4 (same as V_6)
– Left arm
G Anywhere

Summary of Points to Consider in Selecting the Appropriate Monitoring Lead

- Use shoulders and upper arms when possible, keeping the chest clear of electrodes for the following reasons:
  - More closely mimics a real ECG.
  - Chest is clear for defibrillation.
  - Artifact is reduced during CPR.
- **No single lead is ideal for every patient and seldom is a single lead enough for one patient.**
  The choice of lead depends on the following variables:
  - **Arrhythmias.** Monitor on a lead that gives maximum information about the arrhythmia being monitored, (e.g., a patient with premature wide QRSs would best be monitored on V_1 or MCL_1 and V_6 or MCL_6). Use the lead selector switch to obtain as many different "views" of an arrhythmia as necessary.
  - **Age.** QRS axis shifts from right in infancy to left in old age.
  - **Obesity and emaciation.** Obesity may cause low amplitude, misplacement of V leads. Emaciation may make precordial electrode placement difficult.
  - **Thick chest wall.** Often causes low amplitude in frontal plane leads.
  - **Emphysema.** Results in low amplitude and muscle artifact from dyspnea. Do not place electrodes over accessory muscles used for breathing.
  - **Chamber hypertrophy.** Often results in axis shifts.
  - **Cardiac diagnosis.** Ischemia, location of MI, detection of axis shifts require multiple lead evaluation.
  - **Anxiety and restlessness.** Avoid placing electrodes on limbs.
  - **Pacemakers.** Right ventricular placement can usually be verified on leads V_1 and V_6.
  - **Exercise.** Use V_5 or CM_5 in exercise/cardiac rehabilitation to reveal global left ventricular ischemia with J-point and ST-segment depression.

Simultaneous Multiple Leads

In the past, only one ECG lead was continuously displayed and processed. Recent recommendations[34] are to display and analyze at least two and preferably three or more leads. Multilead monitoring permits evaluation of the same PQRST cycle in multiple leads, allows more precise detection and localization of ST-segment shifts, and guards against loss of data from single-channel malfunction.

Other Leads

Telemetry

Telemetry systems are designed for use with two to five electrodes. The two-electrode systems do not require a separate ground electrode. Telemetry units adaptable to the bedside unit have three or more electrodes. The criteria for lead selection are the same as for bedside monitoring.

CM_5 and CC_5

V_5 is the best lead for detecting and monitoring left ventricular (LV) myocardial ischemia, regardless of the site of the coronary artery narrowing. Activity-related myocardial ischemia produces global LV ischemia that is best detected in the lead with the tallest R wave, most often V_5. Therefore it is the lead of choice during inpatient or outpatient cardiac rehabilitation exercise. When it is not possible to obtain a V_5, CM_5 gives a close approximation. The negative electrode is placed on the manubrium and the positive in the V_5 position (Fig. 3-79). CC_5 is another modification of V_5 for detecting left ventricular ischemia. The positive electrode is placed in the V_5 position and the negative electrode is similarly positioned on the right thorax.

Holter

Holter monitors use single, dual, or multiple channel recorders. The single channel recorder is limited to one lead, and lead II is the most popular choice. Dual channel units record two leads simultaneously, and may use four or five electrodes. Dual channels are useful for analysis of arrhythmias and ischemia and for comparative purposes. Moreover, if one lead is lost, one remains. Combination leads include II and MCL_1, and C1 and C5 (similar to V_1 and V_5). Other useful Holter leads are III, CM1 (a modified V_1), CM2 (a modified V_2), and CM5 (a modified V_5)[35] (Fig. 3-80).

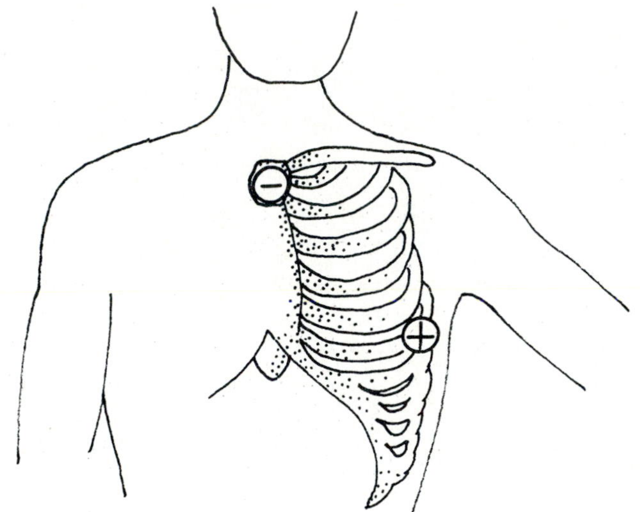

FIGURE 3-79 CM_5 lead

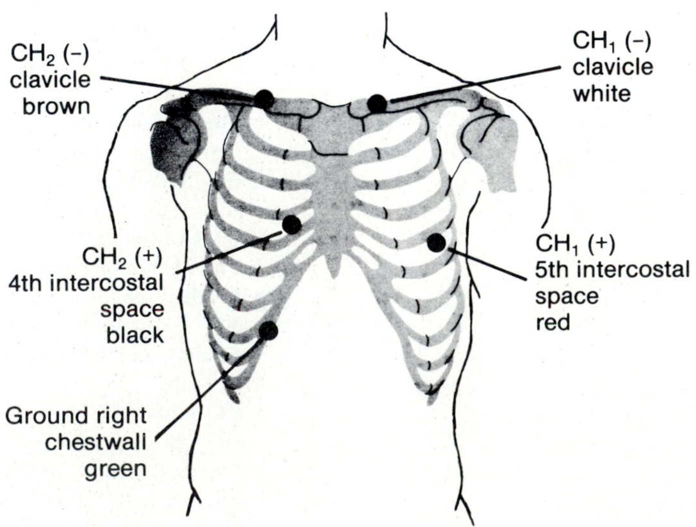

FIGURE 3-80 Example lead placement for Holter recordings. Cardio Data Systems.

The Lewis Lead

A special bipolar chest lead, the Lewis lead[1] is valuable in amplifying the P waves and thereby clarifying the mechanism of an atrial arrhythmia. The two landmarks are the second intercostal space, right sternal border (RSB) and the fourth intercostal space, RSB; the polarity can be interchanged (Fig. 3-81).

The Esophageal Lead

With the advent of clinical cardiac electrophysiology, the use of esophageal leads has lost some of its earlier appeal. It is indicated in the evaluation of supraventricular tachycardias when P waves are obscured.[36] A "pill" electrode attached to an exploring unipolar lead (a V lead) is swallowed until it descends to the level of the atrium. Because the electrode is behind and in close proximity to the left atrium, P waves appear very large.

The S_5 Lead

Another lead that shows P waves well is the S_5 lead. It too is useful in locating P waves obscured by fast ventricular rates. The positive electrode is placed in the fifth intercostal space, RSB, and the negative electrode over the manubrium (Fig. 3-82).

The Right Precordial Leads

Unipolar leads are placed on the right side of the chest in the same locations used for the V leads on the left side of the chest in an effort to gain greater electrocardiographic information about right ventricular disorders, some pediatric arrhythmias, atrial arrhythmias, and congenital heart anomalies (Fig. 3-83).

The diagnosis of right ventricular MI complicating inferior or posterior MI or, less frequently, right ventricular MI occurring in isolation, is aided with the right precordial leads.[37]

The Posterior Leads

Posterior leads V_7 to V_{14} extend from the posterior axillary line on the left to the back. These leads are akin to the anterior V leads and are useful visualizing the posterior aspect of the heart (Fig. 3-84).

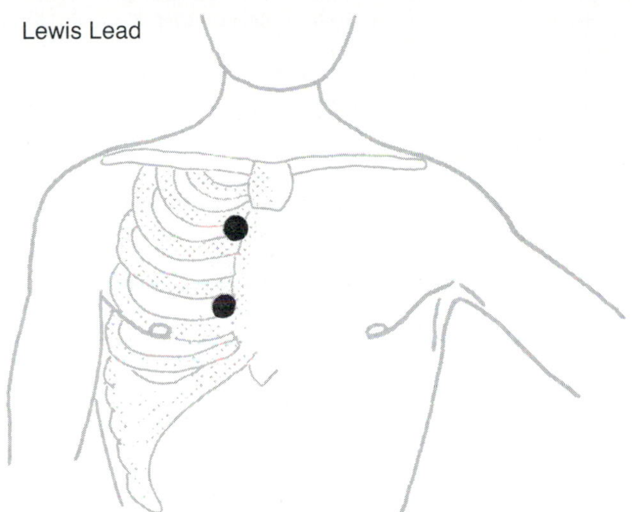

FIGURE 3-81 Lewis lead.

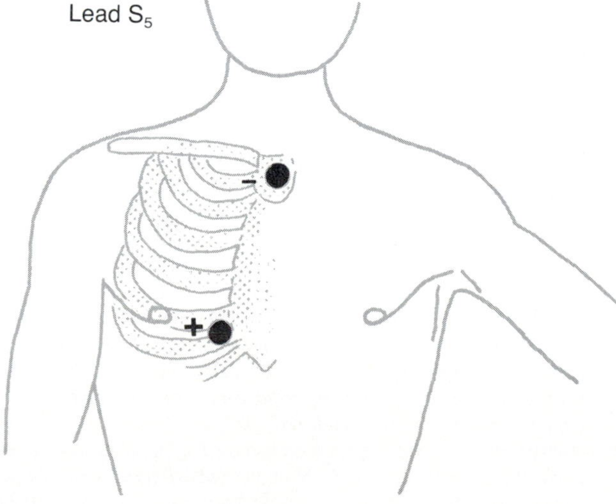

FIGURE 3-82 S_5 lead.

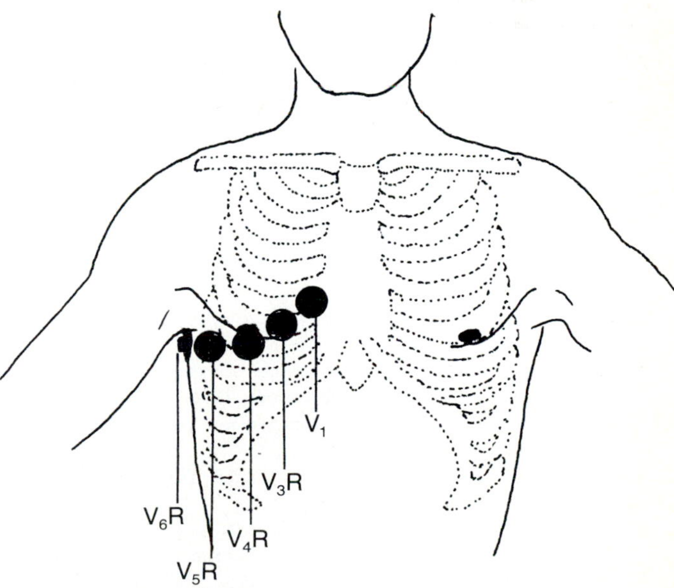

FIGURE 3-83 Right precordial leads. Four additional chest leads course around the right side of the chest in the same anatomic locations as their left counterparts. Lead V_{3R} is equidistant between V_1 (or V_{2R}) and V_{4R}. Lead V_{4R} is in the fifth intercostal space, midclavicular line. V_{5R} is on the same horizontal line as V_{4R} in the anterior axillary line. V_{6R} is in the midaxillary line on the same horizontal line as V_{4R} and V_{5R}.

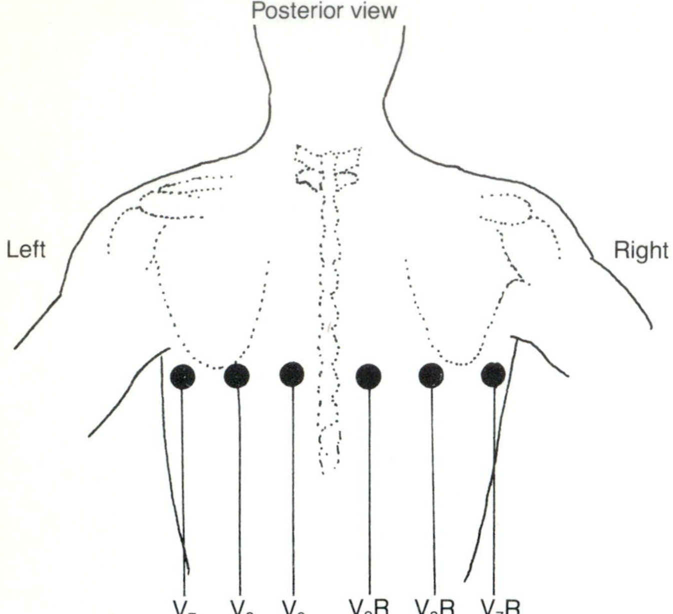

FIGURE 3-84 The posterior precordial leads. These leads are all on the same horizontal line as V_4 to V_6. Leads V_7 and V_{7R} are in the posterior axillary lines. Leads V_8 and V_{8R} are midway between the seventh and ninth electrodes. Leads V_9 and V_{9R} are on the left and right spinal borders.

REFERENCES

1. Goldman MJ. *Clinical Electrocardiography*. 12th ed. Los Altos, CA: Lange Medical Publications, 1986.
2. Donnerstein RL, Scott WA, Lloyd TR. Spontaneous beat-to-beat variation of PR interval in normal children. *Am. J. Cardio.*, Sept., 1990, 66: 753-4.
3. Akhtar M. Electrophysiologic bases for wide QRS complex tachycardia. *PACE*, Jan/Feb., 1983, 6: 83-97.
4. Marriott HJL. *Practical Electrocardiography*. 8th ed. Baltimore: Williams & Wilkins, 1988.
5. Cohen M, Hawkins L, Greenberg S, Fuster V. Usefulness of ST-segment changes in ≥ 2 leads on the emergency room electrocardiogram in either unstable angina pectoris or non-Q-wave myocardial infarction in predicting outcome. *Am. J. Cardiol.*, Jun., 1991, 67: 1368-73.
6. Vinsant MO, Spence MI. *A Commonsense Approach to Coronary Care*. 5th ed. St. Louis: The CV Mosby Co., 1989.
7. Schamroth L. *The Disorders of Cardiac Rhythm*. Vol. I, 2nd ed. London: Blackwell Scientific Publications, 1981.
8. Goldberger AL. Hyperacute T waves revisited. *Am. Heart J.*, Oct., 1982, 104(4): part I, 888-90.
9. Propp DA, Maloney W. Post tachycardia T-wave changes. *J. Emerg. Med.*, Jul/Aug., 1990, 8(4): 463-6.
10. Cowan JC, Yusoff K, Moore M, Amos PA, Gold AE, Bourke JP, Tansuphaswadikul S, Campbell RWF. Importance of lead selection in QT interval measurement. *Am. J. Cardiol.*, 1988, 61: 83-7.
11. Ahnve S. Correction of the QT interval for heart rate: review of different formulas and the use of Bazett's formula in myocardial infarction. *Am. Heart J.*, Mar., 1985, 109(3, part 1): 568-73.
12. Benhorin J, Merri M, Alberti M, Locati E, Moss AJ, Hall WJ, Cui L. Long QT syndrome. *Circ.*, Aug., 1990, 82(2): 521-7.
13. Morganroth J, Brozovich FV, McDonald JT, Jacobs RA. Variability of the QT measurement in healthy men, with implications for selection of an abnormal QT value to predict drug toxicity and proarrhythmia. *Am. J. Cardiol.*, Apr., 1991, 67: 774-6.
14. Ahnve S, Erhardt L, Lundman T, Rehnqvist N, Sjogren A. Effect of metoprolol on QTc intervals after acute myocardial infarction. *Acta Med. Scand.*, 1980, 208(3): 223-8.
15. Hersch C. Electrocardiographic changes in subarachnoid haemorrhage, meningitis and intracranial space-occupying lesions. *Br. Heart J.*, 1964, 26: 785-93.
16. Johnson CT, Cowan M. Relationship between prolonged QTc interval and ventricular fibrillation. *Heart & Lung*, Mar., 1986, 15(2): 141-50.
17. Burch GE, Meyers R, Abildskov JA. A new electrocardiographic pattern observed in cerebrovascular accidents. *Circ.*, May, 1954, 9: 719-23.
18. Reynolds EW, Vander Ark CR. Quinidine syncope and the delayed repolarization syndromes. *Mod. Concepts Cardiovasc. Dis.*, Aug., 1976, XLV(8): 117-22.
19. Vincent GM, Abildskov JA, Burgess MJ. Q-T interval syndromes. *Prog. Cardiovasc. Dis.*, May/Jun., 1974, 16(6): 523-34.
20. Chambers JB, Sampson MJ, Springings DC, Jackson G. QT prolongation on the electrocardiogram in diabetic autonomic neuropathy. *Diabetic Med.*, Feb., 1990, 7(2): 105-10.
21. Perticone F, Ceravalo R, Mattioli P. Prolonged QT interval: A marker of sudden infant death syndrome? *Clin. Cardiol.*, May, 1991, 14: 417-21.
22. Ahnve S, Lundman T. Shoaleh-var M. The relationship between QT interval and ventricular arrhythmias in acute myocardial infarction. *Acta Med. Scand.*, 1978, 204: 17-9.
23. Gorlin RJ, Sedano H. Profound childhood deafness with ECG abnormalities, fainting spells, and sudden death (Jervell and Lange-Nielsen's syndrome, cardio-auditory syndrome, surdo-cardiac syndrome). *Mod. Med.*, Dec. 14, 1970, pp. 138-9.
24. Khan MM, Logan KR, McComb JM, Adgey AAJ. Management of recurrent ventricular tachyarrhythmias associated with Q-T prolongation. *Am. J. Cardiol.*, Jun., 1981, 47: 1301.
25. Schwartz PJ, Periti M, Malliani A. The long Q-T syndrome. *Am. Heart. J.*, Mar., 1975, 89(3): 378-90.
26. Alexopoulos D, Rynkiewicz A, Yusuf S, Johnston J, Sleight P, Yacoub MH. Diurnal variations of QT interval after cardiac transplantation. *Am. J. Cardiol.*, Feb., 1988, 61: 482-5.
27. Laks MM. Long QT interval syndrome. *Circ.*, Oct., 1990, 82(4): 1539-41.
28. Goldberg RJ, Bengtson J, Chen Z, Anderson KM, Locati E, Levy D. Duration of the QT interval and cardiovascular mortality in healthy persons (the Framingham Heart Study experience). *Am. J. Cardiol.*, Jan., 1991, 67: 55-8.
29. Surawicz B, Lasseter KC. Effect of drugs on the electrocardiogram. *Prog. Cardiovasc. Dis.*, Jul., 1970, 13(1): 26-55.
30. Christy JH, Clements SD. Endocrine and metabolic disorders. *In* Hurst JW (ed). *The Heart: Arteries and Veins*. 4th ed. New York: McGraw-Hill, 1978.
31. Horan LG, Flowers NC. Electrocardiography and vectorcardiography. *In* Braunwald E (ed). *Heart Disease; A Textbook of Cardiovascular Medicine*. Philadelphia: WB Saunders, 1980.
32. Jensen JT. *Physics for the Health Profession*. 3rd ed. New York: John Wiley & Sons, 1982.
33. Winsor T. The electrocardiogram in myocardial infarction. *CIBA Clin. Symp.*, 1968, 20(4): 107-33.
34. Mirvis DM, Berson AS, Goldberger AL, Green LS, Heger JJ, Hinohara T, Insel J, Krucoff MW, Moncrief A, Selvester RH, Wagner GS. Instrumentation and practice standards for electrocardiographic monitoring in special care units. *Circ.*, Feb., 1989, 79(2): 464-71.
35. Horner SL. *Ambulatory Electrocardiography: Application and Techniques*. Philadelphia: JB Lippincott, 1983.
36. Arzbaecher R. Long term esophageal recording in the analysis of supraventricular arrhythmias. *In* Stott FD (ed). *International Symposium on Ambulatory Monitoring*. New York: Academic Press, 1982.
37. McMillan JY, Little-Longeway CD. Right ventricular infarction. *Focus Crit Care*. Apr., 1991, 18(2): 158-63.

SELF-ASSESSMENT

MULTIPLE CHOICE

Directions

For each of the questions below, select the correct answer(s) from the choices given. If more than one correct answer is given, mark all that are correct.

Example

The leads comprising the standard ECG are leads
 a. 1, 2, 3, 4, 5, 6, 7, 8, 9, 10, 11, and 12.
*b. I, II, III, aVR, aVL, and aVF.
 c. A, B, C, D, E, and F.
*d. V_1, V_2, V_3, V_4, V_5, and V_6.

An ECG is a diagnostic test to
*a. assess the heart's electrical activity.
 b. measure the strength of the heart's contraction.
 c. assess the patency of the coronary arteries.
 d. determine the competency of the heart's valves.

1. Standard speed for an ECG is
   a. 10 mm/sec.
   b. 25 mm/sec.
   c. 50 mm/sec.
   d. 100 mm/sec.

2. An appropriate method for determining rate of an irregular rhythm is
   a. the box method.
   b. the division method.
   c. the 6-second strip.
   d. counting the rate for a full minute.
   e. reading the digital display on the monitor.

3. On the ECG, atrial depolarization is represented by the
   a. A wave.
   b. P wave.
   c. PR interval.
   d. Ta wave.

4. The normal value for the PR interval is
   a. less than 0.11 seconds.
   b. 0.06 to 0.10 seconds.
   c. 0.12 to 0.20 seconds.
   d. 0.16 to 0.26 seconds.

5. A PR interval that is abnormally long represents delay in
   a. atrial depolarization.
   b. AV junctional conduction.
   c. atrial and ventricular depolarization.
   d. atrial repolarization.

6. The QRS complex represents
   a. depolarization of the atrial myocardium.
   b. repolarization of the atria.
   c. depolarization of the ventricles.
   d. repolarization of the ventricles.

7. The duration of the QRS complex normally measures
   a. 0.10 seconds or less.
   b. 0.10 to 0.16 seconds.
   c. 0.12 to 0.20 seconds.
   d. 0.16 to 0.24 seconds.

8. The ST segment is normally
   a. isoelectric.
   b. elevated.
   c. depressed.
   d. diphasic.

9. Ventricular aneurysm, myocardial injury, left bundle branch block, and pericarditis produce what kind of shift in the ST segment?
   a. Elevation of the ST segment.
   b. Horizontality of the ST segment.
   c. Depression of the ST segment.
   d. An ST segment that is isoelectric or diphasic.

10. The total time required for ventricular depolarization and repolarization is represented on the ECG by the
    a. PR interval.
    b. QRS complex.
    c. ST segment.
    d. QT interval.

11. The leads of the horizontal plane are
    a. the V leads.
    b. I, II, III, V_1, V_2, V_3.
    c. I, II, III, aVR, aVL, aVF.
    d. aVR, aVL, aVF, MCL_1, MCL_6.

12. The hexaxial reference system is an aid for determining
    a. electrical axis on the frontal plane.
    b. electrical axis on the horizontal plane.
    c. determining ventricular force of contraction.
    d. the calibration equivalents of the monitor.

13. Normal axis of the QRS complex is
    a. + 90 to + 180 degrees.
    b. − 90 to − 180 degrees.
    c. 0 to − 90 degrees.
    d. 0 to + 90 degrees.

14. Proper position for the V_1 electrode is
    a. third intercostal space, left midclavicular line.
    b. fifth intercostal space, right midclavicular line.
    c. fourth intercostal space, left sternal border.
    d. fourth intercostal space, right sternal border.

15. Proper electrode placement for V_6 is
    a. midaxillary line, same horizontal line as V_4.
    b. midaxillary line, fifth intercostal space.
    c. posterior axillary line, sixth intercostal space.
    d. anterior axillary line, fifth intercostal space.
    e. anterior axillary line, same horizontal line as V_4.

16. If you have a three-electrode monitor with a lead selector switch for leads I, II, and III, to monitor someone on lead MCL_1, you would put the lead selector switch on
    a. lead I and put the right arm electrode near the left clavicle and the left arm electrode in the fourth intercostal space, right sternal border.
    b. lead II and put the right arm electrode near the left clavicle and the left leg electrode in the V_1 position.
    c. lead III and put the left arm electrode near the left clavicle and the left leg electrode in the fourth intercostal space, right sternal border.
    d. lead I and put the left leg electrode on the V_1 position and the left arm electrode on the left shoulder.

17. Which one statement below is a good criterion for choosing the lead on which you will monitor your patient?
    a. It does not matter which lead is used as long as every staff member uses the same lead. Unit policy should govern which lead is used.
    b. The lead that is used should be determined by several patient variables. No single lead is ideal for every patient.
    c. The lead chosen should be one in which the QRS complex and P wave are positive. Negative complexes are confusing and difficult to interpret.
    d. Patients should be routinely monitored on lead II unless myocardial infarction has occurred. For MI patients, MCL_1 should be used.

MATCHING
Directions

Match each term or phrase in column A with its classification, definition, or synonym in column B. Choices in column B may be used more than once or not at all.

Example

A	B
(A) 1. Telemetry	A. A device used to assess heart rhythm
(A) 2. Holter	B. A telephone for nurses
(A) 3. Bedside monitor	C. An article of clothing
	D. A person who watches a patient at the bedside

A	B
( ) 18. P wave	A. Depolarization of the ventricles
( ) 19. Q wave	B. Repolarization of the ventricles
( ) 20. R wave	C. Depolarization of the atria
( ) 21. S wave	D. Repolarization of the atria
( ) 22. T wave	E. A wave that, when present, follows the T wave
( ) 23. Ta wave	F. The first positive deflection in the P wave
( ) 24. U wave	G. The first positive deflection of the QRS
( ) 25. PR interval	H. If the first deflection of the QRS is negative, it is called this
( ) 26. PR segment	I. A negative deflection in the QRS that occurs after a positive wave
( ) 27. QRS complex	J. An interval measured from the beginning of the QRS to the end of the T wave
( ) 28. QT interval	K. The interval from the end of the P wave to the beginning of the QRS complex
	L. The interval from the beginning of the P wave to the beginning of QRS

A	B
( ) 29.	A. Qr
( ) 30.	B. Qrs
( ) 31.	C. rS
( ) 32.	D. QS
( ) 33.	E. RS
( ) 34.	F. QR
( ) 35.	G. rSR′
( ) 36.	H. rSr′
( ) 37.	I. qRs
	J. R
	K. qR
	L. Rs

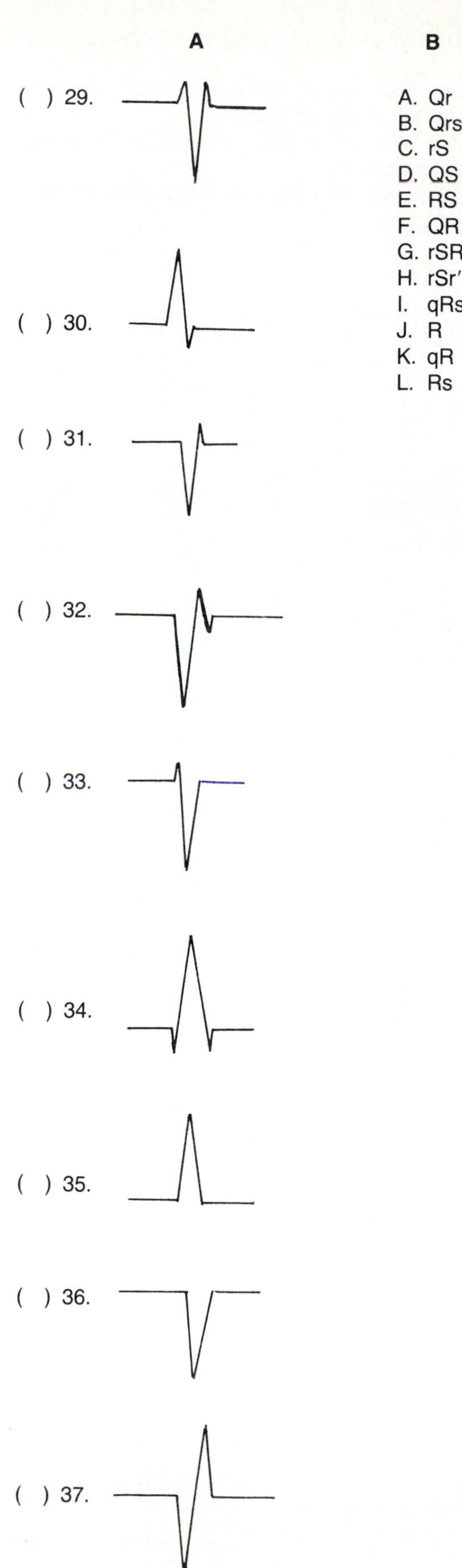

A	B
( ) 38. Left leg +, right arm −	A. I
( ) 39. Fourth intercostal space, right sternal border	B. II
( ) 40. Fifth intercostal space, midclavicular line	C. III
( ) 41. Anterior axillary line	D. aVR
( ) 42. Midaxillary line	E. aVL
( ) 43. Unipolar augmented lead on frontal plane with left arm positive	F. aVF
( ) 44. An "inferior" lead with the left leg + and left arm −	G. V_1
( ) 45. What MCL_6 mimics	H. V_2
	I. V_3
	J. V_4
	K. V_5
	L. V_6

A	B
( ) 46. Normal axis	A. 0 to −90 degrees
( ) 47. Left axis deviation	B. +90 to −90 degrees
( ) 48. Indeterminate axis	C. Also known as *superior right axis*
( ) 49. Right axis deviation	D. 0 to +90 degrees
	E. Also known as *inferior right axis*

TRUE/FALSE
Directions

Determine whether each of the following statements is true or false and indicate with a *T* or *F*.

Example

(F) 1. QRS complexes are always upright.

( ) 50. The leads of the horizontal plane are the V leads.
( ) 51. *Precordial leads* is another term for the V leads.
( ) 52. The leads of the frontal plane are the chest leads.
( ) 53. The anatomic location for the positive electrode in V_6 is the lower left thorax below the nipple.
( ) 54. ST segment elevation may be indicative of myocardial injury.
( ) 55. There is normally an inverse relationship between the heart rate and QT interval: as the rate increases, the QT interval decreases.
( ) 56. Children normally have longer PR intervals than adults.
( ) 57. Leads II, III, and aVF are known as the *inferior leads*.
( ) 58. Leads useful in assessing for septal injury are V_1 and V_2.
( ) 59. Normally in V_1 the QRS complex displays an rSR′ configuration.
( ) 60. The normal QRS in V_6 is a qR configuration.
( ) 61. If the QRS complex is positive in lead I and negative in lead aVF, the QRS axis is superior left.

The remaining questions involve analysis of patient situations and assessment of rhythm strips. Responses required are short answer and essay.

CASE: *DF is a 25-year-old female paramedic. Her 12-lead ECG is displayed here for your analysis.*

62. Analyze DF's heart rhythm using the recommended format.
63. Which method(s) of heart rate determination would be appropriate for this client's ECG?
64. What is the axis of the QRS complex in the frontal plane? Is this normal?
65. Describe any abnormalities you noted. Discuss DF's precordial pattern.

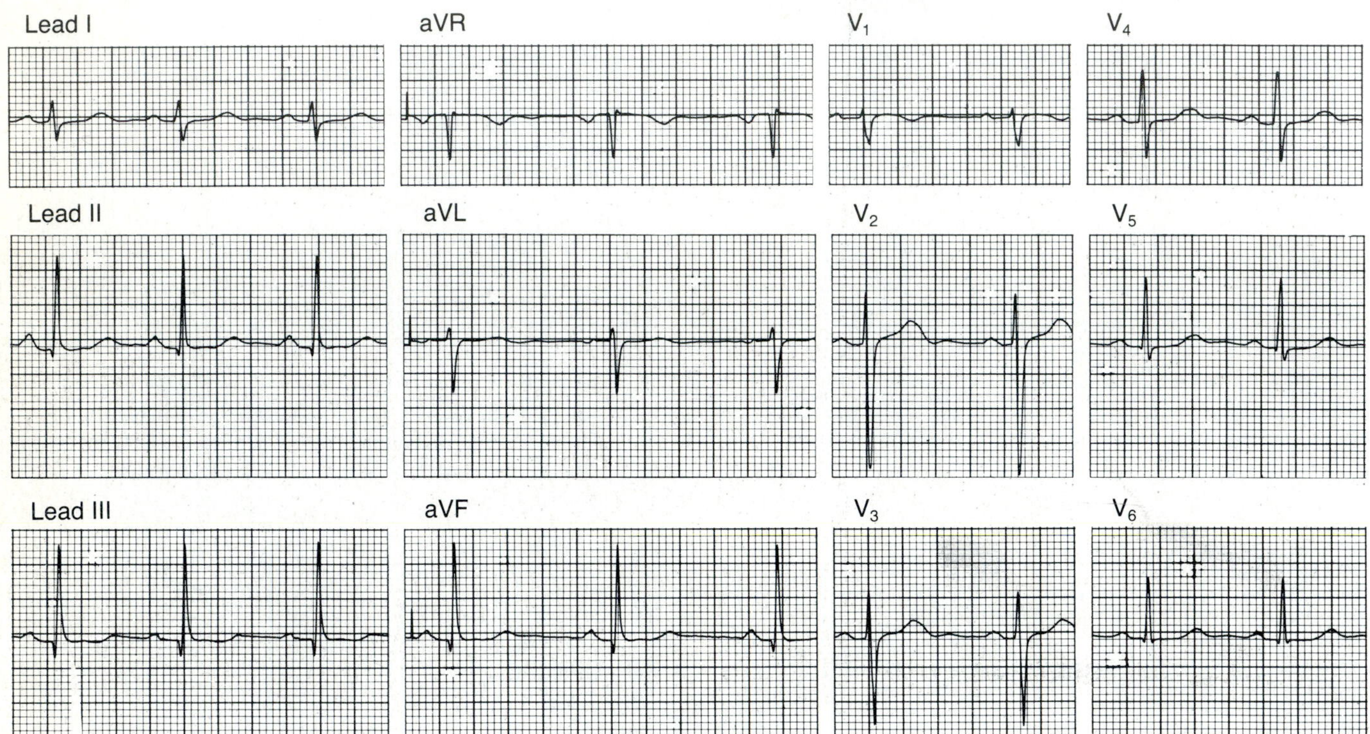

CASE: *Brian is a 6-month-old boy. His ECG is displayed here.*

66. Analyze Brian's heart rhythm and discuss any abnormal findings.
67. Determine the frontal plane axis of Brian's ECG. Is this normal?

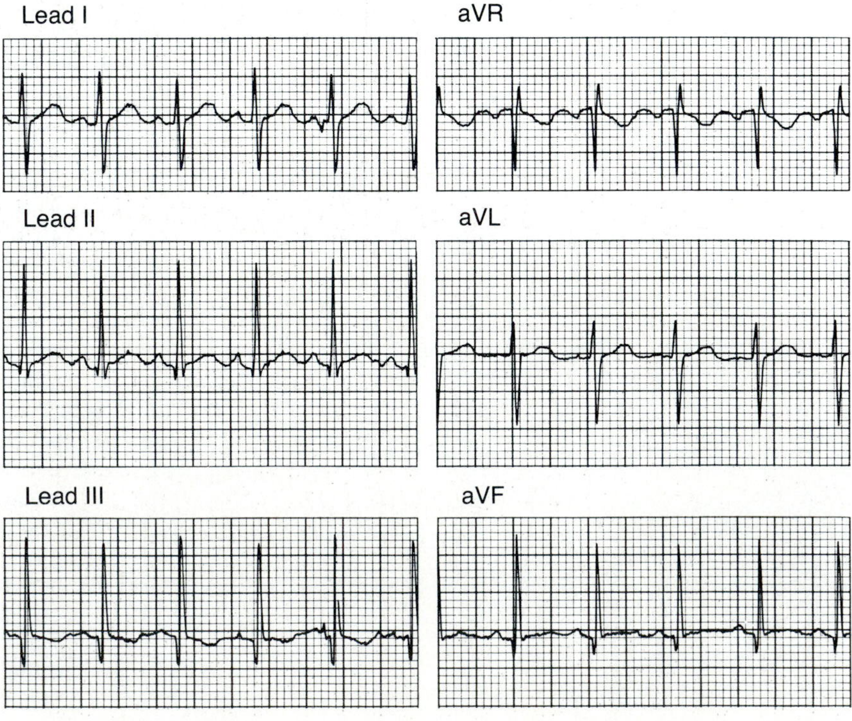

CASE: *Mrs. G is 70 years old and hospitalized with chest pain. She was on the bedside monitor with a five-lead cable so her nurse was able to obtain the six leads of the frontal plane without disturbing her sleep.*

68. Analyze the rhythm and discuss any abnormal findings.
69. What is the axis of the QRS complex?
70. Explain why the P wave and QRS complex are negative on lead aVR.

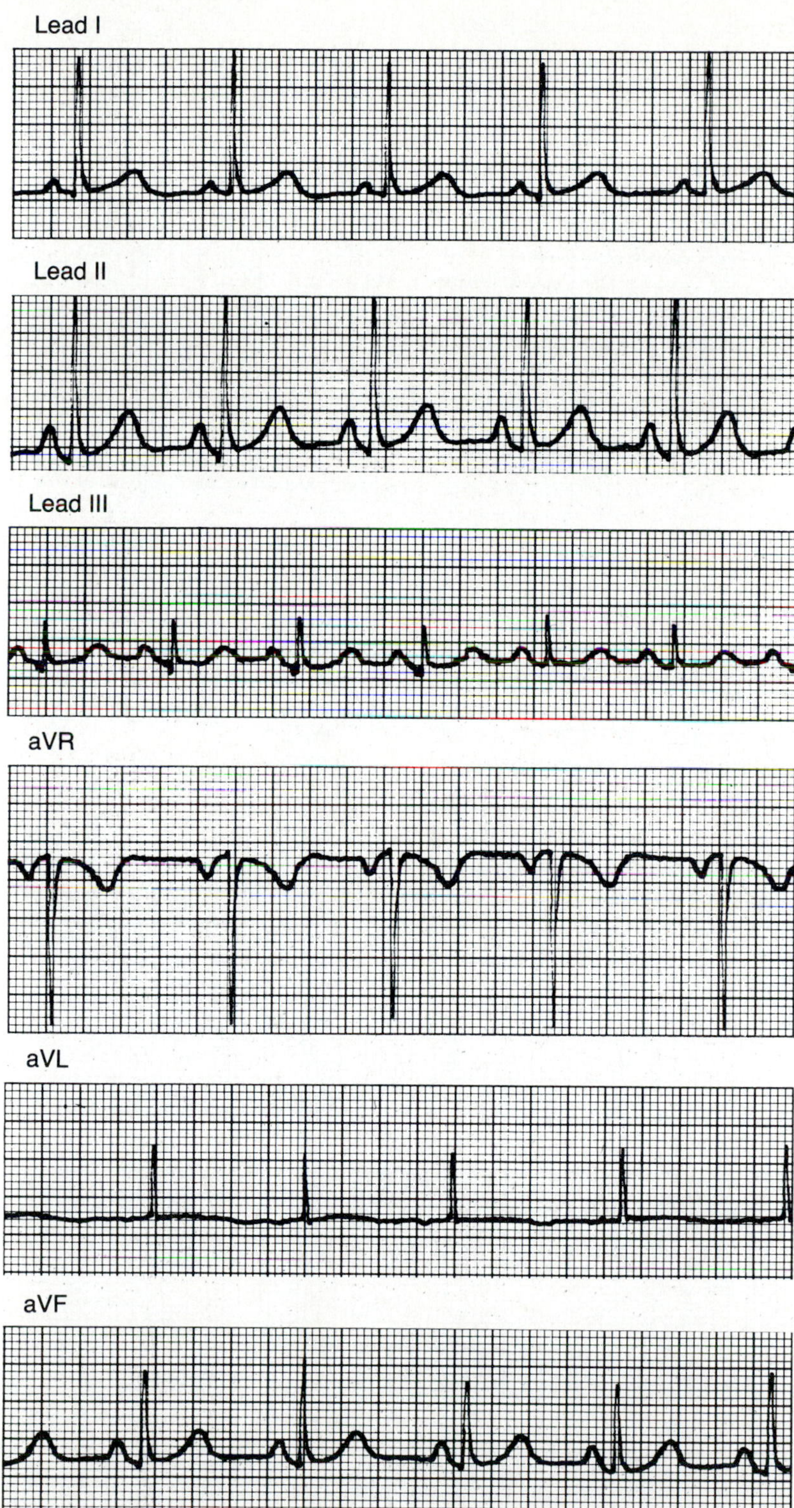

CASE: *SM, a 56-year-old man, is a patient in the coronary care unit. He was admitted for evaluation of severe anterior chest pain radiating to both arms. One of his 12-lead ECGs is presented here for your interpretation.*

71. Interpret SM's rhythm.
72. Determine the QRS axis on the frontal plane.
73. Study the precordial leads and assess the R-wave progression.
74. SM has been diagnosed as having an acute myocardial infarction. Estimate the location of the infarction by interpreting ECG signs. Explain your answer.

Lead I
aVR
V_1
V_4
Lead II
aVL
V_2
V_5
Lead III
aVF
V_3
V_6

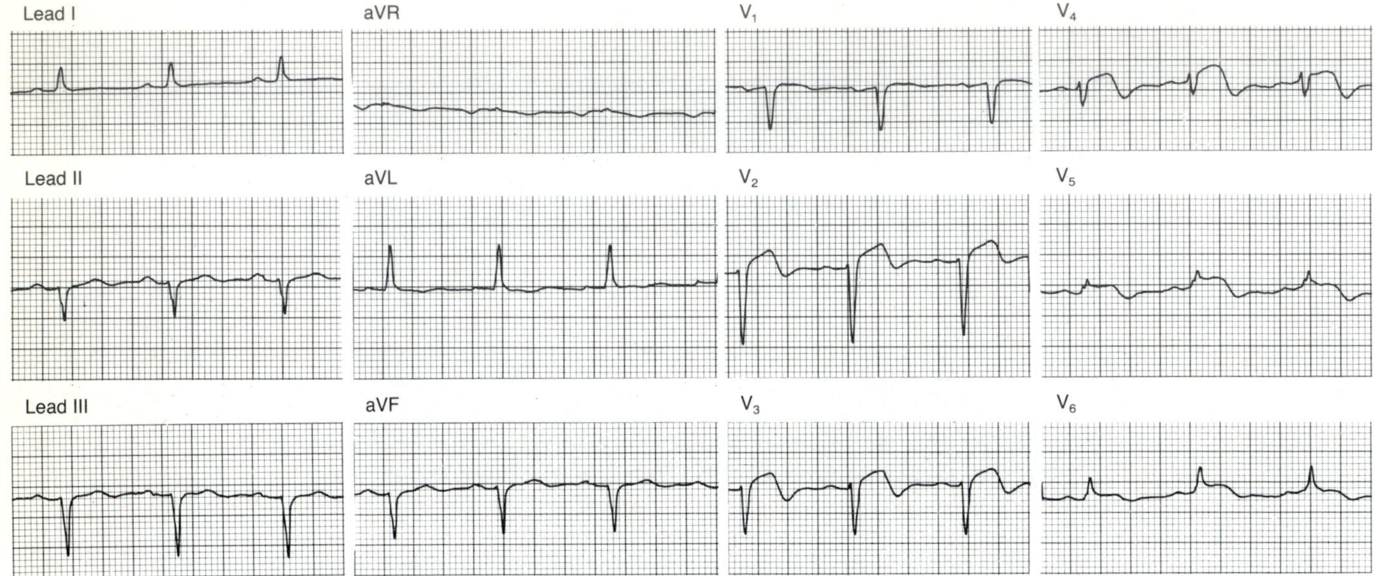

CASE: *JJ, a 42-year-old man, presented to the emergency department (ED) complaining of chest heaviness, nausea, and vomiting. He was pale and diaphoretic. The ED paramedic obtained the following vital signs: BP 108/70, AP 90 bpm, R 20. JJ's 12-lead ECG is submitted for your interpretation.*

75. Interpret JJ's rhythm.
76. Determine the QRS axis on the frontal plane.
77. Study the 12-lead ECG, offer your interpretation, and explain.

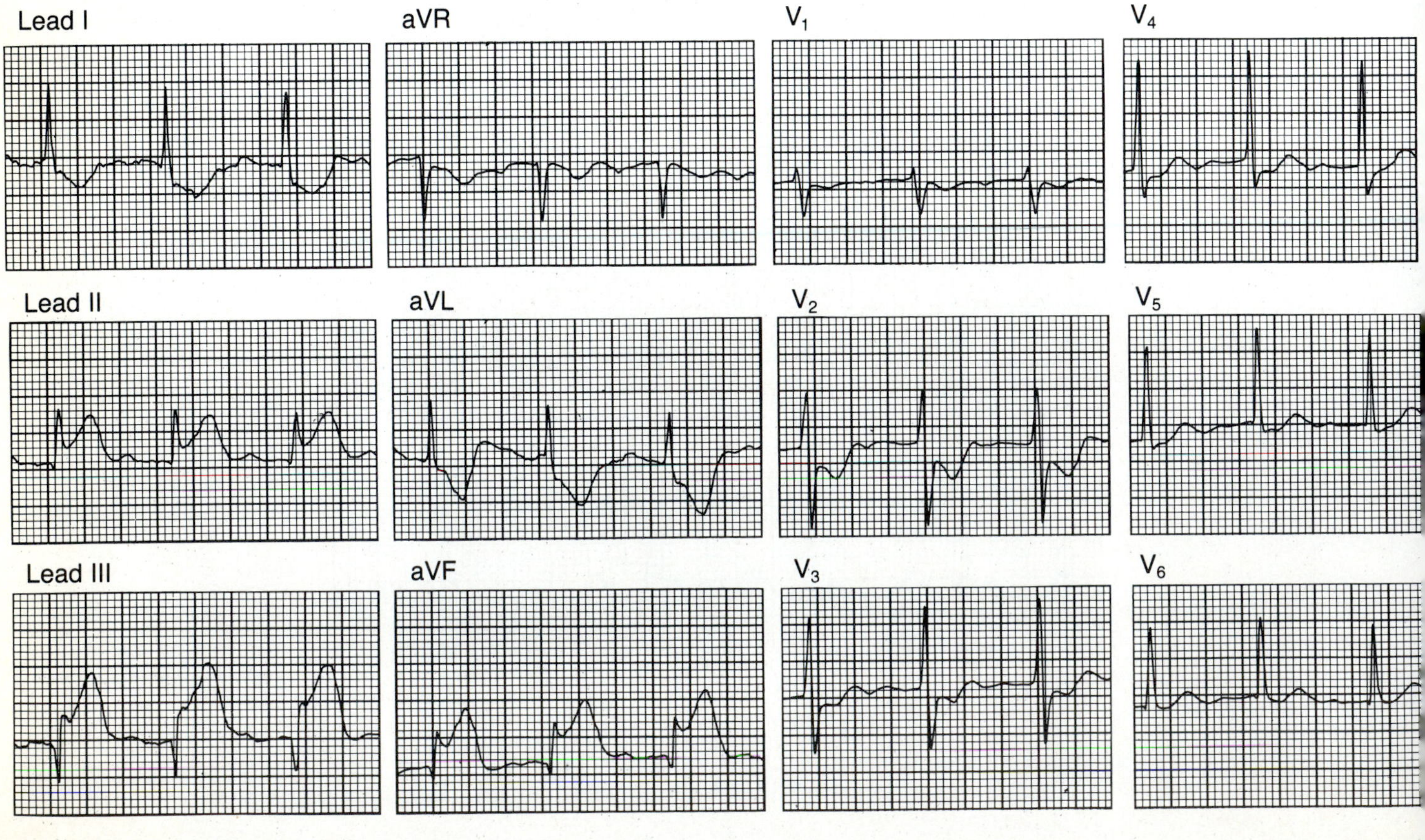

Lead I
aVR
V_1
V_4
Lead II
aVL
V_2
V_5
Lead III
aVF
V_3
V_6

ANSWERS TO SELF-ASSESSMENT

1. b	5. b	9. a	13. d
2. c, d	6. c	10. d	14. d
3. b	7. a	11. a	15. a
4. c	8. a	12. a	16. a, b, c
			17. b
18. C	22. B	26. K	
19. H	23. D	27. A	
20. G	24. E	28. J	
21. I	25. L		
29. H	32. B	35. J	
30. L	33. C	36. D	
31. A	34. I	37. F	
38. B	40. J	42. L	44. C
39. G	41. K	43. E	45. L
46. D			
47. A			
48. C			
49. E			
50. T	53. F	56. F	59. F
51. T	54. T	57. T	60. T
52. F	55. T	58. T	61. T

62. *Rate:* 66 to 75 bpm
    Notice leads I, II, III show the faster rate.
    Rhythm: Regular, based on the limited number of complexes in sequence
    P wave: Normal, one precedes each QRS complex; P wave duration 0.10 seconds, best measured, in this ECG, in lead II or aVF
    PR interval: 0.16 seconds
    QRS Complex: 0.08 seconds, normal;
    QT interval 0.40 seconds; QTc 0.42
    Interpretation: NSR

63. Either the box or division methods.
    The division method:
    For the faster rate, there are 19.5 little boxes between same points of complexes

$$\frac{1500}{19.5} = 76.9 \text{ or } 77 \text{ bpm}$$

For the slower of the two rates, there are 23 small squares between complexes

$$\frac{1500}{23} = 65.2 \text{ or } 65 \text{ bpm}$$

Remember, rate rulers like Dr. Marriott's already have the divisions figured.

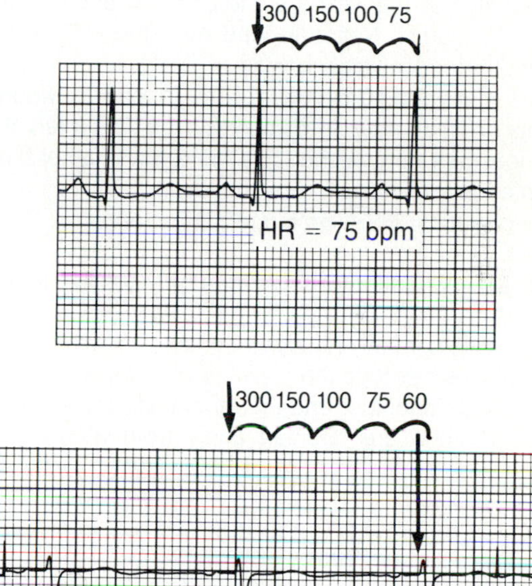

64. For figuring the axis, let us look at lead I first. In this lead the QRS is equally above and below the line, so we know that the axis is perpendicular to lead I. Is it perpendicular going up or down? Look at aVF. The QRS is positive so we know the axis is directed toward aVF's positive pole and, therefore, down. Looking at the circle of degrees, the axis would be +90 degrees, which is normal.

65. This ECG is within normal limits. The precordial pattern begins with an rS pattern in V_1, which is normal. The R wave increases as the S wave decreases, normal R-wave progression.

66. *Rate:* 136 to 150 bpm
    Rhythm: Regular
    P wave: Normal, 0.08 seconds in duration;
    Upright in II, III, aVF
    PR interval: 0.12 seconds, normal
    QRS complex: 0.07 seconds, normal;
    QT interval 0.24 to 0.26 seconds; QTc 0.40 seconds
    Interpretation: Sinus tachycardia, normal for a baby.

67. In lead I, the QRS complex is 6 to 7 mm above and 6 to 7 mm below, so it is essentially an equiphasic QRS complex and therefore perpendicular to lead I. Lead aVF is strongly positive, so the axis is about +90 degrees and normal.

68. *Rate:* 69 to 90 bpm
Rhythm: Regular
P wave: Normal
PR interval: 0.14 seconds
QRS complex: 0.08 seconds
The QRS complex is best measured on a lead that displays all the waves of the complex such as, in this ECG, lead II. Notice in lead aVL, the QRS complex appears deceivingly narrow.
QT interval 0.40 seconds. Note in lead III, where the faster heart rate is displayed, the QT interval also measures 0.40 seconds, is more than half of the R-R interval, and, thus is prolonged.
Interpretation: NSR, prolonged QT interval

69. The axis is normal (positive in lead I, positive in aVF).

70. Lead aVR normally records negative P waves and QRS complexes because the "view" is from the vantage point of the right shoulder and the atrial and ventricular mean vector forces are directed away from aVR's positive pole.

71. *Rate:* 84 to 86 bpm
Rhythm: Regular
P wave: Normal
PR interval: 0.17 seconds
QRS complex: 0.08 seconds;
QT interval 0.36 seconds
Interpretation: NSR

72. In lead I the QRS is positive, so axis is left. In lead aVF the QRS is negative, so axis is superior. Left axis deviation. It is possible to estimate the axis more accurately by looking for a QRS complex that is equiphasic or isoelectric. In this example, aVR is isoelectric. Note the negative P wave preceding the flat QRS complex. Because aVR is isoelectric, the QRS is perpendicular to the lead line of aVR (see Fig. 3-53). Looking at the diagram, this would place the axis at either +120 degrees or −60 degrees. We know the axis is in the superior left quadrant, so rule out +120 degrees. The axis is −60 degrees.

73. There is poor R-wave progression across the precordium. Note that in lead V_1, the initial r wave is not present. Very small r waves appear in V_2, V_3, V_4, and V_5. Taller R waves are expected in all of those leads.

74. The most striking sign is ST-segment elevation in leads V_2 to V_6. This sign, along with the poor R-wave progression across the precordium and the T-wave inversion in leads V_2 to V_5, further supports the diagnosis of anterolateral MI.

75. *Rate:* 94 bpm
Rhythm: Regular
P waves: Present, one precedes each QRS complex and bears constant relationship to QRS
PR interval: 0.24 seconds, prolonged
QRS complex: 0.09 seconds;
QT interval 0.34 seconds
Interpretation: NSR, prolonged PR interval

76. In lead I the QRS complex is positive, so the axis is left; on lead aVF the QRS is positive, therefore inferior. JJ's axis is in the normal quadrant.

77. The most striking feature of this ECG is the ST-segment elevation in the inferior leads, II, III, and aVF. These signs in light of JJ's clinical picture are indicative of an inferior wall myocardial injury pattern. Note also the ST-segment depression in leads I and aVL. These are known as *reciprocal ST-segment changes,* often observed in the leads that are anatomically opposite the area of injury. The ST-segment depression and tall R wave in V_2 may represent involvement of the true posterior wall as well.
Interpretation: probable inferior, inferoposterior myocardial infarction.

PART TWO

THE NURSING PROCESS IN INTERPRETING ARRHYTHMIAS

CHAPTER FOUR

The Nursing Process and Cardiac Arrhythmias

▶ **GOAL**

You will be able to identify patient problems systematically and resolve them, and you will be able to identify the nursing aspects of arrhythmia management.

▶ **OBJECTIVES**

After studying this chapter you should be able to:

1. List the steps of the nursing process.
2. Identify and apply the components of the nursing process: clinical assessment, nursing diagnosis, plan and implementation (patient goal and nursing intervention), and evaluation.

How is the nursing process used in the management of arrhythmias? Traditionally, the study of cardiac rhythm disturbances has centered around the medical diagnosis, which focuses on the pathology, treatment, and cure of the arrhythmia. In contrast a nursing diagnosis is focused on the patient's response or potential response to it. The nursing process enables one to identify patient problems systematically and resolve them.

The nursing aspects of arrhythmia management are important and require special attention, as do the medical aspects. It is the nurse or paramedic who most often assesses the patient, plans the immediate care, intervenes, and evaluates the care before the physician is called. This necessitates a nursing and a medical diagnosis and plan for treatment.

THE STEPS OF THE NURSING PROCESS

Most readers of this volume are already familiar with the nursing process. It is briefly presented here to relate it to the study of arrhythmias. Our intent is not to introduce the subject or teach you how to use it. You have already learned that, and many excellent references are available for that purpose. Rather, we want to assure you that the nursing process is a dependable, systematic method to approach and manage cardiac rhythm disturbances.

Data Base: Problem Identification

Before you can proceed with assessing a problem, you must identify the problem. Establishing a data base, grounded in scientific principles and sound research, enables the practitioner to follow the remaining steps with some degree of competence. You must have a broad, working knowledge of an arrhythmia, its potential for deterioration and, just as important, whether or not it is innocuous. For these reasons, we begin each arrhythmia section with a discussion of definitions, etiology, physiologic mechanisms, and electrocardiographic characteristics.

Assessment

The first, and often the most crucial, step in the nursing process is assessment. The plan of care is based on information gathered in this phase. Data are collected and organized so a plan can be formulated. The nurse collects the information about the patient by three methods: observation, interviewing, and physical examination. How does the patient act during the arrhythmia? How does the patient look? Are there any subjective symptoms such as dizziness, palpitations, or chest pain? Is the patient frightened? What are the vital signs? Urinary output? Peripheral pulses? In summary, how the patient tolerates the arrhythmia is the end result of the assessment phase. This, along with your clinical knowledge of the disorder, will help you define nursing interventions directed at assisting the patient's adaptation.

Nursing Diagnosis

The next step in the nursing process, the nursing diagnosis, is a statement of the patient's actual or potential problem requiring intervention. The diagnosis may be supplemented by describing its relationship to the cause of the problem, if it is known. Therefore it is based on facts, and each diagnostic statement relates to one patient problem. In the study of arrhythmias, there commonly are instances when a diagnosis is shared by both medicine and nursing. Under such circumstances and depending on how emergent the situation, treatment may be the same. An example is when a patient develops ventricular fibrillation, a lethal arrhythmia. In other situations the nursing and medical diagnoses are clearly different. For example, the medical diagnosis might be frequent premature beats; a corresponding nursing diagnosis could be ineffective coping related to emotional stress.

When arrhythmias cause a decrease in cardiac output, which they often do, the nursing diagnostic category into which most of these symptom-producing rhythms fall is "decreased cardiac output." How does the reduced cardiac output affect the patient? Does it cause the person to have chest pain? Shortness of breath? Syncope? Confusion? Decreased urine output? Lowered blood pressure? Pulse deficit? Cold, clammy skin? Lethargy? Additional nursing diagnoses may be identified and based on the response to the decreased cardiac output. For example, when a patient's response to sinus bradycardia (a slow heart rate) is altered mentation, the nursing diagnosis would be: "altered tissue perfusion: cerebral, related to low cardiac output."

What if your young pediatric patient experiences shortness of breath whenever she exercises? The electrocardiogram (ECG) reveals the presence of a paroxysmal supraventricular tachycardia whenever she reaches a certain grade of incline on the treadmill. Her heart rate exceeds 200 beats per minute (bpm) during such episodes. How would the nursing diagnosis be structured? First of all, what is the problem? Shortness of breath during exercise. What is the problem related to? Heart rates in excess of 200 bpm causing a lowered cardiac output because of reduced cardiac filling time. How are the diagnostic statements phrased? "Decreased cardiac output related to paroxysmal supraventricular tachycardia" and "activity intolerance related to shortness of breath secondary to decreased cardiac output."

Other diagnostic categories that consistently apply to rhythm disturbance problems include the following:

1. Altered tissue perfusion: cerebral/cardiopulmonary/peripheral.
2. Chest/anginal pain.
3. Knowledge deficit regarding the arrhythmia and its management.
4. Activity intolerance.
5. Anxiety.
6. Ineffective coping.

Also presented in the text are arrhythmias that, in typical situations, warrant no nursing diagnosis at all. We have therefore omitted the diagnostic statements in these sections. This is not to suggest, however, that a nursing diagnosis could not be formulated in given specific patient situations.

The *ECG diagnosis* is the term by which an arrhythmia is known. Some ECG diagnoses predict patient symptomatology. For example, ventricular fibrillation and ventricular asystole, both resulting in cessation of cardiac pumping, are accompanied by cardiovascular collapse and death, unless corrected. Other ECG diagnoses (e.g., sinus bradycardia, sinus tachycardia) depend on further assessment to plan appropriate patient care. In summary, one ECG diagnosis may have more than one nursing diagnosis, depending on the patient and clinical situation.

Plan and Implementation

Plan

During the planning phase, a plan of care is developed that consists of a goal and interventions. The patient goal is the expected or desired change in the patient's status after receiving these interventions. Successful care of any patient with an arrhythmia depends on the nurse's ability to establish priorities and goals. Setting priorities involves determining whether the arrhythmia poses an immediate threat to the patient's life. For example, a short run of ventricular tachycardia in a patient who has had a myocardial infarction may not produce symptoms of reduced cardiac output. The attending nurse knows, through knowledge gained in establishing a data base, that this is a potentially lethal situation. For this patient, the immediate goal is to restore normal rhythm and prevent subsequent episodes of the arrhythmia. Goals for patients with rhythm disturbances may range anywhere from coping with a chronic arrhythmia to sustaining life during an acute, lethal one.

Implementation

This phase involves administering the care and continuing data collection. What can the nurse do to help solve the patient's problem? What specific interventions will achieve the desired patient outcome/goal? In the management of an arrhythmia, this phase of the nursing process may be closely allied with the medical treatment.

The assessment and intervention statements as written are intended to be instructional guidelines only. They are not prescriptive and are not to be used as a substitute for medical/nursing orders and protocols in your clinical practice. Nor can they be used as a substitute for sound clinical judgment in individual situations. The book's content reflects the authors' knowledge, but this may differ from the standard of clinical practice found in your hospital.

Evaluation

This final phase involves the evaluation of goal achievement and reassessment of the care plan. Has the patient goal been achieved and to what degree? What has been the patient's response to the nursing intervention and medical treatment? Has any progress been made? Is the arrhythmia occurring with less frequency, or has there been a complete return to normal sinus rhythm?

APPLIED NURSING PROCESS

The following care plan generally illustrates the nursing process applied to a specific cardiac rhythm disturbance. Some data base information and electrocardiographic characteristics have been omitted as they would not typically be found in a written plan of care.

MF is a 22-year-old male with a medical diagnosis of paroxysmal supraventricular tachycardia (PSVT) of unknown cause. He is a nonsmoker and is otherwise healthy. There have been multiple episodes of the tachycardia during both exercise and rest. Shortly after onset he develops palpitations with severe chest pain and nausea and becomes quite anxious. He has been admitted to the hospital for observation and treatment.

❖ NURSING DIAGNOSIS 1

Decreased cardiac output related to tachycardia.

❖ ECG DIAGNOSIS

Paroxysmal supraventricular tachycardia.

Clinical Assessment

- Assess for manifestations of reduced cardiac output such as hypotension, neurologic changes (syncope, dizziness, light-headedness), pallor, diaphoresis, and nausea.
- Monitor the peripheral pulses and electrocardiogram.
- Assess for changes in skin color and temperature such as cyanosis and cold, clammy skin.
- Assess for manifestations of congestive heart failure (CHF):
  - Auscultate the lungs for rales.
  - Inspect the external jugular veins for distension.
  - Observe and palpate for peripheral edema.
  - Observe for shortness of breath and cough.
  - Auscultate for a third heart sound (S_3).
- Measure blood pressure.
- Monitor arterial blood gases if necessary.
- Monitor serum potassium, digitalis, and antiarrhythmic drug levels if indicated.
- Assess level of anxiety.

Plan and Implementation

Patient Goal

The patient will demonstrate improvement in cardiac pump performance, reduction in cardiac workload, and will not develop dizziness or syncope.

Nursing Interventions

- Begin intravenous hydration if necessary.
- Prepare for electrical cardioversion if necessary.
- Give oxygen therapy as needed.
- Administer medications as ordered and evaluate their effectiveness.
- Elevate head of bed as needed.
- Provide reassurance and antianxiety measures as needed.
- Initiate Valsalva maneuver if appropriate.

Evaluation

The patient has improved cardiac performance as evidenced by the following:

- Absence of dizziness or syncope.
- Serum drug and electrolyte levels within normal limits.
- Clear lungs.
- Blood pressure within normal range.
- Skin warm and dry.
- No visible or palpable manifestations of fluid retention.
- Nondistended neck veins.
- Absence of feelings of anxiety or panic.

Medical Treatment

- Carotid sinus massage (CSM), Valsalva maneuver
- Electrical cardioversion
- Drugs: propranolol, verapamil, digitalis, quinidine, procainamide, diuretics
- Artificial pacing

❖ NURSING DIAGNOSIS 2

Chest/anginal pain related to imbalance in myocardial oxygen supply and demand.

Clinical Assessment

- Assess the patient's pain for quality, location, intensity, and associated symptoms.
- Assess the level of anxiety related to the tachycardia and angina.
- Question the patient regarding events precipitating the tachycardia and angina (e.g., exercise).
- Monitor the ECG for tachycardia and ischemic changes (ST-segment and T-wave changes).
- Measure cardiac enzymes if indicated.

Plan and Implementation

Patient Goal

The patient will experience relief from anginal pain.

Nursing Interventions

- Administer nitroglycerin or other antianginal agent if measures to terminate the arrhythmia fail.
- Stay with the patient and provide reassurance.
- After resolution of the pain, offer instruction regarding the cause of the chest pain and why the heart's oxygen needs have not been met.

Evaluation

The patient is free of angina and anxiety as evidenced by verbalization of pain relief and a relaxed appearance.

❖ NURSING DIAGNOSIS 3

Knowledge deficit regarding the arrhythmia and its management at home.

Clinical Assessment

Assess the patient's knowledge base.

Plan and Implementation

Patient Goal

The patient will demonstrate methods of arrhythmia recognition and termination and will verbalize information related to the nature and long-term management of the disorder.

Nursing Interventions

- Instruct the patient in the following areas:
  - Appropriate anatomy and physiology.
  - Risk factors (caffeine, alcohol, exercise, stress).
  - Symptoms to report to the physician (nausea, lightheadedness, dizziness, syncope, severe palpitations, chest pain).
  - Complications of the PSVT.
  - Exercise limitations (relationship of the PSVT to type, frequency, and duration of exercise).
  - Pulse taking.
  - Portable monitoring of tachycardia episodes (e.g., the transtelephonic event recorder).
  - Holter monitoring.
  - Medications (name, dose, side effects).
- Instruct the patient in selected techniques to terminate the arrhythmia:
  - Patient-activated radiofrequency pacemaker.
  - Ice water in the face.
  - Valsalva maneuvers.
  - Supine position with legs elevated (results in increased blood volume).
- Provide the patient with Medic Alert literature or jewelry if condition warrants.
- Provide clinic appointment information (i.e., testing of pacemaker function, serum drug levels, physical examination).

Evaluation

- The patient has correctly related the appropriate information regarding management of his rhythm disturbance at home as evidenced by (list the specific criteria used for goal achievement) the ability to:
- Demonstrate Valsalva technique.
- Explain procedure for facial immersion in ice water.
- Recognize onset of the arrhythmia and initiate termination.

Suggestion to the reader. It may also be necessary to consider the nursing diagnoses of "Anxiety" and "Altered tissue perfusion: cardiopulmonary/cerebral/peripheral," in a patient with PSVT. Although some level of anxiety is common to a great many patients with PSVT, it may be a serious problem warranting individual attention. Because reduction in cardiac output may result in significant alteration of systemic perfusion, some patients typically experience manifestations of impending shock instead of angina.

The North American Nursing Diagnosis Association (NANDA), in its continuing effort to achieve consistency and compatibility with the International Classification of Diseases of the World Health Organization and the United States government guidelines for Diagnosis Related Groups (DRGs), has further refined the nursing diagnosis taxonomy. One fundamental change in language is the following: nursing diagnoses formerly prefaced with "potential for . . ." are now stated as "high risk for . . . ."

In studying this book the reader must keep in mind that even though a nursing diagnosis is listed for a particular rhythm disorder, that nursing diagnosis may not necessarily be applicable to every patient with that rhythm disorder. However, it behooves the nurse to consider all the diagnostic categories provided.

BIBLIOGRAPHY

Atkinson LD, Murray ME. *Understanding the Nursing Process*. New York: Macmillan, 1980.

Burke LJ, Gabriel LM, Fischer LE, Zemke SL, Nursing diagnoses, indicators, and interventions in an outpatient cardiac rehabilitation program. *Heart & Lung*, Jan., 1986, 15(1): 70-6.

Caine RM, Bufalino PM. *Critically Ill Adults: Nursing Care Planning Guides*. Baltimore: Williams and Wilkins, 1988.

Carlson JH, Craft CA, McGuire AD, *Nursing Diagnosis*. Philadelphia: WB Saunders, 1982.

Carpenito LJ. *Nursing Diagnosis: Application to Clinical Practice*. Philadelphia: JB Lippincott, 1983.

Dalton J. A descriptive study: defining characteristics of the nursing diagnosis cardiac output, alterations in: decreased. *Image: The Journal of Nursing Scholarship*, Fall, 1985, 17(4): 113-7.

Guzzetta CE, Dossey BM. *Cardiovascular Nursing: Bodymind Tapestry*. St. Louis: The CV Mosby Co., 1984.

Jacoby MK. The dilemma of physiological problems. Eliminating the double standard. *Am. J. Nurs.*, Mar., 1985, 85(3): 281-5.

Kim MF, McFarland GK, McFarlane AM, *Pocket Guide to Nursing Diagnosis*. 4th ed. St. Louis: Mosby-Year Book, 1991.

North American Nursing Diagnosis Association. Classification of Nursing Diagnosis: Proceedings of the eighth conference, North American Nursing Diagnosis Association, Philadelphia: JP Lippincott, 1989.

North American Nursing Diagnosis Association. Taxonomy I revised 1990 with official nursing diagnosis, St. Louis, North American Nursing Diagnosis Association, 1990.

Symposium on nursing diagnosis in critical care. *Heart & Lung,* Sept., 1985, 14(5).

Urden LD, Daire JK, Thelon LA. *Essentials of Critical Care Nursing*. 1st ed, St. Louis: Mosby-Year Book, 1992.

CHAPTER FIVE

The Sinus Rhythms

▶ GOAL

You will be able to distinguish physiologic from pathologic sinus rhythms and use the nursing process in caring for patients with sinus rhythm disturbances.

▶ OBJECTIVES

After studying this chapter and completing the self-assessment exercises, you should be able to:

1. Describe the features of normal sinus rhythm (NSR) for adults and children.
2. Differentiate physiologic from pathologic arrhythmias and identify ECG examples and characteristics of each.
3. List ten etiologic factors associated with sinus tachycardia.
4. Recognize sinus tachycardia on the ECG and assess the patient who is experiencing it. Explain factors you would consider in determining the clinical significance of the arrhythmia.
5. Determine appropriate nursing interventions for the patient with sinus tachycardia.
6. Define sinus bradycardia and compare and contrast its mechanism with sinus tachycardia.
7. Correlate the incidence of sinus bradycardia with myocardial infarction.
8. Identify clinical settings associated with sinus bradycardia and explain the effect of vasovagal reflexes.
9. Recognize sinus bradycardia on the ECG and delineate appropriate assessment measures.
10. Determine nursing interventions in order of priority for the patient with sinus bradycardia and identify criteria to be considered in treating the arrhythmia.
11. Formulate an initial patient teaching plan for the patient with a permanent pacemaker.
12. Differentiate Type II SA block from sinus bradycardia on the ECG, contrast mechanisms and compare nursing interventions.
13. Identify at least two features of sick sinus syndrome.
14. Assess the patient suspected of having sick sinus syndrome and state a common medical treatment.

The sinus rhythms clearly differ from the other anatomic classifications (e.g., the atrial or ventricular arrhythmias) primarily because not all are pathologic rhythm disturbances. Some are known as *physiologic rhythms* or variations of normal sinus rhythm, and are found in healthy people. Although it is important for you to recognize the variations, it is equally important to remember that these arrhythmias are not necessarily harmful or prognostically significant.

NORMAL SINUS RHYTHM

Data Base: Problem Identification

Definitions, Etiology, and Mechanisms

The features of normal sinus rhythm (NSR) have been described in Chapter 3 and are briefly reviewed as an introduction to the physiologic and pathologic rhythms originating in the sinus node. Normal sinus rhythm is the normal rhythm of the heart with impulses generated in the sinus node traveling through the atria, atrioventricular (AV) node, and His-Purkinje system.

The sinus node (SA node) is capable of responding with a wide rate range in response to body demands. Normal heart rate range for adults is 60 to 100 beats per minute (bpm), although physiologic variations outside this range occur in healthy people. This is one reason why we use the terms *physiologic* and *pathologic* to differentiate the array of sinus-originated rhythms. For example, if you were to do 50 push-ups right now, your heart rate would exceed 100 bpm. This would be considered a physiologic tachycardia (because the rate per minute exceeds 100 bpm) rather than a pathologic rhythm disturbance. Likewise a trained athlete at rest might have a heart rate of 35 bpm. Although this is well below 60 bpm, thus classifying it as a bradycardia, it is a physiologic bradycardia, not pathologic. Infants have a normal rate range of approximately 130 to 160 bpm, with the resting heart rate decreasing to 100 bpm or below by age 2 to 3 years[1] (Table 5-1). Fevers and exercise are physiologic variants that may cause tachycardia well in excess of 100 bpm, but this is not a pathologic tachycardia in the sense that it is a product of heart or sinus node disease. Rather, it is a physiologic response to extracardiac factors and, in most cases, this tachycardic response would not produce hemodynamic compromise or require treatment.

What are some other factors causing physiologic variations in heart rate? Generally speaking, rate slows with advancing age,[2,3] although this correlation does not appear to exist in young-to-middle-aged adults.[4] Sinus slowing is frequently found in the elderly and may or may not coexist with the rising incidence of cardiovascular diseases of this age group.[5] Both young[6] and elderly[5] women have been shown to have significantly faster heart rates than men of the same age. Exercise in the healthy young produces rates not exceeding approximately 200 bpm, whereas in the elderly, this maximum exercise rate is approximately 140 bpm.[1] Besides age, sex, and exercise, myriad factors influence heart rate, and these will be discussed in subsequent sections.

Table 5-1 Normal Heart Rates for Infants and Children*

Age	Heart rate (bpm) Resting (awake)	Resting (asleep)	Exercise (fever)
Newborn	100-180	80-160	up to 200
1 week to 3 months	100-220	80-200	up to 220
3 months to 2 years	80-150	70-120	up to 200
2 years to 10 years	70-110	60-90	up to 200
10 years to adult	55-90	50-90	up to 200

*Reprinted with permission from Gillette PC. Cardiac dysrhythmias in infants and children. *In* Engle MA (ed). *Pediatric Cardiovascular Disease. Cardiovascular Clinics,* 11/2. Philadelphia: FA Davis, 1981.

ECG Characteristics

In the adult, NSR heart rate ranges from 60 to 100 bpm and is regular. For infants and children the heart rate ranges are higher (see Table 5-1). There is a P wave preceding every QRS; P waves are rounded, within normal axis range, have a duration of 0.10 seconds or less, and are less than 3 mm in amplitude.

In healthy adults the PR interval is 0.12 to 0.20 seconds, shortening with exercise and its resultant increase in heart rate. Children exhibit shorter PR intervals.

The QRS complexes have a duration of 0.10 seconds or less (refer to Chapter 3), unless an intraventricular conduction delay (IVCD) exists (see Chapter 9). Figs. 5-1 to 5-6 illustrate examples of NSR. The box on this page provides a summary of ECG features of NSR in the adult.

ECG Characteristics
Normal Sinus Rhythm

Rate: 60 to 100 bpm
Rhythm: Regular
P waves: Normal
PR interval: Normal
QRS complex: Normal unless IVCD

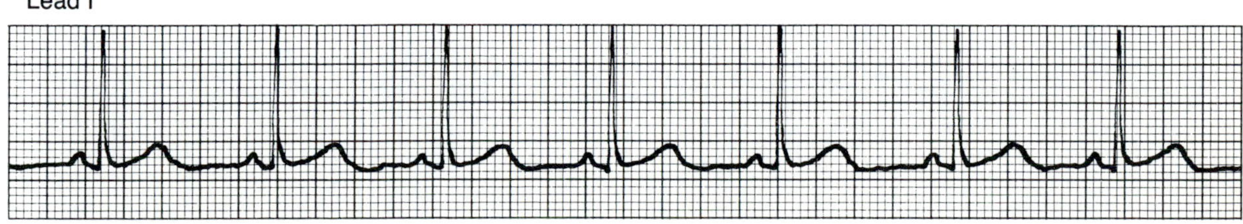

FIGURE 5-1 Normal sinus rhythm. This rhythm strip was obtained from the bedside monitor of an 84-year-old woman.

Rate: 64 to 68 bpm
Rhythm: Regular
P waves: Normal, one precedes each QRS complex
PR interval: 0.14 to 0.16 seconds
QRS complex: 0.07 seconds, R complex, normal
Interpretation: NSR

Lead II

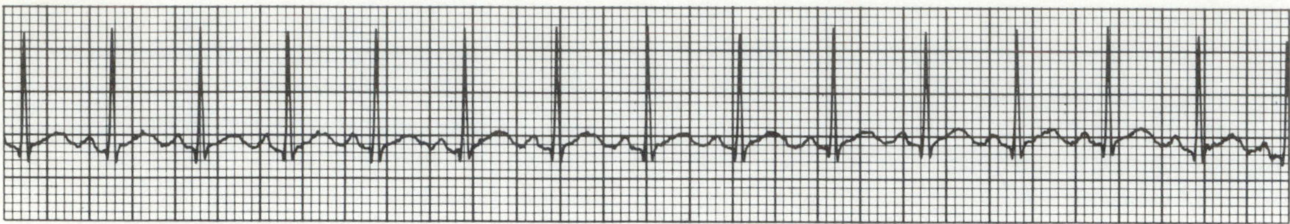

FIGURE 5-2 Normal sinus rhythm. This strip was obtained from a 12-lead ECG of a healthy six-month-old baby boy.

Rate: 136 bpm
Rhythm: Regular
P waves: Normal, one precedes each QRS complex
PR interval: 0.12 seconds, normal
QRS complex: 0.06 seconds, qRs complex, normal
Interpretation: NSR

V_1

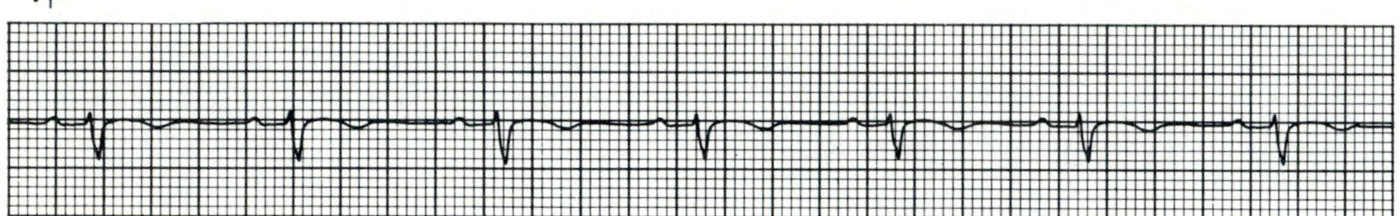

FIGURE 5-3 Normal sinus rhythm. This strip was obtained from a 12-lead ECG of a healthy 26-year-old female.

Rate: 70 bpm
Rhythm: Regular
P waves: Normal, one precedes each QRS complex
PR interval: 0.16 to 0.18 seconds, normal
QRS complex: 0.08 seconds, rS complex, normal
Interpretation: NSR

Lead II

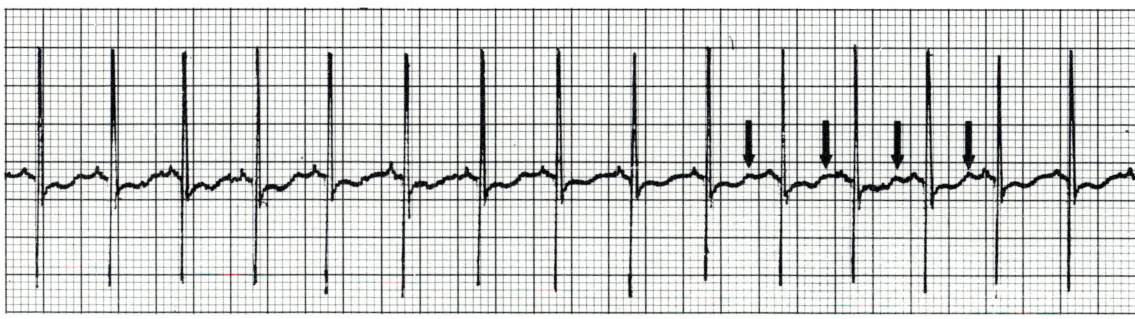

FIGURE 5-4 Normal sinus rhythm in a 1-kg infant with infant respiratory distress syndrome.

Rate: 155 bpm
Rhythm: Regular
P wave: Normal, one precedes each QRS complex
PR interval: 0.08 seconds, normal for infant with heart rate 155 bpm
QRS complex: 0.06 seconds, probable U waves following T waves *(arrows)*
Interpretation: NSR

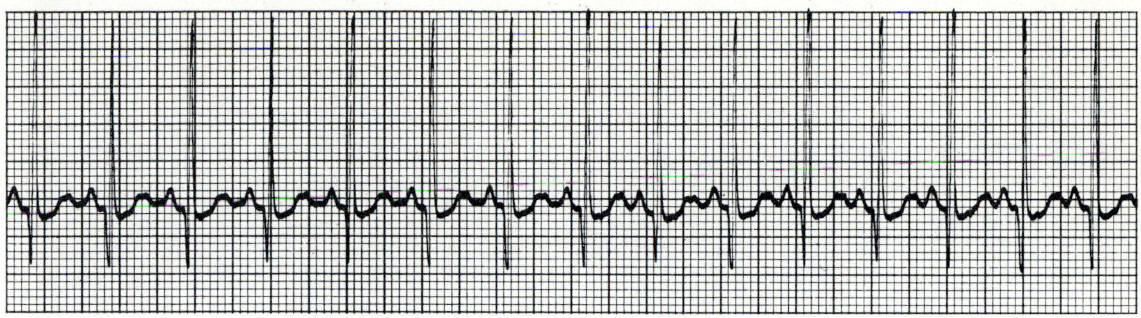

FIGURE 5-5 Normal sinus rhythm in a 2-year-old child with acute Lomotil ingestion.

Rate: 140 bpm
Rhythm: Regular
P wave: Normal, one precedes each QRS complex
PR interval: 0.12 seconds
QRS complex: 0.08 seconds
Interpretation: NSR

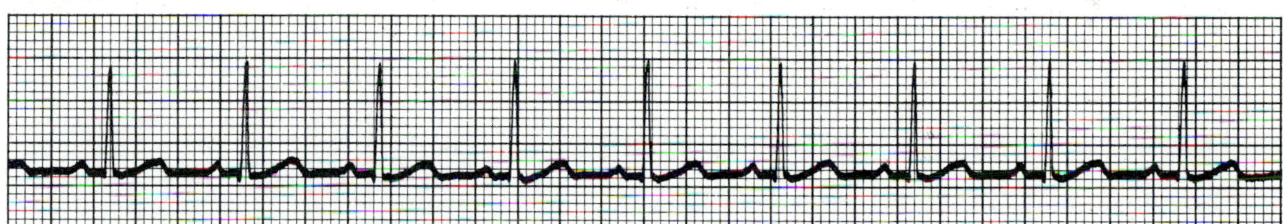

FIGURE 5-6 Normal sinus rhythm in a 15-year-old male.

Rate: 95 bpm
Rhythm: Regular
P wave: Normal, one precedes each QRS complex
PR interval: 0.16 seconds
QRS complex 0.06 seconds
Interpretation: NSR

SINUS ARRHYTHMIA
Data Base: Problem Identification
Definitions, Etiology, and Mechanisms

Sinus arrhythmia is an irregularity of the sinus pacemaker and presents in two patterns: respiratory and nonrespiratory. The respiratory type is a normal finding, influenced by vagal stimulation, and is common in children and young adults.[1,7,8] SA nodal impulse firing varies with phases of respiration, causing an ECG pattern that waxes and wanes with breathing. The heart rate increases with inspiration and decreases with expiration. The nonrespiratory form of sinus arrhythmia appears the same on the ECG, but it is not synchronous with breathing. It has been observed in the elderly and in cases of digitalis toxicity. Digitalis, morphine sulfate, prostigmine, and carotid sinus massage are all known to worsen nonrespiratory sinus arrhythmia.[9]

ECG Characteristics
Sinus Arrhythmia

Rate: Variable
Rhythm: Irregular
P waves: Normal. P-P intervals gradually lengthening and shortening
PR interval: Normal and constant
QRS complex: Normal unless IVCD present

ECG Characteristics

Sinus arrhythmia is a disorder of rhythm, not rate. The rhythm is irregular and may be markedly so. Unless there is an intraatrial conduction delay, the P waves will be normal, and the PR intervals will be normal and remain constant. You will come to recognize the P-to-P intervals (atrial cycle length) gradually lengthening and shortening, and this is the hallmark feature of sinus arrhythmia. Figs. 5-7 to 5-9 are examples of sinus arrhythmia. The box on p. 93 summarizes the ECG features.

Applied Nursing Process

Clinical Assessment

- Detect:
  - An irregular pulse.
  - An irregularity in the ECG.
- Assess the patient and ECG.
  - Determine whether the arrhythmia is respiratory or nonrespiratory in nature.

❖ NURSING DIAGNOSIS

None.

❖ ECG DIAGNOSIS

Sinus arrhythmia.

Plan and Implementation

Patient goal. No specific patient goals are indicated.

Nursing interventions. No specific nursing measures are usually necessary. Sinus arrhythmia does not require treatment.

Evaluation

Because sinus arrhythmia is not one that requires regular evaluation, the patient's adaptive status does not need to be evaluated. Digitalis dosages are not likely to be changed because of the emergence of nonrespiratory sinus arrhythmia.

Medical Treatment

None is required.

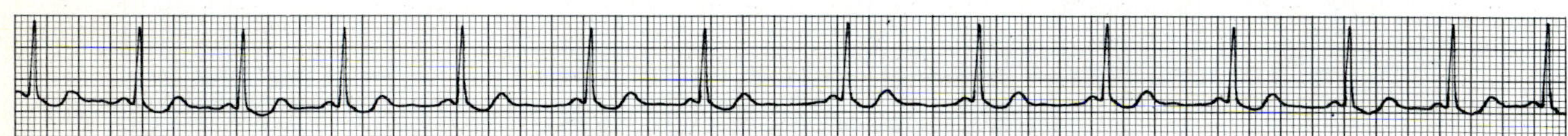

FIGURE 5-7 Respiratory sinus arrhythmia. Note how rhythm waxes and wanes with rate ranging from 100 to as slow as 65 bpm.

Rate: 65 to 100 bpm
Rhythm: Irregular
P wave: Normal, one precedes each QRS complex
PR interval: 0.12 seconds
QRS complex: 0.06 seconds
Interpretation: Respiratory sinus arrhythmia

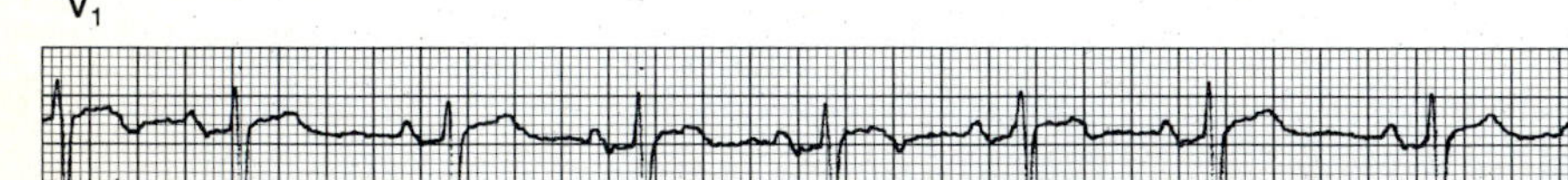
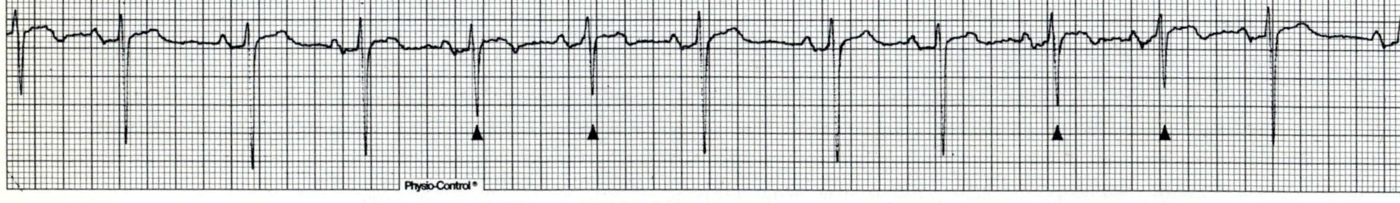

FIGURE 5-8 Respiratory sinus arrhythmia. Note diminution of QRS complexes *(arrows)* with the more rapid phase. In some individuals, movement of the diaphragm causes movement of the heart, resulting in a slight shift of axis correlating with respirations. In this example the rate ranges from 77 to 65 bpm.

Rate: 65 to 77 bpm
Rhythm: Irregular
P wave: Normal, one precedes each QRS complex
PR interval: 0.20 seconds
QRS complex: 0.09 seconds
Interpretation: Respiratory sinus arrhythmia with respiratory axis shift

Lead II

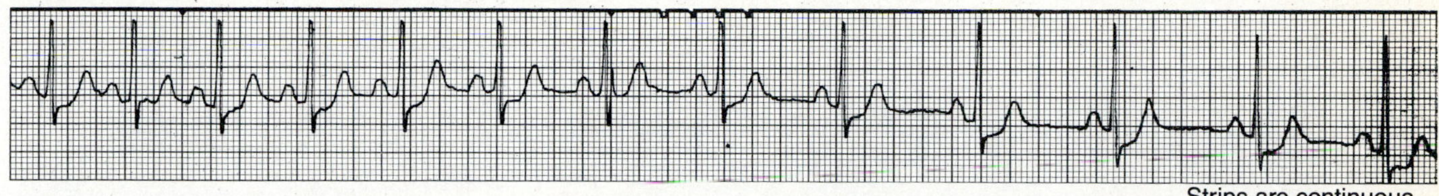

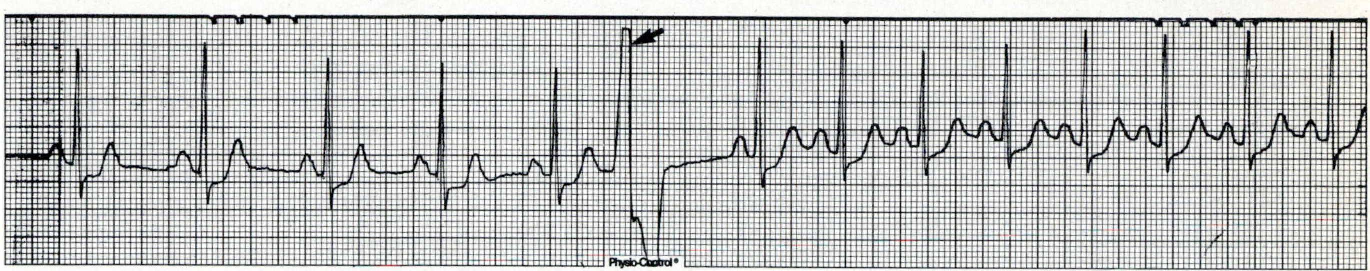

FIGURE 5-9 Nonrespiratory sinus arrhythmia. Waxing and waning of rhythm are not associated with respirations. Rate ranges from 103 to 60 bpm. Large, malformed complex in second tracing *(arrow)* is a premature ventricular beat (see Chapter 8).

Rate: 60 to 103 bpm
Rhythm: Irregular
P wave: 0.13 seconds, too wide, indicates intraatrial conduction delay
PR interval: 0.18 seconds
QRS complex: 0.08 seconds, depressed ST segment
Interpretation: Nonrespiratory sinus arrhythmia with 1 ventricular premature beat

SINUS TACHYCARDIA
Data Base: Problem Identification
Definitions, Etiology, and Mechanisms

Sinus tachycardia is not a primary rhythm but secondary to an underlying cause, and is not necessarily indicative of disease. It is a rhythm of sinus origin with a rate exceeding 100 bpm in the adult. Ordinarily the range of sinus tachycardia is 100 to 150 bpm,[7,10,11] with higher rates during strenuous exercise.[11,12] The rapid sinus discharge is due to enhanced automaticity from a multitude of conditions, many of which cause increased sympathetic tone,[13] and these are listed in the table on p. 97.

Sinus tachycardia occurs in up to 30% of patients with acute myocardial infarction[14] and is often associated with massive myocardial damage.[15] The tachycardia, however, may be a result of pain, anxiety, or, in younger patients, a hyperdynamic state. Such conditions are accompanied by an increase in circulating catecholamines, which is thought to have a negative impact on overall cardiac function, lower the threshold of ventricular fibrillation, and, therefore, significantly worsen the clinical picture.[14,15]

ECG Characteristics

Sinus tachycardia is a regular rhythm with a rate consistently greater than 100 bpm. Unless conduction delays are present, P waves and QRS complexes are of normal duration, and the PR interval is normal and remains constant (Figs. 5-10 to 5-12 and the box on this page).

ECG Characteristics
Sinus Bradycardia

Rate: <60 bpm
Rhythm: Regular
P waves: Normal
PR interval: Normal or prolonged
QRS complex: Normal unless IVCD present

Applied Nursing Process
Clinical Assessment

- Detect:
  - Rapid regular pulse.
  - Regular rhythm on the ECG.
- Assess the patient and ECG.
  - Assess the clinical setting in which the sinus tachycardia is occurring. For example, is the patient febrile? Postoperative? Septic? Has the patient had a recent myocardial infarction? Is the patient in shock? Is the patient in respiratory distress from pulmonary disease?
  - Determine how well the the patient tolerates the rapid heart rate by assessing for signs and symptoms associated with decreased cardiac output.

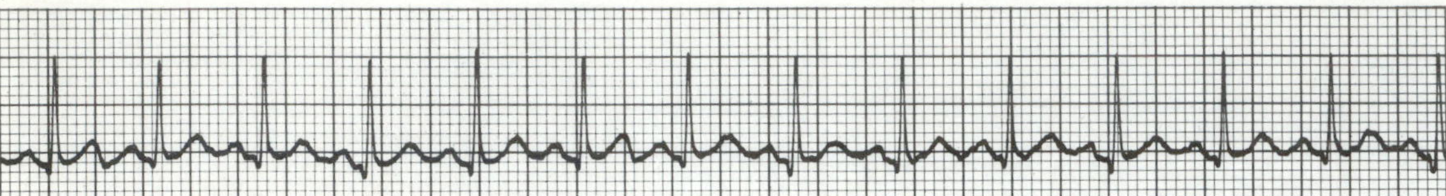

FIGURE 5-10 Sinus tachycardia.

Rate: 136 bpm
Rhythm: Regular
P wave: Normal, one precedes each QRS complex
PR interval: 0.12 seconds
QRS complex: 0.06 seconds
Interpretation: Sinus tachycardia

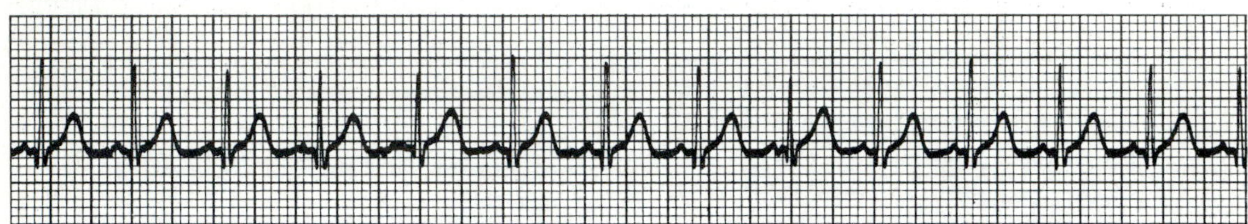

FIGURE 5-11 Sinus tachycardia in a 31-month-old child with thrombocytopenia.

Rate: 132 bpm
Rhythm: Regular
P wave: Normal, one precedes each QRS complex
PR interval: 0.10 seconds, normal for child this age with heart rate 132 bpm
QRS complex: 0.07 seconds
Interpretation: Sinus tachycardia

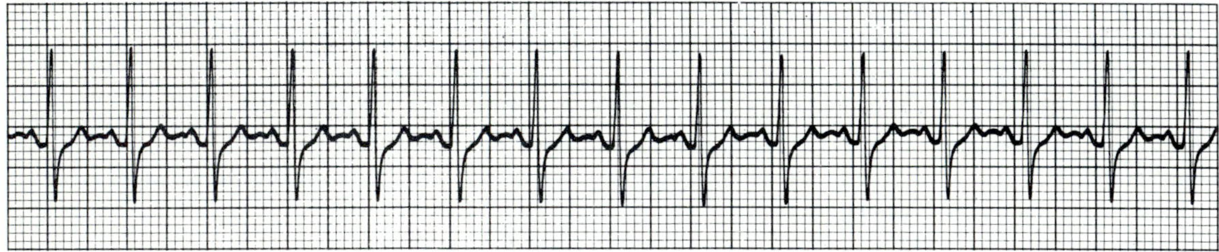

FIGURE 5-12 Sinus tachycardia. This tracing was taken from an 11-year-old female with a 20% body surface area burn. When the tracing was obtained, she was afebrile and on bed rest.

Rate: 150 bpm
Rhythm: Regular
P wave: Normal
PR interval: 0.10 seconds, normal for rate
QRS complex: 0.07 seconds
Interpretation: Sinus tachycardia

Check blood pressure and palpate the peripheral pulses. Are the peripheral pulses weak or bounding?
Assess sensorium.
Assess skin color, temperature, capillary refill.
Measure urinary output.

- In the critically ill patient, measurement of cardiac output and pulmonary wedge pressure may be indicated.
- Assess for adequate hydration.
  Determine tissue turgor.
  Inspect the tongue and mucous membranes.
  Measure the specific gravity of the urine.
  Determine central venous pressure, if indicated.
- Assess for signs and symptoms of congestive heart failure.
  Ask the patient if shortness of breath is present.

Table 5-2 Etiologic Factors in Sinus Tachycardia

Noncardiac	Cardiac	Pharmacologic
Anemia[11,13]	Congestive heart failure[13]	Aminophylline[7]
Anxiety[13]	Left atrial distention[13]	Amphetamines
Burns	Myocardial infarction[8]	Amyl nitrate[8]
Eating[8]	Pericarditis[13]	Atropine[7,8,13]
Emotion, fear[8]	After cardiac transplant	Caffeine[8]
Exercise[8]		Dopamine
Fever[13]		Epinephrine[8]
Hemorrhage or hypovolemia[13]		Isoproterenol[7]
Hypoxemia[11,13]		Nicotine[8]
Infection[8]		Psychotropic drugs[11]
Pheochromocytoma[11]		Quinidine[8]
Pain[13]		
Pulmonary embolus[11,13]		
Shock[8]		
Sympathetic stimulation[13]		
Thyrotoxicosis, hyperthyroidism[8,11]		

Observe for the presence of cough and increased respiratory rate.

Auscultate the lungs for the presence of rales in the bases.

Auscultate the heart for S_3 gallop.

Inspect the neck for external jugular venous distension.

Inspect for peripheral edema.

Record accurate intake, output, and daily weights.

- Assess for signs and symptoms associated with myocardial ischemia (When the heart beats rapidly, its use of oxygen increases. In individuals with compromised coronary circulation, the demand for oxygen may exceed the supply, resulting in decreased myocardial tissue perfusion).

  Question the patient about the presence of chest or arm discomfort.

  Inspect the ECG for ST-segment and T-wave changes.
- Assess diet.

❖ NURSING DIAGNOSIS

(1) Decreased cardiac output related to the factors associated with sinus tachycardia. (2) Altered tissue perfusion: cardiopulmonary, related to tachycardia.

❖ ECG DIAGNOSIS

Sinus tachycardia.

Plan and Implementation

Patient goal. The patient will maintain hemodynamic stability and adequate tissue perfusion and will be free from stressors that can be alleviated.

Nursing interventions.

- Remove the underlying cause of the arrhythmia, if possible.
  - Relieve pain.
  - Combat dehydration.
  - Reduce fever.
  - Allay anxiety.
  - Minimize metabolic expenditure.
  - Prevent physiologic stressors (e.g., shivering).
  - Identify contributing factors that may be eliminated from the patient's environment such as sources of caffeine or medications that may have a stimulant effect, or external stimuli such as visitors, literature, television.
- For acute MI patients, reduce pain with analgesics and anxiety with a muscle relaxant (e.g., diazepam) as ordered. Evaluate patient's response to medication.
- Report to the physician any signs and symptoms suggestive of congestive heart failure. Administer oxygen, digitalis, and diuretics as ordered. Evaluate response.
- Implement medical orders and evaluate their effectiveness.

Evaluation

- The patient exhibits a reduction in heart rate when causative factors are removed.
- The patient maintains hemodynamic stability and adequate tissue perfusion as evidenced by the following:
  - Stable blood pressure.
  - Good peripheral pulses, color, and capillary refill.
  - Normal urine output without weight gain.
  - Absence of ST-segment and T-wave changes on the ECG and no anginal symptoms.
  - Clear lung sounds and an absence of third heart sound.

Medical Treatment

- The underlying cause, such as anemia, drugs, or sepsis, is removed or treated. For example, caffeine is eliminated from the diet, hypovolemia is corrected by fluid replacement, and fever is reduced by a variety of methods.
- If sinus tachycardia is a result of massive myocardial damage and/or congestive heart failure, efforts are made to improve cardiac function and reduce cardiac work load while fluid volume is carefully regulated.
- When hyperdynamic tachycardia is present, cardiac output is above normal. Beta blockade with drugs like propranolol may be used on a short-term basis to control ventricular response. Verapamil may slow the sinus nodal discharge rate.[1]

SINUS BRADYCARDIA

Data Base: Problem Identification

Definitions, Etiology, and Mechanisms

Sinus bradycardia is defined as a rhythm of sinus origin with a rate below 60 bpm. It has long been recognized that asymptomatic, physiologic bradycardia occurs in healthy adults and is considered a normal variant.[16] Sinus bradycardia is frequently observed in athletes engaged in high-performance sports and high levels of training and does not require attention unless symptoms develop or the bradyarrhythmia produces pauses exceeding 4 seconds.[17] In infants and children, it is a common complication of serious systemic illness, such as hypoxemia, acidosis, and increased intracranial pressure; congenital or isolated sinus bradycardia is rare.[18] In all age groups, sinus bradycardia frequently accompanies disorders of inadequate ventilation, such as hypoventilation resulting from airway obstruction.

The bradycardia is due to depressed automaticity and therefore is a disorder of impulse formation, not conduction. Some bradyarrhythmias or bradycardic syndromes, however, may be combined disorders of impulse formation and conduction, where an additional mechanism is operating from a nonsinus origin elsewhere in the conduction system. Like sinus tachycardia, sinus bradycardia has many causes, but what actually depresses the automaticity of the sinus node? It has been suggested that occlusion of the right coronary or left circumflex arteries leading to the SA nodal artery, resulting in ischemia or infarction of the SA node, may affect automaticity,[19] or autonomic imbalance or excessive parasympathetic activity may contribute.[19] Vasovagal reflexes are also thought to play a role in the mechanism of sinus bradycardia.[20] The clinical settings in which sinus bradycardia may occur are listed in Table 5-3.

Sinus bradycardia accompanies acute myocardial infarction in as many as 30% of cases.[23,24] It is associated with a significant percentage of inferior wall infarctions.[8,17] Although a firm correlation has not been established, there is evidence to support the observation that sinus bradycardia during the early postinfarction phase may be a favorable prognostic sign, provided there is not accompanying hemodynamic deterioration.[15,16,20,25-27]

Sinus node dysfunction and sinus bradycardia are common and generally transient findings after cardiac transplantation.[28,29] Ventricular tachycardia may be observed early after orthotopic heart transplantation as well. Sinus node injury or trauma as a consequence of the surgical procedure or acute rejection has anecdotally been linked to the development of bradycardia early after transplantation.[30] Recent clinical studies suggest that disruption of the sinoatrial nodal blood supply may be a predisposing factor in the genesis of bradycardia, and prolonged organ ischemia, surgical trauma, antiarrhythmic drugs, and rejection,

Table 5-3 Etiologic Factors in Sinus Bradycardia

Cardiac (disease of heart or SA node)	Noncardiac (physiologic, neurochemical, or metabolic)	Drugs and electrolytes
Acute MI[7,8]	Elderly[11,16]	Digitalis[8,9,11]
Coronary artery disease[8,11]	Athletes[8,9,11,17]	Hyperkalemia[7,11]
SA node disease[9,11]	Sleep[8]	Beta blockers
Familial sinus bradycardia[21]	Extreme fear[8]	Quinidine[11]
Cardiomyopathy	Carotid sinus sensitivity, massage, stimulation[7,8,11]	Prostigmine[9]
After cardiac transplant	Parasympathetic or vagal stimulation, and Valsalva maneuvers[7,9,11]	Lithium
Congenital long QT syndrome and exercise	Inadequate ventilation and hypoxemia	Amiodarone[1]
	Increased intracranial pressure[8,11]	Clonidine[1]
	Glaucoma[8]	Calcium-channel blockers[1]
	Esophageal diverticula[11]	Parasympathomimetic drugs[1]
	Obstructive jaundice[8,9]	Flecainide
	Sliding hiatal hernia[22]	Propafenone
	Hypothermia[9,11]	Nonionic, hyperosmolar angiography contrast medium
	Hypothyroidism[9,11]	
	Uremia[9]	
	Anorexia nervosa	
	Acidosis	
	Ocular pressure	
	Sleep at high altitude	
	Cervical spine injury	

alone or in combination, may also be important contributing factors.[29,30]

If sinus bradycardia is not an isolated arrhythmia, it is often a component of other sinus node disease or conduction disturbances. In other words, patients with sinus bradycardia often have other conduction abnormalities such as atrioventricular block and sick sinus syndrome (SSS). It may be the first, or only, manifestation of SSS.[8]

ECG Characteristics

Usually a regular rhythm, sinus bradycardia has a rate below 60 bpm. A P wave precedes each QRS complex, and the PR interval is either normal or prolonged. The QRS complexes are of normal duration unless an intraventricular conduction defect is present. Sinus bradycardia is frequently accompanied by some degree of atrioventricular block (described in Chapter 9). Electrocardiographic features of sinus bradycardia are summarized in the box on this page and examples are provided in Figs. 5-13 and 5-14.

ECG Characteristics
Sinus Tachycardia

Rate: >100 bpm
Rhythm: Regular
P waves: Normal
PR Interval: Normal
QRS complex: Normal unless IVCD present

Lead II

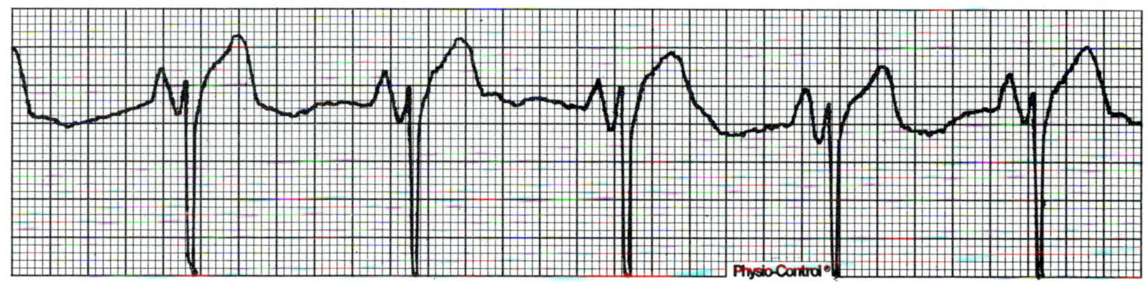

FIGURE 5-13 Sinus bradycardia. QRS complex has an rS configuration because of a left axis deviation. P waves are wide (0.12 seconds in duration) and tall.

Rate: 50 to 56 bpm (rate increases)
Rhythm: Regular
P wave: 0.12 seconds, wide, intraatrial conduction disturbance; 4 to 5 mm tall
PR interval: 0.16 seconds
QRS complex: 0.10 seconds, abnormal axis; elevated ST segment
Interpretation: Sinus bradycardia with intraatrial conduction delay

MCL_1

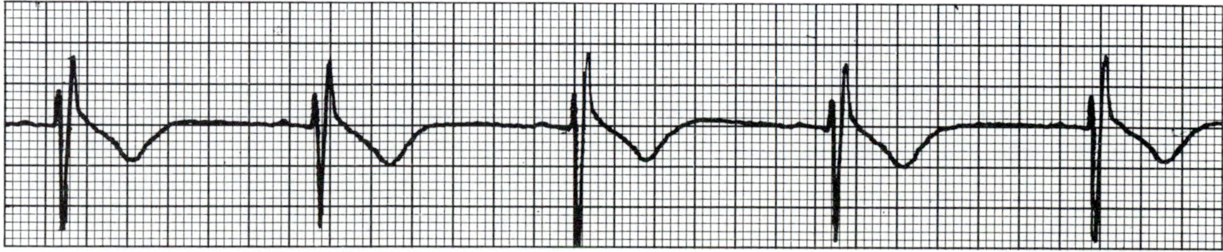

FIGURE 5-14 Sinus bradycardia, QRS complex has an rSŔ pattern, abnormal in lead MCL_1, it is also 0.12 seconds wide, indicative of an intraventricular conduction delay (in this case, right bundle branch block [RBBB]).

Rate: 47 bpm
Rhythm: Regular
P wave: Small
PR interval: 0.18 seconds
QRS complex: 0.12 seconds, RBBB
Interpretation: Sinus bradycardia, RBBB

Applied Nursing Process

Clinical Assessment

- Detect:
  - A slow pulse.
  - A slow, regular rhythm on the ECG.
- Assess the patient and ECG.
  - Assess ventilatory status. Patients who are unable to maintain their own airway patency and ventilation (e.g., those recovering from anesthesia, comatose patients, or those with apneic episodes) are candidates for severe sinus bradycardic episodes. If left to progress, the rhythm often deteriorates to AV block or cardiac arrest.
  - Assess for symptomatic reduction in cardiac output. (In the clinical assessment of sinus bradycardia, it is important to determine if, and to what degree, the rhythm is symptom-producing.)

    Hypotension.

    Weak peripheral pulses.

    Exacerbation of congestive heart failure (CHF) symptoms such as fatigue, dyspnea, cough, rales in the lung bases, distended neck veins, weakness, dependent edema.

    Inadequate cerebral perfusion symptoms such as altered sensorium, light-headedness, dizziness or near syncope, and syncope (loss of consciousness). (Bradycardia-induced syncope is known as a *Stokes-Adams attack.*)
  - Assess for changes in mentation such as a memory lapse, confusion, and sleep disturbances.
  - In the setting of MI or serious coronary artery disease with possible sinus node dysfunction, observe the patient closely for further reduction in heart rate after the administration of opiates and nitrates. Persons with SA nodal dysfunction may not exhibit reflexive tachycardia in the presence of vasodilation or hypotension.
  - If the patient is on digitalis, beta blockers, or potassium, observe for toxicity from these agents such as excessive sinus slowing. More information on these agents is available in Chapter 11 and Chapter 6.
  - Evaluate the patient's response to vagal stimulation: straining at stool, nasopharyngeal and tracheal suctioning, or any activity that elicits the Valsalva maneuver.
  - Monitor for the presence of escape rhythms and "break-through" tachyarrhythmias, and atrioventricular block. These phenomena will be introduced in subsequent chapters.

❖ NURSING DIAGNOSIS

(1) Decreased cardiac output related to bradycardia (2) Altered tissue perfusion: cardiopulmonary/cerebral/peripheral related to low cardiac output. (3) Knowledge deficit regarding management of bradyarrhythmia or pacemaker at home.

❖ ECG DIAGNOSIS

Sinus bradycardia.

Plan and Implementation

Patient goal. The patient will maintain hemodynamic stability with adequate cardiac output and tissue perfusion and will relate appropriate information regarding pulse taking, symptoms of bradycardia and when to report them, and pacemaker management after discharge.

Nursing interventions.

- If the bradycardia is related to inadequate ventilations, open the patient's airway immediately and administer artificial respirations as needed.
- When sinus bradycardia results in hypotension and other signs and symptoms of low perfusion, and a rate of approximately 50 bpm or below the following interventions may be indicated according to hospital policy and/or physician orders:
  - Start an intravenous infusion so medications may be administered.
  - Administer oxygen as needed if not contraindicated.
  - Have atropine available at the bedside and administer it according to degree of symptomatology. For patients who have had a myocardial infarction, administer atropine with extreme caution as significant rate increases may result in dangerous arrhythmias and/or myocardial ischemia.
  - Observe for desired response and tachycardia after atropine administration.
  - Prepare for external pacing or an isoproterenol infusion if atropine is not effective (see Chapters 11 and 13).
  - If the patient has a syncopal episode (a Stokes-Adams attack), flatten the head of the bed, raise the patient's legs, and support ventilation if necessary.
  - Initiate external cardiac pacing if necessary.
- Monitor serum digoxin level and potassium concentration as ordered. Withhold digoxin dosage according to the hospital's policy regarding digoxin level or low heart rate and notify the physician of the actions taken. If serum potassium levels exceed normal, withhold potassium supplements until physician can be notified.
- Instruct the patient as necessary regarding carotid sinus hypersensitivity and the avoidance of vagal maneuvers (e.g., instruct to avoid tight collars, pressure on the neck, straining at stool, and breath-holding associated with such activities as isometric exercises).
- Teach the patient how to take own pulse, what pulse rate needs to be reported to physician, symptoms to be reported such as light-headedness and dizziness. Teach the patient with an implanted pacemaker to take own pulse and to monitor the pacemaker rhythm transtelephonically. See Chapter 13 for more home care guidelines for the pacemaker patient.
- For the patient discharged with a prescription for sublin-

gual isoproterenol, instruct about its use.

- Implement the physician's orders and evaluate the patient's response to any measures taken to correct the arrhythmia.

Evaluation

- The patient is hemodynamically stable as evidenced by the following:
  - Blood pressure within normal range for patient.
  - Warm, dry skin without cyanosis or pallor.
  - Alert sensorium.
- The patient describes the bradycardia and signs and symptoms that warrant notification of the physician.
- The patient's ECG is stable and reflects an adequately perfusing cardiac rhythm.
- The patient knows that continued monitoring for progression of the arrhythmia will be needed as long as symptoms persist.

Medical Treatment

If the patient is asymptomatic, no treatment is required. For short-term management of symptomatic bradycardia, acceleration of the heart rate with atropine, isoproterenol, or external pacing is considered appropriate. Temporary transvenous endocardial pacing is sometimes needed. For long-term management of symptomatic bradycardia, permanent pacing is often indicated.

SINOATRIAL BLOCK

Data Base: Problem Identification

Definitions, Etiology, and Mechanisms

Unlike sinus bradycardia, sinoatrial (SA) block is a disorder of impulse conduction, not formation. In other words the impulse is generated but may not emerge from the nodal region or exhibits delayed conduction to the atrial myocardium (Fig. 5-15). Because of this problem with the

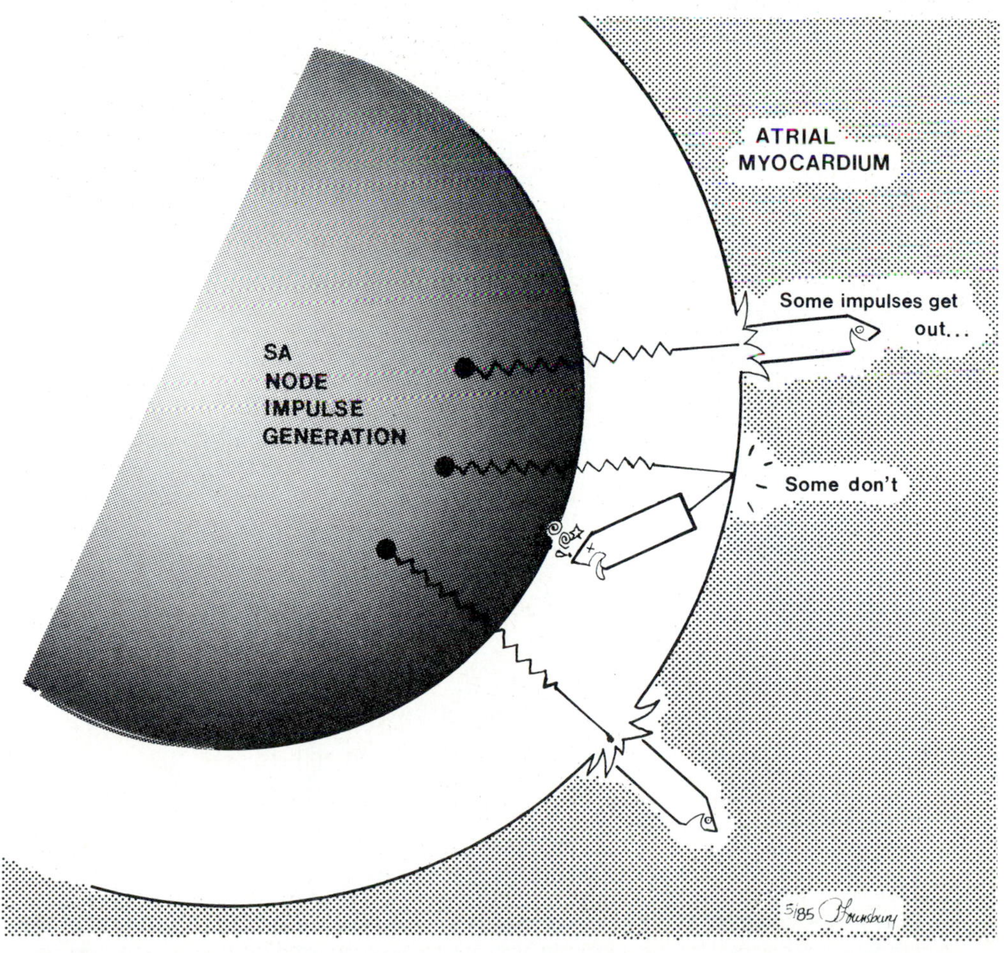

FIGURE 5-15 Sinus exit block. Impulses generated in the SA node do not all exit from the nodal region into the atrial myocardium.

exit of the impulse, the arrhythmia is a type of *exit block*. The degree of block may be incomplete or complete.[8] If the resultant slowing of the rate is great enough, subsidiary pacemakers in the AV junction or ventricles will assume control of the rhythm.

As an isolated rhythm disturbance, SA block is relatively rare.[8] It occurs in people who have sinus node disease,[1] coronary disease,[8] acute infections,[8] carotid sinus sensitivity and increased vagal tone,[8] and in patients taking procainamide,[1] digitalis,[1,8] quinidine,[8] or salicylates.[8]

ECG Characteristics

There are three degrees of SA block: first, second (incomplete), and third (complete).

First degree SA block. In first degree SA block, there is a delay in conduction from the SA node to the atrial tissue. This phenomenon cannot be visualized on the surface ECG and is only presented here for purposes of clarity.

Second degree SA block. Second degree SA block is the most common of these arrhythmias and is classified as either Type I or Type II. Both types exhibit grouped beat-

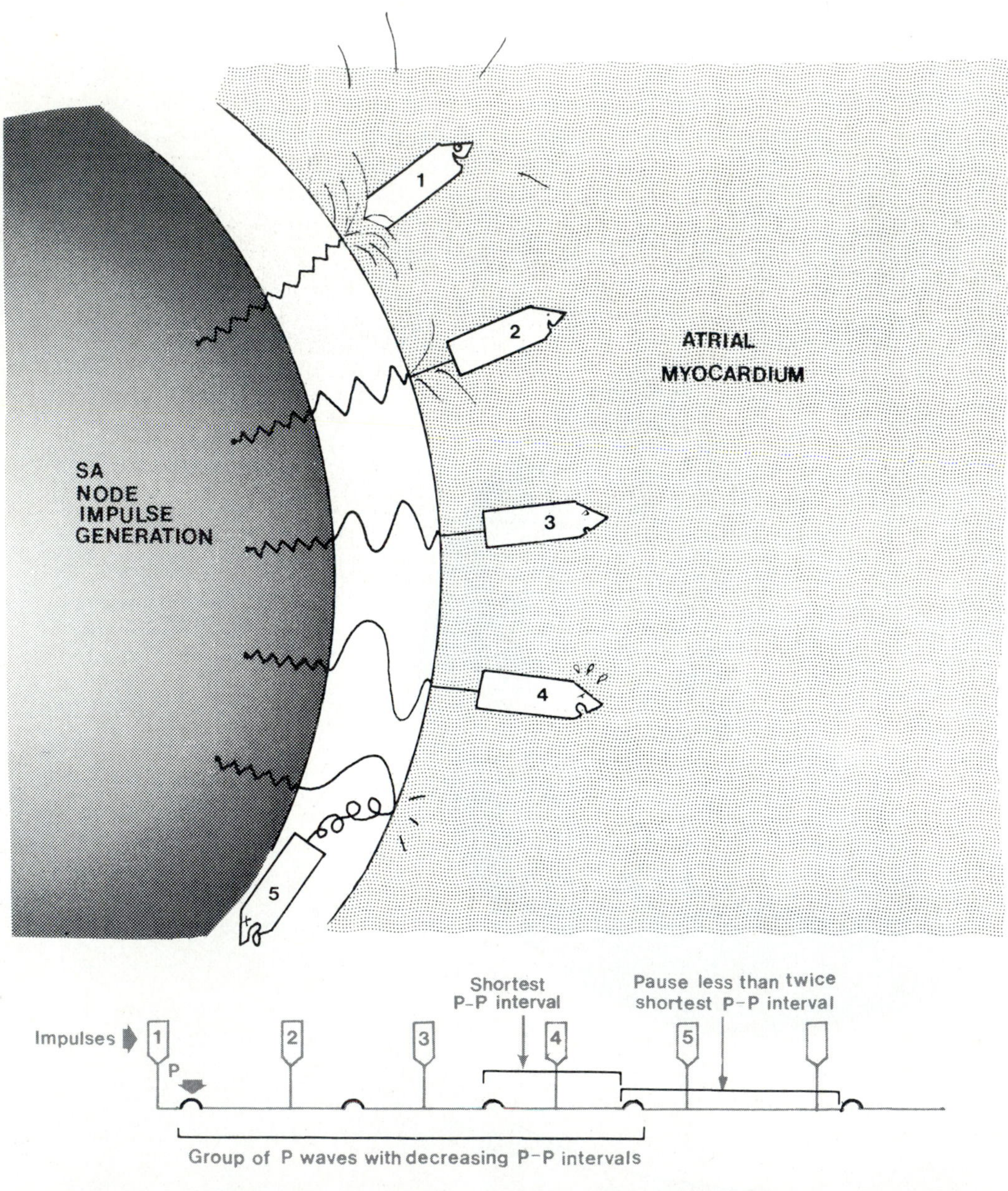

FIGURE 5-16 SA Wenckebach. Sinus impulses (not visible on the surface ECG) generated at regular intervals take increasingly longer to reach the atrial myocardium and produce P waves until one does not emerge. As the SA node impulse-to-P-wave interval lengthens, the P-to-P intervals shorten until a P wave is dropped. This results in groups of beats with the characteristic Wenckebach pattern: decreasing P-P intervals until a P wave is dropped with a pause less than twice the shortest P-P interval.

ing* but with different patterns. In Type I the impulse experiences progressively greater difficulty emerging from the node until one of the impulses does not get through at all (Fig. 5-16). This results in an ECG pattern of P-P intervals that become progressively shorter until one is absent. The longest P-P interval will be less than twice the shortest P-P interval. This periodicity, or progressive change in the length of intervals until a beat is dropped, is known as the *Wenckebach phenomenon,* and is studied again in Chapter 9 (Fig. 5-17 and the box on this page).

Type II second degree SA block also displays periodic dropping of a beat, but there is no progressive shortening of the P-P intervals. Instead, a long P-P interval occurs that is twice the duration of the normal P-P interval, or a multiple thereof. Type II is less common than Type I (Figs. 5-18 to 5-20 and the box on this page).

Third degree SA block. In third degree or complete SA block the P wave is absent, there is sinotrial arrest. No impulses are able to emerge from the SA node, and an escape rhythm (atrial, junctional, or ventricular) takes over (Fig. 5-21). Third degree SA block cannot be documented on surface electrocardiography. A sinus pause is the ECG manifestation, but one cannot be sure of the true mechanism.

*The term *grouped beating* refers to a regularly repeating pattern of beats that signifies progressive delay and block in any conduction pathway (SA or AV nodes and His-Purkinje system), or an association between regular pacemaker impulses and ectopic beats.

Applied Nursing Process

In most cases the SA blocks have slow rates. If the block produces a symptomatic rhythm the clinical assessment, nursing diagnoses, plan, and implementation are the same as for symptomatic sinus bradycardia (see pp. 98 to 101).

ECG Characteristics
Second Degree SA Block, Types I and II

Rate: Variable
Rhythm: Type I: Irregular (Wenckebach periodicity)
Type II: Irregular (with regular grouped beating)
P waves: May be normal or abnormal
P-P interval:
Type I: Irregular with Wenckebach pattern of grouped beating. P waves get closer and closer together until P wave dropped. The longest P-P interval shorter than twice the shortest.
Type II: Regular before and after dropped P wave. Dropped P wave produces a pause that is a multiple of the P-P interval.
PR Interval: Normal or prolonged and constant
QRS complex: Normal unless IVCD present

ML2 telemetry

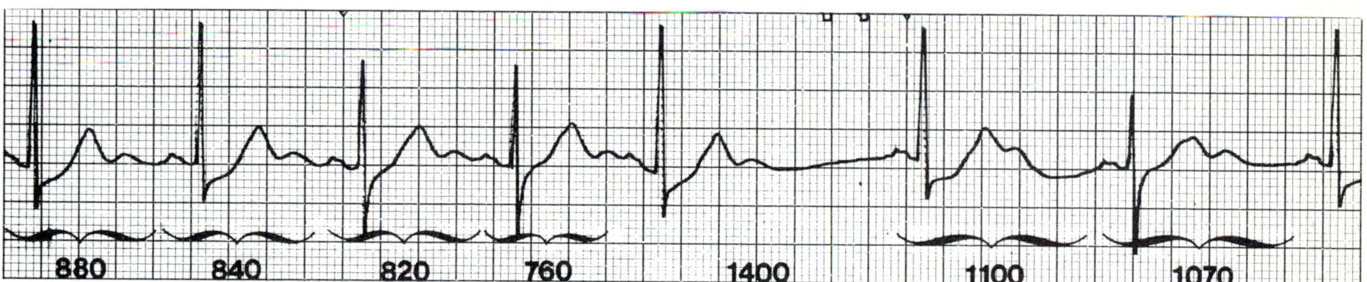

FIGURE 5-17 SA Wenckebach. P-P intervals shorten until a P wave is dropped. The longest P-P interval (1400 msec) is less than twice the shortest (760 msec).

Rate: Approximately 70 bpm
Rhythm: Irregular
P waves: Notched; P-P intervals shorten until a P wave is dropped. One P precedes each QRS complex and bears a constant relation to it.
PR interval: 0.15 seconds, constant
QRS complex: 0.07 seconds; variation in amplitude and axis; U waves present
Interpretation: SA Wenckebach (Type I second degree AV block)

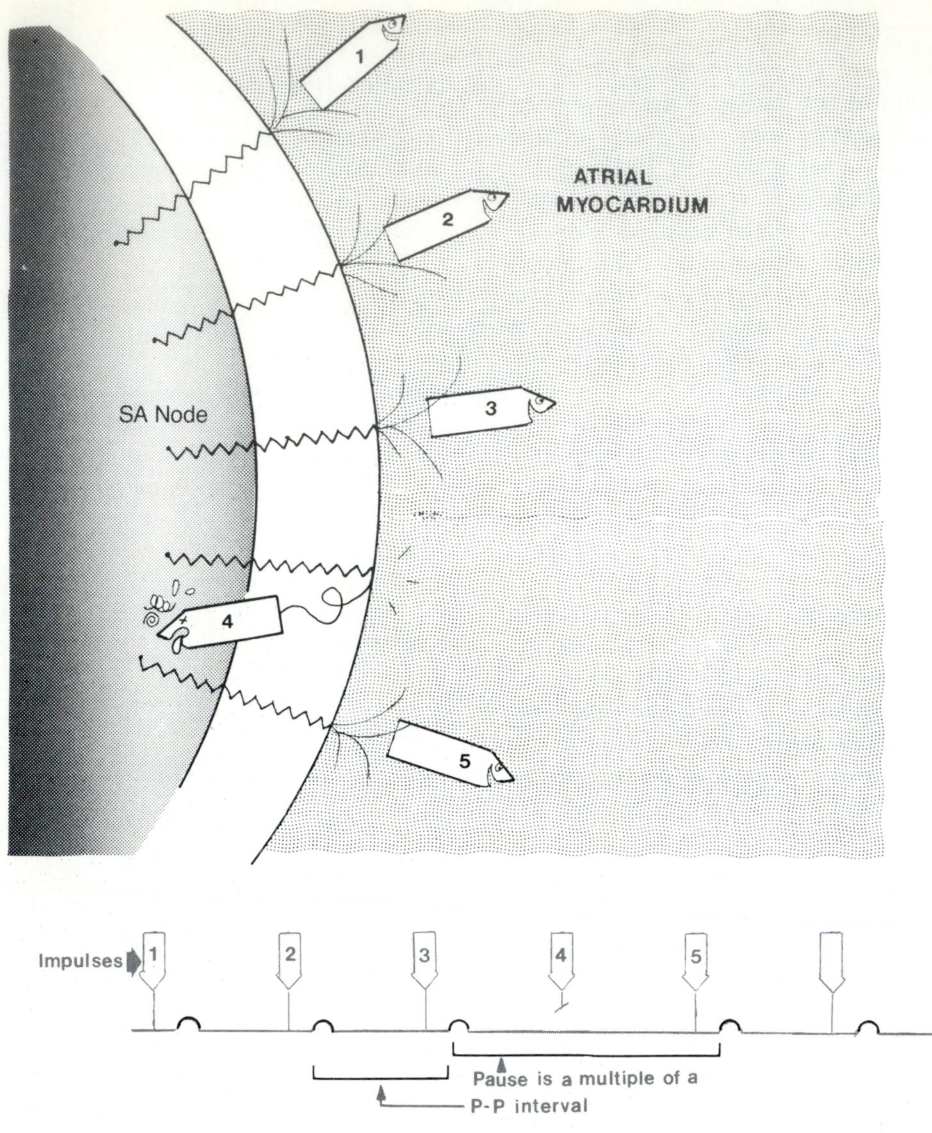

FIGURE 5-18 Type II second degree SA block. Sinus impulses (not visible on the surface ECG) generated at regular intervals do not all reach the atrial myocardium to produce P waves. P-P intervals are regular and pauses are a multiple of the P-P interval.

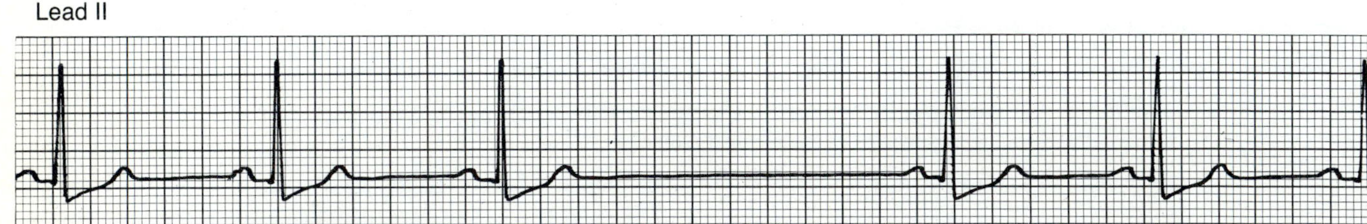

FIGURE 5-19 Sinus bradycardia with 2:1, Type II, second degree SA block. Note pause in rhythm after third complex. This pause is equal to two P-P intervals.

Rate: 50 to 54 bpm (need to count rate for full minute to consider degree to which SA block affects the overall rate per minute)

Rhythm: Irregular with a regular grouped beating pattern

P wave: Normal appearing when present. P-P interval is constant until P wave is dropped, creating a pause that is twice the normal P-P interval.

PR interval: 0.20 seconds, constant

QRS complex: 0.08 seconds

Interpretation: Sinus bradycardia with one episode of 2:1 Type I second degree SA block

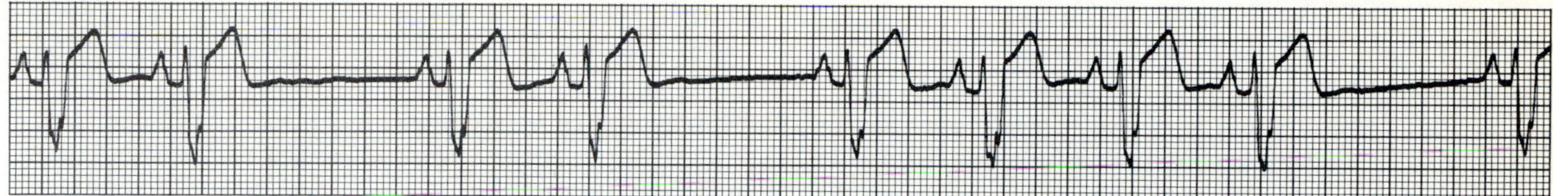

FIGURE 5-20 Second-degree, Type II SA block. This example illustrates 2:1 SA node-to-atrial conduction. Note pauses in rhythm are twice the normal P-P interval. P waves are tall and peaked. There are intraatrial and intraventricular conduction delays present.

Rate: Approximately 50 bpm (count rate for full minute in the presence of SA block)
Rhythm: Irregular with regular grouped beating
P wave: 0.10 to 0.12 seconds, intraatrial conduction delay; tall, peaked; one precedes each QRS complex and bears constant relation to QRS; long P-P intervals are twice the short P-P intervals indicating 2:1 SA block
PR interval: 0.19 seconds, constant
QRS complex: 0.16 seconds (IVCD); elevated ST segment
Interpretation: Sinus rhythm with 2:1 Type II second degree SA block, atrial conduction delay, IVCD

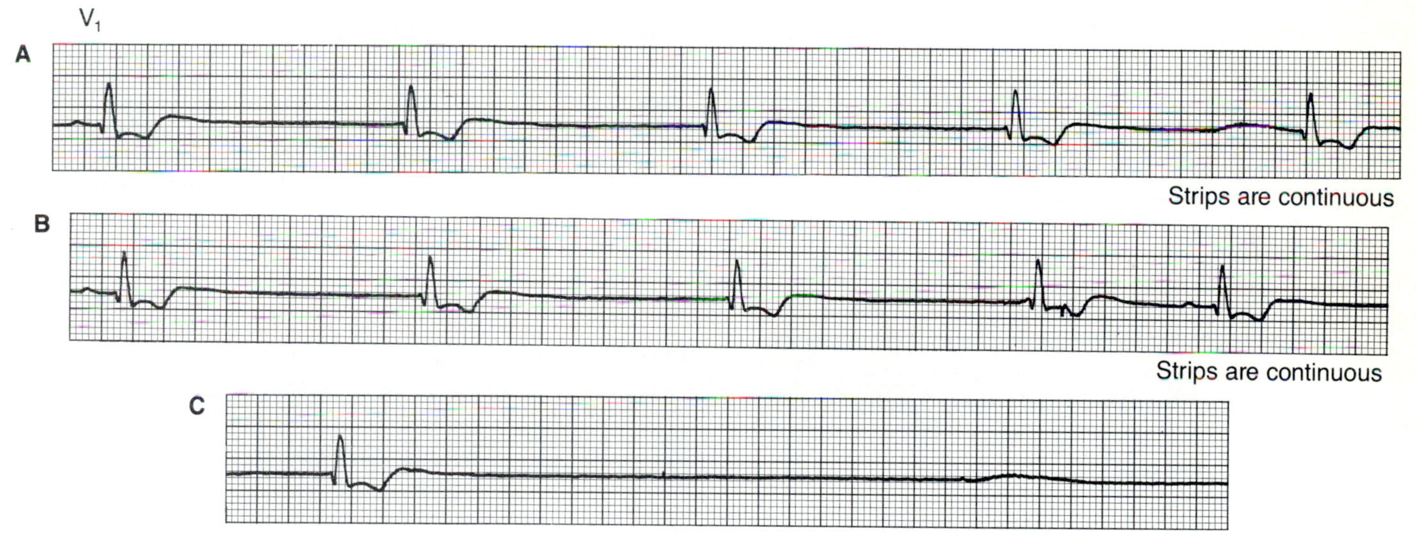

FIGURE 5-21 Sinus arrest. **A,** Note the absence of P waves in all but the first complex. Subsequent complexes are junctional escape beats. **B,** The first and last are sinus captured beats. **C,** The sinus arrest is not accompanied by an escape rhythm of any kind, resulting in asystole.

SICK SINUS SYNDROME

Data Base: Problem Identification

Definitions, Etiology, and Mechanisms

The term *sick sinus syndrome* (SSS) was introduced by Lown[31] to describe failure of the sinus node to fire properly after electrical cardioversion for atrial fibrillation. The label has since become quite popular, if not somewhat inconsistently defined, and has come to represent a constellation of sinus node disorders and abnormalities.

SSS is a disorder of SA nodal impulse formation and conduction and has one or more of the following characteristics:[16]

1. Persistent, severe, and inappropriate sinus bradycardia. The bradycardia is pathologic, not physiologic, and is the most frequently encountered of the arrhythmias comprising this syndrome.[32]
2. Periodic cessation of sinus rhythm, resulting in sinus pause, sinus arrest, and/or sinoatrial block with pos-

sible failure of nonsinus, subsidiary pacemakers.
3. Susceptibility to paroxysmal supraventricular tachycardias, including atrial fibrillation. SSS may initially present as paroxysmal atrial fibrillation.[8]
4. Prolonged suppression of sinus rhythm after electrical or spontaneous conversion of atrial fibrillation or another supraventricular tachycardia, which results in long pauses.
5. Carotid sinus hypersensitivity that may result in prolonged atrial asystole or high degree atrioventricular block.
6. The unifying pathophysiologic alteration is chronic fibrosis of the sinus node.

A clinical subset of SSS is the *bradycardia-tachycardia (brady-tachy) syndrome* in which tachyarrhythmias, often atrial fibrillation, alternate with bradycardia or bradyarrhythmias in a recurrent pattern.[33,34] The lower pacemakers may also be impaired, allowing long asystolic pauses in the absence of sinus impulses. In other words the latent pacemakers do not assume control as they normally would. Brady-tachy syndrome exhibits an array of cardiac and cerebral symptoms, with syncope possibly occurring from the asystole.

SSS may have an acute onset but typically is insidious, progressive, and chronic. A variety of fibrotic, infiltrative, and ischemic conditions may depress pacemaker activity; disease in the sinus node often indicates a conduction problem elsewhere, particularly the AV node.[9,35] Although it occurs in all age groups[8,16] (it has even been recognized in infancy[8]), it is predominantly a primary, idiopathic disorder of the elderly.[8,35] It may occur in children with congenital or acquired heart disease (including post-cardiac surgery) or without demonstrable cardiac abnormalities.[1] However, it must be pointed out that SSS in a child without underlying heart disease is quite rare. Other contributing factors are listed in the box on this page.

The prognosis in SSS is influenced by age, symptoms, prompt treatment, and complicating arrhythmias. The presence and severity of chronic diseases such as hypertension, congestive heart failure, or coronary artery disease are more important prognostic indicators. Generally, the cause of death is not due to artificial pacemaker failure or supraventricular tachycardia (SVT), but myocardial infarction, congestive heart failure, stroke, ventricular arrhythmia, or other complicating medical illnesses such as renal failure or sepsis.

ECG Characteristics

The rate of SSS tends to be slow, except during the tachycardia of brady-tachy syndrome. The rhythm may be regular or irregular. P-wave abnormalities (intraatrial conduction disturbances) are often present, and the PR intervals may be prolonged. Recall that some degree of atrioventricular block is often present in SSS.[1]

Because several arrhythmias comprise this syndrome

Etiologic Factors in Sick Sinus Syndrome

Idiopathic degenerative[8,36,37]
Coronary disease[8,34,36]
Congenital heart defects, with and without surgery[38]
Other surgical injury[8,36]
Drugs: digitalis, aerosol propellants, quinidine, beta blockers,[8,39] procainamide, disopyramide,[39] calcium ion antagonists (except nifedipine),[39] lithium,[39] methyldopa, clonidine, reserpine[39]
Metastatic disease[8,36]
Hemochromatosis[8]
Scleroderma[36]
Cardiomyopathy[8,36,38]
Thyrotoxicosis[36]
Rheumatic fever[36]
Pericarditis[36]
Muscular dystrophies[36]
Collagen disease[8,36]
Amyloidosis[9,36,37]
Sinus node artery disease in acute inferior wall myocardial infarction[40]

ECG Characteristics
Sick Sinus Syndrome

Rate: Tends to be slow: rapid if brady-tachy syndrome
Rhythm: Regular or irregular
P waves: Abnormalities often present, intraatrial conduction delay
PR interval: May be prolonged, may be variable
QRS complex: Normal unless IVCD
Associated rhythm disturbances: Sinus bradycardia
Sinus pauses
Sinus arrest (very long P-P cycle bearing no relationship to the normal P-P intervals)
Sinus arrhythmia
Sinus slowing
Sinoatrial block
Junctional/ventricular escape rhythms
Tachyarrhythmias
AV nodal block
Brady-tachy syndrome

and years may be required to establish a pattern, its course is often not predictable. One or more of the following are included in the diagnosis:

1. Sinus bradycardia.
2. Sinus slowing.
3. Sinus pauses.
4. Sinus arrest (i.e., a prolonged pause or temporary cessation of SA nodal activity; latent subsidiary pacemakers may not activate if there is distal conduction system disease).
5. Sinoatrial block, shifting sinus pacemaker.
6. Junctional, ventricular escape rhythms.
7. Intermittent tachyarrhythmias: sinus tachycardia, atrial fibrillation, atrial flutter, and other SVT.
8. Lone atrial fibrillation.
9. Brady-tachy syndrome: often several SVTs are observed. Tachycardia occurs in brief bouts, ceases, with long pause before NSR, bradyarrhythmia, or escape rhythm ensues. Alternating pattern may occur several times in a few hours.[1]

See Figs. 5-22 and 5-23 for electrocardiographic illustrations and refer to the box on p. 106 for a summary of the ECG characteristics of SSS.

Applied Nursing Process

Clinical Assessment

- Detect:
  - A rapid, slow, or changing pulse rate.
  - An irregular, rapid, slow, or changing pattern in the ECG with the possibility of several different arrhythmias.
- Assess the patient and ECG. Many patients, especially if they are older and are admitted to the hospital with symptoms of altered cerebral function or syncope, will have complete neurologic and thyroid evaluations before

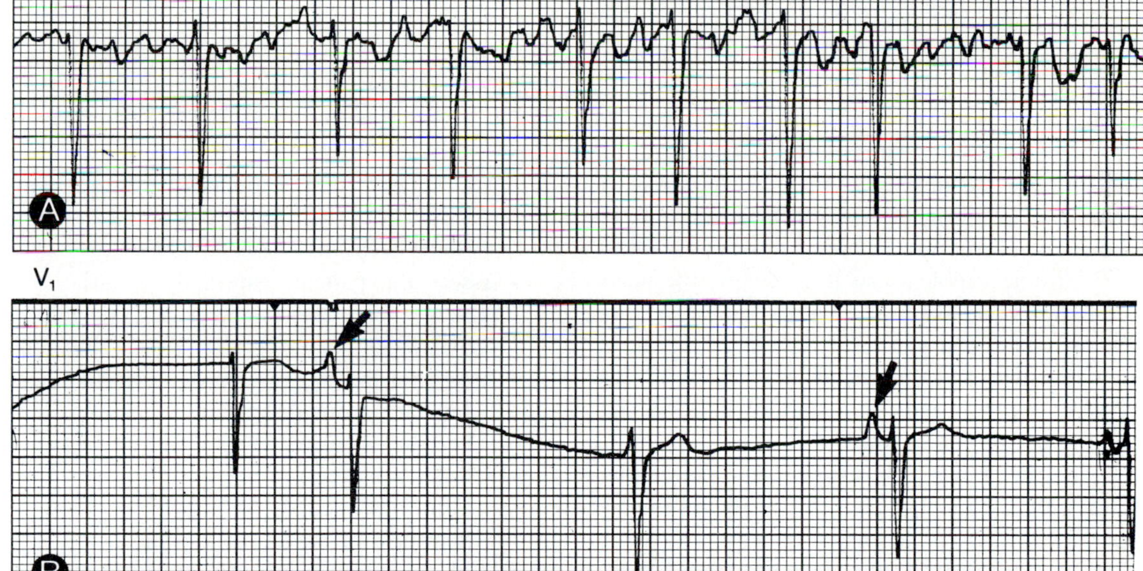

FIGURE 5-22 Sick sinus syndrome (SSS). This 87-year-old male patient was admitted to the hospital for syncopal episodes. **A,** Long periods of atrial fibrillation were interrupted by periods of sinus arrest. **B,** The second strip shows a sinus arrest with junctional escape beats and 2 beats preceded by P waves *(arrows)*. This type of SSS would be classified as a tachy-brady syndrome.

Rate: Atrial: **A,** Too rapid and chaotic to count
B, Approximately 30 bpm
Ventricular: **A,** Approximately 100 bpm
B, Approximately 40 bpm

Rhythm: Irregular

P waves: **A,** Chaotic appearing. **B,** Peaked, irregular, slow; not every QRS is preceded by a P wave

PR interval: 0.13 seconds when present

QRS complex: 0.08 seconds in B, first and third QRS complexes are junctional escape beats.

Interpretation: **A,** Atrial fibrillation, coarse. **B,** Periods of sinus arrest or pauses interrupted by junctional escape beats

Overall impression: brady-tachy syndrome

Lead II

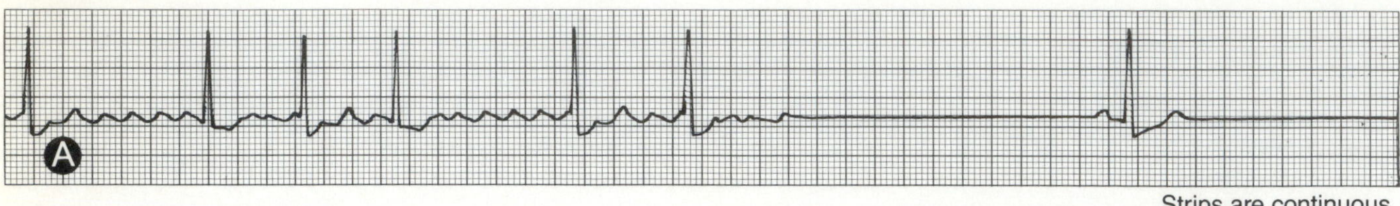

Strips are continuous

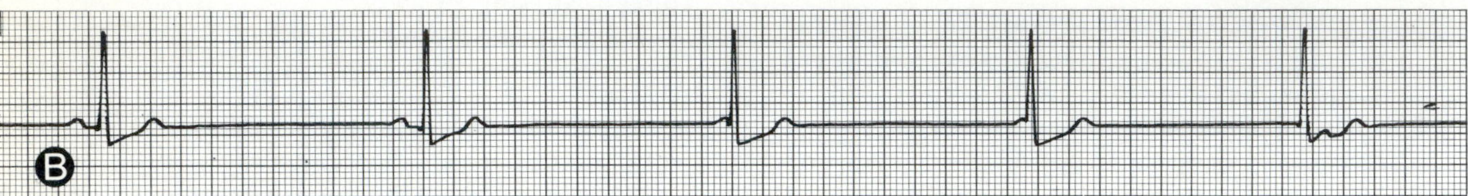

FIGURE 5-23 Sick sinus syndrome (SSS). Atrial flutter/fibrillation alternating with periods of marked sinus bradycardia. Note third QRS complex in strip B initiates a run of slow idiojunctional rhythm (explained in Chapter 7).

Rate: Atrial: Very fast (300+ bpm) initially and slowing to bradycardic rate of 28 bpm

Ventricular: 70 to 80 bpm initially and slowing to 28 bpm

P waves: Initially appear fast and chaotic, suddenly stop and beat at a very slow rate. They do not bear a constant relation to the QRS complex.

PR interval: 0.18 seconds when present in last complex in *A* and first two complexes in *B*

QRS complex: 0.09 seconds

Interpretation: Atrial fibrillation suddenly terminating into a marked sinus bradycardia usurped by a junctional rhythm

Overall impression: brady-tachy syndrome

a diagnosis of SSS is confirmed. Remember to approach your assessment with attention to cerebral, as well as cardiac, changes. Also consider how the patient is tolerating other chronic problems such as congestive heart failure, coronary artery disease, or renal failure. It may be difficult to establish a pattern if the complaints have followed a transient and chronic course. There is increased risk of cerebral and other emboli[1] in SSS, and this possibility should be included in your assessment.

- Monitor and document all arrhythmias, correlating symptoms with rhythm changes. This is always important, but especially so in caring for patients with sinus node disease. This careful documentation helps to establish a relationship between symptoms and rhythm and a clearer clinical picture.
- Assess for additional signs of sinus node depression (e.g., does the heart rate respond appropriately to fever, pain, anxiety?).
- Assess and document all cerebral manifestations: emotional lability, memory lapses, personality change, irritability, lassitude, nocturnal wakefulness, other sleep disturbances, difficulty concentrating, disorientation, impaired judgment, apathy, and paresis.
- Assess and document any cardiovascular manifestations of sinus node dysfunction and reduced cardiac output.
  Dizziness, light-headedness, syncope, and fatigue.
  Palpitations and changes in anginal pattern.
  Blood pressure.
- Assess the patient, especially if atrial fibrillation is present, for manifestations of systemic emboli or stroke, since there is greater risk in this population.[1]
- Assess for the progression of congestive heart failure.
  Jugular venous distension.
  Peripheral edema.
  Rales in lungs.
  Third heart sound.
  Shortness of breath, orthopnea.
- Look for possible adverse drug effects from digitalis, antiarrhythmics, beta blockers (including timolol eye drops), calcium ion antagonists, and antihypertensives.

❖ NURSING DIAGNOSIS

(1) Decreased cardiac output related to bradycardia, tachycardia, and/or loss of atrial contribution to cardiac output. (2) Altered tissue perfusion: cardiopulmonary/cerebral/peripheral related to decreased cardiac output. (3) Knowledge deficit regarding home management of arrhythmia and/or pacemaker.

❖ ECG DIAGNOSIS

Sick sinus syndrome.

Plan and Implementation

Patient goal. The patient's hemodynamic status will remain stable; the patient's heart rate will stabilize within normal range with treatment. The patient will relate appropriate information regarding symptoms that warrant notifying the physician and guidelines for pacemaker care at home. The patient will know how to avoid vagal maneuvers that trigger symptoms in those without a pacemaker.

Nursing interventions.

- Report all cerebral and cardiovascular manifestations of low cardiac output to the physician.
- Evaluate the functioning of the pacemaker and the patient's understanding of it as needed. Refer to sections on sinus bradycardia, Chapter 13, and selected references[41,42] for specific interventions.
- Implement physician's orders and evaluate patient response to measures taken to stabilize the rate. If the patient's tachycardia is treated with antiarrhythmics, note any worsening or exacerbation of bradyarrhythmias (if there is no artificial pacemaker).
- Complete patient teaching as appropriate before discharge. Topics might include permanent pacemaker, drug therapy (digoxin, anticoagulants, antiarrhythmics), activity restrictions, avoidance of vagal maneuvers, and/or carotid sinus hypersensitivity.
- Monitor the patient's behaviors and adaptive status over time because the course of SSS is often chronic and unpredictable; arrange for follow-up evaluations.

Evaluation

- The patient maintains hemodynamic stability as evidenced by the following indicators:
  - Stable blood pressure.
  - No change in sensorium.
  - Warm, dry skin without cyanosis or pallor.
- The patient's heart rate stabilizes after treatment (pacemaker) as evidenced by the following:
  - Heart rate at the prescribed rate.
  - Strong, peripheral pulses without pulse deficit.
- The patient manages own care with pacemaker after discharge as evidenced by the following:
  - Ability to state heart rate ranges indicative of proper pacemaker function.
  - Ability to measure own pulse.
  - Listing symptoms that warrant physician notification.
  - Ability to relate other information concerning individual situation.

Medical Treatment

- If the patient is asymptomatic, no treatment is indicated.[34]
- Reversible causes, such as drugs, are eliminated.
- Electrical cardioversion is generally contraindicated or should be done with great caution.
- The chronic, underlying cause is controlled.
- Permanent artificial pacing for symptomatic SSS is frequently indicated. Sinus node dysfunction is the most common indication for permanent pacemaker implantation.[36] Pacing is also used in children.[38]
- Drug therapy may be indicated for the tachycardia (often atrial fibrillation) of brady-tachy syndrome. Artificial pacing and digitalis are sometimes added to this regimen, and the combination therapy helps to prevent complications of bradyarrhythmias.[34] Pacing may also be necessary if digitalis is used for control of congestive heart failure.[34]
- Warfarin anticoagulation (for atrial fibrillation) may be indicated in selected patients. (Refer to discussion on atrial fibrillation in this chapter.)

REFERENCES

1. Zipes DP. Specific arrhythmias: diagnosis and treatment. *In* Braunwald E (ed). *Heart Disease: A Textbook of Cardiovascular Medicine*. 3rd ed. Philadelphia: WB Saunders, 1988.
2. Dhingra RC. Sinus node dysfunction. *PACE*, Sept., 1983, 6(5): 1062-9.
3. Swiryn S, McDonough T, Hueter DC. Sinus node function and dysfunction. *Med. Clin. North Am.*, Jul., 1984, 68(4): 935-54.
4. Clarke JM, Shelton JR, Hamer J, Taylor S, Venning JR. The rhythm of the normal human heart. *Lancet*, Sept. 4, 1976, 2(7984): 508-12.
5. Fleg JL, Kennedy HL. Cardiac arrhythmias in a healthy elderly population: detection by 24-hour ambulatory electrocardiography. *Chest*, Mar., 1982, 81(3): 302-7.
6. Sobotka PA, Mayer JH, Bauernfeind RA, Kanakis C, Rosen KM. Arrhythmias documented by 24-hour continuous ambulatory electrocardiographic monitoring in young women without apparent heart disease. *Am. Heart J.*, Jun., 1981, 101(6): 753-9.
7. Vinsant M, Spence MI. *Commonsense Approach To Coronary Care: A Program*. 5th ed. St. Louis: The CV Mosby Co., 1989.
8. Marriott HJL. *Practical Electrocardiography*. 8th ed. Baltimore: Williams & Wilkins, 1988.
9. Schamroth L. *The Disorders of Cardiac Rhythm*. Vol. I, 2nd ed. London: Blackwell Scientific Publications, 1981.
10. Goldman MJ. *Clinical Electrocardiography*. 12th ed. Los Altos, CA: Lange Medical Publications, 1986.
11. Fowler NO. *Cardiac Diagnosis and Treatment*. 3rd ed. Hagerstown, MD: Harper & Row, 1980.
12. Andreoli KG, Fowkes VK, Zipes DP, Wallace AG (eds). *Comprehensive Cardiac Care*. 5th ed. St. Louis: The CV Mosby Co., 1983.
13. Hindman MC, Wagner GS. Arrhythmias during myocardial infarction: mechanisms, significance, and therapy. *In* Castellanos A (ed). *Cardiac Arrhythmias: Mechanisms and Management*. Brest AN (ed). *Cardiovascular Clinics*. Philadelphia: FA Davis, Nov. 1, 1980.
14. McIntyre KM, Lewis AJ, Parker MR, Paraskos JA. Myocardial infarction. *In* McIntyre KM, Lewis AJ (eds). *Textbook of Advanced Cardiac Life Support*. Dallas: American Heart Association, 1981.
15. *Textbook of Advanced Cardiac Life Support*. Dallas: American Heart Association, 1987.
16. Dreifus LS, Michelson EL, Kaplinsky E. Bradyarrhythmias: clinical significance and management. *J. Am. Coll. Cardiol.*, Jan., 1983, 1(1): 327-38.
17. Zehender M, Meinertz T, Keul J, Just H. ECG variants and cardiac arrhythmias in athletes: Clinical relevance and prognostic importance. *Am. Heart J.*, Jun., 1990, 119(6): 1378-91.

18. Gillette PC. Cardiac dysrhythmias in infants and children. *In* Engle MA (ed). *Pediatric Cardiovascular Disease*. Brest AN (ed). *Cardiovascular Clinics*, 11/2. Philadelphia: FA Davis, 1981.
19. George M, Greenwood TW. Relation between bradycardia and the site of myocardial infarction. *Lancet*, Oct. 7, 1967, 2(7519): 739-40.
20. Lie KI, Durrer D. Common arrhythmias in acute myocardial infarction. *In* Castellanos A (ed). *Cardiac Arrhythmias: Mechanisms and Management*. Brest AN (ed). *Cardiovascular Clinics*, 11/1. Philadelphia: FA Davis, 1980.
21. Sarachek NS, Leonard JJ. Familial heart block and sinus bradycardia: classification and natural history. *Am. J. Cardiol.*, April, 1972, 29(4): 451-8.
22. Marks P, Thurston JGB. Sinus bradycardia with hiatus hernia. *Am. Heart J.*, Jan., 1977, 93(1): 30-2.
23. Goldreyer BN, Wyman MG. The effects of first hour hospitalization in myocardial infarction (Abstract). Circ., Oct., 1974, 49, 50 (Suppl. III): 121.
24. Rose RM, Lewis AJ, Fewkes J, Clifton JF, Criley JM. Occurrence of arrhythmias during the first hour in acute MI (Abstract). *Circ.*, Oct., 1974, 49, 50 (Suppl. III): 121.
25. Lie KI, Wellens HJJ, Downar E, Durrer D. Observations on patients with primary ventricular fibrillation complicating acute myocardial infarction. *Circ.*, Nov., 1975, 52(11): 755-9.
26. Norris RM, Mercer CJ, Yeates SE. Sinus rate in acute myocardial infarction. *Br. Heart J.*, Sept., 1972, 34(9): 901-4.
27. Epstein SE, Goldstein RE, Redwood DR, Kent KM, Smith ER. The early phase of acute myocardial infarction: pharmacologic aspects of therapy. *Ann. Intern Med.*, June, 1973, 78(6): 918-36.
28. Heinz G, Ohner T, Laufer G, Gasic S, Laczkovics A. Clinical and electrophysiologic correlates of sinus node dysfunction after orthotopic heart transplantation. Observations in 42 patients. *Chest*, Apr., 1990, 97(4): 890-5.
29. Jacquet L, Ziady G, Stein K, Griffith B, Armitage J, Hardesty R, Kormos R. Cardiac rhythm disturbances early after orthotopic heart transplantation: prevalence and clinical importance of the observed abnormalities. *J. Am. Coll. Cardiol.*, Oct., 1990, 16(4): 832-7.
30. DiBiase A, Tse T, Schnittger I, Wexler L, Stinson EB, Valantine HA. Frequency and mechanism of bradycardia in cardiac transplant recipients and need for pacemakers. *Am. J. Cardiol.*, Jun. 15, 1991, 67: 1385-9.
31. Lown B. Electrical reversion of cardiac arrhythmias. *Br. Heart J.*, Jul., 1967, 29: 469-89.
32. Kienzle MG, Doherty JU, Marcus NH, Josephson ME. When do electrophysiologic studies benefit arrhythmia patients? *J. Cardiovasc. Med.*, Jan., 1984, pp. 41-55.
33. Rubenstein JJ, Schulman CL, Yurchak PM, DeSanctis RW. Clinical spectrum of the sick sinus syndrome. *Circ.*, Jul., 1972, 46(1): 5-13.
34. Moss AJ, Davis RJ. Brady-tachy syndrome. *Prog. Cardiovasc. Dis.*, 1974, 16(4): 439-54.
35. Nieminski KE, Kay RH, Rubin DA. Current concepts and management of the sick sinus syndrome. *Heart & Lung*, Nov., 1984, 13(6): 675-81.
36. Gaffney BJ, Wasserman AG, Rotsztain A, Rios JC. Sick sinus syndrome: mechanisms and management. *In* Castellanos A (ed). *Cardiac Arrhythmias: Mechanisms and Management*. Brest AN (ed). *Cardiovascular Clinics*, 11/1. Philadelphia: FA Davis, 1980.
37. Evans R, Shaw DB. Pathological studies in sino-atrial disorder (sick sinus syndrome). *Br. Heart J.*, Jul., 1977, 39(7): 778-86.
38. Gillette PC, Shannon C, Garson A, Porter CJ, Ott D, Cooley DA, McNamara DG. Pacemaker treatment of sick sinus syndrome in children. *J. Am. Coll. Cardiol.*, May, 1983, 1(5): 1325-9.
39. Fenster PE, Kern KB. Office-based management of sinus node disease. *Cardiovasc. Med.*, Apr., 1985, 10(4): 21-3.
40. Alboni P, Baggioni GF, Scarfo S, Cappato R, Percoco GF, Paparella N, Antonioli GE. Role of sinus node artery disease in sick sinus syndrome in inferior wall acute myocardial infarction. *Am. J. Cardiol.*, Jun. 1, 1991, 67: 1180-4.
41. Frye SJ, Yacone LA. Cardiac pacing: a nursing perspective. *In* Hakki A-H (ed). *Ideal Cardiac Pacing. Major Problems in Clinical Surgery*, Vol. 31. Philadelphia: WB Saunders, 1984.
42. Purcell JA, Burrows SG. A pacemaker primer. *Am. J. Nurs.*, May, 1985, 85(5): 553-68.

SELF-ASSESSMENT

MULTIPLE CHOICE

Directions

For each of the questions below, select the correct answer(s) from the choices given. If more than one answer is offered, mark all that are correct.

Examples

The sinus rhythms include those cardiac rhythms and arrhythmias that originate in the

*a. SA node.
b. AV node.
c. Purkinje fibers.
d. bundle of His.

Examples of sinus rhythm disturbances include

*a. sinus tachycardia.
b. atrial fibrillation.
*c. sinus bradycardia.
d. ventricular tachycardia.

1. ECG values of normal sinus rhythm include a
   a. rate of 50 bpm in the adult.
   b. rate of 60 bpm in the adult.
   c. rate of 110 bpm in a 6-month-old baby.
   d. PR interval of 0.06 seconds.

2. Sam, a healthy 42-year-old physician, has normal sinus rhythm with a heart rate of 62 bpm at rest. When he sleeps, his heart rate is as low as 50 bpm and during exercise as high as 170 bpm. Of the statements below, which best describes Sam's heart rate variations?
   a. The heart rate varies from sinus bradycardia to sinus tachycardia, and the rate ranges would be considered extreme, and likely to be due to pathologic sinus node disease.
   b. The heart rate varies from sinus bradycardia to sinus tachycardia. Although the variations in rate may not be pathologic, it is doubtful they are normal.
   c. The heart rate variations of 50 to 170 bpm are well within the range of normal sinus rhythm.
   d. The heart rate range from sinus tachycardia to sinus bradycardia is physiologic, a normal response to exercise and rest.

3. Sinus arrhythmia is characterized by
   a. phasic rate variations in heart rate from below 60 to above 100 bpm.
   b. phasic variations in the rhythm. The rhythm waxes and wanes, gradually increasing and decreasing in rate.
   c. an irregular rhythm that, in its most common form, increases in rate with inspiration and decreases with expiration.
   d. an irregularity in the rhythm that is not affected by such things as respirations and temperature.

4. The ECG features of sinus tachycardia include
   a. a regular heart rate of 100 to 150 bpm (or more with exercise), a P wave that precedes each QRS that is upright in leads II, III, and aVF, and a PR interval of 0.12 to 0.20 seconds.
   b. a regular heart rate of 150 to 200 bpm (higher with exercise), a P wave preceding each QRS that is upright in lead aVR, and a PR interval of 0.06 to 0.12 seconds.
   c. an irregular rhythm with a rate of 100 to 150 bpm with an upright P wave in the inferior leads that precedes each QRS complex with a PR interval of 0.16 to 0.20 seconds.

5. Nursing interventions for the patient with sinus tachycardia include which of the following?
   a. Administer atropine 0.5 mg followed by an intravenous infusion of isoproterenol.
   b. No interventions are indicated for sinus tachycardia.
   c. Remove, or reduce, the underlying cause such as fever, pain, or anxiety.
   d. Notify the physician in the setting of acute myocardial infarction.

6. The incidence of sinus bradycardia is correlated with which of the following clinical settings?
   a. Occlusion of the right coronary artery resulting in an inferior myocardial infarction.
   b. Occlusion of the left anterior descending coronary artery resulting in an anterior myocardial infarction.
   c. Excess vagal tone.
   d. Hypokalemia.
   e. Inadequate ventilation.
   f. Cardiac transplantation.

7. For the patient with sinus bradycardia who is symptomatic, appropriate nursing interventions might include
   a. administration of an intravenous beta blocker such as propranolol.
   b. ventilatory support.
   c. administration of intravenous atropine.
   d. vagal stimulation such as carotid sinus massage.

8. Which criterion below is most important in deciding when sinus bradycardia should be treated?
   a. Whether the patient is symptomatic from the bradycardia.
   b. The rate; if the rate is below 50 bpm, it should be treated.
   c. Ventilatory status; if the bradycardia is due to inadequate ventilations, atropine is indicated.

9. Which statement best compares or contrasts the mechanisms of sinus bradycardia and sinus block?
   a. Sinus bradycardia and sinus block are both disorders of impulse conduction.
   b. Both sinus bradycardia and sinus block are disorders of impulse formation.
   c. Both sinus bradycardia and sinus block may be disorders of either impulse formation or conduction depending on the clinical situation.
   d. Sinus block is a disorder of conduction whereas sinus bradycardia is usually a disorder of impulse formation.

10. Type II SA block produces pauses in the ECG that
    a. are multiples of the P-P interval.
    b. are not multiples of the P-P interval.
    c. are less than twice the shortest P-P interval.
    d. vary with respirations.

11. SSS may include one or more of which of the following?
    a. Heart rate increase above 150 bpm with exercise.
    b. Persistent, severe, and inappropriate sinus bradycardia.
    c. Periodic cessation of sinus rhythm.
    d. Susceptibility to paroxysmal supraventricular tachycardias.

12. A common medical treatment for SSS is
    a. carotid sinus stimulation.
    b. excision of the sinus node.
    c. a permanent transvenous pacemaker.
    d. continued observation; no treatment is usually necessary.

MATCHING

Example

Directions

Match each sinus rhythm in column B with its rate range in column A.

A	B
(B) 1. 60 to 100 bpm	A. Sinus tachycardia
(A) 2. 100 to 150 bpm	B. Normal sinus rhythm
(C) 3. <60 bpm	C. Sinus bradycardia

Directions

Match each sinus rhythm in column B with the clinical setting in column A. Choices in column B may be used more than once.

A	B
( ) 13. Normally present in children	A. Sinus tachycardia
( ) 14. Usually accompanies sleep in the athlete	B. Sinus arrhythmia
( ) 15. Is a normal response to exercise	C. Sinus bradycardia
( ) 16. Accompanies fever	D. Sinus block
( ) 17. Is usually indicative of sinus node disease	E. Sick sinus syndrome
( ) 18. Often accompanies acute inferior myocardial infarction	
( ) 19. Often accompanies congestive heart failure	

TRUE/FALSE

Directions

Determine whether each of the following statements is true or false and indicate with a *T* or *F*.

Example

(T) 1. Normal sinus rhythm is the normal rhythm of the heart.

( ) 20. A normal heart rate for a sleeping newborn is 60 bpm.
( ) 21. The normal sinus rate for a newborn ranges from 80 to 160 bpm.
( ) 22. Nonrespiratory sinus arrhythmia is a normal finding.
( ) 23. SA block is a rhythm that often occurs in the trained athlete.
( ) 24. Type II SA block is characterized by progressive shortening of the P-P interval until a P wave is dropped.

SHORT ANSWER

The remaining questions involve analysis of patient situations and assessment of rhythm strips. Responses required are short answer and essay.

CASE: *JT is a 45-year-old male patient who has greater than 40% body surface area second and third degree burns. He is septic. His rhythm strip is displayed here:*

25. Interpret the rhythm using the standard form suggested for arrhythmia interpretation.
26. Based on what limited information you have about JT's clinical picture, would you interpret his arrhythmia as physiologic or pathologic?
27. Delineate assessment measures and nursing interventions that might be indicated for JT.
28. What factors would you consider in determining the clinical significance of JT's arrhythmia?

Lead II

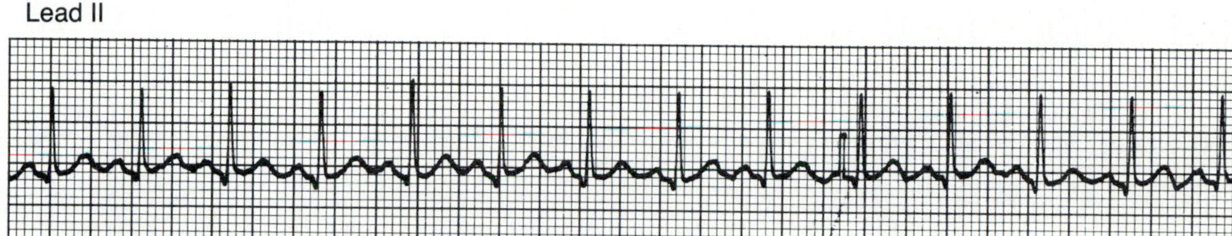

CASE: *Mrs. K, a 62-year-old patient on the surgical unit, is recovering from hip surgery. She had a myocardial infarction 4 years ago and is still bothered by occasional episodes of angina pectoris. Her rhythm strip is displayed here:*

29. Interpret the rhythm and identify any values that are not within normal limits.

V_1

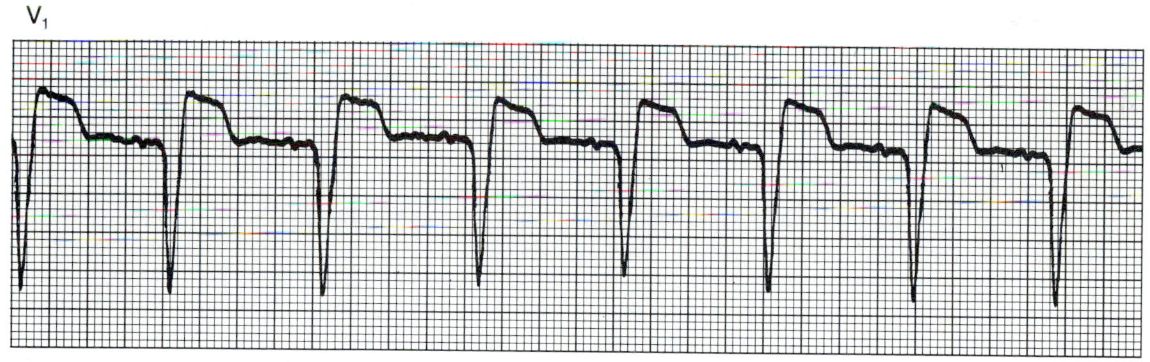

CASE: *Mr. L, 54, is hospitalized on the medical unit for a cerebrovascular accident. He is on telemetry. His rhythm is presented here for analysis.*

30. Analyze the rhythm.

Lead II

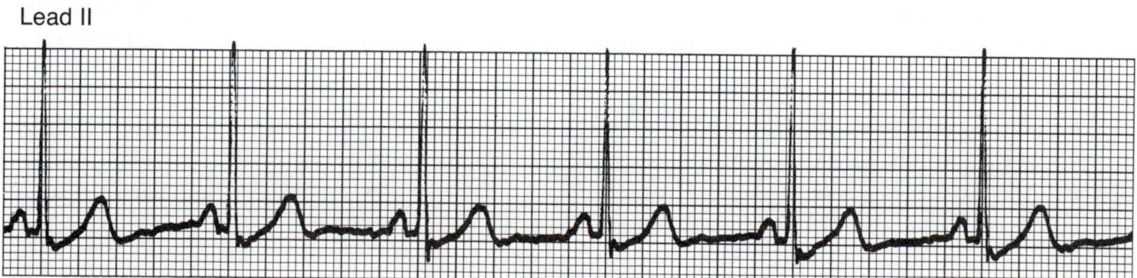

CASE: *Michael is a 16-month-old child in the pediatric intensive care unit with meningitis. During the evening, his high rate alarm sounded, recording a heart rate of 271. His nurse, noting the digital display on the central station, reset the alarm and checked on Michael at the bedside.*

31. Analyze Michael's rhythm.
32. Discuss discrepancies in your findings and the digital display on the monitor. How might you intervene to correct the situation?

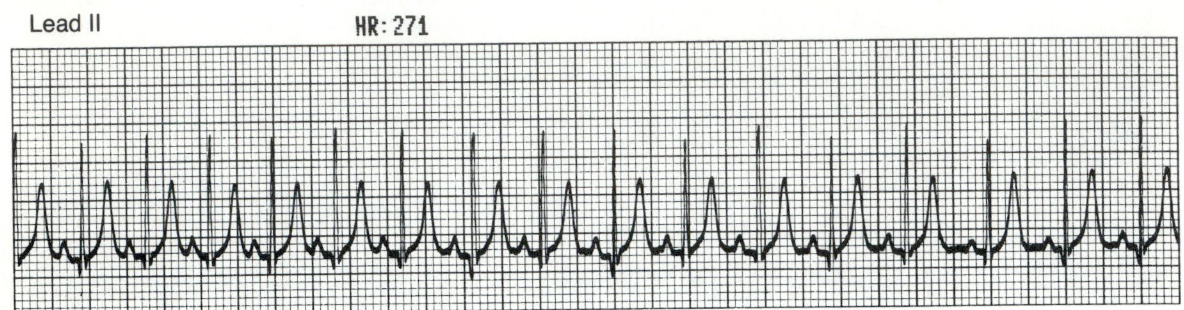

CASE: *This rhythm strip belongs to a 22-year-old female. Variations in the heart rate seem to correlate with respirations.*

33. Analyze the rhythm.
34. Is this a physiologic or pathologic arrhythmia?

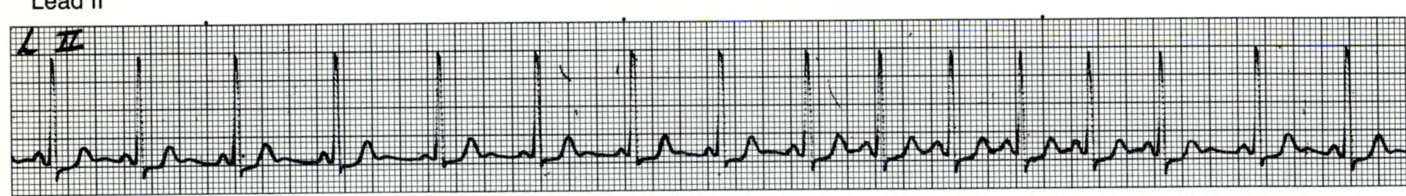

CASE: *Roger B, 66 years old, presented to the emergency room with complaints of severe retrosternal chest pain with radiation to the neck, both shoulders, and left arm. He is pale and diaphoretic with a blood pressure of 106/72. He also appears short of breath and is unable to lie down. The emergency department nurse attaches him to the monitor and obtains this rhythm strip.*

35. Interpret the rhythm.
36. Besides the assessment measures taken above, what others would be appropriate for Mr. B?
37. Describe nursing interventions appropriate for Mr. B in this clinical setting.

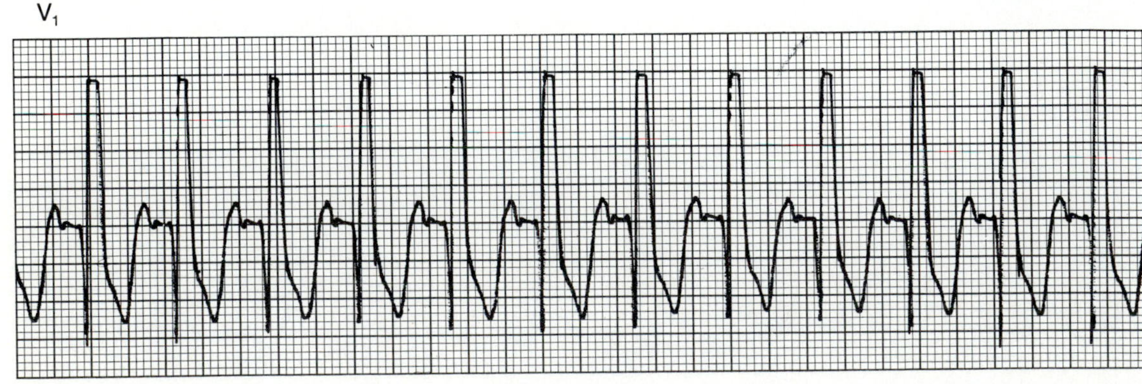

CASE: *Mrs. T. is hospitalized for evaluation of her complaints of light-headedness and a syncopal episode. Her rhythm strip is displayed here.*

38. Analyze the rhythm.
39. In order of priority, list assessment measures and nursing interventions.
40. How might this arrhythmia be treated medically? What factors will your patient teaching plan include for this medical therapy?
41. Compare the mechanism of this arrhythmia with that of sinus bradycardia and explain the term *exit block.*
42. Define syncope.

Lead II

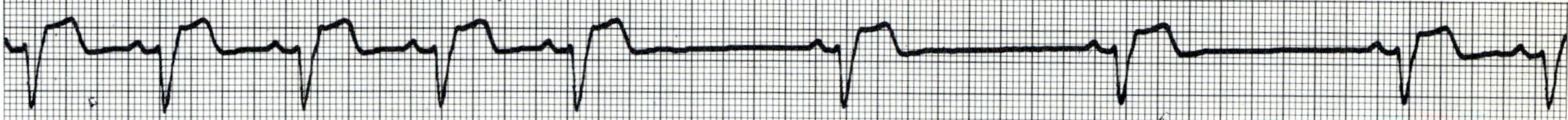

ANSWERS TO SELF-ASSESSMENT

1. b, c
2. d
3. b, c
4. a
5. c, d
6. a, c, e, f
7. b, c
8. a
9. d
10. a
11. b, c, d
12. c

13. B
14. C
15. A
16. A
17. D, E
18. C
19. A

20. F
21. T
22. F
23. F
24. F

25. *Rate:* 136 bpm
    Rhythm: Regular
    P waves: Normal
    PR interval: 0.12 to 0.14 seconds, normal
    QRS complex: qR complex measuring 0.06 seconds, normal
    Interpretation: Sinus tachycardia
26. JT's sinus tachycardia is due to extracardiac factors and is a physiologic response to the burn and infection.
27. Assess temperature, hydration, body weight, blood pressure, peripheral pulses, color of healthy skin and mucous membranes, mentation, and pain level.
    Nursing interventions would include measures directed at correcting the underlying cause, such as reducing fever, if present, preventing shivering, maintaining adequate hydration, and controlling pain.
28. Consider how well the patient is tolerating the tachycardia. If the blood pressure, peripheral pulses, mentation, and color are within normal limits and there are no signs of congestive heart failure, the patient is probably tolerating the tachycardia. In this situation the sepsis and burn are clinically significant, resulting in the tachycardia.
29. *Rate:* 74 to 80 bpm
    Rhythm: Regular
    P waves: Diphasic, normal for V_1
    PR interval: 0.16 seconds, normal
    QRS complex: Qr complex, normal initial r wave is absent, 0.13 seconds, too wide; elevated ST segment
    Interpretation: NSR with IVCD. Elevated ST segment is secondary to IVCD (see Chapter 9).
30. *Rate:* 60 bpm
    Rhythm: Regular
    P waves: Normal for lead II
    PR interval: 0.14 to 0.15 seconds, normal
    QRS complex: Rs complex, normal for lead II
    Interpretation: NSR
31. *Rate:* 150 to 158 bpm
    Rhythm: Regular
    P waves: Normal for lead II
    PR interval: 0.10 to 0.12 seconds, normal for a baby with a heart rate that fast
    QRS complex: qRs complex, 0.05 seconds, normal
    Interpretation: Sinus tachycardia
32. The rate meter indicates the heart rate is 271 bpm. This is an erroneous reading probably due to registering of some of the tall T waves. The situation could be remedied by changing leads or decreasing the gain.

33. *Rate:* 88 to 120 bpm
    Rhythm: Irregular in a phasic pattern with rate waxing and waning with respirations.
    P waves: Normal for lead II
    PR interval: 0.10 to 0.12 seconds, short
    Interpretation: Respiratory sinus arrhythmia, short PR interval
34. Sinus arrhythmia is a normal, physiologic phenomenon common in children and young adults.
35. *Rate:* 125 bpm
    Rhythm: Regular
    P waves: Diphasic in lead V_1, normal
    PR interval: 0.15 to 0.16 seconds, normal
    QRS complex: rSR′, abnormal for V_1, 0.16 seconds in duration, too wide, IVCD present
    Interpretation: Sinus tachycardia with IVCD
36. Mr. B's symptoms are suggestive of possible myocardial infarction. Overt signs of shortness of breath and the presence of sinus tachycardia in this clinical situation should cue the nurse to check for signs of congestive heart failure. Inspect the external jugular veins for distension, auscultate the lungs for the presence of rales, assess peripheral perfusion by inspecting color of extremities, mucous membranes, check for circumoral pallor or cyanosis, check capillary refill, skin temperature.
37. Elevate the head of the bed.
    Administer oxygen by nasal cannula.
    Start intravenous infusion.
    Attempt to alleviate the pain by administering medications according to hospital policy such as nitroglycerin and morphine sulfate.
    Notify the physician immediately.
    Administer prophylactic lidocaine as ordered.
    Obtain a 12-lead ECG.
    While you are caring for this patient, try to reassure him to allay anxiety.
    Sinus tachycardia in the presence of probable myocardial infarction is a significant and possibly ominous arrhythmia. It warrants immediate concern and attention directed at decreasing the ischemic episode.
38. *Rate:* 70 bpm then abruptly halves to 35 bpm
    Rhythm: Irregular (regular grouped beating)
    P waves: Normal for lead II, but rate goes from 70 to 35 bpm
    PR interval: 0.16 seconds, normal
    QRS complex: rS complex, abnormal for lead II; 0.16 seconds, too wide, probable IVCD; elevated ST segment (probably secondary to IVCD)
    Interpretation: Type II second degree SA block, 2:1; IVCD
39. Determine how symptomatic the patient is by checking the level of consciousness, blood pressure, and color. If the patient is symptomatic, as evidenced by altered mentation, light-headedness, or syncope with low blood pressure and pallor, lower the head of the bed, maintain airway patency, notify the physician immediately, administer atropine and/or isoproterenol intravenously according to hospital policy, and prepare for emergency temporary pacemaker insertion.
40. Permanent pacemaker. Initial patient teaching would include the following:
    a. Basic anatomy of the heart and conduction system.
    b. The nature of the patient's arrhythmia.
    c. How a pacemaker works.
    d. The rate ranges within which her pacemaker should function.
    e. How to take her own pulse.
    f. Symptoms that warrant notification of the physician (e.g., signs of infection and pulse values outside prescribed range).
41. The mechanism of sinus bradycardia is usually a disorder of impulse formation, whereas SA block is a disorder of impulse conduction. The term *exit block* describes an impulse that cannot "get out" and cause depolarization. In SA exit block the impulse cannot exit from the SA node to cause depolarization of the surrounding atrial musculature.
42. *Syncope* is a term used for temporary loss of consciousness. It can be the result of a number of pathologic and physiologic disorders. In this chapter, however, it was introduced as a possible complication of low cardiac output resulting from severe sinus slowing or sinus arrest.

CHAPTER SIX

Atrial Rhythm Disturbances and Supraventricular Tachycardias

▶ GOAL

You will be able to distinguish significant atrial rhythm disturbances from normal rhythm variations and use the nursing process in caring for patients with atrial arrhythmias.

▶ OBJECTIVES

After studying this chapter and completing the self-assessment exercises, you should be able to:

1. Explain why atrial arrhythmias are classified as supraventricular, categorize them as either active or passive, list the arrhythmias considered to be supraventricular tachycardias, and define all terms.
2. Explain the clinical significance of each of the atrial arrhythmias and determine which may be found in healthy people and which, when present, are signs of disease.
3. Describe the electrocardiographic features of atrial premature beats (APBs) and their patterns of occurrence, recognize and differentiate them from other supraventricular arrhythmias, and list five causes of APBs.
4. Demonstrate the ability to recognize and distinguish nonconducted APBs, APBs conducted with prolonged PR interval, and aberrantly conducted APBs.
5. Analyze the patient with APBs, appraising clinical status and deciding which assessment measures are indicated, construct a plan for care, and delineate factors to consider in evaluating the plan.
6. Recognize and define multiform atrial tachycardia (MAT) and its most frequently associated finding, differentiate it from other supraventricular tachycardias, and describe its significance.
7. Define paroxysmal supraventricular tachycardia (PSVT), state which age groups are most commonly afflicted, and list five causes or associated findings.
8. Describe and recognize the electrocardiographic characteristics of PSVT and relate the most common mechanism for its initiation and perpetuation.
9. Determine assessment measures for the patient in PSVT, appraise the clinical significance of the arrhythmia, and determine the nursing interventions indicated to terminate it.
10. Decide what level of teaching about the home management of PSVT is appropriate for the patient or the patient's significant others.
11. Explain the electrocardiographic features of atrial tachycardia with block, differentiate it from other supraventricular tachycardias, and relate its most common cause and necessary nursing intervention.
12. Identify and explain the electrocardiographic features of atrial flutter (AFl), list three leads that tend to exhibit flutter waves clearly, and anticipate the ventricular rate in both adult and pediatric patients who have not yet received treatment.
13. Assess the patient in AFl and atrial fibrillation (AF), describe the range of symptoms that may be anticipated, and delineate nursing intervention measures.
14. Differentiate AFl from other supraventricular tachycardias.
15. Compare, contrast, and evaluate the treatment for and progress of AFl and AF.
16. Describe, identify, and explain the electrocardiographic features and initiation of AF before and after treatment.
17. Correlate age with the incidence of AF and list four common causes.
18. Explain the hemodynamic effects of AF and why there is increased risk of thrombus formation.
19. List the atrial arrhythmias for which electrical cardioversion may be indicated and relate two conditions that predispose some patients to dangerous arrhythmias after the shock.

20. Compare, contrast, and explain the electrocardiographic features and clinical significance of wandering pacemaker and atrial escape rhythm, and differentiate both from APBs.

21. After demonstrating the ability to recognize atrial escape rhythm and atrial asystole, decide assessment priorities for the patient with each rhythm and compare and contrast plans of care.

The atrial arrhythmias and supraventricular tachycardias create an interesting group of rhythm disturbances, many of which you will encounter often in your electrocardiographic observations. The major arrhythmias comprising this group are atrial premature beats (APBs), multiform atrial tachycardia (MAT), paroxysmal supraventricular tachycardia (PSVT), automatic atrial tachycardia (AAT), atrial flutter (AFl), atrial fibrillation (AF), wandering pacemaker (WP), atrial escape, and atrial asystole.

Atrial arrhythmias occur as a result of numerous physiologic factors, the most common of which include myocardial infarction, congestive heart failure, hypoxemia, drugs, emotions and stress, pericarditis, disease of the sinoatrial (SA) node, thyrotoxicosis, and electrolyte imbalances.

There are two basic mechanisms responsible for atrial arrhythmias: (1) active, overriding, or *usurping* and (2) a passive, *escape* phenomenon. Therefore the arrhythmias are presented in that order. Recall from previous chapters that the SA node is the primary pacemaker of the heart because its pacemaker cells have the most rapid inherent rate of diastolic depolarization. In other words the SA node is dominant because under normal conditions it fires faster than its subsidiaries (lower pacemakers in the AV node and ventricles). For various reasons, pacemaker cells located elsewhere in the atria may have a more rapid rate of diastolic depolarization than the SA node and will therefore take over or usurp the SA node's dominance. On the other hand, if the SA node's rate slows or fails to depolarize the atria, a passive, escape depolarization normally occurs by default. Throughout the remainder of the book, the word *ectopic* will be used to denote a source of depolarization initiated in an area other than the SA node.

The usurping arrhythmias include the following:

Atrial premature beats.
Multiform atrial tachycardia.
Paroxysmal supraventricular tachycardia.
Automatic atrial tachycardia.
Atrial flutter.
Atrial fibrillation.

Arrhythmias by default include the following:

Wandering pacemaker.
Atrial escape.
Atrial asystole.

Regardless of the mechanism of atrial depolarization, the impulse reaches the AV junctional tissue and is conducted through to the ventricles in the same manner that SA node impulses are. Therefore the QRS complexes will be morphologically similar to the sinus-conducted beats. Exceptions to this generality will be clarified later.

The danger of atrial arrhythmias lies in their potential to result in slow or, more commonly, fast ventricular rates that compromise cardiac output. Slow ventricular rates may cause the patient to have symptoms of decreased perfusion because cardiac output (CO) is diminished due to the slow heart rate (HR). Fast ventricular rates diminish cardiac output because there is inadequate time for ventricular filling, reducing cardiac output by decreasing stroke volume (SV). (Recall the equation: $CO = HR \times SV$.)

The Premature Beat. Before proceeding to the first of the atrial arrhythmias, atrial premature beats, it is helpful to understand some general principles about the premature beat. The atria, junction, and ventricles are all capable of initiating premature beats, which is by far the most common heart rhythm disorder[1] and by no means indicative of heart disease. They occur as a result of sympathomimetic drugs (drugs that mimic stimulation of the sympathetic nervous system), large doses of tobacco or caffeine, and various other drug toxicities.[1] They can occur during periods of emotional excitement or mental stress,[1,2] as a result of blood gas abnormalities and electrolyte disturbances, and as a result of heart transplant rejection and heart diseases such as coronary artery disease and cardiomyopathy. Many times the cause is unknown.

In certain settings a premature beat is significant; under other circumstances, it is irrelevant. It is this distinction that often stimulates debate and is the subject of numerous hospital and prehospital monitoring policies. Skilled patient assessment along with expertise in identifying arrhythmias will be your greatest asset in determining the relevance of a particular patient's arrhythmia. By the time you are finished reading this book, you will have a clear understanding of which of those premature beats (whether atrial, junctional, or ventricular) are relevant. You will also realize that the significance of any premature beat is related to the underlying cardiac abnormality.

ATRIAL PREMATURE BEAT
Data Base: Problem Identification
Definitions, Etiology, and Mechanisms

An atrial premature beat (APB) is defined as an ectopic atrial depolarization that occurs earlier in the cycle than the next expected sinus impulse. As with all the arrhythmias, APBs may be referred to in different ways. The following are some of the references you will encounter:

Atrial premature depolarization (APD)
Atrial premature contraction (APC)
Premature atrial contraction (PAC)
Premature atrial ectopics
Atrial extrasystoles
Atrial ectopy
Atrial ectopic activity (AEA)

These terms are often used interchangeably. In this discussion the term *APB* will be used. It is nevertheless wise to familiarize yourself with the other terms as you will undoubtedly hear them used by colleagues and see them in the literature.

You will recall that atrial pacemaker cells are located not only in the SA node but also in the three atrial internodal pathways. Pacemaker cells are characterized by diastolic depolarization (i.e., they can initiate self-excitation during diastole without external stimulation).[3] In the case of APBs the firing of a pacemaker cell from somewhere in the atria other than the SA node occurs before the next expected sinus impulse, resulting in an early or premature beat.

Significance of APBs. APBs indicate some degree of irritability in the atria. This may be due to many factors. In the presence of acute myocardial infarction, APBs, estimated to occur in 30% of patients,[4] may be a sign of congestive heart failure as distension in the atria results in increased atrial automaticity. Likewise, as the atria increase in size with valvular disorders, the incidence of atrial ectopy increases. They also can occur because of ischemia resulting from hypoxemia or coronary artery disease, pulmonary embolism and infarction, digitalis toxicity, electrolyte imbalance (particularly hypokalemia and hypomagnesemia), metabolic alkalosis, and inflammatory conditions such as pericarditis.[4-6] They occur in heart transplant rejection.

The presence of APBs may forewarn of impending serious atrial arrhythmias such as atrial tachycardia, atrial fibrillation, or atrial flutter.[7] They are clinically significant when their frequency increases the heart rate or, in the case of nonconducted APBs, decreases it, and when their prematurity results in insufficient cardiac filling and reduced cardiac output.[5]

Atrial premature beats also occur in healthy people. Studies of Holter monitoring in nonhospitalized patients have documented atrial ectopy in a significant number of apparently healthy individuals.[8] In a large-scale study of adults, Chiang and coworkers found that premature supraventricular beats are not associated with a higher prevalence of coronary heart disease or an increased risk of sudden death.[8] More recently, continuous ambulatory electrocardiographic monitoring of healthy individuals without apparent heart disease revealed that isolated APBs occurred occasionally (at least once in 24 hours) in 64% of young (aged 22 to 28 years) women[9] and in 13% of young boys (aged 10 to 13 years).[10] It has also been reported that young, male long-distance runners revealed an incidence of 100%,[11] as compared with their untrained counterparts who had an incidence of 56%.[12] The data indicate that the propensity to develop an occasional APB increases with age. In one study of 98 healthy, active 60- to 85-year-old people, 88% had at least one APB per hour and 22% had more than 30/hr.[13] In another recent study of healthy elderly (aged 70 to 81 years) men, atrial ectopic beats were observed in 76.9% of the sample. They were frequent in 15.4% and repetitive in 34.6% of the individuals.[14]

ECG Characteristics

Several features common to most APBs are listed in the box on this page.

- The APB interrupts the rhythmicity of the sinus beat. In other words the interval from the normal sinus P wave to the ectopic P wave (known as the *P prime* or *P′ wave*) is shorter than the intervals between the sinus P waves (P-P′ interval < P-P interval) (Fig. 6-1).
- The early cycle has a QRS complex that is usually the same as the other QRSs.
- The premature P wave (P′) is different from the sinus P waves in at least one lead.
- The P′R interval is 0.12 seconds or longer.
- The APB produces a noncompensatory pause.

In diagnosing APBs, it is helpful to search for P waves in the T waves of the preceding complex, particularly when the rate is fast. It is also helpful to monitor a lead that enables good visualization of P waves (V_1 or MCL_1, II, or S_5).

Morphology of the P′. Since the P′ can arise from nearly any region of the atria, its shape will vary from the sinus P waves depending on where it is initiated. The closer the P′ is to the SA node, the more it resembles the sinus impulses. The farther it is from the SA node, the more different or bizarre the P′ appears (Fig. 6-2).

If the source of the P′ is the left atrium (LA), for example, and the patient is being monitored on lead I (recall: [+] electrode on LA, [−] electrode on RA), the mean vector force of the impulse will be traveling toward the RA, and away from the LA and the positive electrode. There-

ECG Characteristics
Atrial Premature Beats

Early (premature) P′
P′ is different from sinus P in at least one lead
QRS is usually like the sinus-conducted QRS
P′R interval is 0.12 seconds or longer
Noncompensatory pause usually present

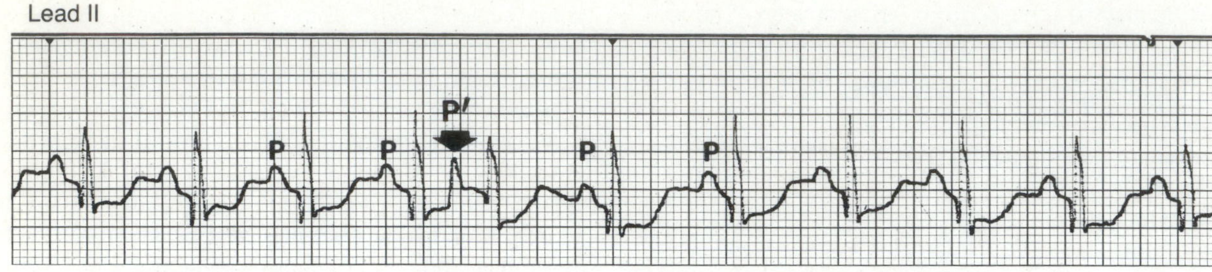

FIGURE 6-1 Atrial premature beat (APB). Note how the rhythm is interrupted by an early P′ wave that is different from the other P waves *(arrow)*.

Rate: 100 bpm
Rhythm: Irregular
P wave: Normal except for P′ wave
PR interval: 0.16 seconds
QRS complex: 0.10 seconds, depressed ST segment
Interpretation: Sinus tachycardia with 1 APB

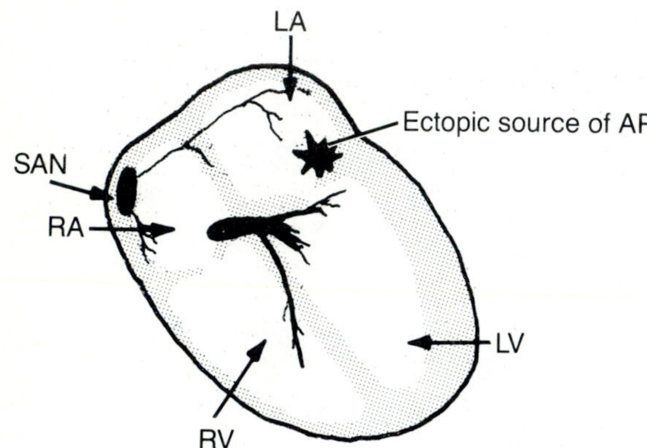

FIGURE 6-2 Schematic representing an ectopic source for an APB. The farther away from the SA node, the more different the P′ wave will appear. SAN = Sinoatrial node. RA = Right atrium. LA = Left atrium. RV = Right ventricle. LV = Left ventricle.

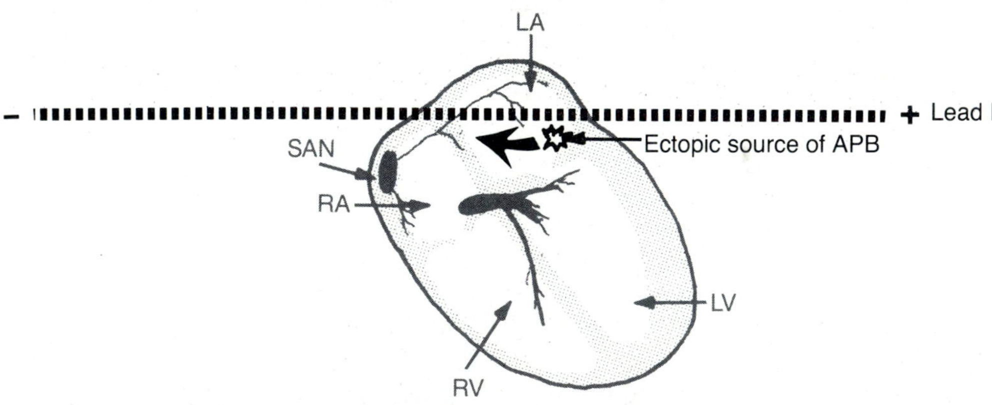

FIGURE 6-3 Ectopic source of atrial depolarization may result in a mean vector force directed from left to right. On lead I, this activation would proceed away from the positive electrode.

fore the P′ will be a negative complex on this lead (Fig. 6-3). The sinus P will appear positive, since the mean vector force will be directed more toward the positive than the negative electrode. The resulting ECG might resemble the schematic and ECG in Fig. 6-4.

If the P′ is near the AV node (AVN), it will depolarize the atria in *retrograde* fashion (i.e., from inferior to superior). On lead II the P′ would appear negative as schematically shown in Fig. 6-5. A P′ located here is difficult or impossible to distinguish from a junctional premature beat

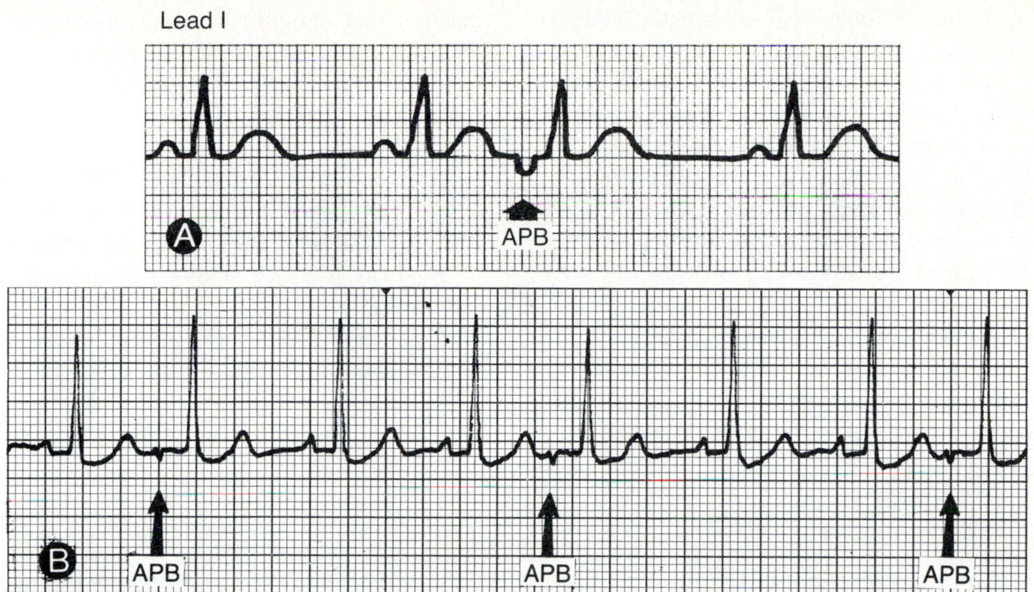

FIGURE 6-4 Appearance of APB on lead I with left to right atrial depolarization. **A,** Graphic representation. **B,** ECG tracing.

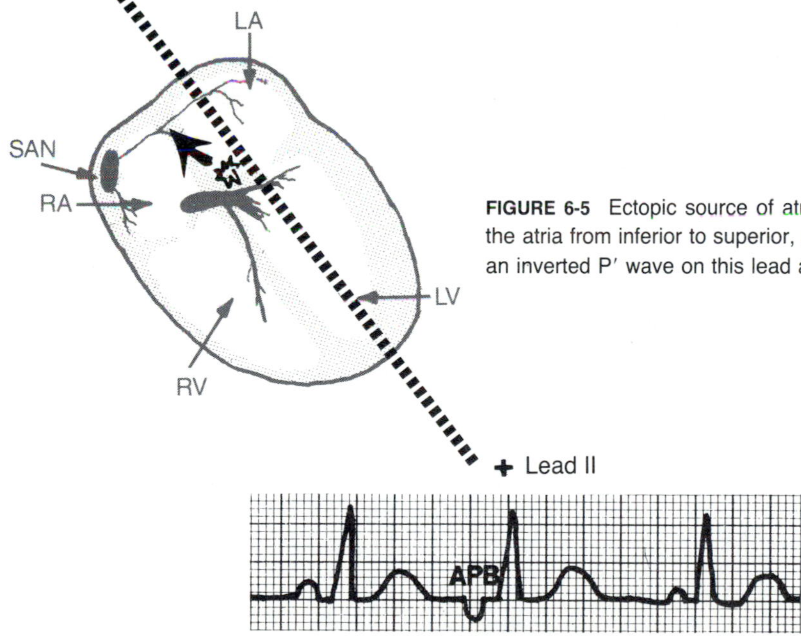

FIGURE 6-5 Ectopic source of atrial depolarization may result in mean vector force of the atria from inferior to superior, away from the positive electrode in lead II resulting in an inverted P′ wave on this lead as illustrated in graphic representation.

(JPB) that produces retrograde atrial depolarization. Thus for the sake of description, some authors have selected 0.12 seconds as a determinative factor in labeling[1]; if the retrograde P′ precedes the QRS by 0.12 seconds or more it is labeled an APB. If the P′ precedes the QRS by less than 0.12 seconds, it is known as a JPB with retrograde atrial depolarization. Keep in mind the only proof of the origin of such a beat is an intracardiac electrophysiologic recording (a diagnostic test where the leads are placed directly in the atrium, AV junction, and ventricle).

Compensatory and noncompensatory pauses. Typically after an APB there is a brief pause in the ECG. The reason for the pause is that the ectopic atrial depolarization also depolarizes the SA node, causing it to "reset". (This resetting is usually not precise because the APB "has a way of stunning the SA node,"[15] delaying the next impulse and resulting in a slightly longer pause than the normal P-P interval.) Thus the P-P′-P interval is shorter than two sinus cycles. It may help to visualize the SA node as a ticking metronome: two "ticks" between which an APB falls comprise two cycles. If beat three occurs when the third tick would occur, it would produce a pause after the APB that would be a compensatory pause. If the third beat falls earlier than the third tick, the pause after the APB is noncompensatory (Figs. 6-6 and 6-7). Most APBs have noncompensatory pauses.

Patterns of occurrence. APBs occur singly or in groups. Their occurrence may be sporadic or frequent, regular or irregular, and these patterns of occurrence are applicable to any of the premature beats. It should be emphasized that definitions vary considerably in the literature. Current, suggested definitions include the following:

1. *Atrial bigeminy or bigeminal APBs.* Every other beat is an APB (Fig. 6-8).
2. *Atrial trigeminy or trigeminal APBs.* APB occurs after every two sinus beats. In other words, every third beat is an APB (Fig. 6-9). (An early definition of the term *trigeminy* was one sinus beat followed by two premature beats.
3. *Atrial quadrigeminy or quadrigeminal APBs.* APB occurs after three sinus beats (every fourth beat is an APB) (Fig. 6-10). (An early definition of the term *quadrigeminy* was one sinus beat followed by three

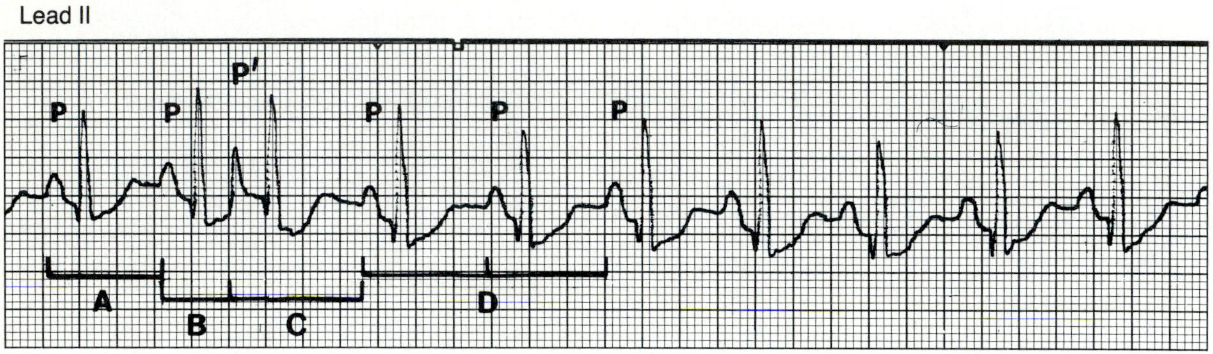

FIGURE 6-6 Noncompensatory pause after APB. Note normal P to P interval *(A)* is longer than the P to P′ interval *(B)* of the APB. Segment D represents the length of time for two P to P intervals to occur and is longer than B + C.

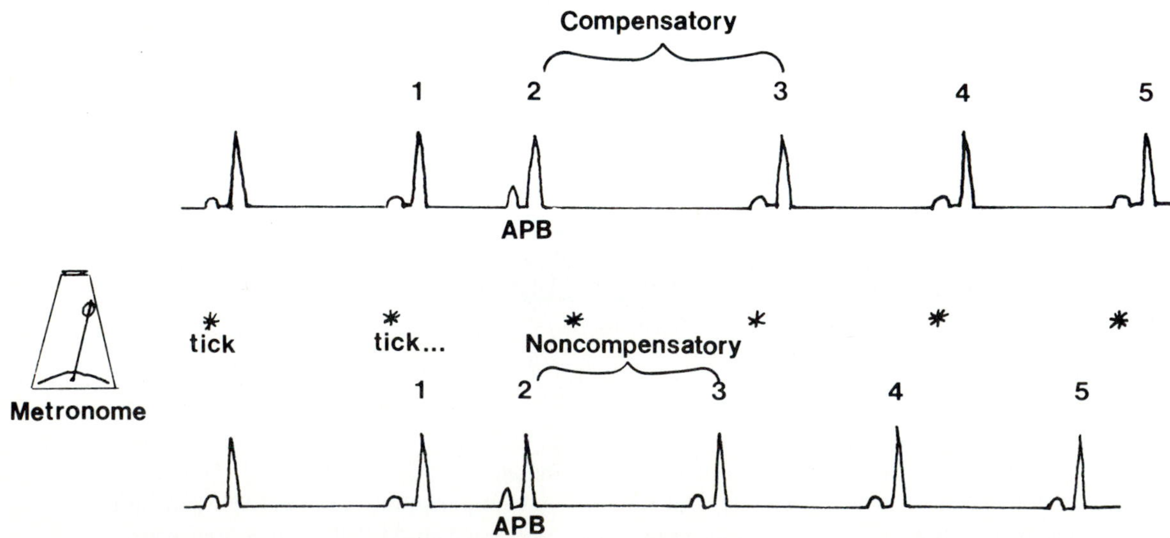

FIGURE 6-7 Compensatory and noncompensatory pauses. A compensatory pause compensates for a beat that normally would have occurred, making the period from beat 1 to beat 3 equal to the period from beat 3 to beat 5. A noncompensatory pause creates a shorter distance from beat 1 to beat 3 than from beat 3 to beat 5.

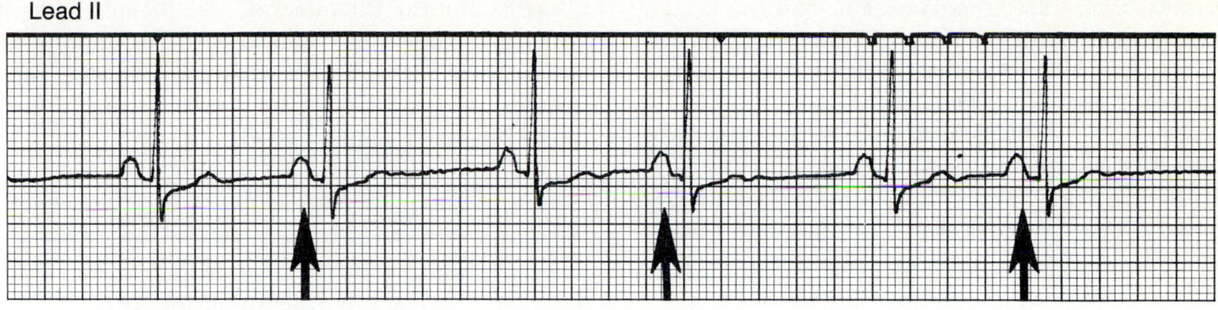

FIGURE 6-8 Atrial bigeminy. Every other complex is early *(arrows).*

Rate: Approximately 70 bpm. Count such irregular rhythms for full minute.
Rhythm: Irregular
P wave: Every other one is premature
PR interval: 0.14 to 0.16 seconds
QRS complex: 0.08 seconds; depressed J point
Interpretation: Atrial bigeminy

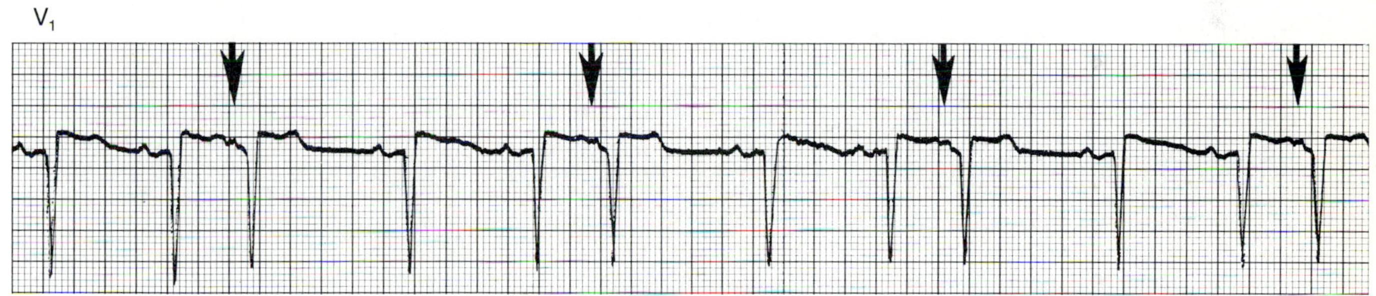

FIGURE 6-9 Atrial trigeminy. Every third complex is early. Each early QRS complex is preceded by an early P′ wave that is different from the other P waves *(arrows).*

Rate: Approximately 75 bpm. Count for full minute.
Rhythm: Irregular
P wave: Normal except for APBs
PR interval: 0.20 seconds
QRS complex: 0.08 seconds
Interpretation: Atrial trigeminy

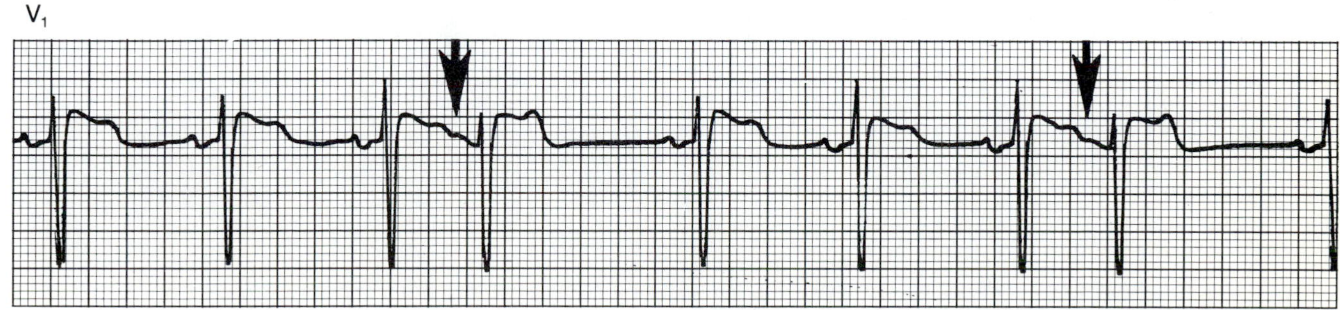

FIGURE 6-10 Atrial quadrigeminy. Note every fourth complex is early.

Rate: 72 bpm
Rhythm: Irregular
P wave: Normal except for APBs
PR interval: 0.17 seconds
QRS complex: 0.09 seconds; elevated ST segment
Interpretation: NSR with atrial quadrigeminy

premature beats; that definition is now obsolete.)

4. *Pair, salvo, or couplet*. Two APBs occurring in succession (Fig. 6-11). When pairs recur in patterns, they represent a form of *grouped beating*.
5. *Triplet, salvo, or three beat run*. Three consecutive APBs. Triplets may also exhibit *grouped beating* (Fig. 6-12).
6. *A run of atrial tachycardia*. Three or more ectopic beats in a row. If they occur in a regular pattern, they may be termed *grouped beating* (Fig. 6-13).
7. *Uniform and multiform APBs*. In describing APBs, remember to note if the ectopic beats are uniform (all the P′ waves are similar in appearance, suggesting they may be unifocal or coming from the same focus), or if they are multiform (the P′ waves are different in appearance and multifocal, or possibly coming from two or more foci) (Fig. 6-14).

APBs and the PR interval. The PR interval in APBs (P′R) is usually within normal limits (0.12 to 0.20 seconds). It can, however, be prolonged (greater than 0.20 seconds); or the APB may be nonconducted (i.e., not followed by a QRS complex at all).

The P′R Interval of the APB

An APB's P′R interval is dependent upon:
- Proximity of the ectopic impulse to the AV junction
- The status of the AV junction
- The degree of prematurity
- The length of the ventricular cycle preceding the APB

Lead II

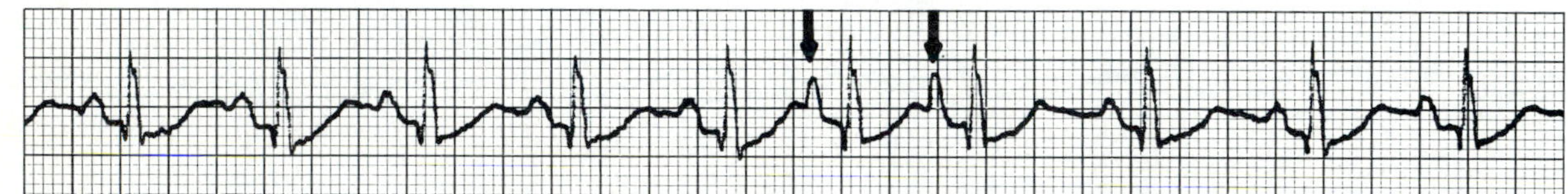

FIGURE 6-11 Pair of APBs. Note rhythm is interrupted by two early complexes occurring in succession *(arrows)*. Both APBs have the same morphology so they are said to be uniform. Pairs are also called salvos or couplets.

Rate: 97 bpm
Rhythm: Irregular
P waves: Normal except for two APBs
PR interval: 0.17 seconds
QRS complex: 0.09 seconds
Interpretation: NSR with pair of APBs

V_1

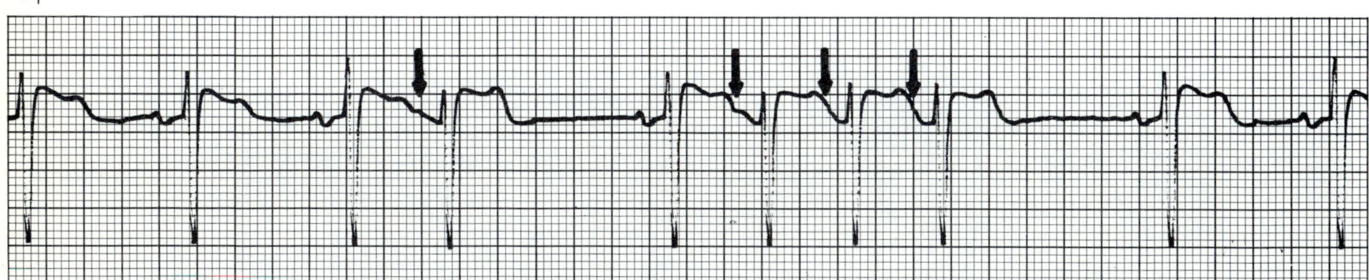

FIGURE 6-12 APB triplet. The rhythm is interrupted by a single APB, then a run of three APBs *(arrows)*.

Rate: 80 bpm. With frequent APBs, rate for full minute may be much higher.
Rhythm: Irregular
P wave: Normal except for APBs
PR interval: 0.16 seconds
QRS complex: 0.08 seconds; elevated ST segment and J point
Interpretation: NSR with frequent APBs occurring singly and in triplets

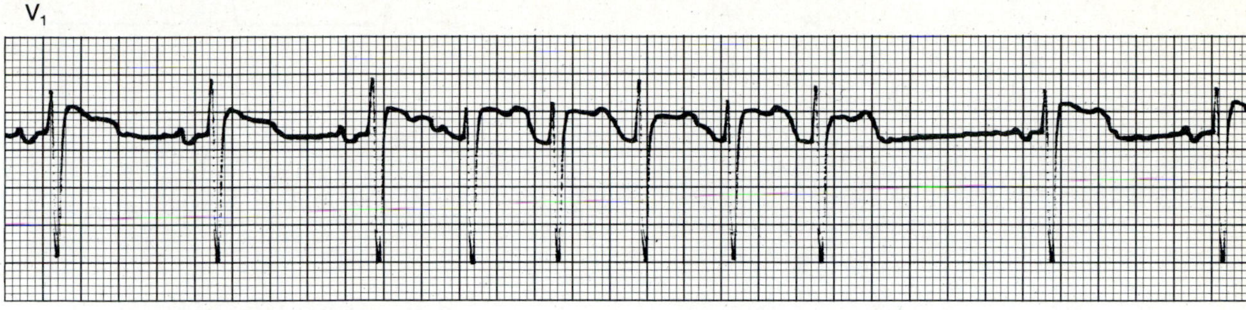

FIGURE 6-13 Run of atrial tachycardia. Note how NSR (first three beats) is interrupted by a run of atrial tachycardia at a rate of 130 bpm.

Rate: NSR rate is 72 bpm; AT rate is 130 bpm. Count rate for full minute.
Rhythm: Irregular because of run of AT
P wave: Normal except for AT
PR interval: 0.16 seconds
QRS complex: 0.08 to 0.09 seconds. Elevated ST segment and J point
Interpretation: NSR with run of AT

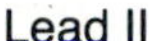

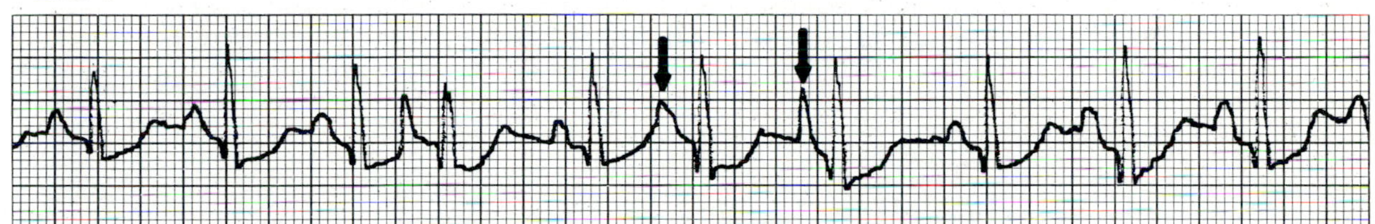

FIGURE 6-14 Multiform APBs. Note two different premature P′ waves (arrows).

Rate: 94 bpm
Rhythm: Irregular
P wave: Tall, irregular in shape
PR interval: 0.16 seconds
QRS complex: 0.10 seconds; prolonged QT interval
Interpretation: NSR with multiform APBs

The P′R interval can vary considerably. Its length depends not only on the proximity of the ectopic atrial impulse to the AV junction (AVJ), as described previously, but also on the ability of the AVJ to conduct impulses. If the junctional cells are slow to recover from their preceding depolarization the subsequent conduction will be delayed, resulting in a P′R interval longer than that of the sinus-conducted beats. This is especially evident when AV conduction is already impaired. The P′R interval is also affected by the previous ventricular cycle length. If the preceding cycle length is prolonged, the subsequent P′R interval may be prolonged as well because the junctional tissue remains partially refractory (recall that the longer the cycle length the longer the refractory period) (Fig. 6-15 and box on p. 124).

Nonconducted APB. If the AV node is still refractory when the premature atrial impulse arrives, the impulse will be blocked and will not be conducted to the ventricles. This nonconducted APB may be due to an exaggeration of the conditions that cause a prolonged PR interval: impaired AV conduction, an APB occurring so early that the AV junction is still refractory, or an APB preceded by a long cycle. (Another cause is a phenomenon known as *con-*

ECG Characteristics
Nonconducted Atrial Premature Beats

Rate: Variable
Rhythm: Irregular, or regular if APBs occur in bigeminy
P waves: Normal except nonconducted APBs will have different shape; nonconducted APB will not be followed by a QRS but will be early.
PR interval: Normal with sinus beats
QRS complex: Normal unless IVCD present

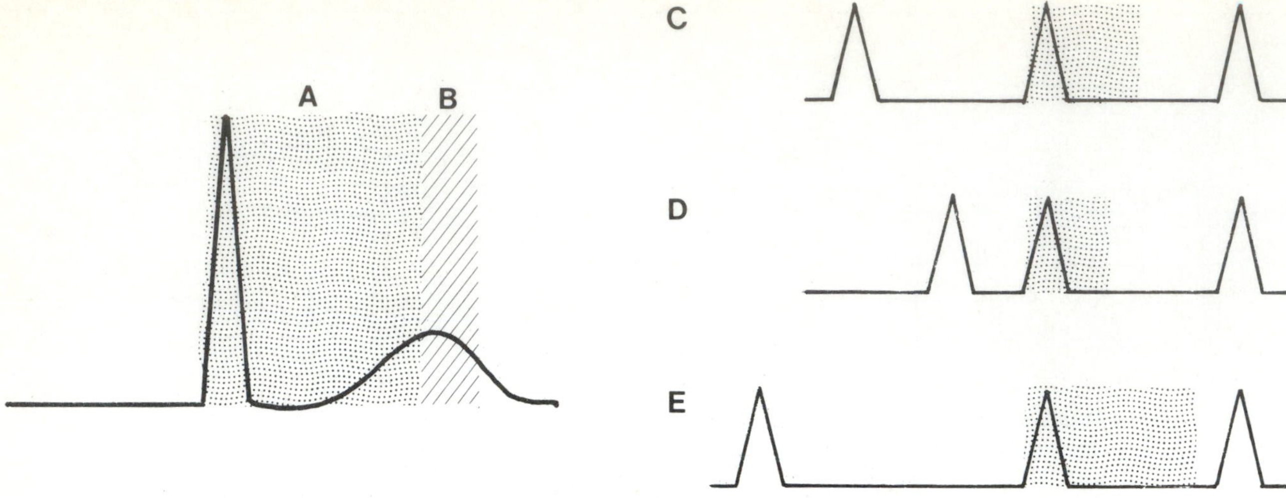

FIGURE 6-15 APBs occurring while the AV junction and bundle branches are still refractory may conduct the QRS complex with a prolonged PR interval or may not be able to conduct a QRS complex at all. The left diagram illustrates hypothetical times during and after the QRS complex when refractory tissue may impede or block conduction of an APB. These periods vary from patient to patient and in the same patient from beat to beat. If an APB occurred during this period, it may not produce a QRS complex *(A)*. An APB occurring during this phase may conduct a QRS after a prolonged PR interval *(B)*. **C, D,** and **E** illustrate how the refractory period is influenced by the preceding R-R interval. If the shaded area represents the refractory period, note how a short preceding R-R interval *(D)* corresponds with a shorter refractory period; a long preceding R-R interval produces a lengthy refractory period *(E)*.

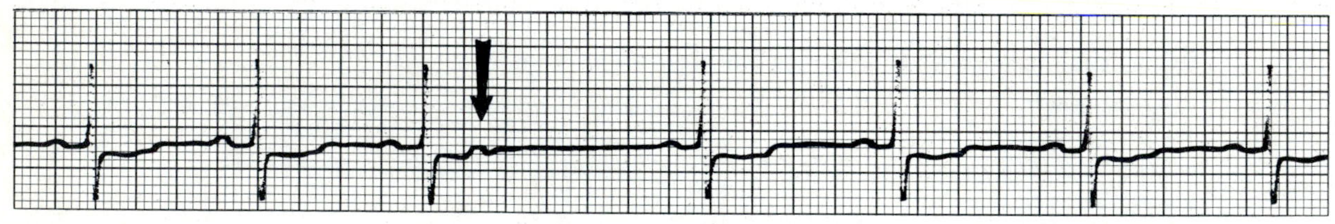

FIGURE 6-16 Nonconducted APB. Note pause in rhythm. Examination of the ST segment and T wave of the complex preceding the pause reveals a P′ wave *(arrow)*.

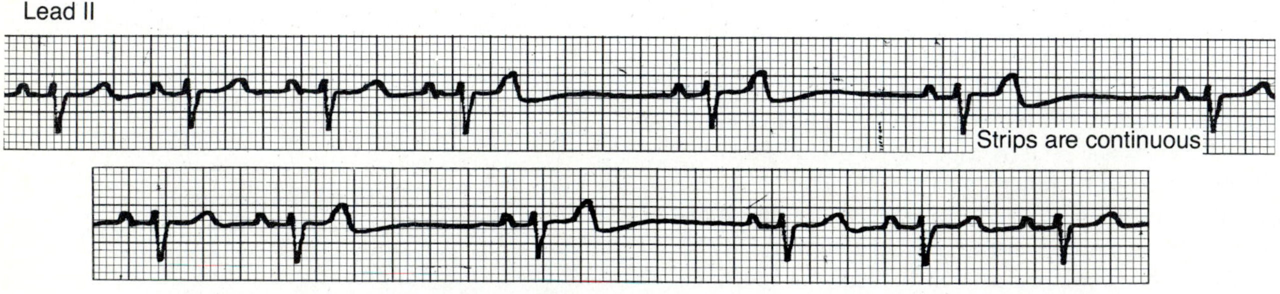

FIGURE 6-17 Sudden decrease in rate due to bigeminal nonconducted APBs. Before each pause in rhythm, note T waves are larger and more peaked because of superimposed APBs.

Rate: 83 bpm with sudden decrease to 46 bpm. Count rate for full minute.
Rhythm: Irregular
P wave: Normal except for APBs
PR interval: 0.17 seconds for P waves that conduct QRS complexes
QRS complex: 0.08 seconds; predominantly negative on lead II resulting from axis shift
Interpretation: NSR with frequent bigeminal nonconducted APBs

cealed AV conduction, a subject reserved for advanced study.)

Nonconducted APBs are often mistaken for potentially serious arrhythmias such as Type II second degree AV block (described in Chapter 9), sinus pause, marked sinus bradycardia, and Type II SA block. In detecting a pause in the ECG rhythm, it is important to search for a P′ wave hidden in the preceding T wave and recall Marriott's aphorism "the commonest causes of pauses are nonconducted APBs"[15] (see the box on p. 125 and Figs. 6-16 and 6-17).

APBs and ventricular aberration. For reasons similar to those that produce a prolonged P′R interval, the APB may find part of the ventricular conduction system still refractory, resulting in *aberrant conduction.* The fascicle of the ventricular conduction system that is slowest to recover is the right bundle branch (RBB). Therefore when an APB finds the RBB refractory, the QRS will be conducted with *RBB block* (RBBB) *aberration.* All the fascicles can produce aberration, but RBBB aberration is by far the most common. Although bundle branch blocks will be discussed later, it is a good idea to familiarize yourself with the characteristic morphology of RBBB at this point because it is frequently encountered in atrial arrhythmias. It is easily identified on lead V_1 or MCL_1. Recall the normal QRS pattern in these leads (rS) (Fig. 6-18). In RBBB there is a terminal R wave on V_1 or MCL_1. The initial deflection is like the other QRSs on that lead (Fig. 6-19). APBs conducted with aberration can be tricky to identify. Remem-

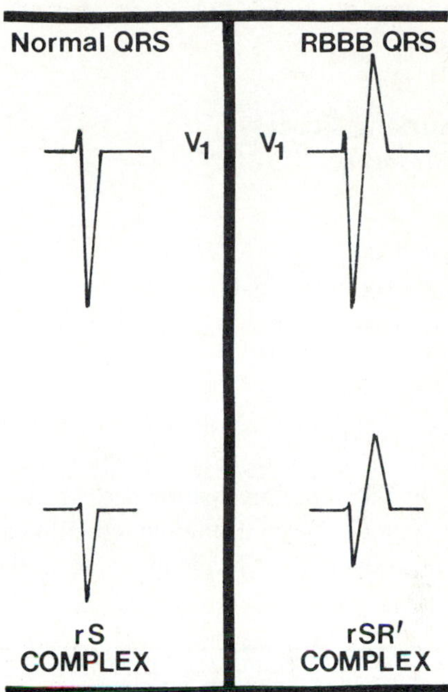

FIGURE 6-18 Comparison of normal QRSs and RBBB QRSs in V_1. A RBBB causes the QRS in V_1 to have a terminal R wave. Bundle branch blocks are discussed in detail in Chapter 9.

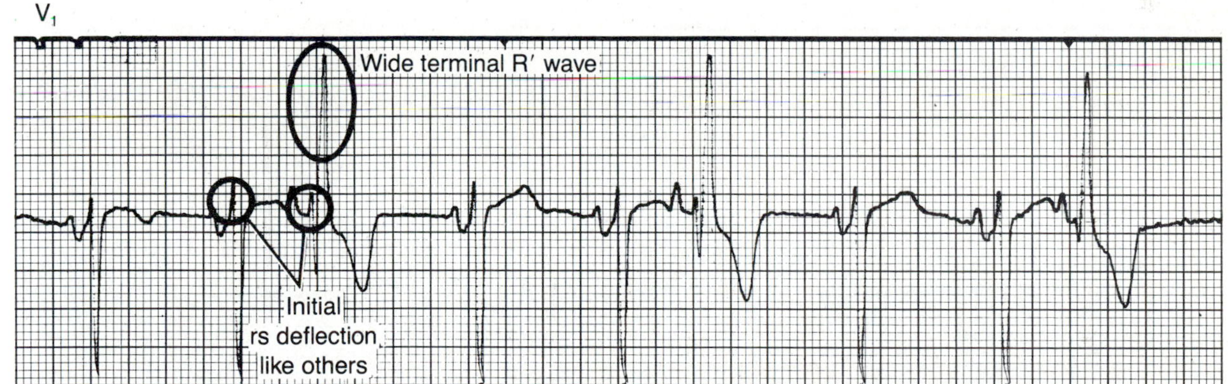

FIGURE 6-19 APBs with RBBB aberration. Note early QRS complexes preceded by early P′ waves. Early QRS complexes have an initial rs configuration closely resembling the normally conducted beats. The wide terminal R′ wave is characteristic of a RBBB on V_1. The aberration also often causes deformation of the T wave.

Rate: 79 bpm
Rhythm: Irregular
P wave: Normal diphasic (+ −) for V_1. P′ wave different from sinus P waves.
PR interval: 0.12 seconds
QRS complexes: 0.08 seconds; APBs with RBBB measure 0.12 seconds
Interpretation: NSR with trigeminal APBs conducted with RBBB aberration

ber, when a premature P′ is not readily detectable, search the preceding T wave.

For a summary of the ECG characteristics of APBs, see the box below.

Applied Nursing Process

Clinical Assessment

- Detect:
  - An irregular pulse.
  - An irregularity in the ECG.
  - A sudden onset of bradycardia (which could be bigeminal nonconducted APBs as illustrated in Fig. 6-20).
- Assess patient and ECG.
  - Assess for symptoms associated with the APBs. Patients with APBs are usually asymptomatic and often unaware of their rhythm disturbance. If the APBs are frequent or nonconducted, the reduction in cardiac output may produce light-headedness or a decrease in blood pressure. Sometimes palpitations and "skipped beats" are experienced.
  - Check the peripheral pulses for the presence of a pulse deficit with the APBs. This can be accomplished by taking the patient's pulse while watching the monitor. If the APB does not produce a pulse, there is a pulse deficit.
  - Obtain blood pressure.
  - Examine neck for external jugular venous distension and other manifestations of congestive heart failure (CHF).
  - Monitor serum electrolytes.
  - Assess respiratory status.
  - Diagnose the arrhythmia using the algorithm in Figure 6-21.
  - Determine the pattern and frequency of the premature beats. Count the number of APBs per full minute three times. Are the beats repetitive (e.g., bigeminy)? Are they alone or in groups (i.e., couplets, triplets)? Is the onset sudden or gradual?
  - Is the arrhythmia related to activity (is the patient asleep?)?
  - Is the arrhythmia related to diet (recent meal? excessive caffeine?)?
  - Is the patient receiving any drugs that may cause APBs? (Digitalis causes enhanced excitability in the atria and impairment of AV conduction. Nonconducted APBs and those with prolonged P′R intervals may be related to its use.[4] APBs may also occur in theophylline toxicity.)
  - Is a central venous catheter being inserted into the patient?

ECG Characteristics
Atrial Premature Beats

Rate: Variable
Rhythm: Irregular resulting from premature beats
P waves: Normal except APB which is different; one P wave precedes each QRS complex; APB is early
PR interval: Normal or prolonged with APB
QRS complex: Normal unless IVCD present

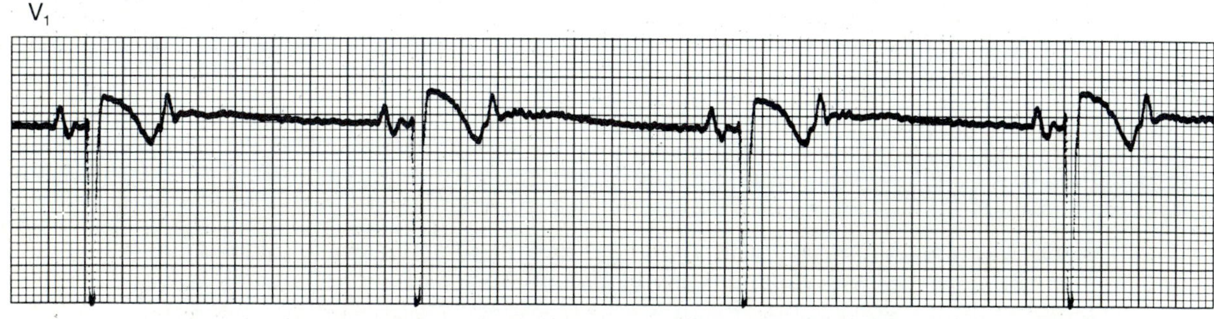

FIGURE 6-20 Bigeminal nonconducted APBs have reduced this ventricular rate to 35 bpm. The atrial rate is 70 bpm. Does the patient need atropine? No! The patient needs antiarrhythmic treatment for the APBs.

Rate: Atrial: 70 bpm
Ventricular: 35 bpm
Rhythm: Atrial: Irregular
Ventricular: Regular
P wave: 0.12 seconds prolonged; bigeminal P′ waves
PR interval: 0.16 seconds
QRS complex: 0.08 seconds
Interpretation: Bigeminal nonconducted APBs with resultant ventricular rate of 35 bpm

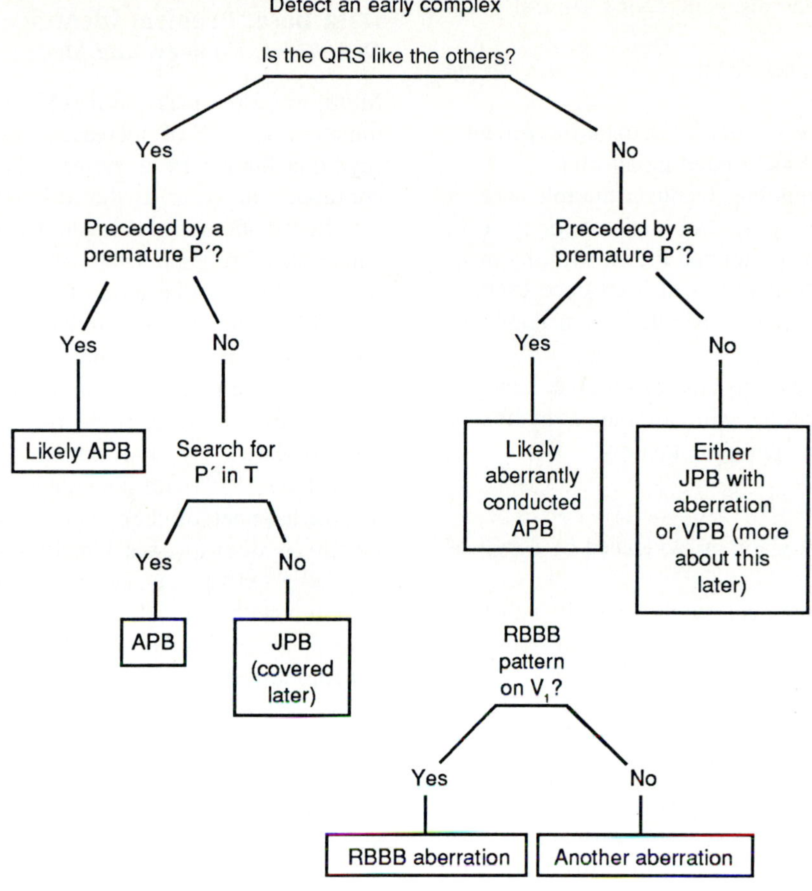

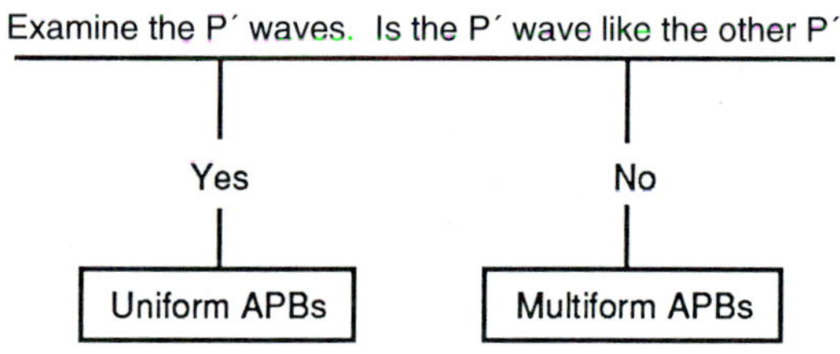

FIGURE 6-21 APB algorithm.

❖ NURSING DIAGNOSIS

Decreased cardiac output related to premature beats.

❖ ECG DIAGNOSIS

Atrial premature beats.

Plan and Implementation

Patient goal. The patient will remain asymptomatic; the underlying cause of atrial ectopy will be corrected.

Nursing interventions.

- If the patient is symptomatic, offer reassurance that the arrhythmia is not life-threatening and that measures will be taken to diminish the symptoms.
- Record the ECG findings. For example, "Monitor showing frequent APBs. 3-8-7 single uniform APBs occurred in three consecutive minutes while sitting in chair. Denies palpitations. No pulse deficit noted with APBs."
- Report significant findings, such as sudden development of frequent APBs (five or more per minute) for several minutes, to the physician. (As a general rule with all the arrhythmias that may be a manifestation of an abnormality, any significant change in the patient's ECG warrants physician notification. Significance is determined on an

individual basis and requires your sound clinical judgment.)

- Instruct the patient to eliminate sources of caffeine and/or alcohol.
- Implement the physician's orders. Evaluate the patient's response to therapy with continued monitoring.
  - For the patient on quinidine, evaluate the tolerance of the drug. Monitor for signs of quinidine toxicity (i.e., prolonged QT interval, prolonged PR interval) by measuring the QT and PR intervals at least once every 8 hours. Notify the physician if the intervals increase significantly.
  - If diarrhea develops, the physician may elect either to administer the medication with aluminum hydroxide gel[16] or to discontinue quinidine therapy.

Evaluation

- The patient is asymptomatic as evidenced by denial of palpitations.
- The patient's hemodynamic status remains stable as evidenced by no change in blood pressure and absence of pulse deficit with the APBs.

Medical Treatment

No treatment is necessary if the APBs are infrequent. When treatment is necessary, the physician treats the underlying cause, such as correction of congestive heart failure, or electrolyte imbalance. Drugs used in the treatment of congestive heart failure (CHF) often include digitalis and diuretics. Rarely, antiarrhythmic drugs such as quinidine or procainamide are used.

THE SUPRAVENTRICULAR TACHYCARDIAS

The supraventricular tachycardias (SVTs) discussed in this chapter—MAT, PSVT, AAT (including AT with block), AFl, and AF—are all rhythms with atrial rates in excess of 100 bpm. They are called *supraventricular tachycardias* because they are tachycardias that originate above the ventricles. Beyond these two characteristics, there are several clinical and electrocardiographic differences that allow these rhythms to fall into the following different categories:

- Clinical presentation
  - Acute or chronic.
  - Paroxysmal or nonparoxysmal (i.e., does it start and stop abruptly?)
  - Sustained or nonsustained.
  - Recurrent or isolated.
- Mechanism
  - Ectopic (automatic) or reentrant.
- ECG features
  - The ventricular and atrial rates.
  - Uniformity of the atrial activity.

MULTIFORM ATRIAL TACHYCARDIA

Data Base: Problem Identification

Definitions, Etiology, and Mechanisms

Multiform atrial tachycardia (MAT) is an uncommon, automatic (because of increased automaticity), ectopic arrhythmia known by a variety of other names and often confused with other rhythm disturbances.* It is characterized by the absence of a single dominant atrial pacemaker[17] and a rate of 100 bpm or greater.[18] MAT may be an underdiagnosed rhythm because of its often transient nature[18,19] and its frequent association with other atrial rhythms (e.g., atrial fibrillation).[18] It should be noted, however, that MAT in some patients is chronic, lasting for months.[19]

This arrhythmia is frequently associated with chronic lung disease[4,18-20] and cor pulmonale.[4,19,20] Coronary heart disease[18-20] with intractable CHF often coexists, and a large number of these patients are diabetic.[4] Digitalis toxicity is often present but does not appear to be causative.[4,19,20] MAT may be a manifestation of theophylline toxicity; reduction of blood levels alone may restore NSR.[21] Although the arrhythmia is not life threatening, patients affected with it are generally over the age of 50 years and seriously ill. There is, therefore, an associated high mortality.[1,4,18,19] Other conditions sometimes associated with MAT include general anesthesia (with hypoxia)[4] and the period immediately after chest or open heart surgery; electrolyte abnormalities such as hypokalemia,[18-20] other metabolic disturbances (acidemia),[20] pulmonary embolism,[4] hypertensive heart disease,[4,20] valvular heart disease,[4,18] infections,[20] and septicemia.[4] On rare occasions, it has been found in normal individuals.[18,22]

*Although the rhythm was described decades earlier, the term *MAT* was coined in 1968.[19] Terms used to describe this rhythm or variations of it include *wandering pacemaker of the atria, chaotic atrial rhythm, chaotic atrial tachycardia, chaotic atrial mechanism,* or *repetitive multifocal paroxysmal atrial tachycardia.*

ECG Characteristics
Multiform Atrial Tachycardia

Rate: 100 bpm or greater
Rhythm: Irregular
P waves: At least three different P′ waves; one precedes each QRS complex; absence of a single dominant pacemaker
PR interval: May vary
QRS Complex: Normal unless IVCD present

ECG Characteristics

There is no agreement concerning the precise mechanism and pathogenesis of MAT, but the mechanism thought to be responsible is some form of triggered automaticity (see Chapter 1). There are several specific ECG features making it a distinctive rhythm. MAT consistently lacks a single dominant pacemaker.[17,20,23] On the ECG, it is characterized by three or more different ectopic P′ waves in the same lead,[19,20,23] an isoelectric baseline between the P′ waves,[6] an atrial rate in excess of 100 bpm[18,19] (occasionally the rate is less than 100 bpm), and an onset that is usually nonparoxysmal.[4] The P′-P′ and P′R intervals are variable[6,18-20,23] (Figs. 6-22 to 6-24 and the box on p. 130).

Applied Nursing Process

Clinical Assessment

The patient will most often exhibit symptoms of the underlying disease (such as chronic obstructive pulmonary disease) rather than the arrhythmia itself.

- Detect:
  - An irregular pulse.
  - An irregularity on the ECG.
  - A heart rate of 100 bpm or greater.
- Assess patient and ECG.
  - Determine the patient's tolerance of the arrhythmia by measuring the heart rate and blood pressure at regular intervals. Assess for pulse deficit.

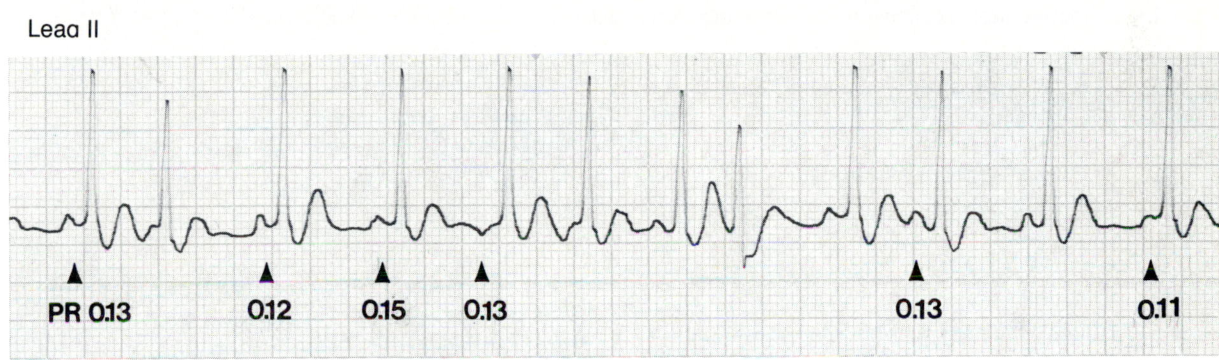

FIGURE 6-22 Multiform atrial tachycardia. Note variation in P waves as well as P′R intervals.

Rate: Approximately 120 bpm. Count for full minute.
Rhythm: Irregular
P wave: Varies in morphology
PR interval: Varies from 0.11 to 0.15 seconds
QRS complex: 0.08 seconds
Interpretation: Multiform atrial tachycardia

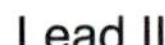

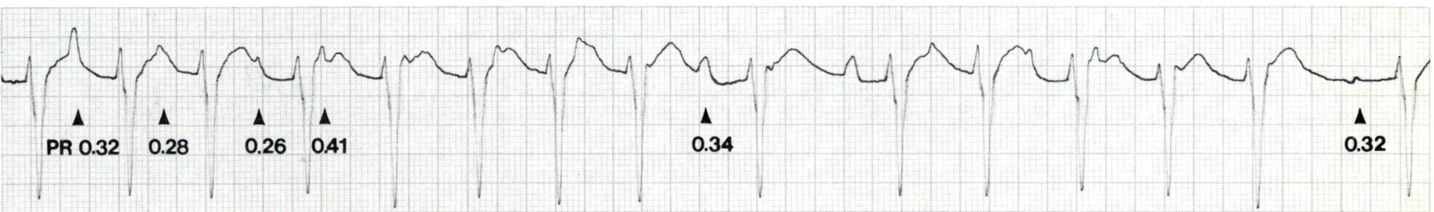

FIGURE 6-23 Multiform atrial tachycardia. Note variable P waves and P′R intervals.

Rate: Approximately 100 bpm. Count for full minute.
Rhythm: Irregular
P wave: Varies in morphology
PR interval: Varies from 0.26 seconds to 0.41 seconds, prolonged
QRS complex: 0.14 seconds, IVCD; negative on lead II because of left axis deviation
Interpretation: Multiform atrial tachycardia

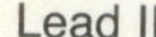

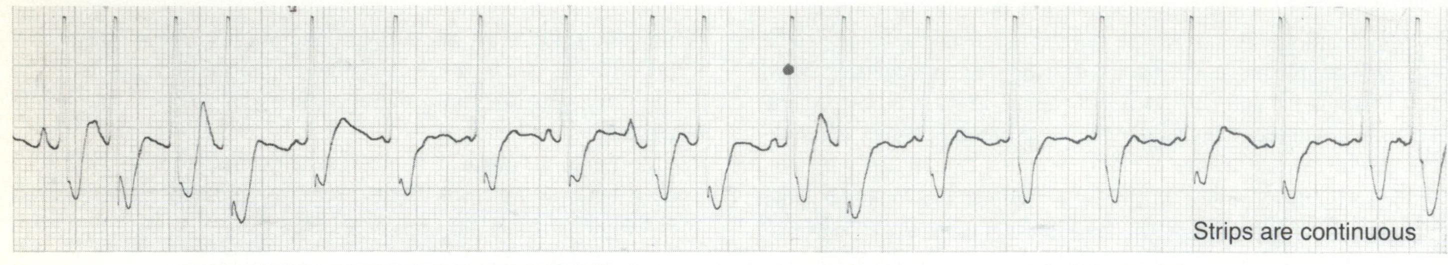

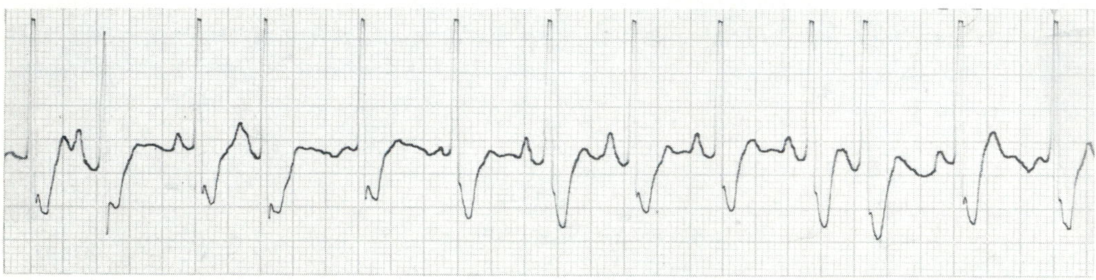

FIGURE 6-24 Multiform atrial tachycardia. Note multiple P wave morphology and variable P′R intervals.

Rate: Approximately 130 bpm. Count for full minute.
Rhythm: Irregular
P wave: Varies in morphology
PR interval: 0.10 to 0.16 seconds
QRS complex: 0.08 seconds
Interpretation: Multiform atrial tachycardia

- Assess the clinical situation in which the arrhythmia is appearing. Does the patient have chronic obstructive pulmonary disease? Is the patient in the early postoperative period? Does the patient have hypertensive or valvular heart disease? Is the patient febrile?
- Assess serum electrolytes.
- Assess respiratory status and arterial blood gases.
- If the patient is febrile, monitor the total and differential white blood cell counts, and obtain blood cultures if indicated.
- Diagnose the arrhythmia. Use the algorithm in Fig. 6-25.

▪ Determine whether patient is receiving theophylline.

❖ NURSING DIAGNOSIS

(1) Decreased cardiac output related to tachycardia. (2) High risk for impaired gas exchange if chronic pulmonary disease is present.

❖ ECG DIAGNOSIS

Multiform atrial tachycardia.

Plan and Implementation

Patient goal. The patient's respiratory status or other primary disorder will stabilize or improve.

Nursing interventions.

▪ Since this arrhythmia often occurs in the presence of hy-

Detect irregularity in the ECG rhythm with all the QRS complexes morphologically similar (that is, the QRS complexes look alike). Differentiate MAT from sinus tachycardia (ST) with multiform APBs and atrial fibrillation (AF).

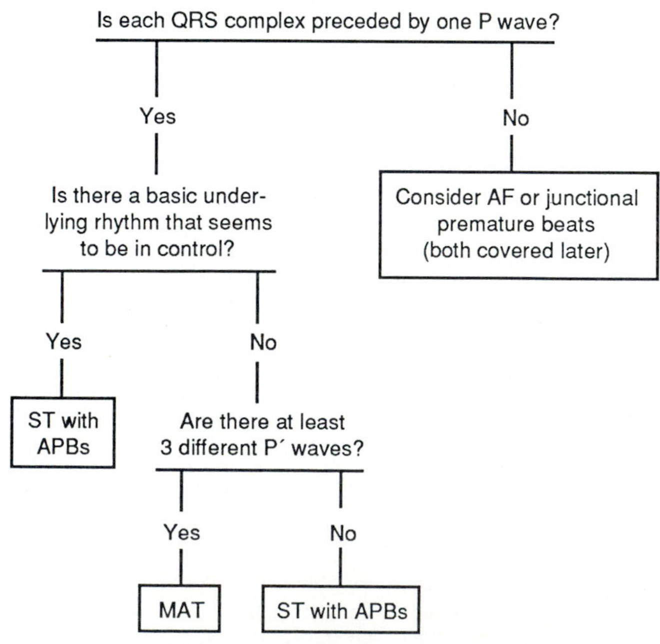

FIGURE 6-25 MAT algorithm.

poxia, hypercapnea, and sometimes with electrolyte disturbances, it is important to periodically monitor these parameters. Appropriate nursing care measures depend on the severity of the patient's condition and nature of the underlying disease.

- The critical nature of the patient's condition requires the nurse to offer emotional support to the patient and significant others and evaluate their adaptation to the clinical situation and prognosis.
- Monitor on a lead that clearly exhibits the P waves. This arrhythmia is often misdiagnosed.
- Carry out the physician's orders and evaluate the patient's response to drug therapy or other intervention. For example, does correction of hypoxemia correlate with stabilization of the arrhythmia?

Evaluation

The patient's respiratory status (or other primary disorder) improves or stabilizes as evidenced by:

- Improved arterial blood gas values.
- Serum electrolytes within normal ranges.
- Improvement in the ECG pattern with less atrial ectopic activity.

Medical Treatment

MAT is often difficult to control with antiarrhythmic agents. Treatment of the underlying condition is more successful in controlling the arrhythmia.[19,20] Recent literature suggests that verapamil may be a useful drug in its management, while the underlying disorder is being corrected.[24] The use of digitalis is evaluated in individual cases, if it is not contraindicated by the underlying condition.

PAROXYSMAL SUPRAVENTRICULAR TACHYCARDIA

Data Base: Problem Identification

Definitions, Etiology, and Mechanisms

The usurping arrhythmias discussed thus far have been predominantly due to automatic phenomena. We now focus on a rhythm disturbance that is more commonly due to what is called a *reentrant* or *reciprocating* impulse. A reciprocating impulse is one that circles and reenters the same area, causing repetitive depolarizations. Although it can occur anywhere in the heart, our discussion in this section is limited to a type that occurs somewhere above the ventricles, above the bifurcation of the His bundle, hence the name *supraventricular*. The term *paroxysmal* connotes the typical, sudden initiation and cessation of the tachycardia. The mechanism of paroxysmal supraventricular tachycardia (PSVT) has long been debated; but it is now believed that the vast majority of PSVTs are a result of reentry involving the AV node as a critical part of the tachycardia circuit. Many cases of PSVT are the result of reentry within the node itself. Other mechanisms that may be responsible for producing this arrhythmia include AV reentry using a concealed bypass tract (that bypasses the AV node), SA nodal reentry, and intraatrial reentry.

PSVT was formerly known as *paroxysmal atrial tachycardia* (PAT). You will see that term used in many textbooks. Recent cardiac electrophysiology studies indicate, however, that the rhythm is not usually a rapid, repetitive firing of an ectopic atrial focus, as had been thought, but rather a circuitous reentry of the impulse involving (most often) the AV node (Fig. 6-26).[6,25] You may be wondering why we are discussing this arrhythmia in the atrial chapter since its source of reentry (circus movement) is usually the AV node. We include it in this chapter because of convention and its historical connection with the atrial arrhythmias.

PSVT is a common arrhythmia in children and young adults (and less common in the elderly). In fact, it is the most common symptom-producing arrhythmia found in children.[26] In infants and children the disorder can be, but often is not, preceded by demonstrable cardiac abnormalities. In the neonate, PSVT is more likely to be caused by a relative immaturity of the conduction system.[27] Supraventricular tachycardias are found in children with congenital heart disease,[28] and may be late sequelae of pediatric heart surgery.[26]

Sometimes the tachycardia is brought on by sympathomimetic drugs, fever, sepsis, myocarditis, or hyperthyroidism. Caffeine intake has been known to induce attacks,[26] and PSVT has been observed after alcohol and tobacco use and during periods of physical or emotional stress in susceptible individuals.

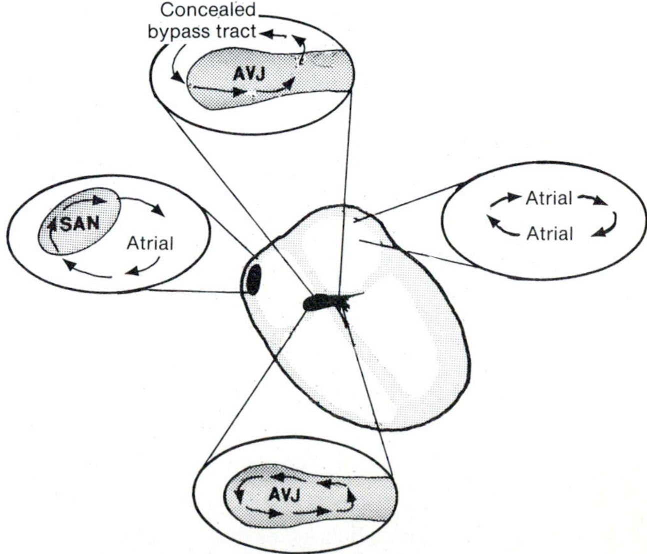

FIGURE 6-26 Possible sites of reentry in supraventricular tachycardia. AVJ = AV junction. SAN = sinoatrial node.

PSVT may be found in healthy adults without heart disease but also can be present in those with rheumatic heart disease, coronary artery disease, thyrotoxicosis, mitral valve prolapse, cardiomyopathy, hypertensive heart disease, chronic or acute cor pulmonale, acute pericarditis, and Wolff-Parkinson-White* (WPW) syndrome.

Less commonly, SVT is found as a chronic disorder. In children it is slower, longer lasting, and less symptom-producing; many have evidence of myocardial dysfunction.[29]

PSVT may be initiated by an APB or ventricular premature beat (VPB). In infants, APBs and sinus acceleration are the most common modes of initiation.[30] This arrhythmia can often be terminated with vagal maneuvers.[17]

Whenever the ventricular rate increases, the period of diastole, or ventricular filling, decreases. When rates exceed 150[31] to 180[32] bpm in normal individuals and 140 bpm in cardiac patients,[32] cardiac output diminishes resulting from decreased stroke volume because of diminished ventricular filling. Tachycardia also increases the myocardial oxygen demand. This, along with diminished coronary artery perfusion related to the shorter period of diastole, may result in decreased myocardial tissue perfusion.

ECG Characteristics

Typically PSVT has an abrupt, or paroxysmal, onset and termination (Fig. 6-27) and is rarely chronic or persistent. (A less common form of SVT displays a comparatively slower rate and may be a chronic disorder lasting for weeks or years.) The adult rate is between 150 and 250 bpm and the rhythm is regular. In infants, the rate ranges are 255 to 320 bpm for neonates, 230 to 350 bpm for infants 1 to 12 months of age, and 180 to 250 bpm for toddlers and children.[27]

The QRS complex is almost always normal in children, but in adults it is not unusual for the QRS complexes to be aberrantly conducted (as APBs can be aberrantly conducted; refer to previous section). Each QRS is associated with a P wave, often obscured by the QRS-T wave forms (Fig. 6-28). When the P wave is visible, it is negative on the inferior leads (II, III, and aVF) (Fig. 6-29). For a summary of the ECG characteristics of PSVT, see the box below.

*Wolff-Parkinson-White (WPW) syndrome, an abnormality in AV conduction, allows atrial impulses to bypass the delay in the AVN. The bypass fibers, known as the *bundles of Kent,* are present only in certain individuals, and do not provide physiologic delay. Hence, rapid atrial arrhythmias produce dangerously rapid ventricular rates.

ECG Characteristics
Paroxysmal Supraventricular Tachycardia

Rate: 150 to 250 bpm (adults and children)
Rhythm: Regular
P waves: Frequently not identified; if seen they bear a constant relationship to the QRS complex and are usually inverted in II, III, aVF.
PR interval: Usually not measurable
QRS complex: Normal unless IVCD present

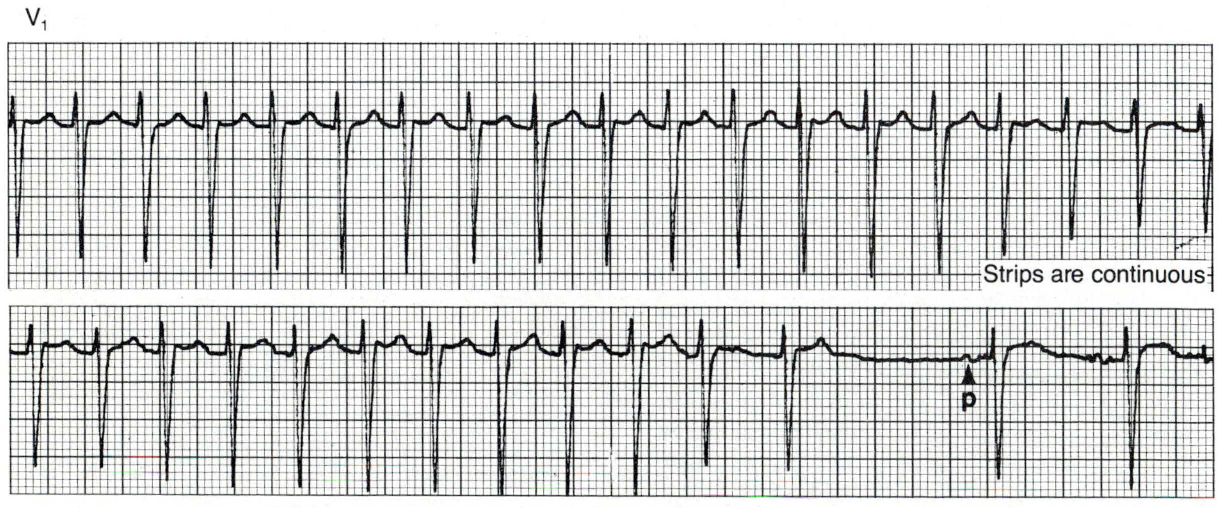

FIGURE 6-27 Paroxysmal supraventricular tachycardia terminating after intravenous verapamil.

Rate: 167 bpm to 86 bpm after conversion
Rhythm: Regular during tachycardia
P wave: Not discernible before conversion. After conversion to NSR, P waves normal for V_1 *(arrow)*
PR interval: 0.15 seconds after conversion
QRS complex: 0.08 seconds
Interpretation: PSVT converting to NSR

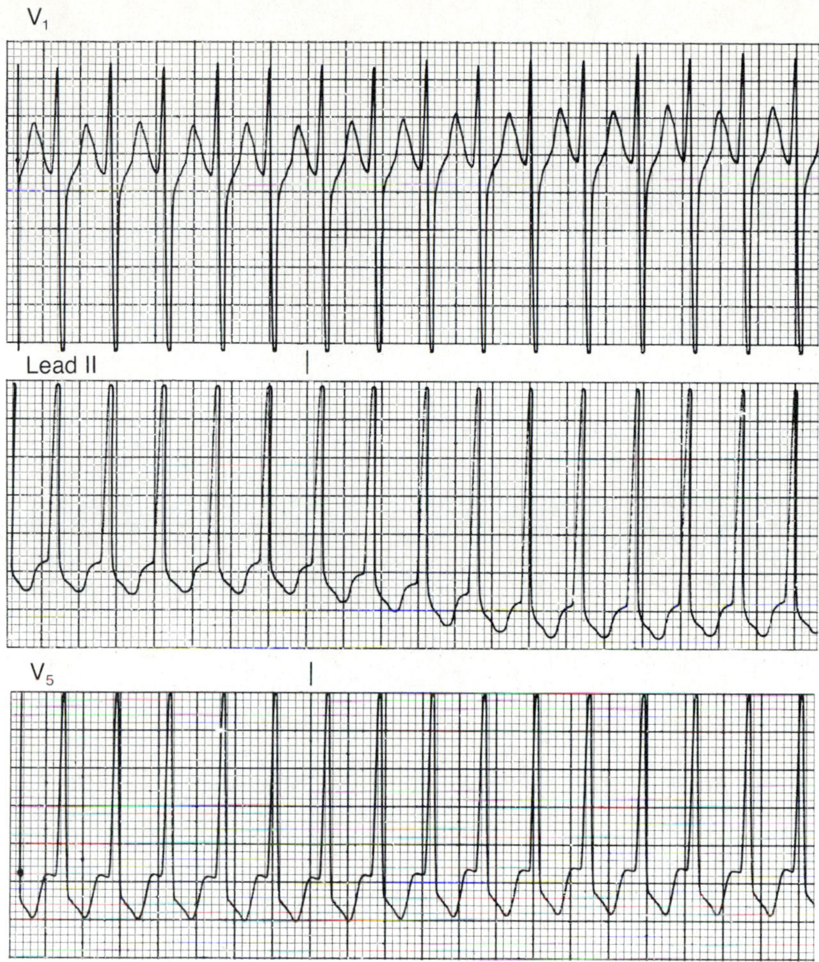

FIGURE 6-28 Supraventricular tachycardia. Simultaneous tracing of three leads, V_1, II, and V_5. Origin of tachycardia cannot be ascertained from this tracing.

Rate: 214 bpm
Rhythm: Regular
P wave: Not discernible
PR interval: —
QRS complex: 0.07 seconds
Interpretation: SVT

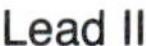

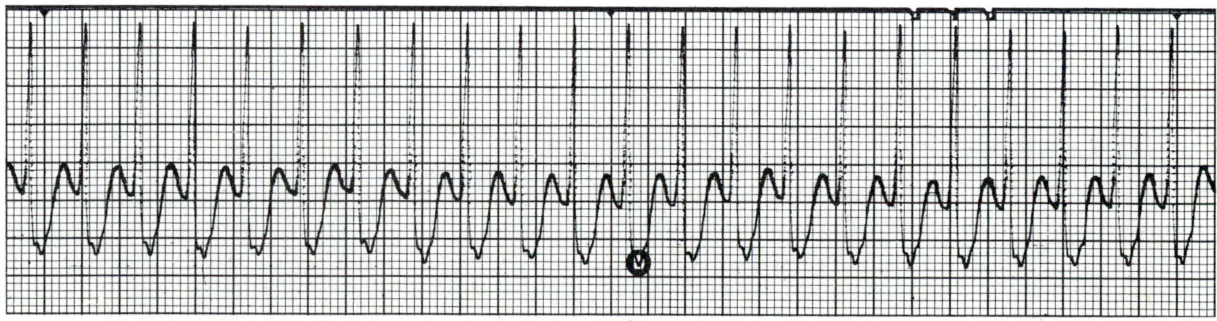

FIGURE 6-29 Supraventricular tachycardia. Inverted P waves (circled) were confirmed on 12 lead ECG.

Rate: 214 bpm
Rhythm: Regular
P wave: Inverted on lead II indicating retrograde atrial depolarization
PR interval: RP interval .08 seconds
QRS complex: 0.06 seconds
Interpretation: SVT, probable AV nodal reentrant

Applied Nursing Process

Clinical Assessment

- Detect:
  - A rapid, regular pulse 150 to 250 bpm.
  - A rapid, regular ECG pattern with (usually) narrow QRS complexes.
  - The sudden onset and abrupt termination of the tachycardia.
- Assess patient and ECG.
  - Assess for symptoms associated with the tachycardia and for symptoms associated with diminished cardiac output:
    Hypotension.
    Syncope, light-headedness or giddiness, altered mentation.
    Pallor, diaphoresis.
  - Assess for symptoms associated with congestive heart failure:
    Shortness of breath.
    Rales in lung bases.
    External jugular venous distension.
    Cough.
    Peripheral edema.
    S_3 heart sound.
  - Assess for signs and symptoms associated with myocardial ischemia:
    Chest and/or arm discomfort.
    Shortness of breath.
    Extreme fatigue.
    ST-segment and T-wave changes.
  - Assess urine output. Many patients with PSVT develop polyuria of up to 3 liters in the first 1 to 2 hours after onset.[33,34]
    Daily weight.
    Accurate intake and output.
  - Assess the patient's level of fear; inquire about symptoms that may be alarming such as palpitations and a feeling that the heart is "racing."
  - Assess the patient's life style and intake of alcohol and caffeine.
  - Diagnose the arrhythmia using the algorithm in Fig. 6-30.

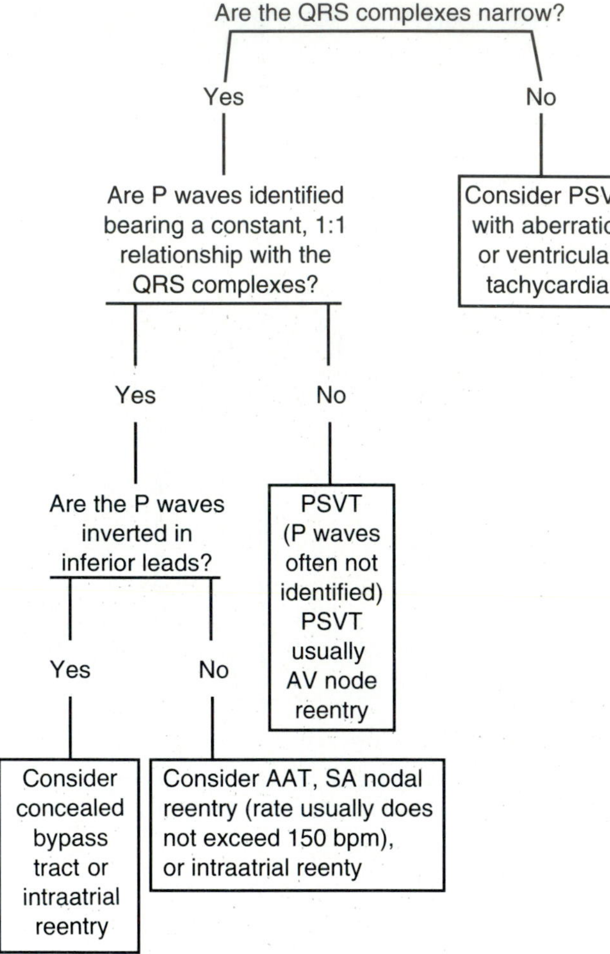

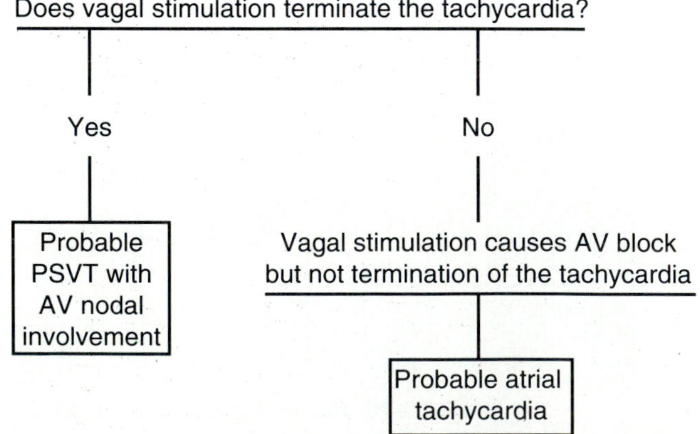

FIGURE 6-30 PSVT algorithm.

❖ NURSING DIAGNOSIS

(1) Decreased cardiac output related to tachycardia. (2) Altered tissue perfusion: cardiopulmonary/cerebral/peripheral, related to reduced cardiac output. (3) Knowledge deficit regarding home management of arrhythmia.

❖ ECG DIAGNOSIS

Paroxysmal supraventricular tachycardia.

Plan and Implementation

Patient goal. The patient will maintain hemodynamic stability, will remain free of pain related to decreased myocardial tissue perfusion, and will relate appropriate information regarding management of the arrhythmia at home.

Nursing interventions.

- Nursing care of the patient in a rapid PSVT involves those interventions directed toward immediate, frequent, and accurate measures to assess the severity of decreased cardiac output and optimize tissue perfusion. Recall that adults are usually able to tolerate this arrhythmia longer than infants, who often show signs of severe compromise and require immediate termination of the arrhythmia.
- Measure blood pressure and assess peripheral pulses and sensorium at frequent intervals to detect deterioration in clinical status. Frequency is determined by the patient's hemodynamic stability and may range from continuous intraarterial pressure monitoring to hourly checks.
- Start an IV as ordered.
- Administer oxygen as needed.
- Take measures to diminish myocardial oxygen demand:
  - Bed rest with commode privileges.
  - Restrict visitors to significant others.
  - Light food intake.
  - Administer tranquilizers/sedatives as ordered.
- Maximize cerebral perfusion.
  - Adjust the head of the bed to flat or low-Fowler's position if there are no signs of congestive heart failure.
- If the patient is severely compromised:
  - Notify the physician at once.
  - Prepare for emergency cardioversion.

    Electrical cardioversion is a procedure in which a direct current electric shock is delivered to the heart through the chest wall. It causes the heart to depolarize, allowing the sinus node to regain control of the rhythm. It is often effective in terminating PSVT but is *contraindicated* in the patient who is digitalis toxic, since it may elicit lethal ventricular arrhythmias such as ventricular fibrillation.

    For this procedure the patient will require short-term sedation such as an antianxiety agent, a muscle relaxant, or a sedative. Airway management is a priority. (See Chapter 12 for "Nurse's Role in Countershock Therapy.") (See "Medical Treatment.")
- Instructing the patient to perform the Valsalva maneuver may terminate the arrhythmia by reflex vagal stimulation,[35] which increases delay in the AV node, thereby interrupting the reentry circuit.
  - Instruct the patient to take a deep breath and try to exhale against a closed glottis, bearing down as if having a bowel movement. This method may be contraindicated if the patient is experiencing angina with the PSVT. (See "Medical Treatment".)
- Record and document the arrhythmia at frequent intervals (as often as every five minutes in the unstable patient) and any changes in rhythm.
- Monitor heart rate and blood pressure during intravenous administration of digitalis, beta blockers, calcium-channel blockers, or Type I or Type III agents.
- If the patient is receiving antiarrhythmic drugs, evaluate their effectiveness while assessing for specific signs of toxicity (see Chapter 11).
- Submersion of the patient's face in cold or ice water for a few seconds may terminate the arrhythmia. This method is not used for the patient with a history of coronary artery disease or PSVT-induced angina, since it may cause reflex constriction of the coronary arteries. It is a popular method of conversion for children. (See "Medical Treatment," below.) Before performing such a procedure, check with the physician or the institutional policies.
- Reassure the adult patient that, with early recognition and treatment, the arrhythmia is not life-threatening.
- The arrhythmia may be life-threatening in infants. Reassure the parent(s) that the baby's condition will improve when the arrhythmia is brought under control.
- If the arrhythmia is a common occurrence, teach the patient about its mechanism, and methods of termination (Valsalva maneuver and/or facial submersion in ice water).
- If the arrhythmia is precipitated by caffeine and/or alcohol, instruct the patient to avoid them.
- Implement physician's orders and evaluate the effectiveness of methods used to abolish the arrhythmia. Make frequent assessments of the ECG to evaluate the patient's tolerance of antiarrhythmic drugs and to detect early signs of toxicity. (See Chapter 11.)

Evaluation

- The patient exhibits stable hemodynamic status during the arrhythmia as evidenced by the following:
  - Maintenance of consciousness.
  - Palpable peripheral pulses with adequate blood pressure.
  - Clear breath sounds with no complaints of shortness of breath.
  - Absence of peripheral edema.
  - Maintenance of comfort without ECG signs of myocardial ischemia.
- The patient performs activities of daily living without interference from the arrhythmia.

Medical Treatment

Reflex vagal stimulation is often among the first medical interventions for the older child[36] and adult because it can rapidly extinguish the tachycardia. Vagal stimulation is generally achieved with carotid sinus massage (CSM)[35,36] or the Valsalva maneuver.[36] A seemingly innocuous procedure to the casual observer, CSM is performed only by physicians and nurses who are specially trained. Since it can result in sequelae such as atrial fibrillation, ventricular arrhythmias, asystole, and stroke, it is performed only when resuscitative equipment is available. It is done carefully in the elderly because of the relatively high incidence of obstructive atherosclerotic disease and the tendency for a profound response.[37] In infants, vagal maneuvers are difficult to perform and are not effective.[29]

A physical conversion technique that occasionally succeeds is *thump version* or a *precordial thump*. Delivered with the fleshy portion of the fist, it can cause depolarization sufficient to abolish the arrhythmia. Another physical conversion technique is elicitation of the diving reflex, in which the patient's face is submerged in cold water.[33] Some authors believe that the elicitation of the diving reflex is the safest method of terminating PSVT in an infant younger than 6 months, or in children old enough (8 years or older) to cooperate.[26,36] In the newborn, a cloth soaked in ice water may be held over the nose and mouth for 10 to 15 seconds to terminate the tachycardia.[36]

Drug therapy is directed toward interrupting the reentrant circuit, usually by increasing the delay in the AV node. Verapamil or adenosine are often used initially. Propranolol[38] or esmolol are also choices of emergency treatment. Edrophonium chloride and phenylephrine[38] have been used successfully in the past for initial treatment but are no longer primary choices.

Chronic therapy is designed to prevent subsequent attacks. Initial therapy usually consists of drug(s) with AV nodal blocking capability, such as digitalis, beta blockers, or calcium blockers. Type I or Type III drugs may be needed in selected refractory cases.[39]

Cardioversion is occasionally used to terminate PSVT. When cardioversion is the preferred treatment (and it is when the patient's condition is critical[38]), low energy (50 joules for an adult) is used for the precordial shock. Cardioversion is the treatment of choice for infants (¼ joule/pound); since they are usually severely compromised, necessitating immediate treatment.[29]

Overdrive pacing is frequently successful in terminating reentrant PSVTs and may be successful if other measures fail. This procedure involves placing a pacing catheter into the right atrium or on the epicardial surface and stimulating the atria at high rates, resulting in termination of the arrhythmia. In postoperative coronary artery bypass patients, temporary epicardial pacemakers are often inserted prophylactically. Overdrive pacing is then the treatment of choice in these patients (see Chapter 13). Some of these devices are patient activated.

AUTOMATIC ATRIAL TACHYCARDIA AND ATRIAL TACHYCARDIA WITH BLOCK

Data Base: Problem Identification

Definitions, Etiology, and Mechanisms

As discussed previously, some of the supraventricular tachycardias have atrial origins and are due to abnormal automaticity, and some (such as PSVT) are due to a reentrant mechanism. As explained in the last section, the term *paroxysmal atrial tachycardia* (PAT), now known as *PSVT*, is outmoded. Likewise, the arrhythmia about to be studied is also known by another term; *PAT with block* is currently known by the name *AT with block*. This arrhythmia is a manifestation of an automatic atrial tachycardia (AAT). The terms *PAT* and *PAT with block* are still commonly used, but they are antiquated and do not reflect the mechanism of the arrhythmia. Recent electrophysiologic research has indicated that few of the PATs are truly atrial as their name would imply; most are AV reentrant tachycardias. Automatic atrial tachycardias are not always paroxysmal; indeed, they are often nonparoxysmal. Clinical electrophysiology studies (EPS) have revealed important information correlating the origins, clinical features, and electrocardiographic criteria of the SVTs.

Unlike PSVT, automatic atrial tachycardia results from abnormal atrial automaticity rather than reentry, has a comparatively slower rate (less than 200 bpm), and often exhibits varying degrees of AV nodal block. An uncommon arrhythmia, AAT often exhibits signs of AV block; thus the term *AT with block*. (*AAT with block* would be an acceptable synonym.) Since AT with block is the most frequently encountered form of AAT, our discussion is limited to it.

AT with block may be a result of digitalis toxicity (and less commonly, acute myocardial infarction), although it comprises only a small percentage of the rhythm disturbances found in these two disorders. Hypokalemia seems to provoke the arrhythmia.[6] Other conditions that may be associated with it include chronic obstructive pulmonary disease, hypoxia, various metabolic abnormalities, amphetamines, and alcohol ingestion.[6]

ECG Characteristics

Initiation of AT with block may be paroxysmal (starting abruptly) but more commonly is nonparoxysmal (onset is more gradual), exhibiting what is known as a *warm-up phenomenon*. *Warm-up* is a term used for automatic rhythms that gradually, rather than abruptly, increase in rate. In this respect, AT with block is unlike PSVT, which is usually initiated by a premature beat.

The atrial rate is between 100 to 200 bpm, often less than 175. The P waves are small but visible and may be uniform or multiform.

Because not all of the atrial impulses conduct to the ventricles and AV conduction is unpredictable, the resultant ventricular rate and rhythm may be regular, irregular, or regularly irregular (another term for grouped beating in which the irregularity occurs in a pattern). The PR interval may be normal or prolonged with the impulses that are conducted. The important thing to remember is that not every P wave results in a QRS complex. (Patterns of conduction and AV block will be discussed in Chapter 9.)

When the atrial rate is around 150 to 160 bpm, it may

be confused with sinus tachycardia. To help differentiate the two, consider the clinical picture and remember that in sinus tachycardia the P waves will be uniform, regular, and slightly larger (Fig. 6-31 and the box on this page).

Applied Nursing Process

Clinical Assessment

- Detect:
  - A regular or irregular pulse.
  - More P waves than QRS complexes on the ECG.
- Assess patient and ECG.
  - Patients are often unaware of this arrhythmia, but nevertheless should be assessed for their tolerance of it. Assess blood pressure and pulse. The patient should be monitored.
- Assess for clinical signs of digitalis toxicity (see Table 6-1).
  - Anorexia, nausea, vomiting.
  - Yellow vision, tinting, or halos.
  - ECG manifestations of digitalis toxicity (in addition to AT with block).
    - Progressive AV block (increasing PR interval and P waves not conducted to the ventricles with resultant decrease in ventricular rate).
    - Increased automaticity throughout the heart (atria, junction, and ventricles).
  - Monitor serum digoxin level and potassium.
  - Diagnose the arrhythmia. Detect more P waves than QRS complexes with atrial rate 100 to 200 bpm and all QRS complexes morphologically similar.

❖ NURSING DIAGNOSIS

Decreased cardiac output related to tachycardia.

❖ ECG DIAGNOSIS

Atrial tachycardia with block.

Plan and Implementation

Patient goal. The patient will be asymptomatic during the arrhythmia and will relate appropriate information concerning precautions and symptoms of toxicity if receiving digitalis. The arrhythmia will abate with correction of the underlying cause.

Nursing interventions.

- Notify the physician.

ECG Characteristics
Atrial Tachycardia with Block

Rate: ≥100 bpm (atrial); ventricular rate ≤atrial rate
Rhythm: Regular or slightly irregular (atrial); often irregular (ventricular)
P waves: Often small, one or more precedes each QRS
PR interval: Normal or prolonged with conducted P waves
QRS complex: Normal unless IVCD present

TABLE 6-1 Adverse and Toxic Reactions to Digitalis

Electrocardiographic	Physical
Sinus bradycardia	Anorexia*
SA and AV blocks	Nausea*
Ectopy (atrial, junctional, ventricular*)	Vomiting*
	Diarrhea
Tachycardia (atrial, junctional, ventricular*)	Yellow vision or tinting
Accelerated junctional rhythm	

*Rare in children.

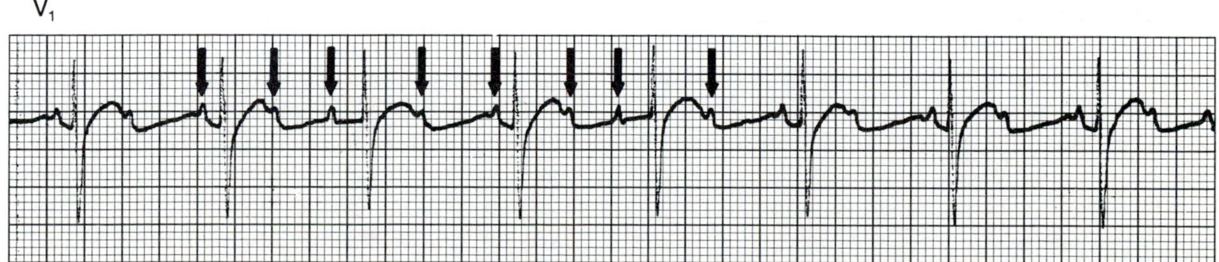

FIGURE 6-31 Atrial tachycardia with block. Note small P waves, irregular in rhythm *(arrows).*

Rate: Atrial: 160 bpm
Ventricular: 80 bpm
Rhythm: Irregular
P wave: More P waves than QRS complexes; P waves small, irregular
PR interval: 0.11 to 0.18 seconds
QRS complex: 0.08 seconds
Interpretation: Atrial tachycardia with block (2:1 conduction)

- Hold digoxin until physician is notified and serum digoxin and potassium levels are obtained.
- If the patient is digitalis toxic, hold until serum level is within normal limits. If the arrhythmia is related to digitalis toxicity, it should show signs of improvement within 24 to 48 hours after the drug is withheld, unless renal failure is present.
- Initiate patient teaching for those receiving digitalis including the following instructions:
  - How to take own pulse.
  - Signs and symptoms of digitalis toxicity.
  - The importance of precise compliance with prescription directions. (Many patients hold the mistaken belief that if a "little is good, more must be better.")
  - The importance of having digoxin blood levels drawn on a regular basis.
- Implement physician's orders. Evaluate measures taken to correct the underlying cause and correct the arrhythmia. For example, evaluate the response to beta blockers and the degree of arrhythmia control.

Evaluation

- The patient is asymptomatic during episodes of AT with block as evidenced by the following:
  - No change in blood pressure.
  - No complaints of palpitations.
- The arrhythmia disappeared with correction of underlying cause as evidenced by the following:
  - Return to normal sinus rhythm.
- The patient shows evidence of understanding dosages and precautions associated with digitalis use.

Medical Treatment

Medical treatment often includes administration of a beta blocker such as esmolol or propranolol,[41] which reduces automaticity (see Chapter 11). Type I drugs have occasionally been effective. The site of origin of the tachycardia can be mapped and surgically resected in selected cases. AT with block does not respond well to overdrive pacing, cardioversion,[4] or increased vagal tone.[17]

When AT with block is due to digitalis toxicity, serum potassium must be maintained at high normal levels. In more severe cases, diphenylhydantoin may be helpful. Antidigitalis antibodies are available for life-threatening cases when rapid and complete reversal of the arrhythmia is mandatory.

ATRIAL FLUTTER

Data Base: Problem Identification

Definitions, Etiology, and Mechanisms

Atrial flutter (AFl), another of the supraventricular tachycardias, is characterized by atrial depolarizations occurring at rapid (250 to 350 bpm), regular rates displaying characteristic flutter waves. Its mechanism of perpetuation is controversial but is likely a form of reentry within the atria.[6,25,42] The ventricles are protected from such high atrial rates by the AV node, which delays and blocks impulses, thereby preventing extremely high ventricular rates.

Although it is a frequently encountered rhythm disorder, AFl is far less common than AF. Occurring in all age groups, AFl is almost always associated with some form of heart disease, usually coronary artery disease or rheumatic heart disease but can occur with pulmonary embolism, pericarditis, myocarditis, acute myocardial infarction, cardiomyopathy, and thyrotoxicosis. It may appear in WPW syndrome, one of the AV nodal bypass arrhythmias (impulses from the atria bypass the AV node en route to the ventricles and, thus, are not delayed).[4] When it occurs in children, AFl is frequently associated with congenital heart disease,[28] and it is far more rare than junctional tachycardia (JT) or PSVT.[27] Alcohol abuse has been implicated as an etiologic factor in some individuals.[43] It has also occurred after cardiac surgery,[44] including orthotopic heart transplantation.[45]

AFl is initially paroxysmal and maybe short lived, lasting hours or days. It may, however, be chronic and last months or years. It is often seen as a transitional rhythm in the course of AF.

Patients who have AFl exhibit symptoms ranging from mild palpitations to overt cardiac failure and cardiogenic shock, depending on the ventricular rate and the underlying cardiac status.[37] As mentioned, the intact AV node usually protects the ventricles from excessive rate increases. In cases of WPW syndrome and after certain pediatric cardiac surgical procedures (such as the Mustard procedure or corrective surgery for transposition of the great vessels), conduction to the ventricles may be 1:1, resulting in dangerously high ventricular rates and shock.[46]

The prognosis of AFl is variable, depending on the etiology and the underlying cardiac disorder. The presence of AFl during the course of an acute myocardial infarction or recurrent congestive heart failure is a poor prognostic sign.

ECG Characteristics

The striking feature that distinguishes AFl from other rapid atrial rhythms is the characteristic flutter waves ("saw-tooth" or "picket fence" appearance of the P waves) on the ECG (Fig. 6-32). As ventricular rates accelerate, it becomes more difficult to detect the presence of AFl (Fig. 6-33) obscured by QRS complexes. AFl waves will most likely not appear on every lead; a 12-lead ECG may reveal their presence on only one or two leads, often an inferior lead such as II, III, or aVF.[42] V_1 is also good for detection of flutter waves.

Close inspection of the flutter wave (the F wave) will frequently reveal an asymmetric, pointed complex in which the negative component is more pronounced than

Lead II

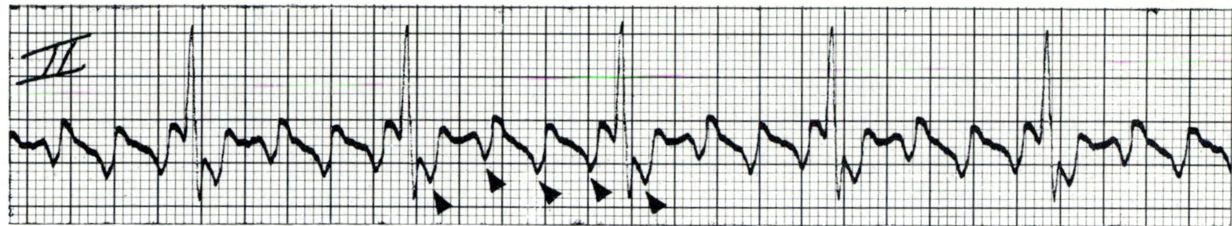

FIGURE 6-32 Atrial flutter. Note precise regularity of F waves. Since there are four flutter waves for every QRS complex, it is termed AFl with 4:1 conduction.

Rate: Atrial: 250 bpm
Ventricular: 60 bpm
Rhythm: Atrial: Regular
Ventricular: Regular
P wave: Flutter waves
PR interval: Not measured in AFl
QRS complex: 0.08 seconds
Interpretation: AFl with 4:1 conduction

Lead II

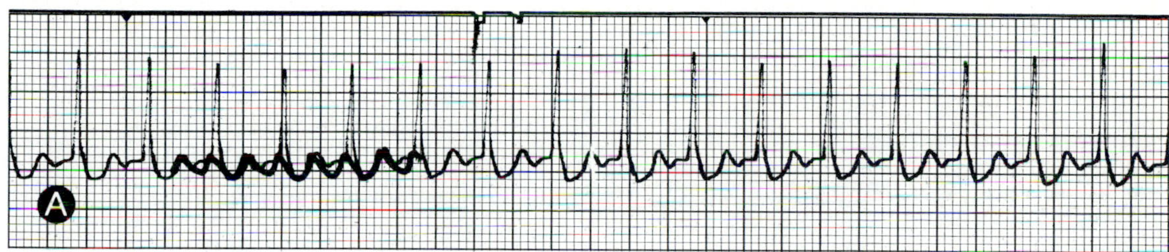

MCL_1

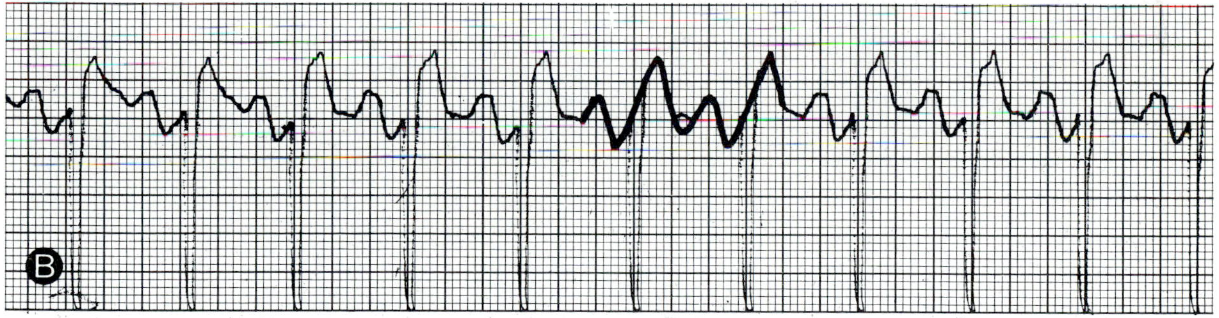

FIGURE 6-33 Two examples of atrial flutter with 2:1 conduction, both confirmed by 12-lead ECG. Flutter waves are highlighted to aid otherwise obscure atrial activity.

A.

Rate: Atrial: 334 bpm
Ventricular: 167 bpm
Rhythm: Atrial: Regular
Ventricular: Regular
P wave: Flutter waves at 2:1 ratio to QRS complex are obscured
PR interval: —
QRS complex: 0.06 seconds
Interpretation: Atrial flutter with 2:1 conduction

B.

Rate: Atrial: 200 bpm
Ventricular: 100 bpm
Rhythm: Atrial: Regular
Ventricular: Regular
P wave: Large flutter waves at 2:1 ratio to QRS complexes; flutter rate is unusually slow and flutter waves unusually large.
QRS complex: 0.09 to 0.10 seconds
Interpretation: "Slow" atrial flutter with 2:1 conduction

the positive (Fig. 6-32). Typically, the flutter rate is 300 ± 10 bpm[42] but may be less than 250 bpm or as high as 425 bpm. In newborns, it can approach 500 bpm.[36]

Fortunately, not all the atrial impulses reach the ventricles because of physiologic delay in the AV node. The ratio of flutter waves (F) to QRS complexes before medical treatment is usually 2:1 (Fig. 6-33), resulting in a ventricular rate of 150 bpm.[37] With treatment directed at prolonging AV conduction the ratio widens to 4:1. The QRS-to-F-wave ratio is more often even than odd. The R-R interval is variable since ratios are not always constant, except when 2:1 conduction is present (Fig. 6-34).

Since AV conduction delay is less developed in infants, 1:1 atrial flutter is not unusual (Fig. 6-35). This 1:1 conduction may also be observed in the adult when AV conduction delay is diminished as a result of exercise or following initiation of quinidine or procainamide therapy. When 1:1 conduction is observed in the quinidine or procainamide-treated adult, the flutter rate is relatively slow (i.e., <250 bpm).

Characteristically, the rhythm of the flutter waves is precisely regular (Fig. 6-32). However, administration of certain antiarrhythmic drugs may result in slower, slightly irregular flutter cycles.

Problems in the electrocardiographic differential diagnosis sometimes occur if the QRS is widened due to a bundle branch block (BBB) and the rate is rapid, obscuring the flutter waves (Fig. 6-36). Diagnosing atrial flutter and differentiating it from arrhythmias such as ventricular tachycardia (described in Chapter 8) will be aided by inspection of the ECG on different leads. Vagal stimulation may also assist in the diagnosis. By increasing the delay in the AV node, vagal stimulation results in slowing of the ventricular rate, allowing the F waves to be revealed.

Fig. 6-37 illustrates an unusual form of AFl, occurring in paroxysms.

Lead II telemetry

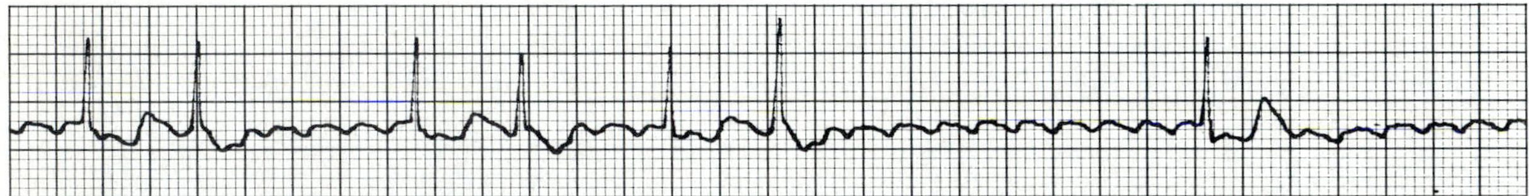

FIGURE 6-34 Atrial flutter. Note saw-tooth appearance of flutter waves and variable R-R intervals.

Rate: Atrial: 330 bpm
Ventricular: about 70 bpm
Rhythm: Atrial: Regular
Ventricular: Regular
P wave: Flutter waves
PR interval: —
QRS complex: 0.06 seconds
Interpretation: Atrial flutter with ventricular response 70 bpm

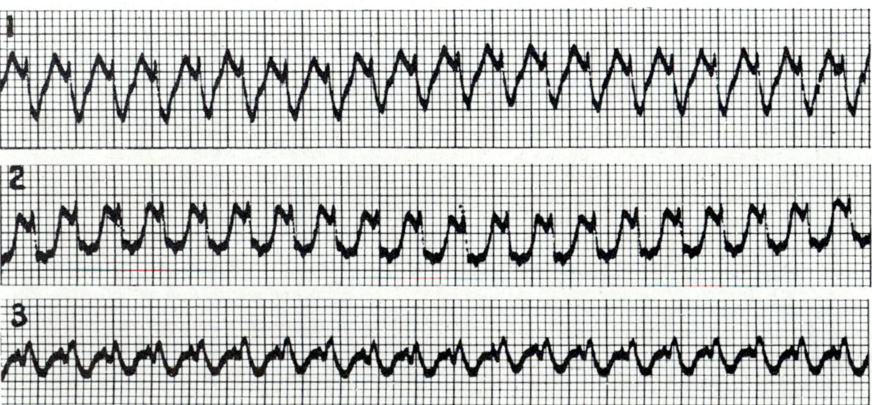

FIGURE 6-35 Atrial flutter at a rate of 256 bpm with 1:1 AV conduction and an incomplete right bundle branch block pattern. From Marriott HJL. *Practical Electrocardiography.* 8th ed. Baltimore: Williams & Wilkins, 1988, p. 187.

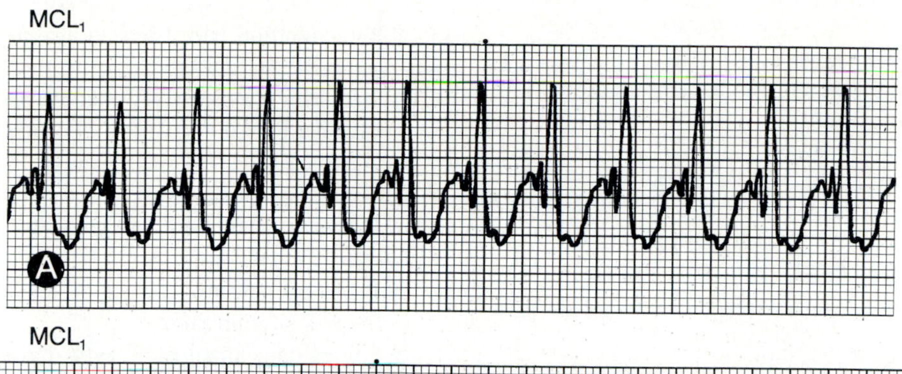

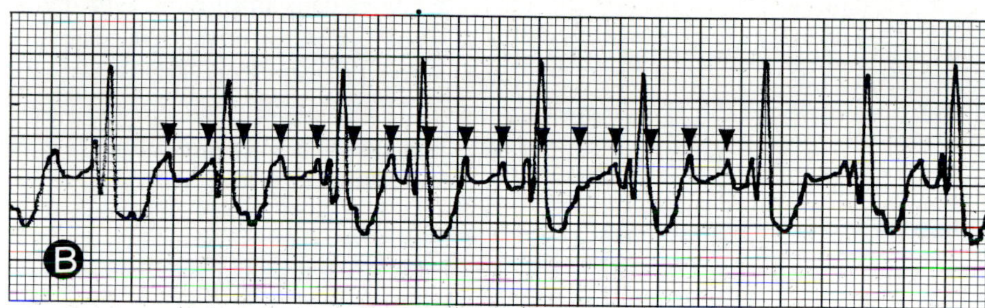

FIGURE 6-36 Atrial flutter in the presence of bundle branch block. **A,** This tracing is difficult to interpret. The wide QRS complexes obscure the underlying atrial flutter. **B,** When the R-R intervals lengthen, the underlying atrial flutter is revealed.

Rate: Atrial: 300 bpm
Ventricular: 150 to 120 bpm
Rhythm: Atrial: Regular
Ventricular: Regular in A, irregular in B
P wave: Flutter waves with 2:1 conduction in A and 2:1 and 3:1 conduction in B
PR interval: —
QRS complex: 0.12 seconds, rsR′ morphology in V_1 consistent with RBBB
Interpretation: AFl with 2:1 and 3:1 conduction

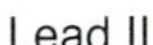

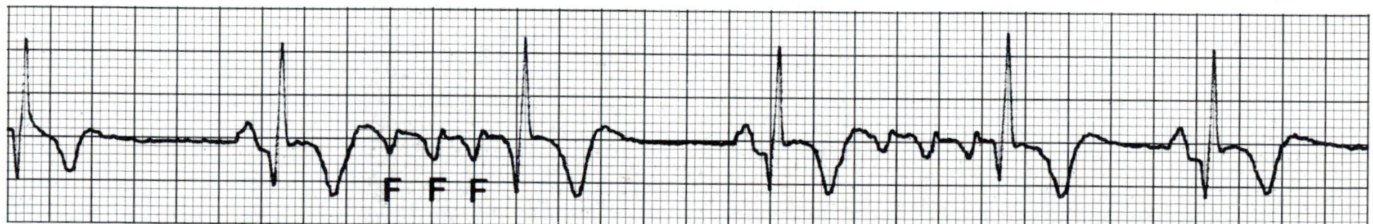

FIGURE 6-37 Intermittent atrial flutter. Note paroxysmal appearance of flutter waves *(F)*.

Rate: Atrial: 60 to 300 bpm
Ventricular: 52 to 63 bpm
Rhythm: Irregular
P wave: Flutter waves present in paroxysms; sinus P waves slightly notched
PR interval: 0.16 seconds with sinus-conducted impulses
QRS complex: 0.09 seconds, significant Q wave present in lead II; T wave inverted
Interpretation: NSR with intermittent atrial flutter

ECG Characteristics
Atrial Flutter

Rate: 250 to 350 bpm (atrial);
150 bpm or below (ventricular)—in adult (usually)
Rhythm: Regular (atrial);
regular or irregular (ventricular)
P waves: Flutter waves—"saw tooth" appearance; two or more precede each QRS
PR interval: Not measured
QRS complex: Normal unless IVCD present

See the box above for a summary of the ECG features of AFl.

Applied Nursing Process

Clinical Assessment

- Detect:
  - A regular or irregular pulse 150 bpm or less.
  - A regular supraventricular tachycardia with a ventricular rate of 150 ± 10 bpm, a regular ventricular rhythm at a rate of 75 bpm with AFl waves apparent, or an irregular ventricular rhythm (of any rate) with AFl waves apparent.
- Assess the patient and ECG.
  - Assess the patient's tolerance of the arrhythmia and for signs of decreased cardiac output.
    Measure blood pressure and pulse.
    Assess for pulse deficit.
  - Assess the patient's skin color and temperature.
  - In rapid AFl with 1:1 conduction to the ventricles, cardiac output will decrease and perfusion may become seriously compromised. Hypoperfusion resulting in light-headedness or syncope, hypotension, pallor, and cool, diaphoretic skin is an emergency requiring immediate intervention.
  - Regarding the clinical manifestations of AFl, one must consider the underlying or coexisting disorders. Since CHF is often present in patients with AFl, assessment of the cardiovascular and pulmonary parameters is indicated. Check for signs and symptoms of CHF: rales in the lower lung fields, external jugular venous distension, cough, shortness of breath, and peripheral edema.
  - If the patient has coronary artery disease with a history of chest pain, assess for the development or progression of angina during the flutter. The pain may be rate dependent, related to imbalance in myocardial oxygen supply and demand.
  - Determine if the patient is experiencing palpitations.
  - Monitor the patient and assess the ECG, noting the ventricular rate, the ratio of flutter waves to QRS complexes, and the stability and consistency of the rhythm. If recognition and differential diagnosis of the rhythm are difficult, attempt to slow the ventricular rate momentarily (to identify flutter waves) by having the patient perform the Valsalva maneuver, if it is not contraindicated.
  - Monitor serum electrolytes, especially potassium.
  - Monitor serum drug levels such as digoxin and quinidine.
  - If the patient has CHF or prosthetic valves, assess for the risk of embolism.
  - For patients medicated with digoxin, assess for signs and symptoms of digoxin toxicity (see Table 6-1).
  - For patients receiving other antiarrhythmics, assess ECG for signs of drug toxicity (see Chapter 11).
  - Diagnosis of the arrhythmia is usually not difficult unless the AV conduction ratio is 2:1. Use the algorithm in Fig. 6-38 to assist in the differential diagnosis.

❖ NURSING DIAGNOSIS

(1) Decreased cardiac output related to tachycardia. (2) Altered tissue perfusion: cerebral/cardiopulmonary/peripheral, related to reduced cardiac output.

❖ ECG DIAGNOSIS

Atrial flutter.

Plan and Implementation

Patient goal. The patient's arrhythmia will convert to normal sinus rhythm (NSR) or to AFl with a controlled ventricular response. For the patient in whom AFl is a chronic arrhythmia, the ventricular rate will be controlled within normal limits.

Nursing interventions.

- The nursing management is guided by the patient's history and the severity of the arrhythmia. Much depends on the ventricular rate and degree of reduction in cardiac output.
- If the cardiac output is compromised significantly, take measures to improve cerebral perfusion and decrease myocardial oxygen demand.
  - Lower the head of the bed if not contraindicated.
  - Encourage rest.
  - Avoid intake of stimulants.
  - Administer oxygen if indicated.
- If electrical cardioversion is the selected therapy, see Chapter 12 and selected references[47,48] for a discussion of the nurse's role during cardioversion therapy.
- For patients receiving digoxin, teach the action of the drug, dosages, and symptoms of toxicity. Instruct that digoxin is not a "PRN" drug and, if palpitations are noted, that additional doses are unnecessary and poten-

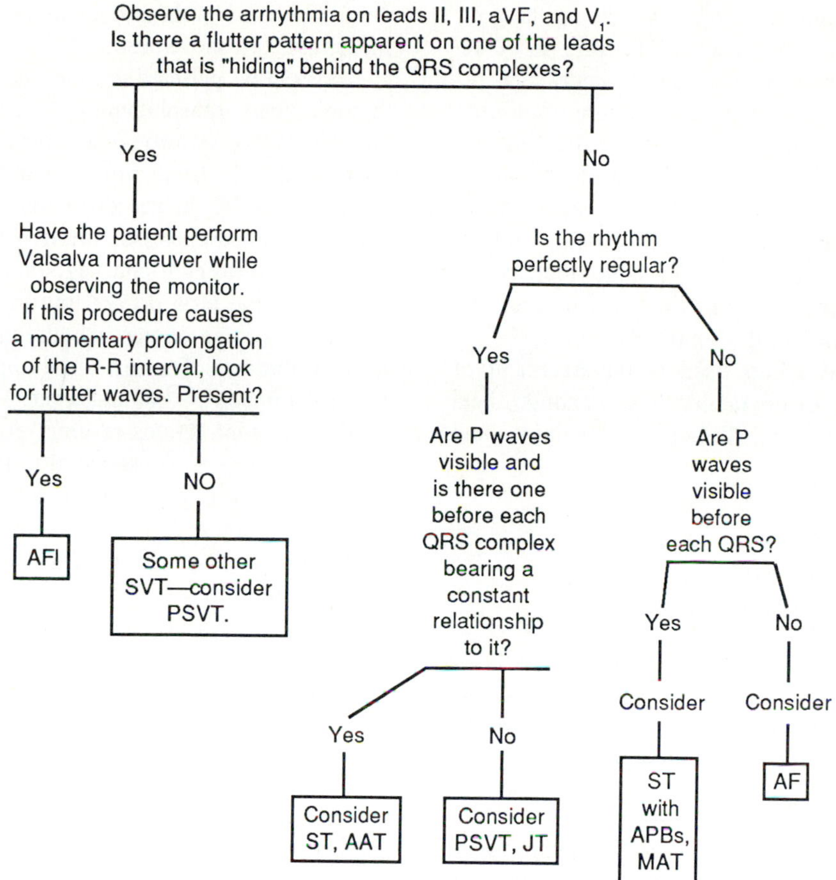

FIGURE 6-38 Atrial flutter algorithm.

tially harmful. Instruct the patient to seek medical attention if such symptoms appear.

- Implement physician's orders.
- Administer antiarrhythmic drugs as ordered; evaluate patient response to the drugs and their effectiveness in controlling the arrhythmia. See Chapter 11 for specific information on the electrocardiographic effects of antiarrhythmic agents.

Evaluation

- The patient's rhythm converts to a stable rhythm as evidenced by NSR (or, as the case may be, AF with a controlled ventricular rate) on the monitor.
- Or the patient remains in AFl with a controlled ventricular rate.
- The patient remains hemodynamically stable as evidenced by the following:
  - Stable vital signs.
  - Clear lung fields.
  - Full orientation.
  - Absence of dizziness, light-headedness, or syncope.

Medical Treatment

Nonpharmacologic

Electrical cardioversion is a frequently successful therapeutic approach. The initial energy requirement is 25 joules (see p. 356).[6,37]

Atrial overdrive pacing[37] (see Chapter 13) may be indicated. It is more successful with AFl rates less than 360 bpm. Pacing will frequently convert the arrhythmia to a sinus rhythm. Occasionally atrial pacing is obtained via the esophagus, especially in children.

Pharmacologic

The goal of pharmacologic therapy is to reduce the ventricular rate and, if possible, convert the AFl to NSR. Since the immediate goal is to control ventricular response, drugs such as verapamil or esmolol are often used initially. Then digitalization is instituted to increase the delay at the AV node. Formerly the combination of digoxin and quinidine were popular therapeutic choices. Since quinidine (1) causes a decrease in the flutter rate and (2) has an initial vagolytic effect on the AV node, thereby improving AV conduction, it is always started after the digoxin to avoid increases in the ventricular rate.

Other antiarrhythmic agents used in the treatment of AFl include verapamil, disopyramide, procainamide, beta blockers, sotalol, amiodarone, flecainide, encainide, and propafenone.

ATRIAL FIBRILLATION

Data Base: Problem Identification

Definitions, Etiology, and Mechanisms

One of the most common arrhythmias encountered in the adult population, atrial fibrillation (AF) can be an isolated event or a chronic, lifelong rhythm disturbance. It rarely affects children but when it does, congenital heart disease,[4,28] rheumatic heart disease, or cardiomyopathy[27] is almost always present.

In AF, orderly atrial depolarization is lost and replaced with rapid, chaotic quivering. Effective atrial contraction is sacrificed and, hence, the atrial contribution to cardiac output (the *atrial kick*) is lost. Loss of the atrial kick can reduce cardiac output by as much as 30%.

The physiologic mechanism responsible for AF is not entirely clear. It has traditionally been thought to be due to multifocal ectopic atrial impulse formation. More recently, multiple reentry has been advanced as the probable major mechanism. Numerous small areas in the atria at various stages of depolarization and repolarization excite adjacent tissue groups in different stages of refractoriness, perpetuating the chaos. Atrial enlargement with increased atrial pressure and wall tension may be structural factors involved in the mechanism of AF.[49]

AF can be initiated by either (1) an atrial stimulus occurring during the vulnerable period of atrial repolarization (e.g., an APB or a stimulus from an atrial pacemaker) or (2) the deterioration of one of the rapid atrial arrhythmias into AF. For example, AFl often degenerates from an orderly flutter into disorderly fibrillation.

There are four major underlying conditions associated with atrial fibrillation: rheumatic or mitral disease, ischemic heart disease, hypertension, and hyperthyroidism[15,37] (approximately one third of hyperthyroid patients have AF[50]). Of these causes, hypertensive cardiovascular disease is the most common.[49] Other causes include pulmonary embolism,[51] cor pulmonale, atrial septal defect, and hypertrophic cardiomyopathy.[49] However, AF can accompany any cardiac disease and has been documented in patients without demonstrable disease as well.[15,37,52]

Constrictive pericarditis, cardiac surgery (including orthotopic heart transplantation),[45] congestive heart failure, and the WPW syndrome are sometimes complicated by AF,[53] and it is frequently a manifestation of sick sinus syndrome (SSS). It has also been associated with alcohol abuse, sustained exercise, emotional upset, gastrointestinal disturbances, fatigue, and vagotonic activity.[54-56]

Because the atria do not uniformly contract and empty during the course of the arrhythmia, patients are prone to develop thrombi. The left atrial appendage is a site noted for their formation.[51] If and when AF is terminated and orderly atrial contractions resume, emboli may enter the arterial circulation. Consequently, thromboembolic events are a serious complication of AF and pose a risk which cannot be ignored.[57]

The prognosis of AF depends on the associated cardiac disease and degree of thromboembolic activity.[49] When AF complicates acute myocardial infarction, which it does in 6% to 16% of cases,[4] it tends to be associated with a larger infarction and a poor prognosis.

ECG Characteristics

The atrial rate and rhythm in this arrhythmia are so disorganized they defy analysis. Fibrillatory waves replace discrete P waves. These f waves may appear to be fine or coarse but they are always disorganized and so rapid (350 to 600 cycles/min) that they cannot be counted (Fig. 6-39). When the f waves are coarse, short bursts of flutter waves can often be identified. Some call this kind of coarse AF *fib-flutter* (Figs. 6-39 and 6-40). Because the AV junction is bombarded with impulses that penetrate it in varying degrees, portions of the junction remain refractory and unable to respond to impulses in any orderly way. This is a form of what is known as *concealed conduction* (the AV junction is refractory due to conduction of an impulse that does not result in a QRS complex). The resultant ventricular response is always irregular, unless AV dissociation exists, a phenomenon discussed in Chapter 9.

The ventricular rate in untreated AF is above 100 bpm and is often labeled *uncontrolled atrial fibrillation*. When accompanied by a rapid ventricular response (greater than 150 bpm), AF is associated with complications such as myocardial infarction, hypotension, and congestive heart failure.[57] Conditions that shorten the refractory period in the AV junction, allowing the ventricular rate to increase, include sympathetic nervous system stimulation from administration of sympathomimetic drugs (e.g., epinephrine, norepinephrine, or isoproterenol), emotional stress, exer-

Lead II

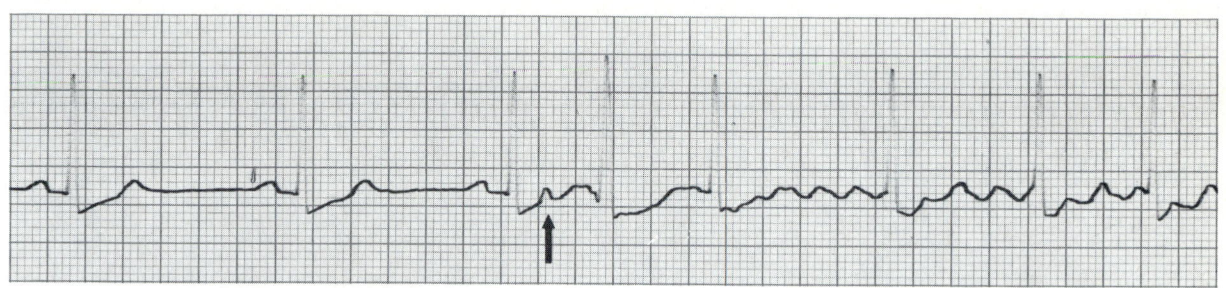

FIGURE 6-39 Initiation of atrial fibrillation. Note APB initiating atrial fibrillation *(arrow).* Flutter waves are also apparent. When both flutter and fibrillatory waves are present in the same tracing, some call it *flutter-fib.* Others prefer to call it *coarse fibrillation* unless flutter waves are consistent.

Rate: 50 bpm both atrial and ventricular then
Atrial: Too rapid to count
Ventricular: Approximately 80 bpm
Rhythm: Regular, becomes irregular
P wave: Normal until atrial fibrillation
PR interval: 0.20 seconds when in sinus bradycardia
QRS complex: 0.06 seconds
Interpretation: Sinus bradycardia going into atrial fibrillation

V_1

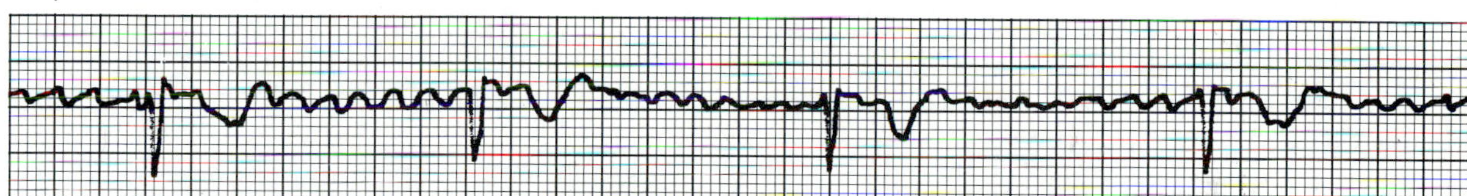

FIGURE 6-40 Atrial flutter-fib. Note the presence of both flutter and fibrillatory waves.

Rate: Atrial: Too rapid to count
Ventricular: Approximately 45 bpm. Count for full minute.
Rhythm: Irregular
P wave: F waves and f waves present
PR interval: —
QRS complex: 0.06 to 0.07 seconds
Interpretation: Atrial flutter-fib, controlled

Lead II

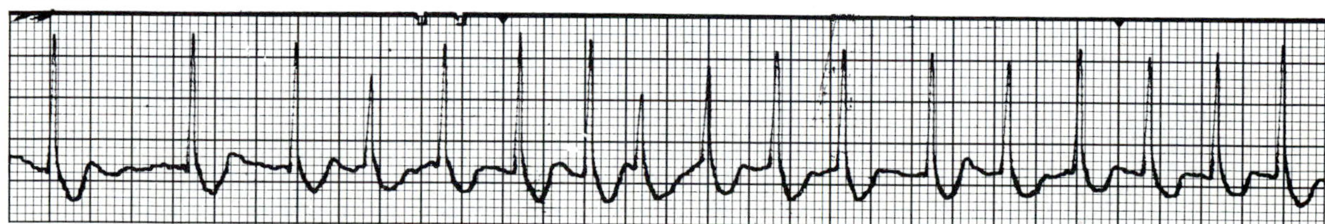

FIGURE 6-41 Uncontrolled atrial fibrillation. Note as rate increases, less irregularity is apparent in the ventricular response.

Rate: Atrial: Too rapid to count
Ventricular: Approximately 180 bpm
Rhythm: Irregular
P wave: f waves
PR interval: —
QRS complex: 0.06 seconds
Interpretation: Uncontrolled atrial fibrillation

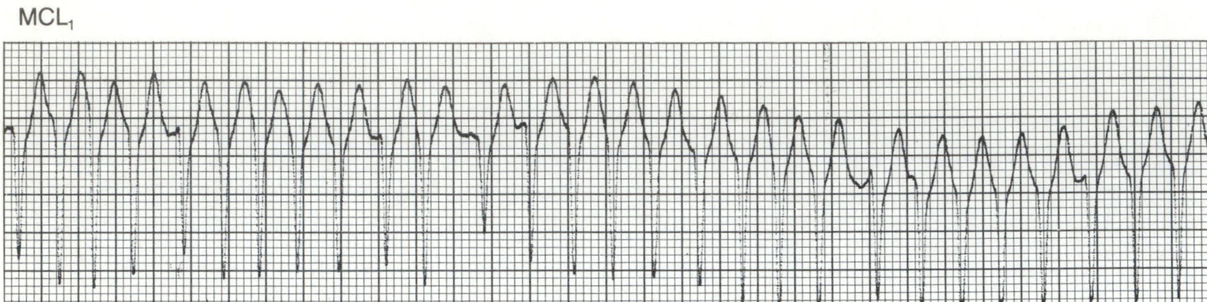

FIGURE 6-42 Atrial fibrillation in the presence of WPW syndrome. Note the ventricular rate reaches 300 bpm, making atrial fibrillation in this clinical situation a potentially lethal arrhythmia. Note characteristic irregular ventricular response.

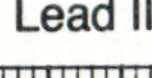

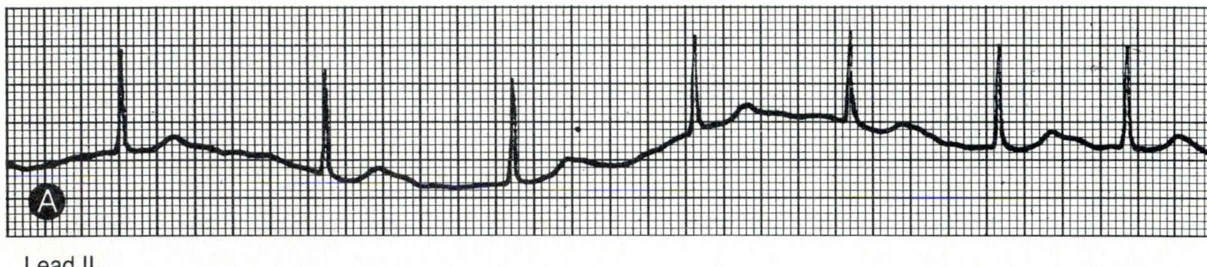

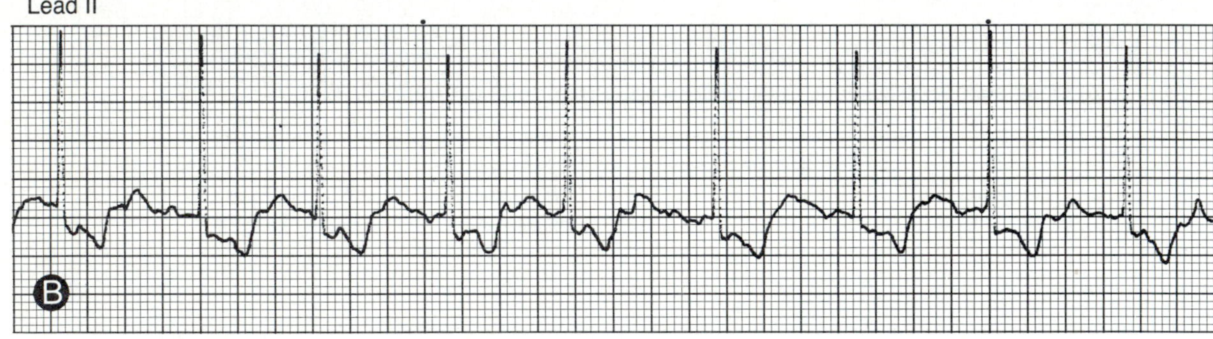

FIGURE 6-43 **A,** Fine atrial fibrillation. Note absence of obvious fibrillatory waves. Diagnosis is based on irregularity of ventricular rhythm and absence of P waves. **B,** Atrial fibrillation. Fibrillatory waves much more apparent. Diagnosis is based on irregular ventricular response and chaotic looking P waves.

A.

Rate: Approximately 65 bpm. Count for full minute.
Rhythm: Irregular
P wave: Nonidentifiable
PR interval: —
QRS complex: 0.06 seconds
Interpretation: Fine, controlled atrial fibrillation

B.

Rate: Approximately 90 bpm. Count for full minute.
Rhythm: Irregular
P wave: Chaotic appearing
PR interval: —
QRS complex: 0.06 seconds; depressed ST segment; inverted T wave
Interpretation: Controlled atrial fibrillation

cise, fever, and hypotension. Persons with WPW syndrome (an arrhythmia in which conduction from the atria to the ventricles is spread via a tract that bypasses the AV junction) are at grave danger of extremely rapid ventricular rates because the AV node is not available to slow impulses reaching the ventricles (Figs. 6-41 and 6-42).

Conversely, factors that increase the refractory period in the AV junction will result in a decrease of the ventricular response or rate. Increasing vagal tone and decreasing sympathetic stimulation will bring about such a response. Ventricular rates less than 100 bpm are usually the result of treatment and are therefore known as *controlled atrial fibrillation*. In all cases the ventricular rhythm is *irregular*. Irregularity becomes more difficult to detect, however, when the ventricular rate increases; there is less time in the cycle for irregularities to be apparent (see Figs. 6-41 and 6-42).

Fibrillatory waves are usually most evident on leads V_1 and the inferior leads (II, III, and aVF), but this varies with patients. Some leads on the 12-lead ECG may appear to have no f waves at all. The baseline between QRS complexes will be flat. The clue to the presence of AF in such a situation is the irregular ventricular rhythm and unidentifiable P waves (Fig. 6-43, *A*).

Contour of the QRS complexes often varies from beat to beat when fibrillatory waves are coarse. This is because the surface ECG is the algebraic sum of all electrical events; positive fibrillatory waves superimposed on positive QRS complexes will increase the amplitude of the QRS and vice versa (see Fig. 6-41).

When the ventricular rate is less than 60 bpm, there is pronounced delay in the AV node (see Fig. 6-40). Detection of *regular* QRS complexes at a slow rate in the presence of AF suggests the possibility of high degree (third degree) AV block. The rhythm is regular because all the impulses from the atria are blocked and the ventricular rhythm is under the control of a lower pacemaker.

Ventricular ectopy and right and left bundle branch blocks often occur in the presence of AF and will be addressed in more detail in subsequent chapters.

Always be aware of the possibility of artifact masquerading as AF. Fig. 6-44 illustrates such an example.

A summary of the ECG characteristics of AF is presented in box on p. 150.

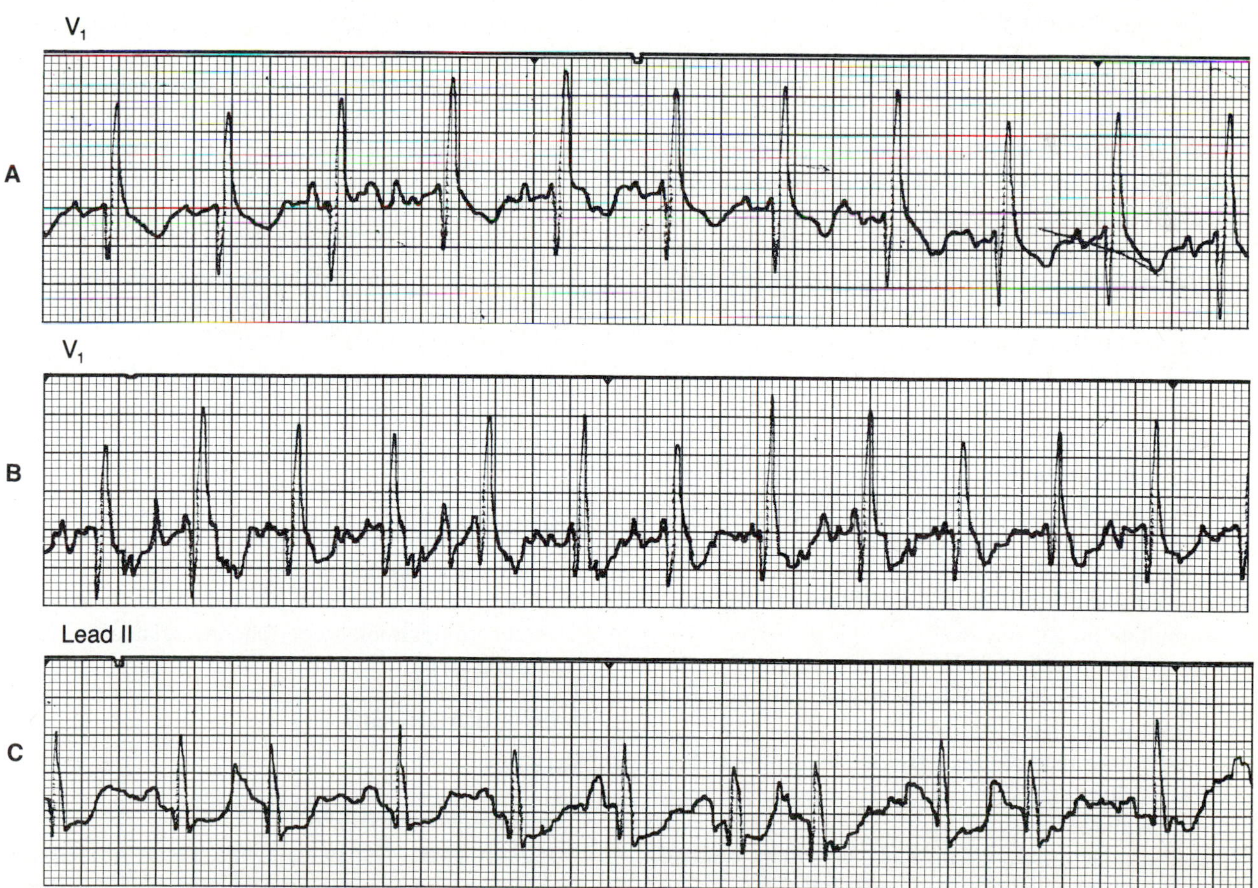

FIGURE 6-44 Artifact. In each tracing, movement artifact distorts the appearance of the rhythm. Familiarize yourself with the mask of artifact. **A,** Sinus tachycardia with IVCD (RBBB). **B,** Sinus tachycardia with RBBB. **C,** NSR with frequent APBs.

ECG Characteristics
Atrial Fibrillation

Rhythm: Irregular (both atrial and ventricular)
Rate: Atrial (too rapid to determine); ventricular—variable
P waves: Not identifiable or chaotic looking
PR interval: Not measurable
QRS complex: Normal unless IVCD present

Applied Nursing Process
Clinical Assessment

The patient in AF may or may not be symptomatic. The development of symptoms will have much to do with the ventricular response (rate) and the underlying disorder.

- Detect:
  - An irregular pulse.
  - An irregularity on the ECG.
  - Chaotic looking or no identifiable P waves on the ECG.
- Assess the patient and ECG.
  - Closely monitor the patient's adaptation to the arrhythmia. Since loss of the atrial kick accompanies atrial fibrillation, a decrease in cardiac output is present even with a controlled response. This may lower blood pressure and produce other symptoms of decreased perfusion.
    Measure blood pressure.
    Assess quality of peripheral pulses, detecting pulse deficits.
    Check skin color and temperature.
  - Assess mentation and the presence of symptoms such as light-headedness, dizziness, near-syncope, or syncope.
  - Measure intake and output.
  - Assess for manifestations of congestive heart failure.
    Auscultate breath sounds.
    Check for external jugular venous distension.
    Inspect for peripheral edema located in dependent areas of the body.
    Question the patient about feeling short of breath.
    Observe for cough.
    Auscultate the heart for S_3.
  - Whenever a tachycardia is present, the patient is at risk of decreased myocardial tissue perfusion.
    Question the patient regarding the presence of chest discomfort suggestive of myocardial ischemia.
    Study the 12-lead ECG for signs of myocardial ischemia such as depressed ST segments or T-wave changes.
  - Assess the ECG.
    Fibrillatory waves are often best seen in leads V_1, II, III, and aVF.
    Monitor the ventricular response. Slow responses in the absence of treatment may signal the presence of conduction system disease.[58]
  - Be on the alert for thromboemboli. The risk is greatest during the period of conversion from AF to NSR (or NSR to AF).[51]
    Assess mentation.
    Evaluate pulmonary status.
    Assess peripheral pulses and skin color.
  - Monitor serum potassium and digoxin levels as ordered.
  - If the patient is receiving anticoagulants, monitor the prothrombin time (usually two times normal is the desired level[51]).
    For patients on long-term anticoagulation, teach the necessary precautions to avoid accidental bleeding. Instruct the patient to have prothrombin time tests done according to the physician's direction.
  - For the patient receiving digoxin, assess for signs and symptoms of adverse digitalis effects (refer to Table 6-1 on p. 139.)
    One of the ECG signs of digitalis toxicity is accelerated junctional rhythm which, in the presence of AF, displays itself as a *regular* ventricular rhythm.
    Another ECG sign of digitalis toxicity is AV conduction delay, which results in slowing of the ventricular response. With a high degree of AV block, all the fibrillatory impulses will be blocked and the ventricles will be controlled by a lower pacemaker.
  - Diagnose the arrhythmia using Fig. 6-45.
  - Evaluate effectiveness of antiarrhythmic drugs while assessing for specific signs of toxicity (see Chapter 11).

❖ NURSING DIAGNOSIS

(1) Decreased cardiac output related to loss of atrial kick and/or tachycardia. (2) Altered tissue perfusion: cerebral/cardiopulmonary/peripheral, related to decreased cardiac output.

❖ ECG DIAGNOSIS

Atrial fibrillation.

Plan and Implementation

Patient goal. The patient will maintain adequate cardiac output and tissue perfusion and will not develop a thromboembolism.

Nursing interventions.

- Notify the physician immediately if the heart rate is rapid

Differentiate coarse atrial fibrillation from multiform atrial tachycardia and irregular rhythms with ventricular rates 100 bpm or more. Detect an irregular ventricular rhythm.

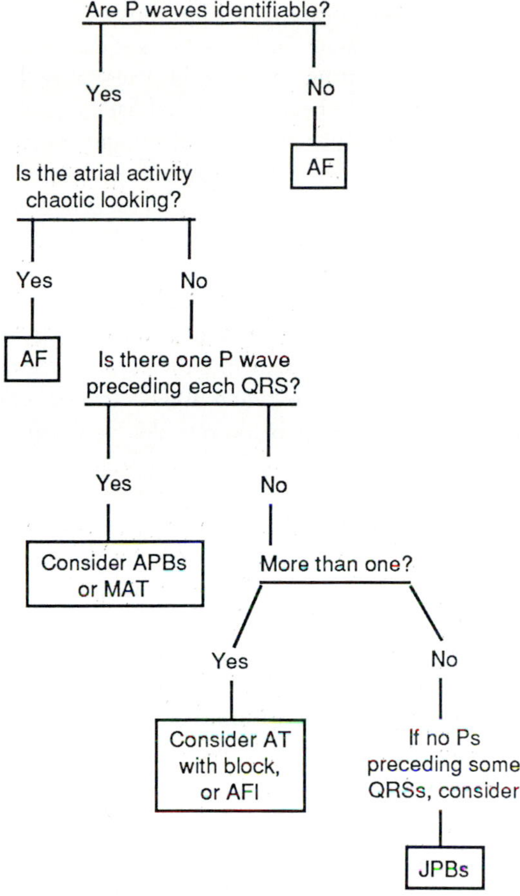

FIGURE 6-45 Atrial fibrillation algorithm.

and the patient is hemodynamically compromised.

- Administer oxygen if indicated.
- If the patient is aware of a change in rhythm, reassure that the arrhythmia is usually amenable to treatment.
- Obtain serum potassium and digoxin levels as ordered.
- If the patient is receiving anticoagulation therapy, obtain prothrombin time.
- If elective cardioversion is planned, digoxin is usually discontinued 24 hours before.
- If cardioversion is to be performed, explain the procedure and reassure the patient. Refer to Chapter 12 for the nurse's role in countershock therapy. Also refer to Medical Treatment, nonpharmacologic, for additional information concerning cardioversion.
- Provide appropriate patient teaching regarding digitalis preparations, quinidine, beta blockers, verapamil, or warfarin (refer to Chapter 11). For the patient receiving a digitalis preparation, teach the following:
  - How to take own pulse.
  - The signs and symptoms of toxicity.
  - The importance of periodic serum digoxin levels.
  - The importance of taking the medication as prescribed.
- Implement physician's orders.
- Evaluate the electrocardiographic and hemodynamic response to antiarrhythmic drugs and any adverse effects. For example, patients receiving drugs that exert a negative inotropic effect (beta blockers, disopyramide) may show signs and symptoms of congestive heart failure.

Evaluation

- The patient has an adequate cardiac output and remains hemodynamically stable as evidenced by
  - Stable blood pressure in normal range for patient.
  - Warm, dry skin without pallor or cyanosis.
  - No complaints of dizziness or light-headedness.
- The patient maintains electrolyte balance and therapeutic serum digoxin blood level as evidenced by the following:
  - Serum potassium (and other electrolytes) within normal range.
  - Digoxin level in therapeutic range.
  - An irregular ventricular response within normal range (60 to 100 bpm). A ventricular response that becomes regular in the presence of AF may indicate digitalis toxicity manifested by accelerated idiojunctional rhythm or advanced AV block.
- The patient maintains adequate tissue perfusion as evidenced by the following:
  - The absence of chest discomfort.
  - Stable ST-segment and T-wave configurations without evidence of ischemia on the 12-lead ECG.
  - No signs of thromboembolism.
  - Full orientation.
  - Normal respirations.
- The patient shows no signs of congestive heart failure as evidenced by the following:
  - Clear lung fields on auscultation.
  - No jugular venous distension.
  - A normal respiratory pattern.
  - The absence of an S_3 heart sound.

Medical Treatment

Pharmacologic

Treatment of AF is directed at controlling the ventricular response by increasing the delay in the AV junction. Therapy may also be directed at restoring normal sinus rhythm. Drugs that have been used in the treatment of AF include digitalis, quinidine (after digitalization), procainamide, disopyramide, amiodarone, sotalol, flecainide, encainide, propafenone, beta blockers (alone or with digitalis), and verapamil. Anticoagulants are often administered prophylactically, and both warfarin and aspirin have been shown to reduce risk of embolic stroke compared with placebo.

Nonpharmacologic

Cardioversion is more effective in the termination of AF of relatively recent onset (less than 1 year), especially in younger patients.[59] Once the arrhythmia becomes chronic, transient conversion to NSR is possible, but generally cannot be maintained.[49,57]

In many settings the energy dosage begins at 25 to 50 joules or watt-seconds (w-s),* and increases by increments of 50 to 100 w-s if subsequent shocks are necessary. The energy requirement for an adult is variable and depends on several factors. Energy requirements are greater in patients with chronic, long-standing AF, alcoholism, cardiomyopathies, WPW syndrome, severe coronary heart disease, acute myocardial infarction, and congestive heart failure with rapid ventricular rates.[6] Studies have indicated the average energy required to convert AF is approximately 100 w-s; cardioversion at 100 to 200 w-s initially is successful in 78% to 90% of cases.[6,60,61]

Electrical cardioversion is inadvisable in the presence of SSS, digitalis toxicity, and electrolyte imbalances. Failure to sustain NSR after previous conversions,[57] advanced mitral valve disease or mitral valve replacement, and left atrial enlargement[6] reduce the likelihood of successful treatment. Digitalis toxicity and electrolyte imbalances predispose the patient to dangerous arrhythmias following countershock. In the presence of SSS, termination of the AF may result in slow atrial activity. The other conditions mentioned are associated with chronic AF that is not amenable to sustained conversion.

The risk of embolism increases after both electrical and pharmacologic conversion.[47]

Medically refractory AF, especially when associated with a rapid ventricular response, may be managed by surgical or catheter ablation of the AV junction combined with permanent cardiac pacing.[62,63] Surgical ablation is accomplished via scalpel or laser excision, and catheter ablation is either by direct current (DC) or radiofrequency (RF).

WANDERING PACEMAKER

Data Base: Problem Identification

Definitions, Etiology, and Mechanisms

Wandering pacemaker (WP), still referred to in much of the literature as *wandering atrial pacemaker,* is clouded by a plethora of definitions. WP should be thought of as a helpful rhythm, since it generates beats from the AV junction, as well as throughout the atria, when normal sinus impulses have been disturbed. Thus, it is a rhythm by default, one of the escape rhythms. It presents when sinus impulses are slowed due to sinus bradycardia or relative sinus slowing.[64] Therefore it is a phenomenon secondary to disorders such as sinus arrhythmia or sinus bradycardia, and often results from changes in vagal tone. The supraventricular escape beats are variable and come from the atria or junction, whichever generates impulses first.

WP is not considered an abnormality in most circumstances. Investigators have found it to be common in children and young adults.[12,65] It is postulated that the arrhythmia in this age group is related to excess vagal tone rather than heart disease. Brodsky et al[12] observed WP at least once in over half the young male adults in their study. It is frequently noted in athletes. WP does not appear to be as common in aging adults. Indeed, one study of a healthy elderly population revealed no episodes.[13]

ECG Characteristics

Since WP is a rhythm by default and occurs as a result of sinus slowing, the P-P′ intervals are longer than the P-P intervals. The P′ waves will appear morphologically different from the sinus P waves, ranging in shape from upright to inverted (inverted in the inferior leads if the impulse is originating from the junctional area or the bottom of the atria). Because of differing proximity of the impulse to the AV junction, the P′R interval may vary (Fig. 6-46 and the box on this page.)

Applied Nursing Process

Clinical Assessment

- Detect:
  - A possible slight irregularity in pulse and ECG.
  - Different P waves on the ECG.
- Assess the patient and ECG.
  - With the initial display of the arrhythmia, assess blood pressure and peripheral pulses to be certain the patient is tolerating the arrhythmia. Subsequent episodes of the arrhythmia do not require assessment if the patient was

ECG Characteristics
Wandering Pacemaker

Rate: Variable, often slow, <100 bpm
Rhythm: Irregular
P waves: Vary from normal to inverted; one P wave precedes each QRS complex; P-P′ interval > P-P interval
PR interval: Variable
QRS complex: Normal unless IVCD present

*The strength of a countershock is expressed in energy (joules (j) or watt-seconds (w-s)), which is the product of power and duration:

$$\underset{\text{(Joules)}}{\text{Energy}} = \underset{\text{(Watts)}}{\text{Power}} \times \underset{\text{(Seconds)}}{\text{Duration}}$$

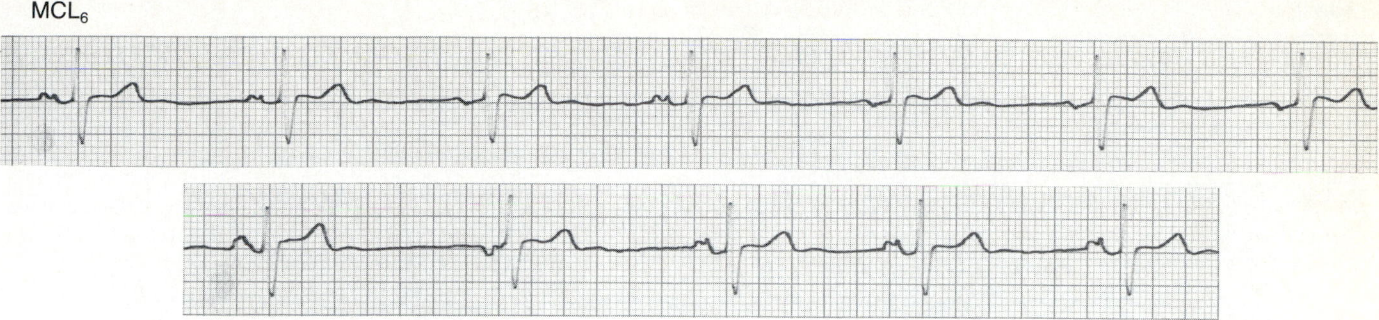

FIGURE 6-46 Wandering pacemaker. Note five different p′ waves, none of which are premature.

Rate: 41 to 48 bpm
Rhythm: Irregular (bottom strip)
P wave: 5 different morphologies
PR interval: 0.12 to 0.20 seconds
QRS complex: 0.09 seconds
Interpretation: Wandering pacemaker

asymptomatic with the initial episode unless there is a significant change in the character of the arrhythmia.

- Diagnose the arrhythmia. Differentiate it from APBs; detect a rhythm with variable P waves and possibly variable rhythm and PR interval. Do the P′ waves appear prematurely? If so, the P′ waves are APBs.

❖ NURSING DIAGNOSIS

Decreased cardiac output related to bradycardia.

❖ ECG DIAGNOSIS

Wandering pacemaker.

Plan and Implementation

Patient goal. The patient will remain hemodynamically stable during the arrhythmia.

Nursing intervention.

- Since WP is secondary to sinus slowing, it is never a primary diagnosis and therefore has no primary significance. The significance is always that of the underlying sinus bradycardia which, in most cases, is benign, requiring no treatment.[53]
- Record the arrhythmia and note when it occurs in relation to activity or medications.

Evaluation

- The patient remains hemodynamically stable as evidenced by the following:
  - No change in blood pressure, color, or sensorium.

Medical Treatment

Treatment of the primary sinus bradycardia may be necessary if the patient is symptomatic.

ATRIAL ESCAPE RHYTHM

Data Base: Problem Identification

Definitions, Etiology, and Mechanisms

Atrial escape rhythms (idioatrial rhythms) are fairly common and emerge when a sinus impulse defaults through slowing or SA block[66] or after ectopic atrial activity. The default may be due to a depression of sinus impulse formation or conduction. Atrial escape beats are a symptom or feature of the underlying cause.

ECG Characteristics

The P wave is altered and late, as opposed to APBs that are premature. The atrial rate is slow (below 60 bpm) and the rhythm is regular. The P′ waves may be uniform or multiform (Fig. 6-47 and the box on p. 154).

Applied Nursing Process

Clinical Assessment

- Detect:
  - A slow pulse.
  - Different P waves.
- Assess patient and ECG.
  - The clinical assessment is the same as for sinus bradycardia.
    - Measure the blood pressure.
    - Determine the patient's tolerance of the arrhythmia.
    - Question patient about symptoms associated with a markedly slow heart rate such as syncopal episodes or periods of light-headedness.
  - Ask if the patient has been taking any antiarrhythmic drugs that cause sinus slowing.
  - Diagnose the arrhythmia using the algorithm in Fig. 6-48.

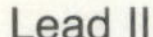

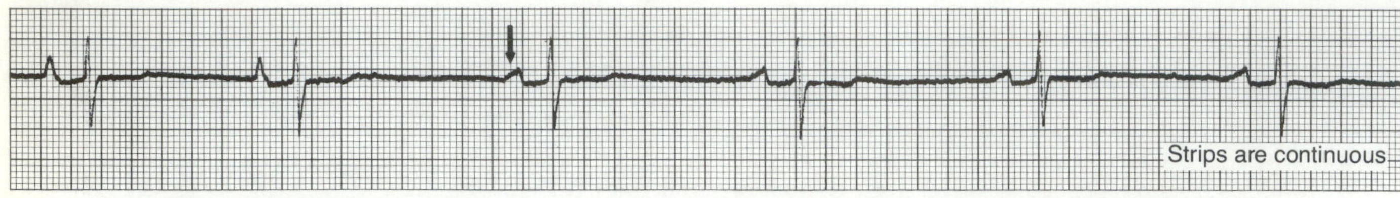

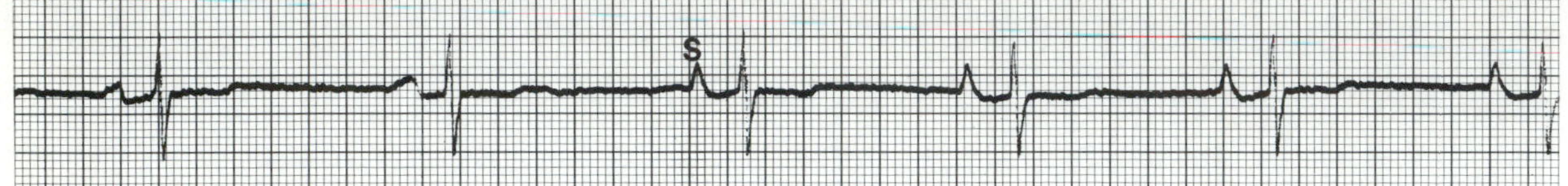

FIGURE 6-47 Atrial escape rhythm. First two complexes in top strip represent sinus bradycardia at rate 43 bpm. After the second complex, the sinus rhythm either stops or slows, allowing an atrial escape rhythm *(arrow)* to assume temporary control by default (at a slower rate of 38 bpm) until sinus rhythm again resumes control in the third complex, bottom strip *(s)*.

Rate: 38 to 43 bpm

Rhythm: Regular but varies with two different pacemakers

P wave: Sinus P waves are tall and peaked; atrial escape P′ waves are 0.12 seconds wide and different in shape

PR interval: 0.26 seconds with sinus conducted impulses, 0.23 seconds with atrial escape rhythm, both prolonged

QRS complex: 0.08 seconds

Interpretation: Sinus bradycardia with prolonged PR interval and intermittent atrial escape rhythm resulting from sinus slowing or arrest

---

ECG Characteristics
Atrial Escape Rhythm

Rate: Any—but usually slow

Rhythm: Irregular due to late-in-cycle escape beats

P waves: Normal except for atrial escape beats; one P wave precedes each QRS complex; atrial escape P′ waves are later than expected; sinus P waves and are of different shape

PR interval: Normal

QRS complex: Normal unless IVCD present

Differentiate from wandering pacemaker and APBs. Detect a slowing sinus rhythm with subsequent QRS complexes preceded by P′ waves different from the sinus P waves.

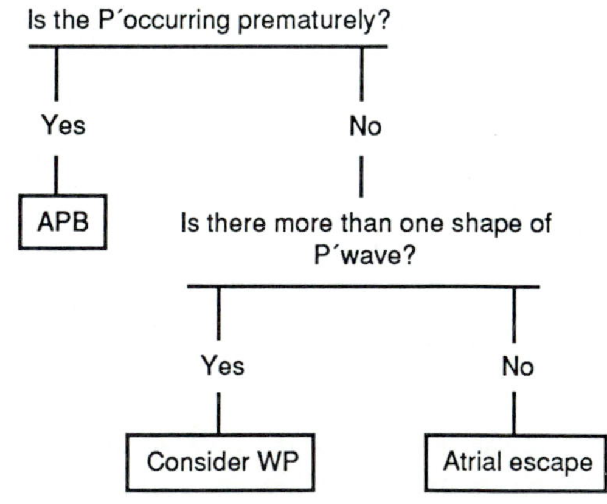

FIGURE 6-48 Atrial escape rhythm algorithm.

❖ NURSING DIAGNOSIS

Decreased cardiac output related to bradycardia.

❖ ECG DIAGNOSIS

Atrial escape rhythm.

Plan and Implementation

Patient goal. The patient will maintain hemodynamic stability.

Nursing interventions.

- Since this is a default rhythm, it will disappear once normal sinus node function is restored. If the patient is sleeping, simply awakening him/her may be all that is necessary to abolish the arrhythmia.

- If the patient is symptomatic consider the following interventions based on clinical judgment, physician orders, and institutional policy:
  - Start an IV infusion.
  - IV atropine may be indicated.
  - An isoproterenol infusion may be necessary if atropine is not effective.
  - Consider external pacing.
  - Administer oxygen if not contraindicated.
  - Place the patient in a low-Fowler's or flat position if cardiac output is sufficiently compromised to result in cerebral insufficiency.
- Implement the physician's orders; evaluate the patient's response to measures taken to correct the rhythm disturbance.
- Determine if correction of the suspected underlying cause is correlated with improvement of the arrhythmia by continued ECG monitoring.

Evaluation

- The patient remains hemodynamically stable as evidenced by the following:
  - Stable or no change in blood pressure.
  - Warm, dry skin with good color.
  - Full orientation.

Medical Treatment

Treatment is directed towards correcting the underlying problem. If the patient is symptomatic and correction of the underlying problem does not alleviate the arrhythmia, pacemaker therapy may be necessary.

ATRIAL STANDSTILL

Data Base: Problem Identification

Definitions, Etiology, and Mechanisms

Atrial standstill, or atrial asystole, is defined as the absence of atrial activity on the ECG. When this occurs, junctional or ventricular escape rhythms will likely take control of the rhythm. The most common cause of atrial standstill is digitalis or quinidine toxicity.[4] Other cardioactive drugs or sinus node disease can also cause this condition, as can hyperkalemia.

ECG Characteristics

There is no visible atrial activity. The ventricular rate is variable but should be regular. The configuration of the QRS complexes depends on the site of the lower pacemaker assuming control of the rhythm. If the junction becomes the pacemaker, the QRS complexes will be narrow and normal appearing. A ventricular focus that functions as the pacemaker will produce a wide QRS complex that is different from the normal, sinus-conducted QRS complexes since the impulse does not traverse the conduction system in the ventricles. Irregularity of the ventricular response would lead one to suspect that fine AF is present (Fig. 6-49 and the box above).

ECG Characteristics
Atrial Asystole

Rate: Ventricular rate will likely by 70 bpm or less (controlled by either a junctional or ventricular escape rhythm)
Rhythm: Regular
P waves: Absent
PR interval: None
QRS complex: Normal if site of pacemaker is AV junction; wide if site is in the ventricles or if there is IVCD present

Applied Nursing Process

Clinical Assessment

- Detect:
  - A regular pulse of (probably) not over 70 bpm.
  - Absence of P waves on the ECG.
- Assess patient and ECG.
  - With atrial standstill, there is no atrial contribution to the cardiac output. Assess the patient's tolerance to the arrhythmia by doing the following:
    Measuring the blood pressure frequently.
    Checking for signs and symptoms of hypoperfusion including mentation, skin color and temperature, and urinary output.
  - Monitor serum potassium and appropriate serum drug levels.
  - Since there is no atrial contraction to empty the atria sufficiently, the possibility exists that thrombi may form in the atria. Assess for indications of thromboembolism if atrial activity returns.
    Check sensorium, color, peripheral pulses.
    Assess respirations.
  - Diagnose the arrhythmia. Differentiate it from fine atrial fibrillation. Detect a slow ventricular rhythm with no P waves visible anywhere on the ECG. Is the ventricular rhythm regular? If not, consider AF.

❖ NURSING DIAGNOSIS

Decreased cardiac output related to loss of the atrial kick and bradycardia.

❖ ECG DIAGNOSIS

Atrial asystole with junctional or ventricular escape rhythm.

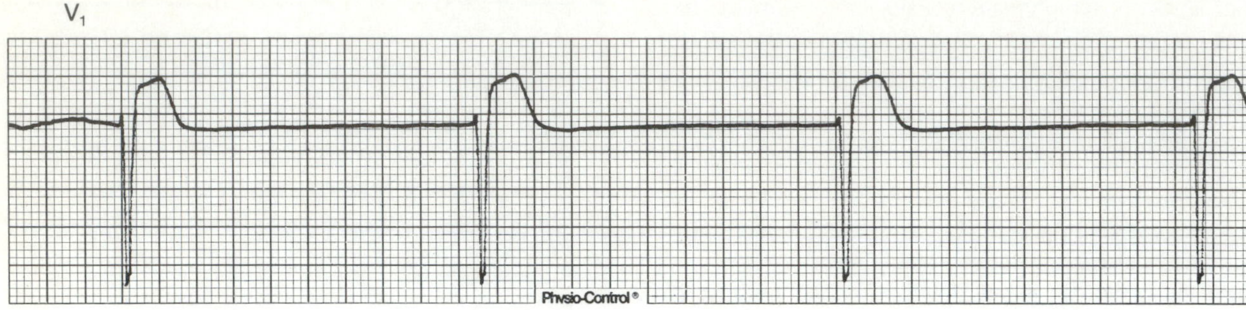

FIGURE 6-49 Atrial asystole. There is no evidence of atrial activity. The junction is in control with an **idiojunctional** pacemaker at a rate of 32 bpm.

Rate: Ventricular: 32 bpm
Rhythm: Regular
P wave: None identified
PR interval: —
QRS complex: 0.08 to 0.10 seconds; elevated ST segment
Interpretation: Atrial asystole with idiojunctional escape rhythm

Plan and Implementation

Patient goal. The patient will maintain adequate cardiac output for the duration of the arrhythmia. The patient's arrhythmia will subside after causative factors have been removed.

Nursing interventions.

- If the patient is symptomatic consider the following interventions based on physician orders, institutional policy, and clinical judgment:
  - Notify the physician at once.
  - Administer oxygen.
  - Start an IV infusion.
  - Administer atropine IV if indicated (see Chapter 11).
  - Lower the head of the bed to a flat or low-Fowler's position to facilitate cerebral perfusion.
  - If atropine is ineffective, an isoproterenol infusion may be indicated. Administer slowly, according to institutional policy.
  - Initiate external pacing if indicated (see Chapter 13).
- Obtain order for serum electrolytes.
- Hold medications that may further potentiate the arrhythmia, such as digoxin or quinidine, and be sure the physician is notified of such actions.
- Obtain appropriate serum drug levels such as digoxin or quinidine, as ordered.
- Implement physician's orders; evaluate the patient's response to measures taken to correct the arrhythmia.
- Correlate correction of the suspected underlying cause with improvement of the ECG pattern and the patient's condition. Watch for the return of atrial activity.
- If the patient has had a pacemaker inserted, evaluate the response to the increase in heart rate, and any adverse effects such as thromboemboli. Refer to Chapter 13 for additional information concerning the nurse's role in pacemaker therapy.

Evaluation

- The patient's arrhythmia has been corrected as evidenced by the following:
  - A return of normal atrial activity on the ECG or
  - An appropriate response to artificial pacing.
- The patient remains hemodynamically stable with adequate cardiac output as evidenced by the following:
  - Blood pressure within normal range for patient.
  - Full orientation.
  - Warm, dry skin without cyanosis or pallor.

Medical Treatment

If correction of the underlying cause does not alleviate the arrhythmia, pacemaker therapy may be indicated (see Chapter 13).

REFERENCES

1. Fowler NO. *Cardiac Diagnosis and Treatment*. 3rd ed. Philadelphia: Harper & Row, 1980.
2. Lown B, DeSilva RA. Roles of psychologic stress and autonomic nervous system changes in provocation of ventricular premature complexes. *Am. J. Cardiol.*, May, 1978, 41(6): 979-85.
3. Vassalle M. Automaticity and automatic rhythms. *Am. J. Cardiol.*, Sept., 1971, 28: 245-52.
4. Chung EK. *Principles of Cardiac Arrhythmias*. Baltimore: Williams & Wilkins, 1983.
5. Bleifer SB, Bleifer DJ, Hansmann DR, Sheppard JJ, Karpman HL. Diagnosis of occult arrhythmias by Holter electrocardiography. *Prog. Cardiovasc. Dis.*, May/June, 1974, 16(6): 569-99.
6. Antman EM. *Supraventricular Arrhythmias*. Upper Montclair, NJ: Health Scan, 1981.
7. Meltzer LE, Pinneo R, Kitchell JR. *Intensive Coronary Care: A Manual for Nurses*. 4th ed. Bowie, MD: RJ Brady, 1983.
8. Chiang BN, Perlman LV, Ostrander LD, Epstein FH. Relationship of premature systoles to coronary heart disease and sudden death in the Tecumseh epidemiologic study. *Ann. Intern. Med.*, Jun., 1969, 70(6): 1159-66.

9. Sobotka PA, Mayer JH, Bauernfeind RA, Kanakis C, Rosen KM. Arrhythmias documented by 24 hour continuous ambulatory electrocardiographic monitoring in young women without apparent heart disease. *Am. Heart J.*, Jun., 1981, 101(6): 753-9.
10. Scott O, Williams GJ, Fiddler GI. Results of 24 hour ambulatory monitoring of electrocardiograms in 130 healthy boys aged 10-13 years. *Br. Heart J.*, 1980, 44: 304-8.
11. Talan DA, Bauernfeind RA, Ashley WW, Kanakis C, Rosen KM. Twenty-four hour continuous ECG recordings in long distance runners. *Chest*, Jul., 1982, 82(1): 19-24.
12. Brodsky M, Wu D, Denes P, Kanakis C, Rosen KM. Arrhythmias documented by 24-hour continuous electrocardiographic monitoring in 50 male medical students without apparent heart disease. *Am. J. Cardiol.*, Mar., 1977, 39: 390-5.
13. Fleg JL, Kennedy HL. Cardiac arrhythmias in a healthy elderly population: Detection by 24-hour ambulatory electrocardiography. *Chest*, Mar., 1982, 81(3): 302-7.
14. Wajngarten M, Grupi C, Bellotti GM, Da Luz PL, Azul LG, Pileggi F. Frequency and significance of cardiac rhythm disturbances in healthy elderly individuals. *J. Electrocardiol.*, Apr., 1990, 23(2): 171-6.
15. Marriott HJL. *Practical Electrocardiography*. 8th ed. Baltimore: Williams & Wilkins, 1988.
16. Wilkerson RD (ed). *Cardiac Pharmacology*. New York: Academic Press, 1981.
17. Graboys T. The treatment of supraventricular tachycardias. *N. Engl. J. Med.*, Jan. 3, 1985, 312(1): 43-4.
18. Lipson MJ, Naimi S. Multifocal atrial tachycardia (chaotic atrial tachycardia): Clinical associations and significance. *Circ.*, Sept., 1970, 42(3): 397-407.
19. Shine KI, Kastor JA, Yurchak PM. Multifocal atrial tachycardia; clinical and electrocardiographic features in 32 patients. *N. Engl. J. Med.*, Aug. 15, 1968, 279(7): 344-9.
20. Anderson JL. Multifocal atrial tachycardia, atrial flutter, atrial fibrillation. *In* Winkle RA (ed). *Cardiac Arrhythmias: Current Diagnosis and Practical Management*. Menlo Park, CA: Addison-Wesley, 1983.
21. Sessler CN, Cohen MD. Cardiac arrhythmias during theophylline toxicity. A prospective continuous electrocardiographic study. *Chest*, Sept., 1990, 98(3): 672-8.
22. Gaughan GL, Gorfunkel HJ. Physiologic and biologic variants of the electrocardiogram. *In* Rios JC (ed). *Clinical Electrocardiographic Correlations*. Brest AN (ed). *Cardiovascular Clinics*, 8/3. Philadelphia: FA Davis, 1977.
23. Phillips J, Spano J, Burch G. Chaotic atrial mechanism. *Am. Heart. J.*, Aug., 1969, 78(2): 171-9.
24. Levine JH, Michael JR, Guarnieri T. Treatment of multifocal atrial tachycardia with verapamil. *N. Engl. J. Med.*, Jan. 3, 1985, 312(1): 21-5.
25. Josephson ME, Seides SF. *Clinical Cardiac Electrophysiology Techniques and Interpretations*. Philadelphia: Lea & Febiger, 1979.
26. Garson A, Gillette PC, McNamara DG. Supraventricular tachycardia in children: Clinical features, response to treatment, and long term follow-up in 217 patients. *J. Pediatr.*, Jun., 1981, 98(6): 875-82.
27. Roberts N, Moss J, Edelman E, Hartman K. Cardiac arrhythmias in children. Part I. Tachyarrhythmias. *J. Cardiovasc. Pulm. Tech.*, Aug. 9, 1980, 8(5): 53-60.
28. Dance D, Yates M. Nursing assessment and care of children with complications of congenital heart disease. *Heart & Lung*, May, 1985, 14(3): 209-14.
29. Gillette PC. Cardiac dysrhythmias in infants and children. *In* Engle MA (ed). *Pediatric Cardiovascular Disease*. Brest AN (ed). *Cardiovascular Clinics*, 11/2. Philadelphia: FA Davis, 1981.
30. Dunnigan A, Benditt DG, Benson DW. Modes of onset ("initiating events") for paroxysmal atrial tachycardia in infants and children. *Am. J. Cardiol.*, Jun., 1, 1986, 57(15): 1280-7.
31. Benchimol A, Liggett MS. Cardiac hemodynamics during stimulation of the right atrium, right ventricle, and left ventricle in normal and abnormal hearts. *Circ.*, Jun., 1966, 33(6): 933-44.
32. Samet P. Hemodynamic sequelae of cardiac arrhythmias. *Circ.*, Feb., 1973, 47(2): 399-407.
33. Villadares BK, Lemburg L. Use of the "diving reflex" in paroxysmal atrial tachycardia. *Heart & Lung*, Mar., 1983, 12(2): 202-5.
34. Fujii T, Kojima S, Imanishi M, Ohe T, Omae T. Different mechanisms of polyuria and natriuresis associated with paroxysmal supraventricular tachycardia. *Am. J. Cardiol.*, Aug. 1, 1991, 68: 343-8.
35. Waxman MB, Wald RW, Sharma AD, Huerta F, Cameron DA. Vagal techniques for termination of paroxysmal supraventricular tachycardia. *Am. J. Cardiol.*, Oct., 1980, 46: 655-64.
36. Garson A. The six most common acute cardiac dysrhythmias in children. Part 2. *Appl. Cardiol.*, Jun./Jul., 1984, 12(4): 13-23.
37. Rae AP. Supraventricular tachyarrhythmias: Atrial flutter and atrial fibrillation. Horowitz L (series ed). Interpreting an ECG. *Geriatrics*, Mar., 1985, 40(3): 93-108.
38. Sung RJ, Castellanos A. Supraventricular tachycardia: Mechanisms and treatment. *In* Castellanos A (ed). *Cardiac Arrhythmias: Mechanisms and Management*. Brest AN (ed). Cardiovascular Clinics, 11/1. Philadelphia: FA Davis, 1980.
39. Jordaens L, Gorgels A, Stroobandt R, Temmerman J. Efficacy and safety of intravenous sotalol for termination of paroxysmal supraventricular tachycardia. *Am. J. Cardiol.*, Jul. 1, 1991, 68: 35-40.
40. Yeh SJ, Kou HC, Lin FC, Hung JS, Wu D. Effects of oral diltiazem in paroxysmal supraventricular tachycardia. *Am. J. Cardiol.*, Aug., 1983, 52(3): 271-8.
41. Sung R. Beta blockade in the treatment of arrhythmias. *Cardio.*, Sept., 1985, pp. 37-9.
42. Boineau JP. Atrial flutter: A synthesis of concepts. *Circ.*, Aug., 1985, 72(2): 249-57.
43. Engel TR, Luck JC. Effect of whiskey on atrial vulnerability and "holiday heart." *J. Am. Coll. Cardiol.*, Mar., 1983, 1(3): 816-8.
44. Kurer CC, Tanner CS, Vetter VL. Electrophysiologic findings after Fontan repair of functional single ventricle. *J. Am. Coll. Cardiol.*, Jan., 1991, 17(1): 174-181.
45. Jacquet L, Ziady G, Stein K, Griffith B, Armitage J, Hardesty R, Kormos R. Cardiac rhythm disturbances early after orthotopic heart transplantation: Prevalence and clinical importance of the observed abnormalities. *J. Am. Coll. Cardiol.*, Oct., 1990, 16(4): 832-7.
46. Gillette PC. Supraventricular arrhythmias in children. *J. Am. Coll. Cardiol.*, Jun., 1985, 5(6): 122B-9B.
47. De Silva RA, Graboys TB, Podrid PJ, Lown B. Cardioversion and defibrillation, Part 1. *Am. Heart J.*, Dec., 1980, 100(6): 881-95.
48. American Heart Association. *Textbook of Advanced Cardiac Life Support*. Dallas: American Heart Association, 1987.
49. Savage DD, Abbott RD, Kannel WB. Chronic atrial fibrillation in the general population. *Primary Cardiol.*, Apr., 1983, pp. 49-51; 59-62; 64.
50. Roberts WC (ed). *Cardiology 1985*. New York: Yorke Medical Books, 1985.
51. Kerber RE. When and how to perform cardioversion. *Hosp. Ther.*, Mar., 1985, pp. 44-53.
52. Peter RH, Gracey JG, Beach TB. A clinical profile of idiopathic atrial fibrillation. *Ann. Intern. Med.*, Jun., 1968, 68(6): 1288-95 1296.
53. Schamroth L. *The Disorders of Cardiac Rhythm, Vol. I.* 2nd ed. London: Blackwell Scientific Publications, 1981.

54. Lamb LE, Pollard LW. Atrial fibrillation in flying personnel: Report of 60 cases. *Circ.*, May, 1964, 29(5): 694-701.
55. Luria MH. Selective clinical features of paroxysmal tachycardia: A prospective study in 120 patients. *Br. Heart J.*, May, 1971, 33(3): 351-7.
56. Peter RH, Gracey JG, Beach TB. A clinical profile of idiopathic atrial fibrillation. *Ann. Intern. Med.*, Jun., 1968, 68(6): 1288-95.
57. Willoughby ML, Dunlap DB. The treatment of atrial fibrillation and flutter: A review. *Heart & Lung,* Sept., 1984, 13(5): 578-84.
58. Rosen KM, Loeb HS, Sinno MZ, Rahimtoola SH, Gunnar RM. Cardiac conduction in patients with symptomatic sinus node disease. *Circ.*, Jun., 1971, 43(6): 836-44.
59. Van Gelder IC, Crijns HJ, Van Gilst WH, Verwer R, Lie KI. Prediction of uneventful cardioversion and maintenance of sinus rhythm from direct-current electrical cardioversion of chronic atrial fibrillation and flutter. *Am. J. Cardiol.*, Jul. 1, 1991, 68: 41-46.
60. Halmos PB. Direct current conversion of atrial fibrillation. *Br. Heart J.*, May, 1966, 28(3): 302-8.
61. Lown B. Electrical reversion of cardiac arrhythmias. *Br. Heart J.*, Jul., 1967, 29: 469-89.
62. Scheinman MM, Laks MM, DiMarco J, Plumb V. Current role of catheter ablative procedures in patients with cardiac arrhythmias. A report for health professionals from the subcommittee on electrocardiography and electrophysiology, American Heart Association. *Circ.*, Jun., 1991, 83(6): 2146-53.
63. Singer I, Kupersmith J. Nonpharmacological therapy of supraventricular arrhythmias: Surgery and catheter ablation techniques. *PACE,* Aug., 1990, 13: 1045-58.
64. Schamroth L, Goldberg LH. The concept of a wandering pacemaker. *Heart & Lung,* Jul./Aug., 1972, 1(4): 519-22.
65. Fosmoe RJ, Averill KH, Lamb LE. Electrocardiographic findings in 67,375 asymptomatic subjects. II. Supraventricular arrhythmias. *Am. J. Cardiol.*, Jul., 1960, 6(1): 84-95.
66. Garlick I, Schamroth L. Sinus bradycardia leading to atrial escape. *Heart & Lung,* Sept./Oct., 1975, 4(5): 791.

SELF-ASSESSMENT

MULTIPLE CHOICE

Directions

For each of the questions below, select the correct answer(s) from the choices given. If more than one correct answer is given, mark all that are correct.

Examples

Atrial arrhythmias originate in which structure of the heart?
a. Sinus of Valsalva.
*b. Atria.
c. Junction.
d. Ventricles.

Examples of atrial rhythm disturbances include:
a. Sinus arrhythmia.
b. Sinus bradycardia.
*c. Automatic atrial tachycardia.
d. Wandering pacemaker.

1. Supraventricular arrhythmias are so named because
   a. they involve the atria.
   b. they are initiated by APBs.
   c. they originate above the ventricles.
   d. they do not involve the ventricles.

2. Causes of APBs include all of the following *except:*
   a. congestive heart failure.
   b. ischemia resulting from hypoxemia or coronary artery disease.
   c. digitalis toxicity.
   d. hypothyroidism.
   e. pulmonary embolism.

3. APBs are significant
   a. when their frequency increases the heart rate.
   b. whenever they occur, since they represent myocardial ischemia.
   c. if they result in a decrease in cardiac output.
   d. when they occur in children.

4. ECG features of APBs include
   a. a premature P′ wave that is different from the sinus P wave in at least one lead.
   b. the QRS after the premature P wave is usually wider than 0.12 seconds.
   c. the P-P′ interval is longer than the P-P interval.
   d. A P′R interval of 0.20 seconds or greater.

5. MAT is often associated with
   a. hyperkalemia.
   b. sudden infant death syndrome.
   c. myocardial infarction.
   d. chronic obstructive pulmonary disease.

6. Which statement below most closely describes MAT?
   a. At least three different P′ waves are identifiable in addition to the dominant sinus rhythm.
   b. A single dominant pacemaker cannot be identified.
   c. The atrial activity is chaotic with nonidentifiable P waves.
   d. There are at least two P′ waves before each QRS complex.

7. The mechanism responsible for PSVT in most cases is
   a. increased atrial automaticity.
   b. excessive AV junctional irritability.
   c. SA nodal/atrial reentry.
   d. AV nodal reentry.

8. Correlated with age, which of the following statements is most accurate?
   a. The incidence of PSVT increases with age.
   b. PSVT is a common arrhythmia in children.
   c. There is no consistent correlation of PSVT with age groups.
   d. The incidence of PSVT is common in all age groups.

9. The following may be associated findings of PSVT:
   a. caffeine intake.
   b. tobacco use.
   c. ingestion of alcohol.
   d. emotional stress.

10. Electrocardiographic features of PSVT include which of the following statements?
    a. The onset and termination of the arrhythmia are abrupt.
    b. The onset exhibits the warm-up phenomenon.
    c. The rhythm is usually slightly irregular.
    d. The rhythm is regular.

11. The following methods may be successful in terminating PSVT:
    a. administration of sympathomimetic drugs.
    b. having the patient perform the Valsalva maneuver.
    c. submersion of the patient's face in ice water.
    d. electrical cardioversion.

12. AT with block is a type of
    a. automatic atrial tachycardia.
    b. paroxysmal supraventricular tachycardia.
    c. reentrant atrial tachycardia.
    d. AV nodal automatic tachycardia.

13. A common cause of AT with block is
    a. caffeine ingestion.
    b. digitalis toxicity.
    c. emotional stress.
    d. hyperthyroidism.

14. The adult patient in AFl who has not been treated with antiarrhythmic medication will most often experience which of the following conduction ratios?
    a. 1:1.
    b. 2:1.
    c. 3:1.
    d. 4:1.
    Such a ratio of atrial to ventricular beats will likely result in a ventricular rate of approximately:
    a. 75.
    b. 100.
    c. 150.
    d. 200.
    e. 300.

15. Three leads that tend to exhibit flutter waves well are
    a. II, III, and aVF.
    b. I, V_1, and V_6.
    c. aVR, aVL, and aVF.
    d. V_4, V_5, and V_6.

16. Electrocardiographic features of AFl include:
    a. atrial rate of 100 to 200 bpm.
    b. atrial rate of 250 to 350 bpm.
    c. undulating, chaotic baseline.
    d. saw-tooth baseline on at least one lead.

17. Electrical cardioversion may be indicated for termination of certain atrial arrhythmias. Which of the following may be converted by cardioversion?
    a. Frequent APBs.
    b. PSVT.
    c. AFl.
    d. AF.
    e. WP.

18. The following arrhythmias result in loss of the atrial component to cardiac output (the atrial kick):
    a. WP.
    b. AF.
    c. atrial asystole.
    d. atrial escape rhythm.

19. Two conditions that may predispose a patient to dangerous arrhythmias after cardioversion include:
    a. hyperkalemia.
    b. hypokalemia.
    c. digitalis toxicity.
    d. hypothyroidism.

20. Patients in AF are at increased risk for thromboembolism. The reason for this is:
    a. in AF the contents of the atria are not sufficiently expelled, allowing thrombi to form.
    b. AF is often accompanied by platelet aggregation.
    c. AF so diminishes cardiac output that patients' inactivity results in thrombus formation in the lower legs and pelvic regions.
    d. AF is nearly always a symptom of underlying valvular heart disease, a common site for thrombus formation.

21. The four most common causes of AF are:
    a. hypertensive cardiovascular disease, rheumatic or mitral disease, hyperthyroidism, ischemic heart disease.
    b. myocardial infarction, hypertensive cardiovascular disease, Marfan's syndrome, hypokalemia.
    c. WPW syndrome, pericarditis, hyperthyroidism, gastrointestinal bleeding.
    d. systemic hypertension, myocardial infarction, hypomagnesemia, metabolic alkalosis.

22. Of the statements below, which most closely describes the incidence of atrial fibrillation in various age groups?
    a. Common in all age groups.
    b. Rare in the adult population, common in children.
    c. Common in the adult population, rare in children.
    d. Rare in all age groups.

23. AF is initiated by
    a. an automatic ectopic atrial pacemaker exhibiting the warm-up phenomenon.
    b. multiform atrial tachycardia.
    c. deterioration of one of the rapid atrial arrhythmias.
    d. an APB falling in the vulnerable period of the atria.

MATCHING

Directions

Match each arrhythmia in column A with its correct classification in column B. Choices in column B may be used more than once or not at all.

Example

A	B
(A) 1. An SA nodal arrhythmia	A. Sinus bradycardia
(C) 2. An atrial arrhythmia	B. VPBs
(B) 3. A ventricular arrhythmia	C. Atrial tachycardia
	D. Junctional tachycardia

A	B
( ) 24. Atrial escape rhythm	A. Active or usurping
( ) 25. Atrial fibrillation	B. Passive or escape
( ) 26. Atrial flutter	C. Can be either
( ) 27. Atrial premature depolarizations	D. Is neither
( ) 28. Automatic atrial tachycardia	
( ) 29. Paroxysmal supraventricular tachycardia	
( ) 30. Wandering pacemaker	

A	B
( ) 31. Atrial asystole	A. May be found in healthy people
( ) 32. Atrial escape rhythm	B. Rarely found in healthy people
( ) 33. Atrial fibrillation	
( ) 34. Atrial flutter	
( ) 35. Atrial premature beats, occasional	
( ) 36. Atrial tachycardia with block	
( ) 37. Multiform atrial tachycardia	
( ) 38. Paroxysmal supraventricular tachycardia	
( ) 39. Wandering pacemaker	

A	B
( ) 40. Bigeminy	A. Every other beat is APB
( ) 41. Couplet	B. Every third beat is APB
( ) 42. Pair	C. Every fourth beat is APB
( ) 43. Run of atrial tachycardia	D. Two APBs in succession
( ) 44. Trigeminy	E. Three APBs in succession
( ) 45. Triplet	F. Four or more APBs in a row
( ) 46. Quadrigeminy	
( ) 47. Salvo of three	

TRUE/FALSE

Directions

Determine whether each of the following statements is true or false and indicate with a *T* or *F*.

Example

(F) 1. The presence of APBs is a poor prognostic sign.

( ) 48. APBs in healthy individuals are associated with a higher incidence of sudden cardiac death.

( ) 49. PSVT may be life-threatening in an infant.

( ) 50. AFl with 1:1 conduction is more common in infants than adults.

( ) 51. Bigeminal nonconducted APBs often cause significant reduction in cardiac output because the heart rate is nearly halved.

( ) 52. PSVT is a common arrhythmia associated with digitalis toxicity.

( ) 53. The condition that MAT is most often associated with is valvular heart disease.

( ) 54. A fast ventricular rate results in decreased cardiac output because the ventricles do not have adequate time to fill.

The remainder of the questions involve analysis of patient situations and assessment of rhythm strips. Responses required are short answer and essay.

CASE: *Your patient, a 30-year-old female elementary school teacher, came to the emergency room with complaints of palpitations, rapid heart action, and near-syncope. By the time she arrived, she said her symptoms had abated. Her vital signs on admission were: T 97.8; AP 78; R 16; BP 118/74. Suddenly she developed the rhythm below. She said, "Oh, I feel that way again."*

55. Analyze the rhythm. How is the arrhythmia classified? What is the nursing diagnosis?
56. What will you include in your assessment of this patient?
57. Is the arrhythmia clinically significant? Why?
58. Establish nursing intervention priorities.
59. What factors will you consider in deciding whether patient teaching is indicated? Develop a patient teaching plan for management of this arrhythmia at home.

V_1

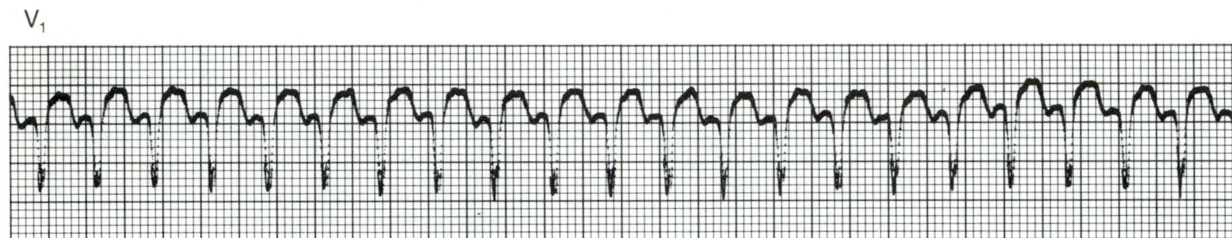

CASE: *Ms. S is a 76-year-old patient admitted to the medical wing with a medical diagnosis of congestive heart failure.*

60. Analyze the rhythm.
61. What factors will you consider in assessing this patient? What is a common cause of this arrhythmia? The admission orders are:
    1. Admit.
    2. 2 gm sodium diet.
    3. CBC, electrolytes stat.
    4. Heparin lock IV.
    5. Digoxin 0.50 mg IV stat.
62. What will your care plan priorities be for this patient?

Lead II

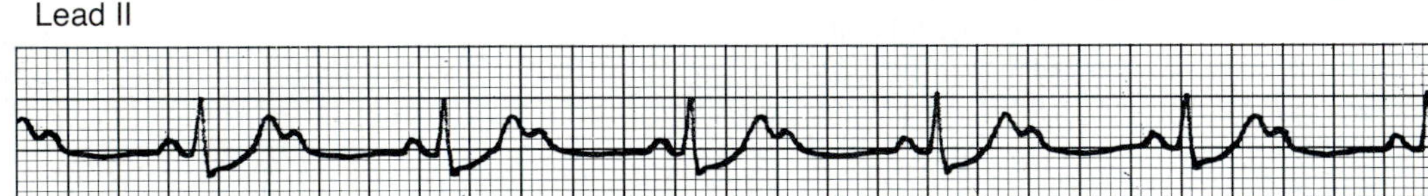

CASE: *Mr. G., a 57-year-old patient in the coronary care unit, was admitted for evaluation of chest pain and shortness of breath. He has had a myocardial infarction in the past. His rhythm strip is displayed below.*

63. Analyze the rhythm.
64. Describe the ECG features of the arrhythmia diagnosed in question 63.
65. Discuss the variability of the PR intervals displayed with the early beats.
66. Besides assessing the rhythm, what else will you include in your assessment?
67. Based on your findings, describe nursing intervention measures.
68. What factors will you consider in evaluation of this patient?

Lead II

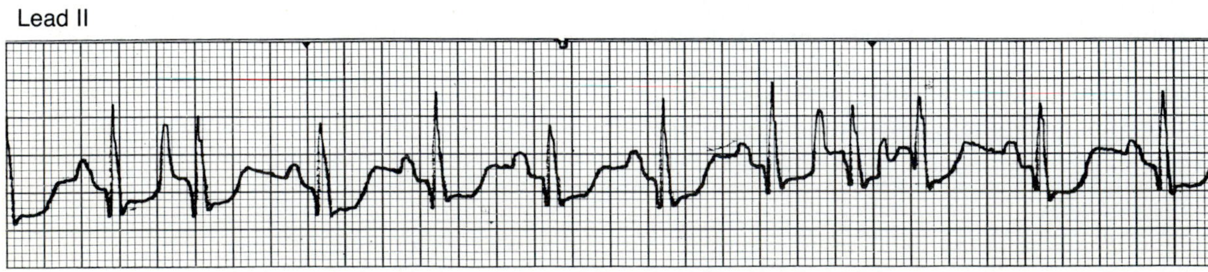

CASE: *Mrs. L is a 43-year-old patient who is in the recovery room after a hysterectomy. She is known to have hypertensive cardiovascular disease. Her monitor pattern is displayed below. Her admission ECG showed normal sinus rhythm.*

69. Analyze the rhythm.
70. Plan your nursing intervention after delineating assessment measures.

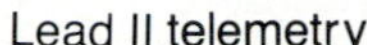

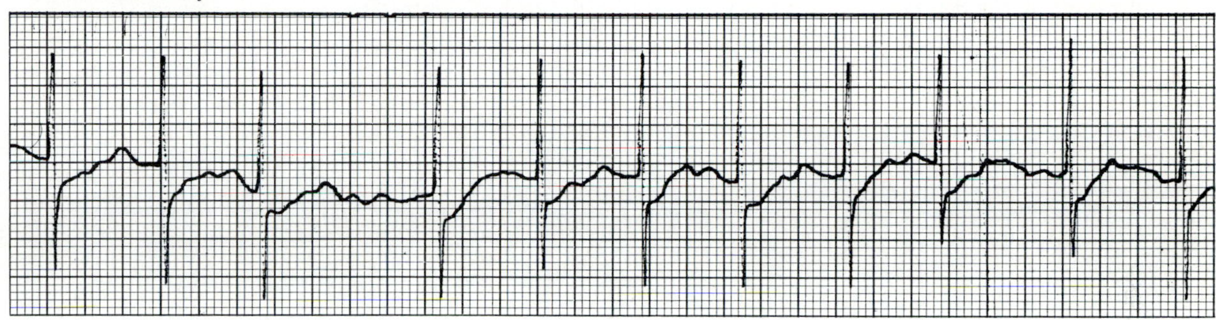

CASE: *GT, a 58-year-old male patient, has a history of heart disease. He is in the intensive care unit recovering from a car accident in which he suffered a fractured pelvis. His rhythm strip is below.*

71. Analyze the rhythm. Explain the beats that interrupt the rhythmicity. Is this rhythm encountered often?

V_1

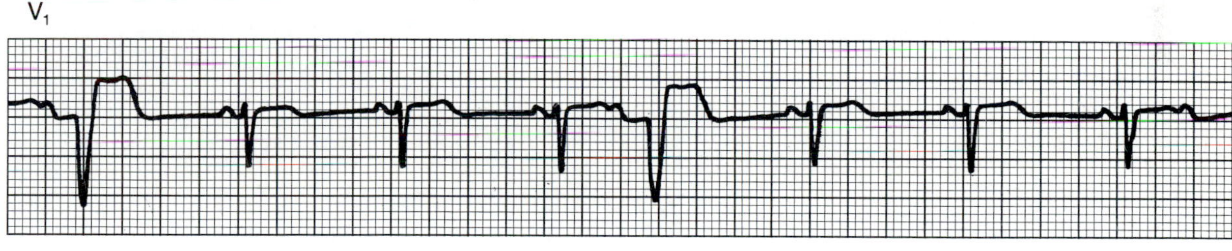

CASE: *Mr. R., 42 years old, has had a large myocardial infarction. Approximately 24 hours after admission, he developed the rhythm below.*

72. Analyze the rhythm.
73. How is the arrhythmia clinically significant?
74. List assessment measures.
75. Compare the treatment of AFl with AF.

Lead II

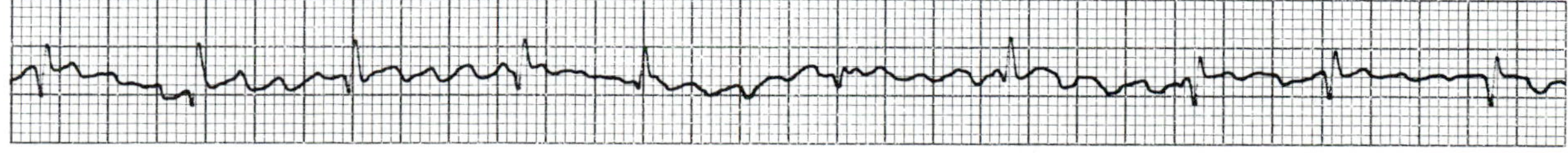

CASE: *MK is an 86-year-old male on your telemetry unit. His rhythm strip follows:*

76. You have just arrived. MK is your patient. The monitor pattern below is representative of the pattern he has been showing since admission. Interpret the rhythm. Explain how the rhythm is clinically significant.
77. Describe additional measures to assess this patient.
78. Plan intervention and explain what factors you considered in making your decision.

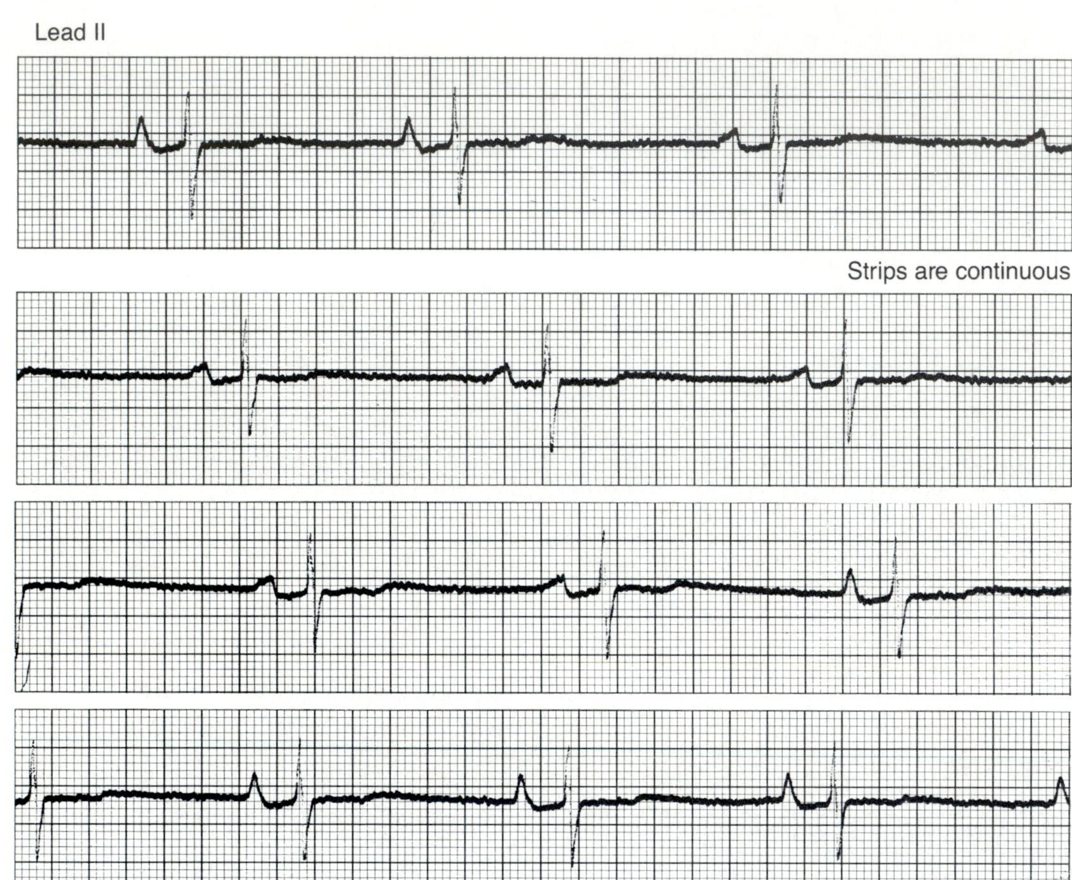

CASE: *Mr. N. is a 60-year-old patient in the intensive care unit with a medical diagnosis of chronic obstructive pulmonary disease, respiratory distress. His ECG pattern is presented below.*

79. Interpret the arrhythmia and describe its clinical significance.

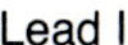

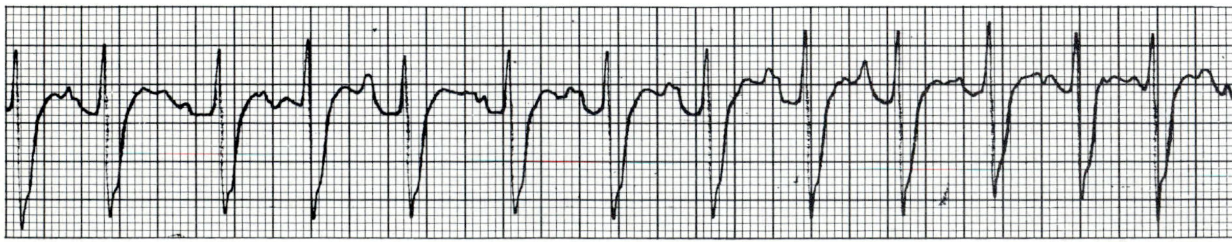

The remainder of the self-assessment is devoted to arrhythmia interpretation. Analyze the arrhythmias and answer any additional questions.

80. Interpret the rhythm and describe it as you would on a patient's record.

How is the rhythm clinically significant?
Are any emergency medications indicated?
How else might this arrhythmia be manifested electrocardiographically?

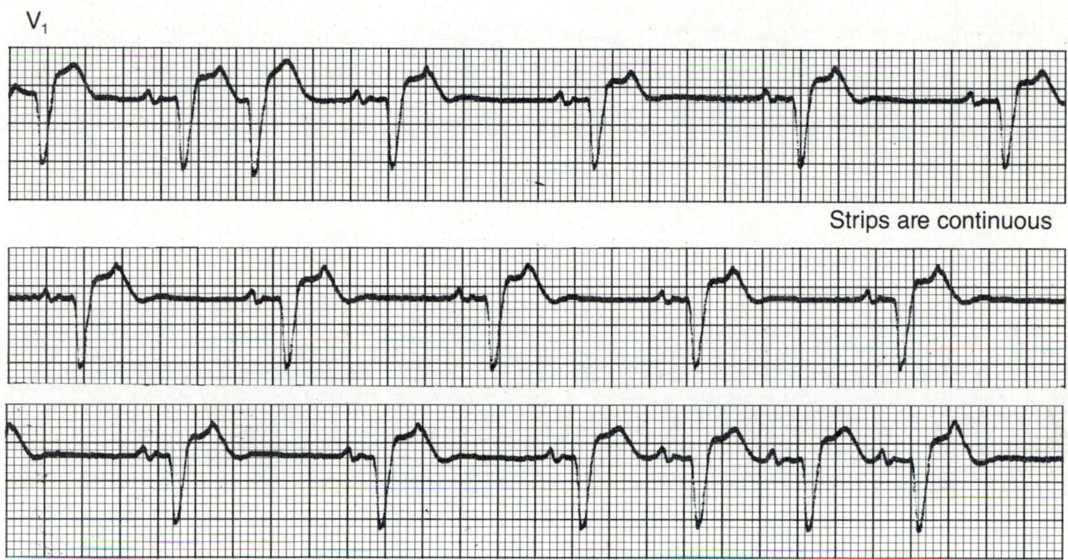

81. Interpret the rhythm.

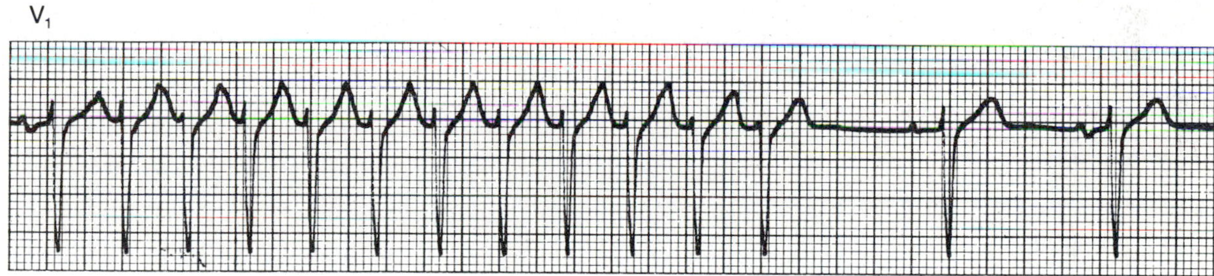

82. Interpret the rhythm and describe it as you would on the patient's record.

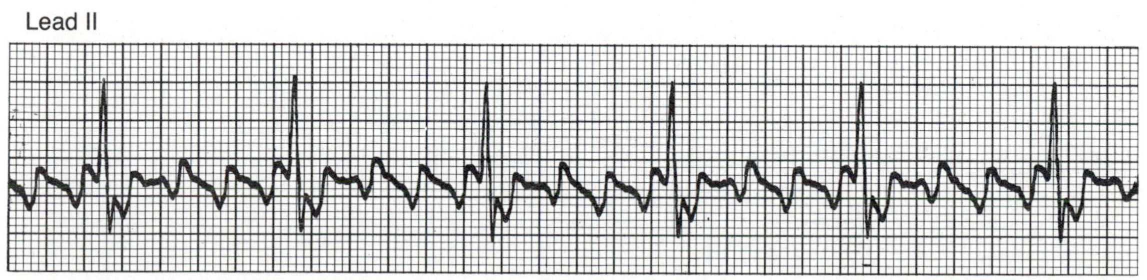

83. Interpret the rhythm.

Lead III

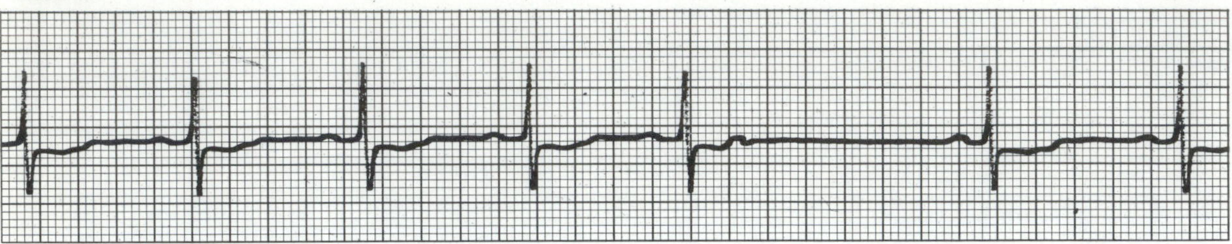

84. Interpret the rhythm. Be careful.

Lead II

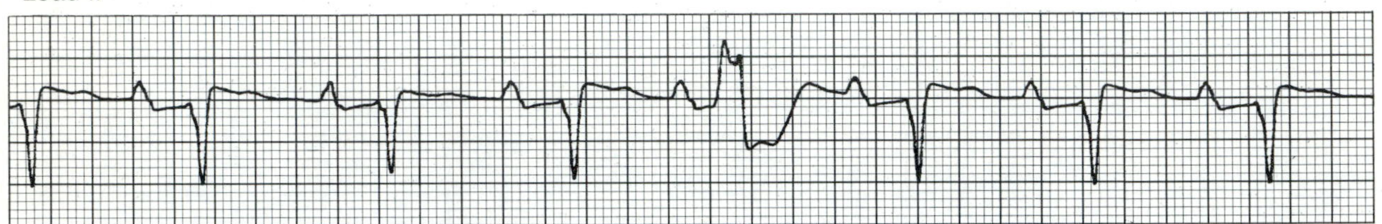

85. Explain what is happening in this rhythm strip.

Lead II

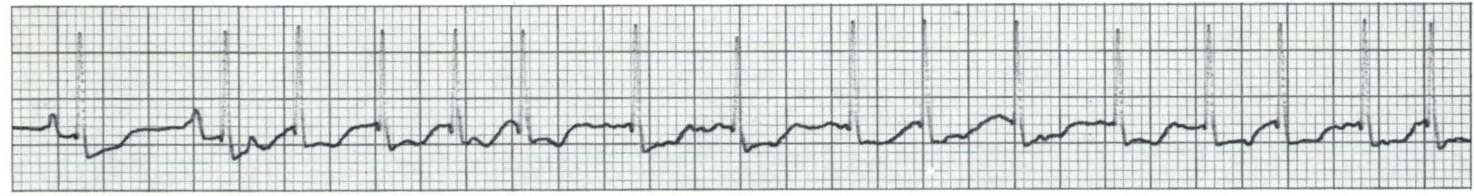

86. Interpret the rhythm.

MCL_1

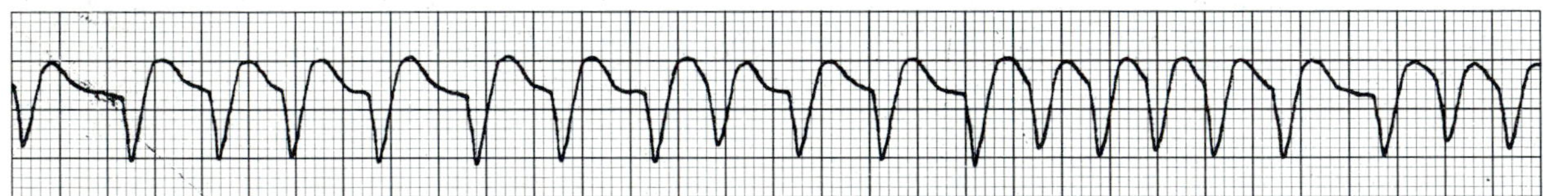

87. Interpret the rhythm.

MCL_1

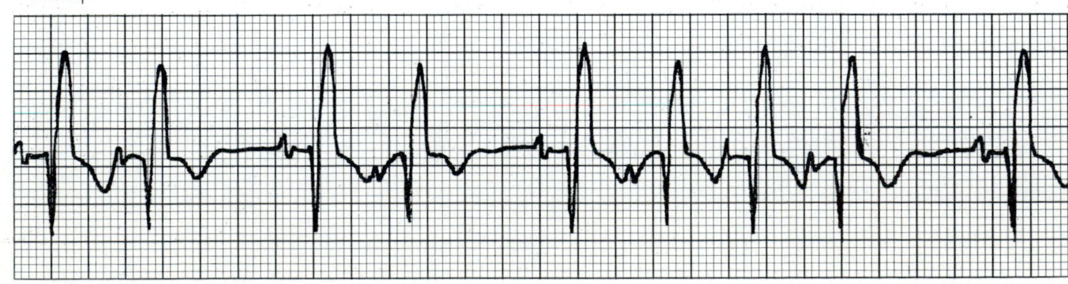

ANSWERS TO SELF-ASSESSMENT

1. c
2. d
3. a, c
4. a
5. d
6. b
7. d
8. b
9. a, b, c, d
10. a, d
11. b, c, d
12. a
13. b
14. b, c
15. a
16. b, d
17. b, c, d
18. b, c
19. b, c
20. a
21. a
22. c
23. c, d

24. B
25. A
26. A
27. A
28. A
29. A
30. B
31. B
32. B
33. B
34. B
35. A
36. B
37. B
38. A
39. A
40. A
41. D
42. D
43. E, F
44. B
45. E
46. C
47. E
48. F
49. T
50. T
51. T
52. F
53. F
54. T

55. *Rate:* 200 bpm
 Rhythm: Regular
 P waves: Present but not clearly delineated. On each T wave there is evidence of a P wave.
 PR interval: Approximately 0.14 seconds
 QRS complex: 0.08 to 0.09 seconds
 Interpretation: Because the rhythm started suddenly, it is named *paroxysmal supraventricular tachycardia.* The rhythm is classified as one of the supraventricular tachycardias.
 Nursing diagnosis: Decreased cardiac output related to tachycardia.
56. Immediately assess skin color and warmth, sensorium, blood pressure, peripheral pulse, presence of other symptoms such as shortness of breath, chest discomfort, light-headedness. After symptoms are alleviated, assess history and life style.
57. Yes! With such a rapid ventricular rate, the ventricles do not have adequate time to fill, resulting in a diminished cardiac output.
58. If the patient is sitting, assist her to a supine or low-Fowler's position. Elevating both legs may help improve blood pressure. Assign your assistant to do this.
 Reassure the patient.
 Have her perform the Valsalva maneuver.
 According to institutional policy, other methods that may be attempted by the nurse include brief submersion of the face in ice water and administration of intravenous verapamil.
 Notify the physician.
 Prepare for administration of other medications and/or cardioversion.
59. In deciding whether this patient should be taught to manage this arrhythmia at home, you would consider such factors as age, maturity, level of apprehension, and ability to comprehend. This patient is a school teacher and she will probably be able to comprehend the nature of the arrhythmia. You need to assess the other factors. The teaching plan should include:
 a. Assessment of knowledge base.
 b. Explanation of the arrhythmia and the nature of the rhythm disturbance.
 c. Instructions for medication use, if prescribed.
 d. Instructions and demonstration of selected methods for self-termination of the arrhythmia. If the Valsalva maneuver was successful, she should try this first.
 e. Evaluate her comprehension by having her return the demonstration.
60. *Rate:* Atrial 120 bpm
 Ventricular 60 bpm
 Rhythm: Atrial regular
 Ventricular regular
 P waves: two P waves for every QRS. Bear constant relationship to QRS.
 QRS complex: 0.08 seconds; depressed ST segment
 QT interval: Approximately 0.40 seconds
 Interpretation: AT with block, 2:1 conduction
61. In addition to checking how well she is tolerating the rhythm (e.g., color, sensorium, blood pressure), check the medications that she was taking at home. If she is on digoxin, assess for signs of toxicity. Digoxin toxicity is a common cause of this arrhythmia.
62. Hold the digoxin. Obtain the serum potassium as soon as possible. Notify physician for digoxin level, if indicated.
63. *Rate:* 100 to 110 bpm
 Rhythm: Irregular
 P waves: Underlying rhythm, P waves are normal. Frequent P′ waves that are premature and are different in shape to the sinus P wave. P wave precedes each QRS complex.
 PR interval: 0.16 seconds
 QRS complex: 0.10 seconds, qRs complex
 QT interval: Not discernible on this lead. You would need to view on another lead.
 Interpretation: NSR with rate 96 to 100 bpm; frequent APBs increase rate to 110 bpm
64. APBs: Premature P′ wave that is different from the sinus P in at least one lead. PR interval of APB > 0.12 seconds. Noncompensatory pause, usually.
65. The PR intervals of the APBs are 0.14 to 0.16 seconds. The PR interval of APBs depends on the following:
 - the proximity of the ectopic atrial focus to the AV junction.
 - the condition of the AV junction.
 - how premature the APB is.
 - the length of the cycle preceding the APB.

66. Check for signs of congestive heart failure (e.g., shortness of breath, rales in the lung bases, distended external jugular veins). Also check electrolytes, other medications he is receiving, the pattern of the arrhythmia with regard to the consistency with which it manifests in relation to diet, sleep, stress, etc.
67. If the patient has symptoms of congestive heart failure, the physician should be notified. Also request serum electrolytes if indicated. If the patient is experiencing palpitations with the APBs, reassure him that the arrhythmia is not serious.
68. Check the effect of the medications used to treat the congestive heart failure. Evaluate progress of lung sounds and other symptoms, as well as frequent and consistent sampling of the rhythm to determine if the number of APBs per minute is increasing or decreasing. Watch for development of AFl or AF.
69. *Rate:* 100 bpm
    Rhythm: Irregular
    P waves: Chaotic
    PR interval: —
    QRS complex: 0.06 seconds
    QT interval: Not able to determine on this lead
    Interpretation: Uncontrolled AF
70. Assess how well the patient is tolerating the arrhythmia. Check for signs and symptoms of congestive heart failure. Notify the physician.
71. *Rate:* 75 bpm.
    Rhythm: Irregular
    P waves: One precedes each normal QRS; one precedes each abnormal QRS. They all bear constant relationships to their respective QRS complexes. The P′ waves that precede the two wide QRS complexes are premature. There is one premature P wave (end of strip) that is not followed by a QRS complex.
    PR interval: 0.11 seconds with normal QRS complexes; 0.18 seconds with abnormal QRS complexes.
    QRS complex: 0.08, rS complex in V_1 is normal; elevated ST segment; abnormal QRS complexes are 0.10 to 0.12 seconds.
    QT interval: 0.32 seconds
    Interpretation: NSR with two aberrantly conducted APBs and one nonconducted APB
    The aberrantly conducted QRS complexes are a result of insufficient recovery of a portion of the bundle branch system in the ventricles. This pattern of aberration is unusual. The more common pattern is a rSR′ pattern of RBBB.
72. *Rate:* Atrial: 300+ bpm
    Ventricular: 90 bpm
    Rhythm: Atrial: Regular with some periods of irregularity
    Ventricular: Irregular
    P waves: Mostly saw-tooth configuration
    PR interval: —
    QRS complex: 0.06 seconds
    QT interval: Not measurable on this lead
    Interpretation: Atrial flutter-fib, controlled
73. The cardiac output may be diminished. In the presence of an acute myocardial infarction, the arrhythmia tends to indicate a poorer prognosis. It may be an indication of atrial distension resulting from congestive heart failure. It also may be an indication of atrial involvement in the infarction.
74. Determine how well the patient is tolerating the arrhythmia. Assess for signs of diminished cardiac output and possible causes by measuring: blood pressure, lung sounds, sensorium, external jugular venous distension, skin color and temperature, and serum electrolytes.
75. The treatment for these two arrhythmias is very similar.
76. The first two complexes with the peaked P waves represent a sinus bradycardia at a rate of 42 bpm. After the second complex, the rate slows, the P waves are different with a rate of 37 bpm. The slower rhythm is an atrial escape rhythm and persists until the faster one again takes control.
    The rhythm is clinically significant because it may result in diminished cardiac output due to the slow rate. It may also be an indication of SA node dysfunction.
77. The patient should be assessed for his tolerance of the arrhythmia. Measure blood pressure, check peripheral pulses, skin temperature and color, and assess for signs of congestive heart failure.
78. Intervention for an arrhythmia such as this may range from continued observation to emergency treatment with atropine, isoproterenol, and/or preparation for transvenous pacing. The intervention depends on your assessment findings. If the patient is asymptomatic, continued observation and being sure the physician is aware of the rhythm disturbance may be all that are indicated.
79. There appear to be four different P waves with none appearing to be the dominant rhythm. The rate is 120 bpm. One P wave precedes each QRS complex. The rhythm is likely multiform atrial tachycardia. Since it usually accompanies a poor physical state, it tends to be associated with a poor prognosis. The arrhythmia itself is not potentially lethal, however.
80. Monitor showing bigeminal APBs, most of which are nonconducted, reducing the overall ventricular rate to 56 to 60 bpm. Short four beat run of NSR with rate 100 bpm shows a PR interval of 0.16 to 0.18 seconds. QRS 0.12 seconds, IVCD with a QS configuration and elevated ST segment.
    The rhythm is clinically significant because the patient's heart rate is suddenly nearly halved. Diminished cardiac output is likely.
    There are no emergency medications indicated as nursing intervention. If you were contemplating administering atropine, think about the consequences. Would you want the atrial rate to increase (it is already 100 bpm)?
    With improved AV nodal conduction, there is a good chance the patient would conduct every complex. What the patient needs is treatment directed at decreasing the APBs. Notify the physician, check for signs of decreased cardiac output and congestive heart failure. Other ways APBs can be manifested are with prolonged PR intervals and/or with ventricular aberration.
81. The strip starts with a sinus beat. There is an APB that initiates a burst of PSVT at a rate of 188 bpm. The PSVT ends abruptly, is followed by an atrial escape beat, then a sinus beat.

82. Monitor showing AFl with 4:1 conduction. Ventricular response is regular at 60 bpm. AFl rate 240 bpm. QRS 0.10 seconds.
83. NSR with rate 66 bpm. One nonconducted APB, PR interval 0.20 seconds, P wave 0.12 seconds indicating possible intraatrial conduction disturbance. QRS complex 0.08 seconds.
84. Sinus rhythm with rate 66 to 72 bpm, prolonged PR interval at 0.28 seconds. QRS is a QS complex on lead II and measures 0.11 seconds. The rhythmicity is interrupted by an early, wide QRS complex that is preceded by a P wave. Did you call this an aberrantly conducted APB? Is the P wave premature? No, it is not. This is a VPB, which we have not yet studied. We included this here to remind you of the criteria for diagnosing APBs.
85. The patient is having APBs and goes into uncontrolled AF.
86. Ventricular rhythm irregular with no identifiable P waves—AF, uncontrolled, IVCD.
87. Atrial bigeminy, four beat run of atrial tachycardia at rate 125 bpm. PR interval 0.16 seconds and up to 0.18 seconds with APBs. IVCD present (specifically RBBB). Overall rate approximately 90 bpm.

CHAPTER SEVEN

AV Junctional Rhythm Disturbances

▶ GOAL

You will be able to identify atrioventricular (AV) junctional rhythm disturbances, differentiate them from dangerous, life-threatening arrhythmias, and use the nursing process in caring for your patients.

▶ OBJECTIVES

After studying this chapter and completing the self-assessment exercises, you should be able to:

1. Demonstrate knowledge of which leads are most helpful in assessing junctional arrhythmias.
2. Differentiate junctional from atrial premature beats, and compare nursing interventions.
3. Categorize the junctional arrhythmias as passive or usurping.
4. Identify two situations in which a junctional arrhythmia may be lethal.
5. Compare and contrast the ECG features of, and nursing interventions for, junctional automatic tachycardia and paroxysmal AV nodal reentrant tachycardia.
6. Recognize accelerated idiojunctional rhythm, differentiate it from junctional automatic tachycardia, and determine nursing interventions based on assessment.
7. Explain the ECG characteristics of AV dissociation, and demonstrate ability to recognize its presence. Define isorhythmic AV dissociation.
8. Identify at least four conditions that may provoke junctional arrhythmias.
9. Explain how an echo beat occurs.
10. Determine assessment measures in order of priority for the patient in an idiojunctional rhythm. Discuss factors you would consider before initiating nursing interventions, and list in order of priority.

Recall from Chapter 1 that the atrioventricular junction (AVJ) is the portion of the conduction system that includes the AV node (AVN) and the bundle of His. The AVN has three sections: the region where atrial fibers enter the AVN (A-N), the AVN itself (N), and the portion of the AVN extending into the bundle of His (N-H). The term *junctional* encompasses all areas of the AVN and bundle of His. Since junctional tissue contains cells capable of spontaneous depolarization, it is capable of automaticity and any of its areas can act as pacemakers or sites of ectopic discharge[1] (Fig. 7-1). Junctional arrhythmias comprise a relatively small group that are not seen as often as their atrial or ventricular counterparts.

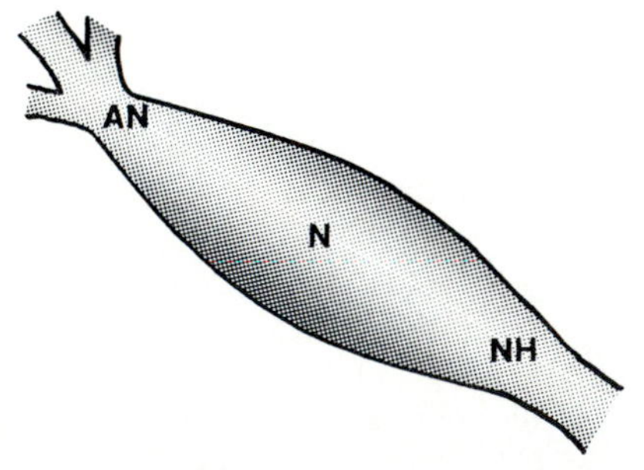

FIGURE 7-1 The AV node.

JUNCTIONAL PREMATURE BEATS

Data Base: Problem Identification

Definitions, Etiology, and Mechanisms

Premature beats arising from the junctional area (junctional premature beats [JPBs]) probably result from increased automaticity. Their occurrence may or may not be related to organic heart disease.[2] They may be a manifestation of ischemia and/or digitalis toxicity and, like atrial premature beats (APBs), may be associated with congestive heart failure (CHF), myocardial infarction (MI), rheumatic heart disease, or increased sympathetic tone.[3] They have the same clinical significance as APBs.[1]

JPBs are much less common than either APBs[4,5] or

ventricular premature beats (VPBs). Also referred to as *junctional extrasystoles,*[6] JPBs appear in about 9% of hospitalized patients.[7]

ECG Characteristics

JPBs resemble atrial extrasystoles in two respects: they occur earlier in the cycle than the next expected impulse, and the QRS complex resembles those of the sinus beats (unless there is aberration). Both APBs and JPBs are considered supraventricular in origin. JPBs may be preceded by a P wave that is also premature, but the P wave is conducted retrogradely (backwards) through the atria, resulting in a P′ wave that is negative rather than positive in the inferior leads (II, III, and aVF) (Fig. 7-2 and Table 7-1). (Recall APBs are always preceded by a premature P′ wave that is different from the sinus P waves.).

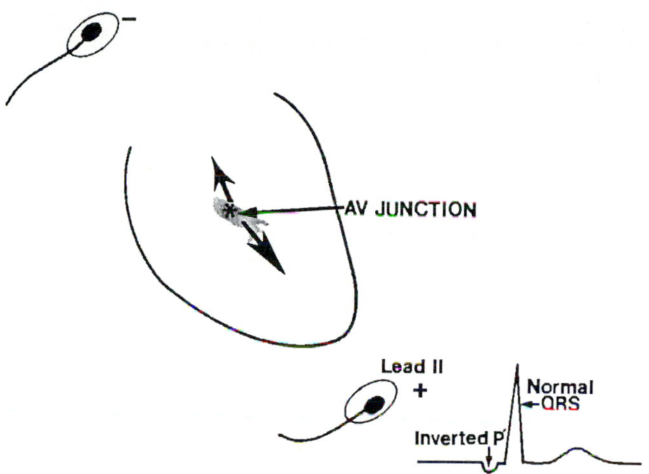

FIGURE 7-2 An impulse originating in the AV junction causes ventricular depolarization in the normal manner, but atrial depolarization is retrograde resulting in an inverted P′ wave in inferior leads that may occur before, during, or after the QRS complex.

Retrograde atrial depolarization. Regardless of whether the source of the JPB is the A-N, N, or N-H region, retrograde atrial depolarization is common. Since the impulse is traveling from the junction superiorly through the atria, the resultant atrial inscription is negative on leads II, III, aVF, V_5, and V_6, upright in leads aVR and aVL, almost flat in I, and variable but often predominantly upright in V_1[6] (Figs. 7-3 and 7-4). When the P′ wave is diphasic in V_1 it is a negative-positive, as opposed to the normal positive-negative, diphasic pattern.[6]

Because the JPB can activate the atria either before, during, or after ventricular depolarization, its superiorly directed P′ wave may be inscribed on the ECG before, during, or after the QRS complex.[6] When the P′ wave appears before the QRS, the P′R interval is usually shorter than the PR in sinus rhythm, usually 0.10 seconds or less[4] (Figs. 7-3 and 7-4). How can a JPB with retrograde atrial depolarization be distinguished from a low atrial APB on the surface ECG? This is frequently impossible, but some[4] suggest diagnosing JPB if the P′R interval is 0.10 seconds

Table 7-1 Comparison of APBs and JPBs

APBs	JPBs
Early QRS always preceded by early P′ wave	Early QRS may or may not be preceded by early P′ wave. If it is, P′ is inverted in inferior leads (II, III, and aVF).
P′R interval 0.12 seconds or greater	P′R interval 0.10 seconds or less P′ wave may follow QRS within 0.20 seconds and will be inverted in inferior leads.
QRS normal unless IVCD	QRS normal unless IVCD

Lead II

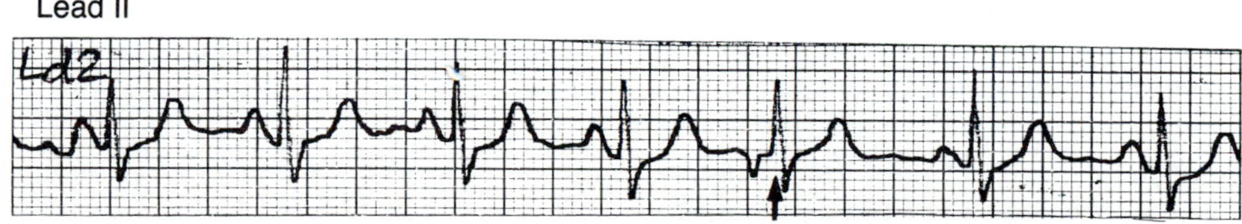

FIGURE 7-3 NSR with one JPB *(arrow).* Note early QRS complex preceded by an inverted P′ wave, indicating retrograde atrial depolarization. The early QRS complex is like the others and the P′R interval is 0.10 seconds.

Rate: 85 bpm
Rhythm: Irregular (resulting from early complex)
P waves: One precedes each QRS. The P′ preceding the early QRS is inverted on lead II.
PR interval: 0.14 seconds, P′R interval 0.10 seconds
QRS complex: 0.10 seconds
Interpretation: NSR, one JPB with retrograde atrial depolarization

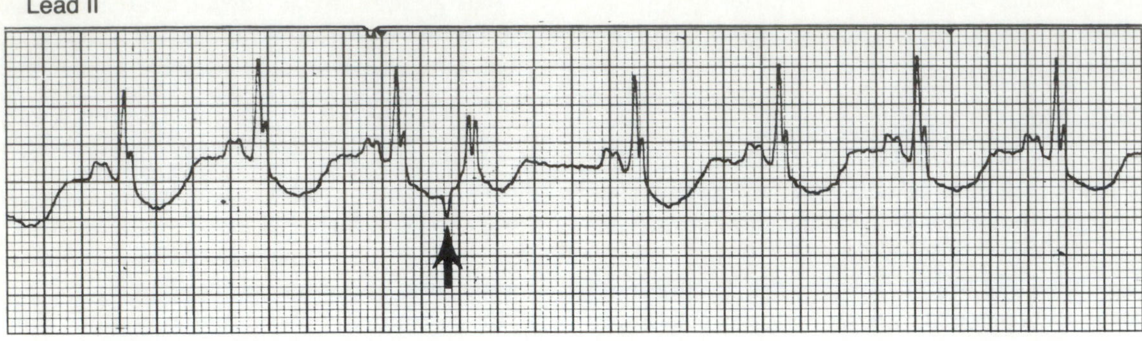

FIGURE 7-4 NSR with one JPB. Again, note early QRS complex preceded by inverted P′ wave on lead II *(arrow)*. The early QRS complex is slightly different from the others but has their same basic morphology. The P′R interval is 0.08 seconds.

Rate: 83 bpm
Rhythm: Irregular (resulting from early complex)
P waves: One precedes each QRS. The P′ preceding early QRS is inverted on lead II. Except for this early P′, the P waves are wide (0.12 seconds) and notched.
PR interval: 0.14 seconds, P′R interval 0.08 seconds
QRS complex: 0.10 seconds, early QRS is 0.12 seconds
Interpretation: NSR, one JPB with retrograde atrial depolarization, probable intraatrial conduction defect

or less. When the P′ wave follows the QRS, it usually does so within 0.12 seconds, causing the P′ to be located in the ST segment[4] (Fig. 7-5). When retrograde atrial depolarization and ventricular depolarization occur simultaneously or when there is no retrograde atrial depolarization (retrograde block), a P′ wave is not visible. In such situations it is either not present or buried within the QRS complex. (Figs. 7-6 and 7-7).

It would seem likely that the position of the P′ wave in relation to the QRS complex could give clues regarding its anatomic site of origin (e.g., if the P′ appears before the QRS complex, the origin is likely the A-N region). This is not the case. The position of the P′ in relation to its QRS cannot be used to locate the ectopic focus. Speed of conduction depends on the conduction properties of the AV junction in the retrograde and anterograde directions, and the P′-QRS relationship depends on the differences between anterograde and retrograde conduction times.[6]

Reciprocal or echo beats. When the P′ follows the QRS by a fairly long interval, it may find the AV node, bundle of His, and bundle branches no longer refractory from the preceding depolarization, thus allowing the atrial impulse to reactivate the ventricles and produce another QRS complex of normal configuration.[1,8] This is known as an *echo beat* (Fig. 7-8).

Patterns of occurrence. Like APBs and VPBs, JPBs can occur in bigeminy, trigeminy, and quadrigeminy and in salvos, couplets, and runs (Fig. 7-9). You may need to review "Patterns of Occurrence" in Chapter 6 before proceeding.

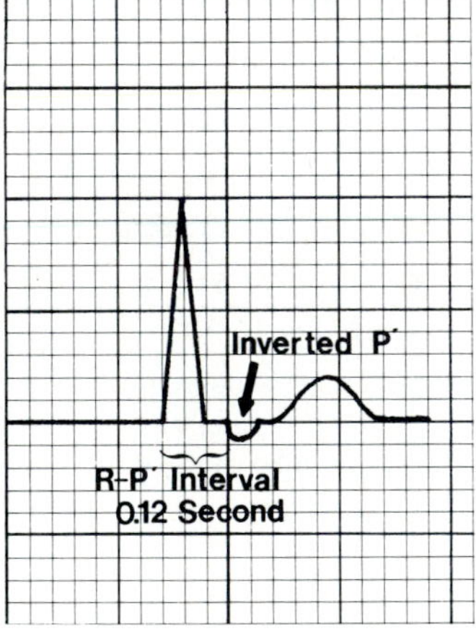

FIGURE 7-5 Schematic of junctional complex with retrograde atrial depolarization occurring after the QRS complex. Retrograde atrial depolarization produces a negative P′ wave in inferior leads. R-P′ interval is 0.12 seconds in this example.

Coupling interval. Like APBs and VPBs, JPBs often display fixed coupling intervals; intervals from preceding QRSs to premature beats are consistent.[5] Like APBs, JPBs usually do not have compensatory pauses. Retrograde atrial depolarization also depolarizes the SA node, resulting in a "resetting".

QRS complex. Although most often resembling the sinus-conducted QRS complex, a peculiarity of a junctional

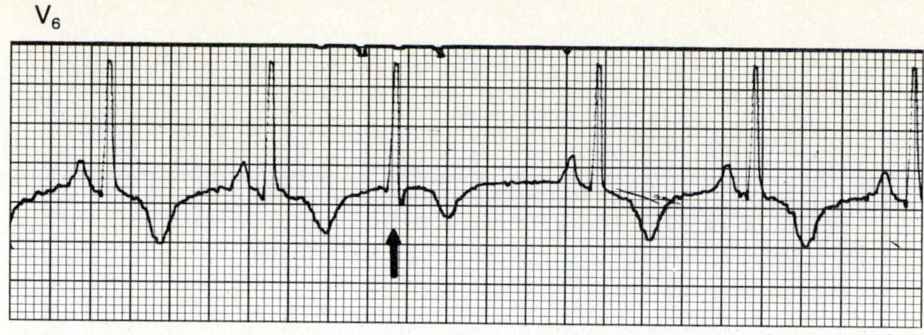

FIGURE 7-6 NSR with one JPB *(arrow).* Note prematurity of QRS complex and absence of P wave. What appears to be a terminal s wave in the JPB may be the last portion of an inverted P′ wave.

Rate: 75 bpm
Rhythm: Irregular (resulting from early complex)
P waves: One precedes all but the early QRS; P waves large.
PR interval: 0.15 seconds
QRS complex: 0.08 to 0.10 seconds; inverted T waves
Interpretation: NSR with one JPB

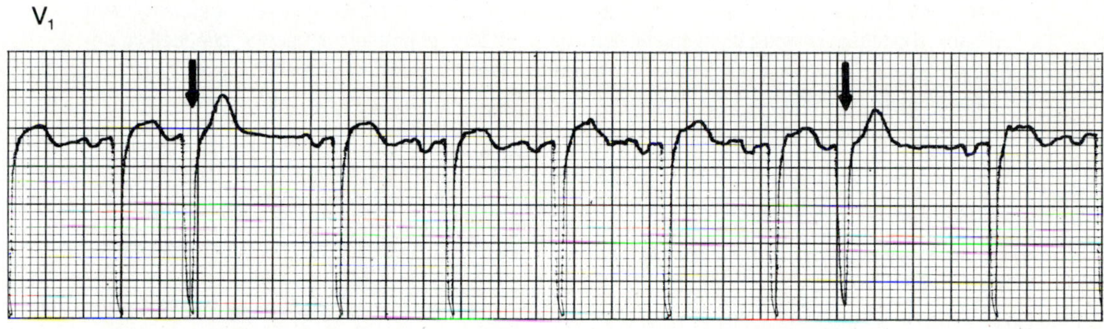

FIGURE 7-7 Sinus tachycardia (ST) with two JPBs *(arrows).* Note prematurity of QRS complexes and absence of preceding P waves. JPBs are often conducted with slight aberration. It is wise to analyze such complexes on several leads.

Rate: 106 bpm
Rhythm: Irregular (resulting from two early complexes)
P waves: One precedes each QRS except for two early complexes. P waves are diphasic, normal for V_1.
PR interval: 0.15 seconds
QRS complex: 0.09 seconds. The two JPBs are slightly wider and their T waves slightly taller. The presence of a P wave in the T waves of the JPBs cannot be ruled out. Multilead analysis is indicated in such situations.
Interpretation: ST with two JPBs

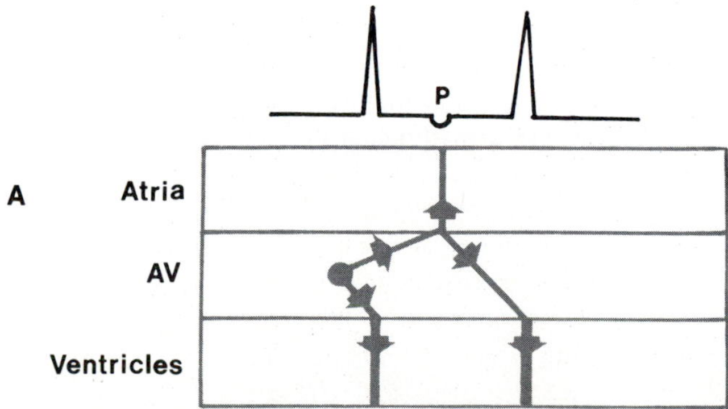

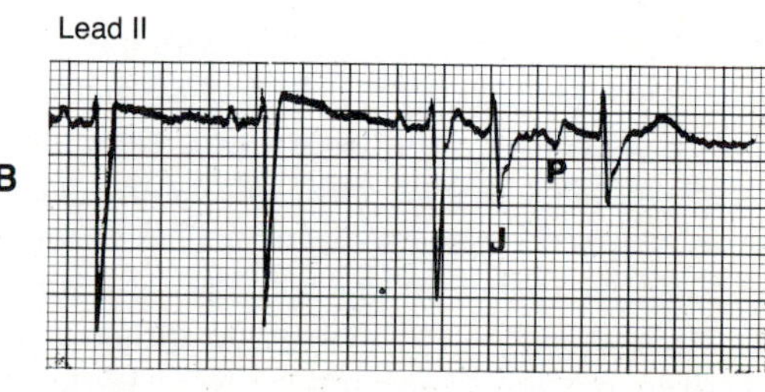

FIGURE 7-8 Junctional echo beat: **A,** A junctional beat *(J)* causing retrograde atrial depolarization *(P)* that may be delayed sufficiently to allow the impulse to reactivate the ventricles. **B,** The resultant tracing on an inferior lead resembles the graphic illustration *(A).* Note in the ECG tracing *(B)* after three sinus-conducted impulses, a JPB appears and is followed by a retrogradely conducted P′ wave. After activating the atria, the impulse again activates the ventricles.

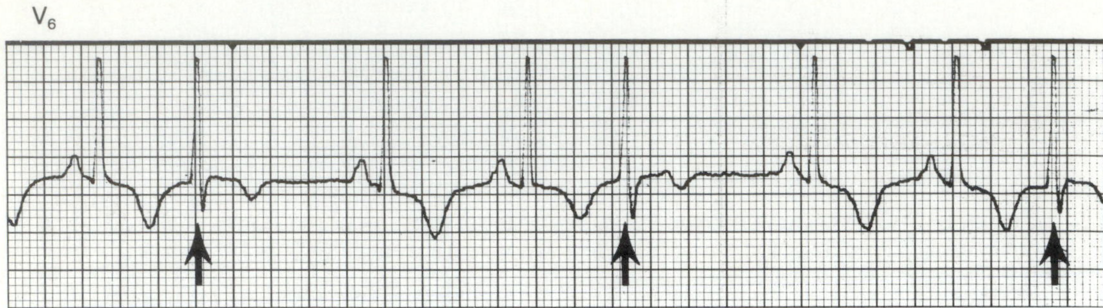

FIGURE 7-9 JPB in trigeminy *(arrows)*. Note junctional complexes occur every third complex and have an Rs configuration, making them slightly different morphologically from the sinus conducted beats. This slight aberration is of the RBBB type. Changing the lead to V_1 would confirm this.

Rate: 85 bpm
Rhythm: Irregular
P waves: One precedes each QRS except for three early complexes. P waves are large, probably because of intraatrial conduction delay.
PR interval: 0.16 seconds
QRS complex: 0.07 to 0.08 seconds sinus complexes; 0.10 to 0.12 seconds JPB, probable RBBB aberration
Interpretation: NSR, junctional trigeminy with RBBB aberration, intraatrial conduction defect

ectopic beat is its propensity to display minor (usually) aberration of the QRS complex regardless of whether it is early or late (escape).[6] Marriott[6] attributes this to either of the following two possibilities: the origin of the impulse is in close proximity to a Mahaim fiber (one of the AV nodal bypass tracts), resulting in at least partial conduction to the ventricles via this tract; or the origin of the ectopic junctional focus is located so the impulse is distributed asynchronously to the bundle branches.

The box on this page summarizes the ECG features of junctional ectopy.

ECG Characteristics
Junctional Premature Beats

Rate: Variable, within normal range
Rhythm: Irregular
P wave: If present, before or after QRS and inverted
PR interval: 0.10 seconds or less if present
QRS complex: Normal, unless IVCD. Often slight aberration

Applied Nursing Process
Clinical Assessment

- Detect:
  - An irregular pulse.
  - An irregularity in the ECG.
- Assess the patient and ECG.
  - Assess for symptoms associated with the JPBs. Although most patients with JPBs are asymptomatic and unaware of their rhythm disturbance, some may experience symptoms ranging from palpitations, or the feeling of "skipped beats", to signs and symptoms of reduced cardiac output. When the JPBs are frequent and early enough in the cycle, cardiac filling is reduced. Moreover, the atrial kick may be lost and this may decrease cardiac output as well. Symptoms associated with diminished cardiac output include light-headedness, pulse deficit, and lowered blood pressure.
  - Appraise the clinical setting in which the JPBs are occurring. For example, has the patient had a myocardial infarction?
  - Is the arrhythmia related to activity or diet?
  - Monitor serum electrolytes.
  - Assess factors that may contribute to the increase in automaticity (such as digitalis).
  - Diagnose the arrhythmia using the algorithm in Fig. 7-10.
  - Determine the frequency of the JPBs. Document the number per minute at frequent (e.g., hourly) intervals to determine consistency of occurrence.
  - Assess for progression of the arrhythmia to junctional tachycardia.

❖ NURSING DIAGNOSIS

Decreased cardiac output related to reduced ventricular filling.

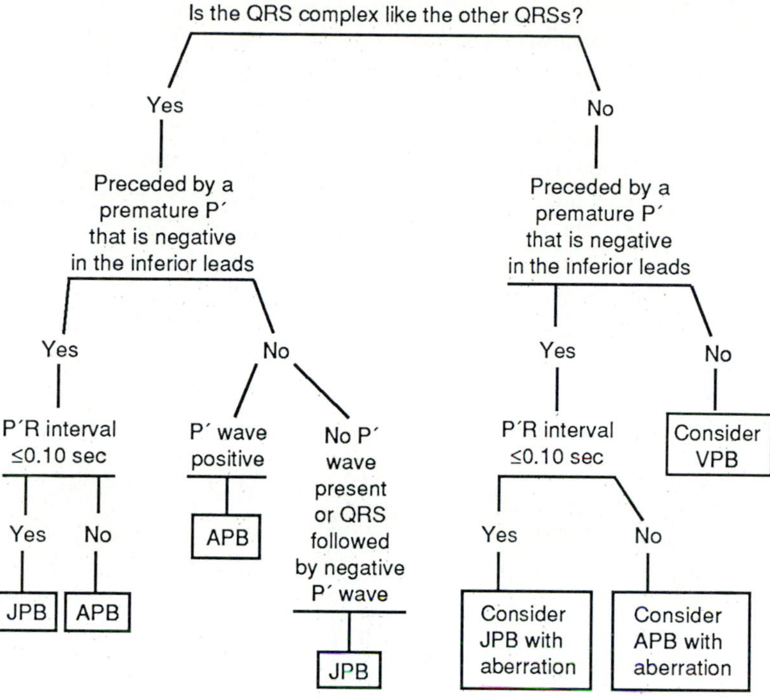

FIGURE 7-10 JPB algorithm.

❖ ECG DIAGNOSIS

Junctional premature beats.

Plan and Implementation

Patient goal. The patient will remain asymptomatic or will regain asymptomatic status.

Nursing interventions.

- If the patient is symptomatic take the following steps:
  - Reassure the patient that measures will be taken to diminish the symptoms.
  - Inform the patient that the arrhythmia will not pose a threat to his/her well-being.
  - Evaluate the patient's response to the arrhythmia on a continuing basis.
- Record the frequency of JPBs and any change in the pattern of occurrence.
- Monitor on a lead that allows differentiation of JPBs from APBs (e.g., one of the inferior leads that will display a negative P′ wave) or V_1, which will display a positive or a negative-positive diphasic P′ wave.
- Report significant findings to the physician. As a general rule, notify the physician of any change in rhythm that may indicate an abnormality. Your judgment of the patient's clinical situation will dictate the immediacy of such notification.
  - If the patient suddenly develops frequent JPBs (five or more per minute) for several minutes, the physician should be notified. Immediate notification is indicated if the patient's cardiac output is compromised or the JPBs cause discomfort.
  - If the patient has exhibited only an occasional JPB, you may elect to wait to inform the physician until the next visit.
- Observe for progression of the arrhythmia to junctional tachycardia.
- Implement medical orders and evaluate the patient's response.

Evaluation

- The patient does not develop junctional tachycardia or arrhythmia-related symptoms as evidenced by the following:
  - Stable blood pressure and heart rate.
  - Absence of pulse deficit.
  - Denial of light-headedness and palpitations.

Medical Treatment

Treatment is directed toward stabilizing the underlying cause.

JUNCTIONAL AUTOMATIC TACHYCARDIA

Data Base: Problem Identification

Definitions, Etiology, and Mechanisms

Junctional tachycardia (JT) is an arrhythmia that is rarely encountered. It is defined as three or more JPBs in succession[4] at a rate of 100 bpm or greater and is due to enhanced automaticity. A more common tachycardia involving a circuitous reentry in the AV node is paroxysmal supraventricular tachycardia (PSVT), which is discussed in Chapter 6.

The significance of JT is best judged in light of the associated clinical condition.[4] Seen in all age groups, in adults it is associated with the same conditions as JPBs and is not considered a dangerous arrhythmia. In children, however, rapid JT is considered life-threatening,[9] since ventricular dysfunction and congestive heart failure occur soon after onset of the tachycardia.[10] It is not an unusual form of SVT in this population[9,11,12] and tends to run in families.[10] Occurring in 15% of patients who have undergone corrective surgery for tetralogy of Fallot, JT is noted less frequently in other pediatric corrective cardiac procedures,[13] occurring in about 8%.[14]

ECG Characteristics

If the arrhythmia begins as a succession of JPBs, its onset and termination will be abrupt,[4] but characteristically it gradually accelerates.[12] The rate ranges from 100 to 200 bpm in adults. In a recent study by Bär et al [15] a mean rate of 167 bpm, with a range of 118 to 231 bpm, was found. In children the rate is often less than 200 bpm[10] but sometimes approaches 250 to 300 bpm.[13] JT usually has a consistently regular rhythm (Fig. 7-11).

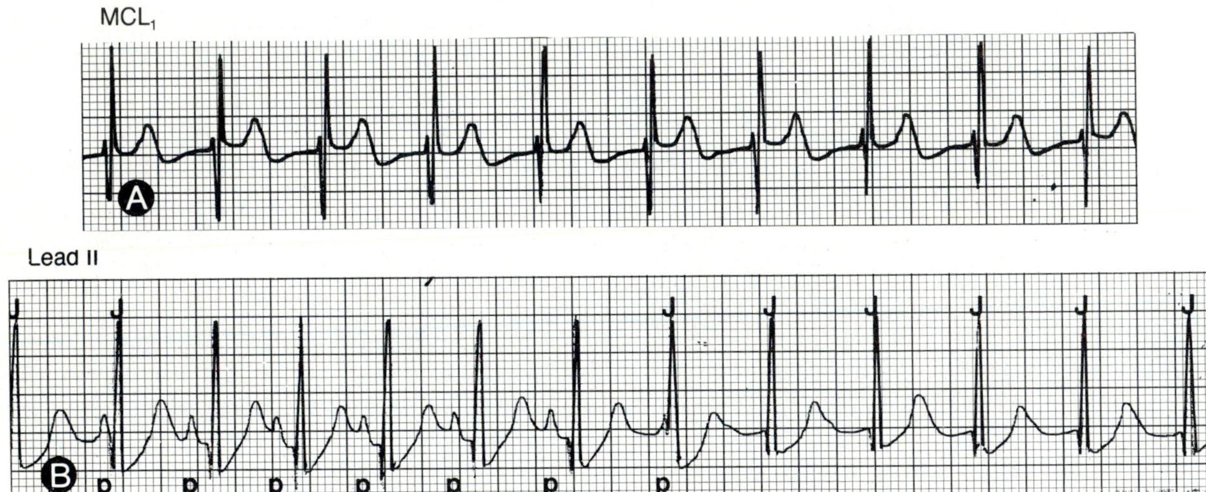

FIGURE 7-11 Two examples of junctional tachycardia (JT).

A.

Rate: 104 bpm
Rhythm: Regular
P waves: None visible
PR interval: None
QRS complex: rSR′ 0.08 seconds with RBBB morphology
Interpretation: JT

B.

This tracing is a sample of a persistent intermittent junctional tachycardia taken from a 12-year-old boy. As the slow phase of his sinus arrhythmia appeared, an ectopic junctional pacemaker usurped *(J)* and became the dominant pacemaker. The atria *(P)* presumably continued to beat independently of the ventricles resulting in a phasic AV dissociation. Although not shown in this short sample, when the sinus rate increased, the P wave emerged and captured the ventricles. When atrial and ventricular rates are the same during dissociation, the dissociation is said to be *synchronized.* Further discussion of AV dissociation is presented later in this chapter and Chapter 9.

Rate: 108-112 bpm
Rhythm: Irregular
P waves: Normal. During slow phase of sinus arrhythmia, atria and ventricles become dissociated.
PR interval: 0.12 to 0.13 seconds with sinus conducted beats
QRS complex: qR 0.06 to 0.07 seconds; junctional pacemaker usurps at a rate of 108 bpm when sinus rate slows to 100 bpm.
Interpretation: Sinus tachycardia slowing to allow usurpation by junctional tachycardia

P′ waves. Most of the time the P′ wave is buried in the QRS complex.[15] In children, this may be the case, but more often the P′ wave is found after the QRS complex.[13] When a P′ wave is visible, its axis is superior.[15] Usually one P′ wave per QRS complex will be seen, a ratio of 1:1.

QRS complex. The QRS complex will appear normal, since the impulse traverses normal intraventricular conduction pathways. There may be aberration at rapid rates resulting from temporary abnormal intraventricular conduction, a result of unequal refractoriness of the bundle branches.[4]

For a summary of the ECG features of JT, see the box below.

On the surface ECG, differentiating JT from other supraventricular tachycardias such as atrial tachycardia, atrial flutter, and PSVT is sometimes impossible. In such cases, electrophysiology studies may be necessary.[15]

Applied Nursing Process

Clinical Assessment

- Detect:
  - A rapid, regular pulse of 100 to 200 bpm in the adult; 130 to 300 bpm in the infant.
  - A rapid, regular ECG pattern with (usually) narrow QRS complexes.
- Assess the patient and ECG.
  - Assess for symptoms associated with the arrhythmia.

    Since the rate is rapid, ventricular filling time is reduced. Also, the atrial contribution to cardiac output is lost. These factors contribute to reduced cardiac output. Thus the most important assessment is the patient's tolerance of the arrhythmia. Assess the patient's blood pressure, sensorium, skin color, and temperature.

    Rapid heart rates also increase the myocardial oxygen demand. In certain individuals the oxygen demand may exceed the supply, resulting in decreased myocardial tissue perfusion. Assess for signs of myocardial ischemia such as chest discomfort or ST-segment and T-wave abnormalities on the ECG.

    Assess for signs and symptoms of developing congestive heart failure: subjective signs such as dyspnea, or cough; auscultate the lung fields for presence of rales; auscultate the heart for presence of S_3; examine the external jugular veins for distension.
  - Assess the patient's and/or parents' (in the case of the child) level of anxiety.
  - Diagnose the arrhythmia using the algorithm in Fig. 7-12.

ECG Characteristics
Junctional Automatic Tachycardia

Rate: 100 to 200 bpm adults
130 to 300 bpm children
Rhythm: Regular
P wave: Buried in QRS (in children, appears after QRS). When present, inverted in inferior leads.
PR interval: Not applicable
QRS complex: Normal unless IVCD

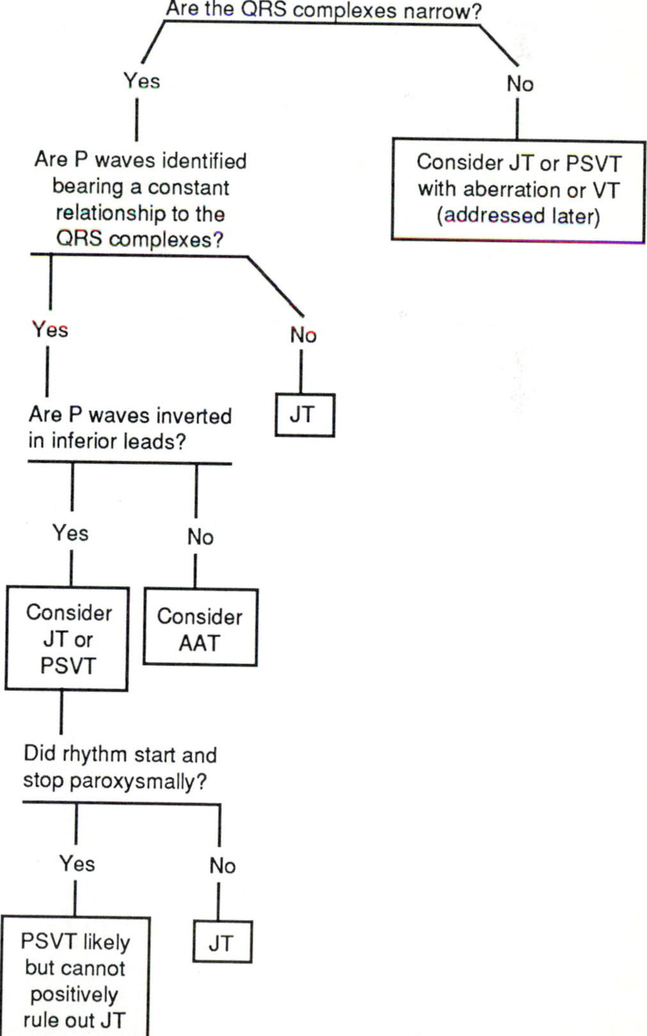

FIGURE 7-12 JT algorithm.

❖ NURSING DIAGNOSIS

(1) Decreased cardiac output related to tachycardia. (2) Altered tissue perfusion: cardiopulmonary/cerebral/peripheral, related to tachycardia and low cardiac output.

❖ ECG DIAGNOSIS

Junctional tachycardia.

Plan and Implementation

Patient goal. The patient will maintain hemodynamic stability and sufficient cardiac output until the arrhythmia is terminated and a normal rhythm ensues.

Nursing interventions.

- Nursing care of the patient in a tachycardia of any kind involves those interventions directed toward frequent, immediate, and accurate assessment and actions that improve cardiac output to prevent decreased tissue perfusion. An adult is usually able to tolerate this arrhythmia for longer periods than an infant. Infants often show signs of severe compromise and require immediate termination of the arrhythmia.
- If the patient is severely compromised, notify the physician at once. Be prepared for emergency cardioversion and/or artificial pacing (see Chapters 12 and 13).
- Ask the patient to perform the Valsalva maneuver if it is not contraindicated.
- Take measures to diminish myocardial oxygen demand and maximize cerebral perfusion.
  - Promote physical and emotional rest.
  - Restrict visitors to significant others.
  - Provide light food intake.
  - Administer tranquilizers/sedation as ordered.
  - Keep the head of bed in flat or low-Fowler's position if signs of CHF have not yet manifested.
- Start an IV infusion as ordered.
- Administer oxygen PRN.
- Record and document the arrhythmia at frequent intervals (as often as every 5 minutes in the unstable patient), as well as any changes in rhythm.
- Choose a lead that allows maximum visualization of P′ waves, if present.
- Provide appropriate patient teaching if pacing or electrical cardioversion is to be used.
- Monitor heart rate and blood pressure during intravenous administration of antiarrhythmic agents such as propranolol.
- If the patient is receiving antiarrhythmic drugs, evaluate effectiveness and assess for specific signs of toxicity (see Chapter 11).
- Carry out medical orders as directed and evaluate the patient's response.

Evaluation

- The patient maintains adequate cardiac output and remains hemodynamically stable as evidenced by the following:
  - Stable blood pressure in normal range for patient.
  - Warm, dry skin without pallor or cyanosis.
  - Full orientation.
- The patient maintains sufficient coronary perfusion as evidenced by the following:
  - Absence of angina.
  - Absence of ST-segment T-wave changes on the ECG.
- The patient shows no signs of congestive heart failure as evidenced by the following:
  - Clear lung fields on auscultation.
  - No external jugular venous distension.
  - Normal respirations without cough or complaints of shortness of breath.
  - Normal heart sounds.
- The method of terminating the patient's arrhythmia is effective as evidenced by the following:
  - Return to normal sinus rhythm.
  - No further episodes of JT.

Medical Treatment

- Vagotonic measures such as carotid sinus compression and the Valsalva maneuver[5] may terminate the arrhythmia.
- Remove secondary causes of increased sympathetic tone.[13]
- Artificial pacing and/or electrical cardioversion is often instituted in children[13] (see Chapters 12 and 13). Other successful methods of treatment in children include catheter ablation or surgical His-bundle ablation.[10]
- Medications sometimes used in the treatment of JT include digitalis[4] if the patient is not digitalis toxic, intravenous propranolol,[13,14] or esmolol, a short-acting beta blocker.

JUNCTIONAL ESCAPE BEATS AND IDIOJUNCTIONAL RHYTHM

Data Base: Problem Identification

Definitions, Etiology, and Mechanisms

Escape beats are protective in that they take over when the primary pacemaker, the SA node, slows or fails.[1] As a fairly dependable secondary pacemaker, junctional escape beats are not unusual and are considered a normal finding, especially in children and young adults, more often in males than females. The overall incidence for all age groups is roughly 9%,[16] but up to 45% of young healthy children[17,18] and about 22% to 40% of young adult males[19,20] exhibit junctional escape beats during their slowest heart rates.[17] The incidence for young women appears to be much less,[21] and in the elderly it is rare.[22]

Junctional escape beats do not always occur as a normal phenomenon, however. Sometimes their presence is attributable to excessive digitalis that enhances automaticity in the junctional tissue while indirectly decreasing sinus rate.[1] Other causes include quinidine, toxic reactions to beta- or calcium-channel blockers, rheumatic fever, other acute infectious myocarditides, coronary artery disease,[1] acute myocardial infarction, hypoxemia, and hyperkalemia.[23] Junctional escape rhythms may appear in virtually any setting that causes sinus node function to diminish. Thus they are not uncommon during the early postoperative period after orthotopic heart transplantation when SA node dysfunction, antiarrhythmic drugs, or surgical trauma, alone or in combination, occur.[24]

ECG Characteristics

Junctional escape beats occur by default (i.e., they end a cycle longer than the previous R-R intervals). When two or more occur in succession at the junction's own inherent rate of diastolic depolarization, 40 to 70 per minute, the rhythm is known as *idiojunctional rhythm* (IJR). The prefix *idio* is used when there is no retrograde atrial depolarization; the junctional pacemaker is controlling only the ventricles. If retrograde atrial depolarization accompanies the junctional rhythm, the prefix is dropped (Figs. 7-13 to 7-15).[6] When the junctional rhythm occurs at a rate less than 40 bpm, it is termed *junctional bradycardia*.

AV dissociation. When the sinus rate slows sufficiently to allow an IJR to ensue, often the two rates are very much alike. A junctional rhythm takes over control of the ventricles whereas the sinus rhythm still controls the atria. This results in what is known as *AV dissociation* (the atria and ventricles beat independently). When the rates of these two rhythms are the same, or nearly so, the dissociation is labeled *synchronized* or *isorhythmic AV dissociation*. The IJR is regular. Fig. 7-16 illustrates such an instance. As the sinus rate slows, the junction takes control of the ventricular rhythm. In the top strip, it looks as though the P waves are moving closer and closer to the QRS. What has happened is the sinus rate has slowed and the junction is depolarizing independently at a slightly faster rate. The junctional rhythm therefore assumes and maintains control until the fourth complex in the second

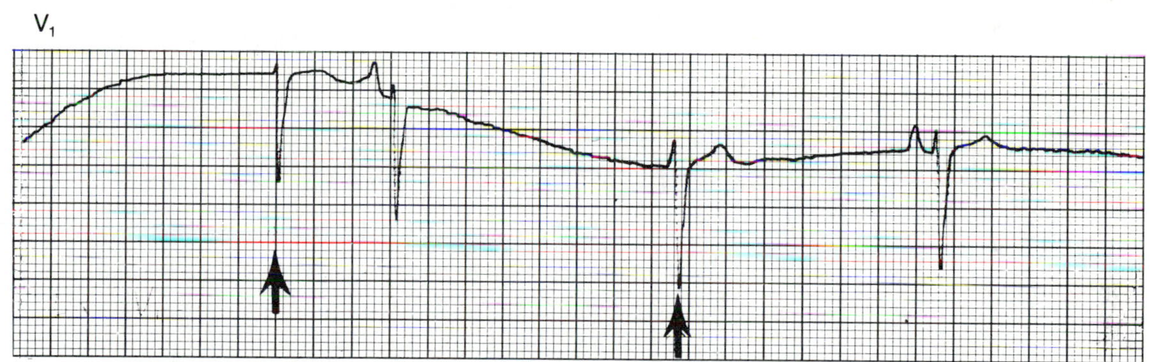

FIGURE 7-13 Junctional escape beats. Sinus slowing leads to two junctional escape beats (first and third QRS complexes). This slow rhythm is the bradycardia counterpart of a patient with brady-tachy syndrome.

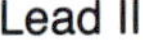

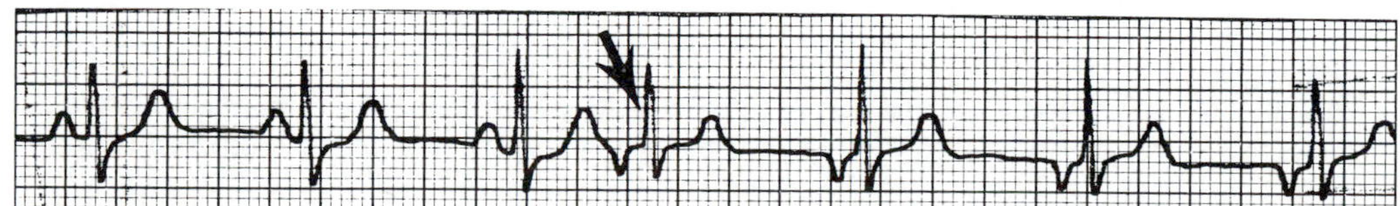

FIGURE 7-14 JPB initiating a run of junctional rhythm *(arrow)*.

Rate: NSR 71 bpm, junctional rhythm 68 bpm
Rhythm: Irregular
P waves: One precedes each QRS. P′ waves are inverted in lead II indicating retrograde atrial depolarization.
PR interval: 0.15 seconds, P′R interval 0.10 seconds
QRS complex: 0.08 to 0.10 seconds
Interpretation: NSR interrupted by a usurping junctional rhythm with retrograde atrial depolarization

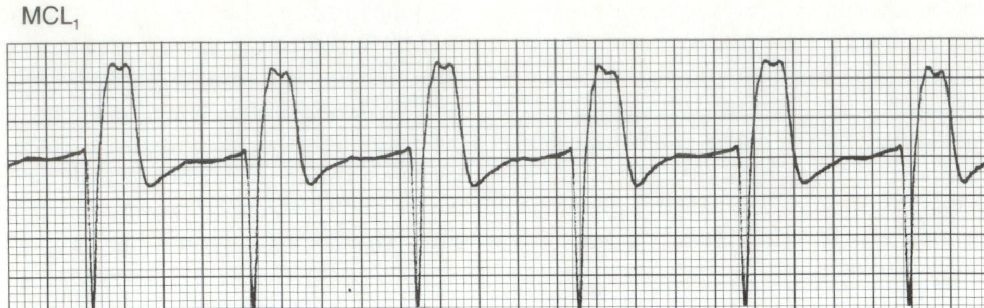

FIGURE 7-15 Idiojunctional rhythm. This rhythm strip is from a patient with chronic renal disease and hyperkalemia.

Rate: 70 bpm
Rhythm: Regular
P waves: None visible
PR interval: None
QRS complex: Approximately 0.10 seconds; elevated ST segments
Interpretation: IJR

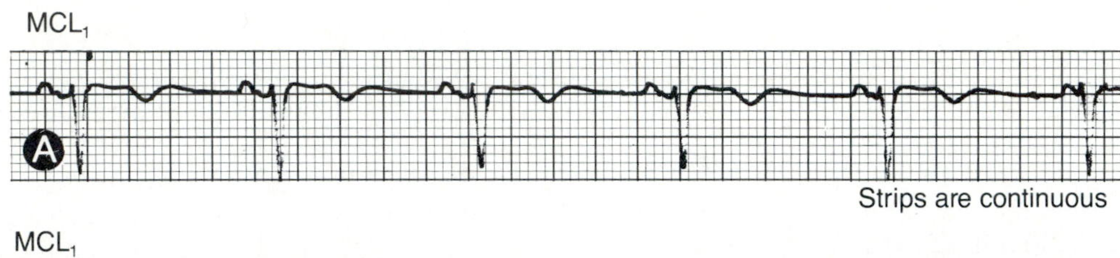

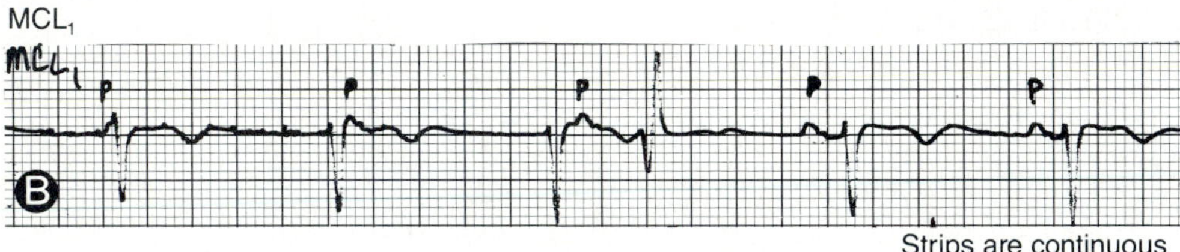

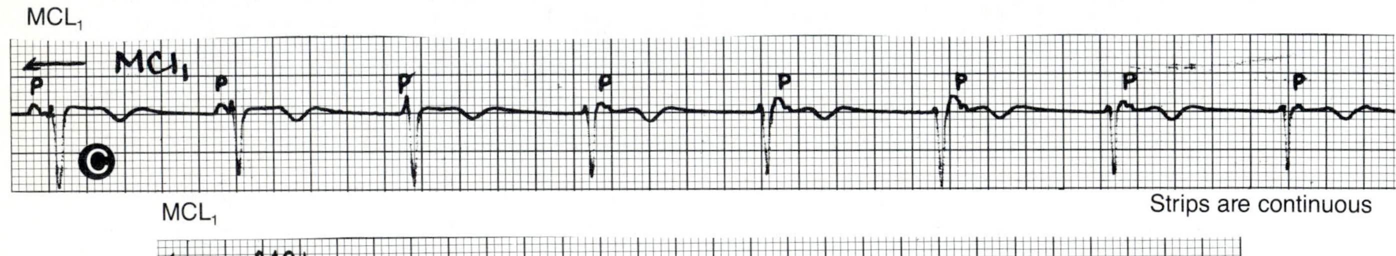

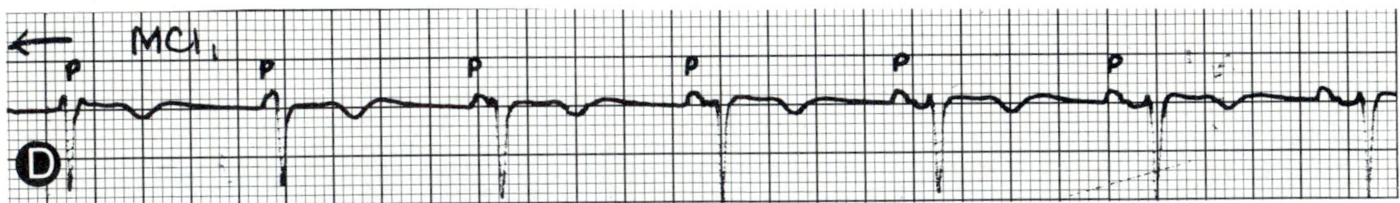

FIGURE 7-16 Isorhythmic AV dissociation as a result of IJR. **A,** At the end of the strip the sinus rate slows to 61 bpm, allowing an idiojunctional rhythm to emerge. Notice how the P waves seem to migrate closer to the QRS complexes. This is because the atria and ventricles are beating independently of one another (AV dissociation). **B,** IJR with AV dissociation continues until the fourth QRS complex, a sinus capture with RBBB aberration. **C,** The next beat is sinus rhythm, which is then usurped by the slightly faster IJR. NSR again emerges at the end of strip **D.**

Rate: 63 bpm slowing to 61 bpm
Rhythm: Predominantly regular
P waves: P wave does not bear a constant relationship to QRS. Atrial rhythm is regular and is independent of the ventricular rhythm.
PR interval: 0.17 seconds for sinus-conducted beat (next to last complex in second strip), 0.26 seconds for sinus capture (third to last complex in second strip)
Interpretation: NSR with sinus slowing resulting in IJR with isorhythmic AV dissociation

ECG Characteristics
Idiojunctional Rhythm

Rate: 40 to 70 bpm
Rhythm: Regular
P wave: May or may not be present
AV dissociation may occur
If retrograde atrial depolarization present, P waves occur before, during, or after QRS and are inverted on inferior leads.
PR interval: Same as JPB; none in AV dissociation
QRS complex: Normal unless IVCD

strip. This complex is early and conducted with a right bundle branch block (RBBB). It is early because it is a sinus-conducted complex; the sinus impulse was able to conduct because it found the AV junction and bundle branches nearly recovered from their previous depolarization—all except for the right bundle branch, which was still refractory (hence the RBBB). The PR interval is also prolonged. The fifth QRS is also sinus-conducted but then the P waves migrate toward the QRS complexes (note the last PR interval in the second strip is shorter than the previous one). The synchronized AV dissociation continues until it appears that the sinus is in control of the rhythm at the end of the last strip where the PR interval is again 0.16 seconds. Take your calipers and plot the P′ waves as they phase in and out of the QRS complexes. Refer to Fig. 7-11, *B* for an example of AV dissociation in the presence of JT.

Junctional rhythm with retrograde atrial depolarization. When the junctional pacemaker causes depolarization of the atria in retrograde fashion, P′ waves may appear before, during, or after the QRS complexes. Remember the P′ waves will be inverted (usually) in the inferior leads when retrograde atrial depolarization occurs.

See the box above for a summary of the ECG features.

Applied Nursing Process

Clinical Assessment

- Detect:
  - Possible slight irregularity and slight slowing of the patient's pulse and ECG.
  - P waves not bearing a constant relationship to QRS complexes or inverted (on inferior leads) P waves before or after QRS complexes.
- Assess the patient and ECG.
  - Assess the patient's tolerance of the arrhythmia by determining blood pressure, mentation, skin color and temperature.
  - Determine the cause of the arrhythmia. An escape rhythm is never a primary diagnosis but is secondary to another event.

    If, for example, a young, athletic male with a sleeping heart rate of 34 bpm develops IJR, it is likely a normal phenomenon secondary to sinus bradycardia.

    If an elderly individual displays IJR after a three-second period of asystole, it is necessary to determine the nature of the asystolic pause. Was it due to sinus arrest? AV block? This patient will require immediate attention.
  - Diagnose the arrhythmia; differentiate from JPBs and APBs.

❖ NURSING DIAGNOSIS

Decreased cardiac output related to bradycardia, if present, and loss of atrial contribution to cardiac output.

❖ ECG DIAGNOSIS

Junctional rhythm or idiojunctional rhythm. A note to the purist: when the junctional rhythm is not accompanied by retrograde atrial depolarization, the prefix *idio* is used. When retrograde atrial depolarization occurs, the rhythm is termed simply *junctional rhythm*.

Plan and Implementation

Patient goal. The patient will remain asymptomatic with sufficient cardiac output and will not develop complications from sinus slowing.

Nursing interventions.

- Evaluate the significance of the arrhythmia. Because it is secondary to sinus slowing, IJR is never a primary diagnosis. Rather, the significant rhythm is the underlying sinus bradycardia, with possible hemodynamic compromise related to the loss of atrial kick.
- Record and document the frequency and duration of escape episodes.
- If the patient is symptomatic, it may be necessary to administer atropine, according to hospital policy or physician orders.
- Lower the head of the bed if the patient feels lightheaded or has low blood pressure (providing the patient is not in congestive heart failure).
- Evaluate the patient's response to any measures taken to ameliorate the arrhythmia or to improve the patient's tolerance of the arrhythmia.
- Carry out medical treatment as ordered.

Evaluation

The patient remains hemodynamically stable as evidenced by the following:

- No change in blood pressure during escape episodes.
- Palpable peripheral pulses.
- Warm, dry extremities without pallor or cyanosis.

- Denial of light-headedness.
- Full orientation.

Medical Treatment

- If necessary, the primary rhythm disturbance is treated.
- Treatment may not be required (since the rhythm appears to be a normal phenomenon in the young).
- If hemodynamically compromised, atropine, isoproterenol, or external pacing may be necessary to increase the rate sufficiently until a transvenous pacemaker can be inserted.

ECG Characteristics
Accelerated Idiojunctional Rhythm

Rate: 70 to 100 bpm
Rhythm: Regular
P wave: Same as IJR
PR interval: Same as JPB; none in AV dissociation
QRS complex: Normal unless IVCD

ACCELERATED IDIOJUNCTIONAL RHYTHM

Data Base: Problem Identification

Definitions, Etiology, and Mechanisms

Since the inherent rate of diastolic depolarization of the AV junction is 40 to 70 bpm, a junctional rhythm faster than 70 bpm yet slower than tachycardia (100 bpm) is known as *accelerated idiojunctional rhythm* (AIJR).[25] Other labels for this rhythm not used in this text include *nonparoxysmal AV nodal tachycardia,*[4] *idionodal tachycardia,*[4] and *accelerated AV junctional escape rhythm.*[26]

AIJR is seen in patients with digitalis toxicity,[1,8] acute inferior myocardial infarction, acute carditis, and postoperatively after open heart surgery. It is a fairly common postoperative arrhythmia in children after Fontan repair.[27] Occasionally it is seen in apparently healthy individuals,[22] including children.[12] It is thought to be induced by delayed after-depolarizations[26] or enhanced automaticity.

Usually the rhythm causes trivial hemodynamic changes, but the atrial kick is lost and, if a patient has serious preexisting hemodynamic impairment, cardiac output may be significantly compromised.

ECG Characteristics

AIJR generally emerges when its rate just exceeds that of the sinus rate, and therefore will likely be *end-diastolic,*[4] occurring just before the expected sinus-conducted impulse. Since the rates of the AIJR and sinus rhythm are similar, simultaneous discharge is a common development resulting in *AV dissociation*[4] (recall that AV dissociation exists when the atria and ventricles beat independently). When the sinus rate exceeds that of the AIJR, the latter will be abolished.[4] During periods of AV dissociation P waves and QRS complexes will be regular, but the P waves will not bear a constant relationship to the QRS complexes. Thus the PR intervals will not be consistent.

AV dissociation need not always be present in an accelerated junctional rhythm. The junction may also pace the atria producing retrograde atrial depolarization, resulting (most often) in negative P waves in the inferior leads (II, III, and aVF) that precede or follow the QRS complex. When they precede the QRS complex the P′R interval is often short (0.10 seconds or less); when the P′ wave follows the QRS complex the RP′ interval is often 0.20 seconds or less. Retrograde atrial depolarization may also occur simultaneously with ventricular depolarization, resulting in a P′ wave hidden within the QRS complex. When the junction controls the entire heart, including the atria, drop the *idio* prefix and call the arrhythmia *accelerated junctional rhythm.*

The QRS complex will appear normal unless an intraventricular conduction defect is present (Fig. 7-17). Refer to the box above for a summary of the electrocardiographic characteristics of AIJR.

Applied Nursing Process

Clinical Assessment

- Detect:
  - A regular ECG with possibly a weaker peripheral pulse.
  - A change in the PR interval, AV dissociation, disappearance of P waves, or inverted P′ waves in inferior leads.
- Assess the patient and ECG.
  - Since the atrial kick is often lost, assess the patient for symptoms of diminished cardiac output associated with the AIJR; the patient will likely be asymptomatic. Check the blood pressure, peripheral pulses, skin color, and mentation.
  - Assess the clinical situation in which the arrhythmia occurs. For example, does it occur during sleep? Does waking the patient alleviate the arrhythmia?
  - Obtain the serum digoxin level, if indicated.

❖ NURSING DIAGNOSIS

Decreased cardiac output related to loss of atrial contribution to cardiac output.

❖ ECG DIAGNOSIS

Accelerated idiojunctional rhythm.

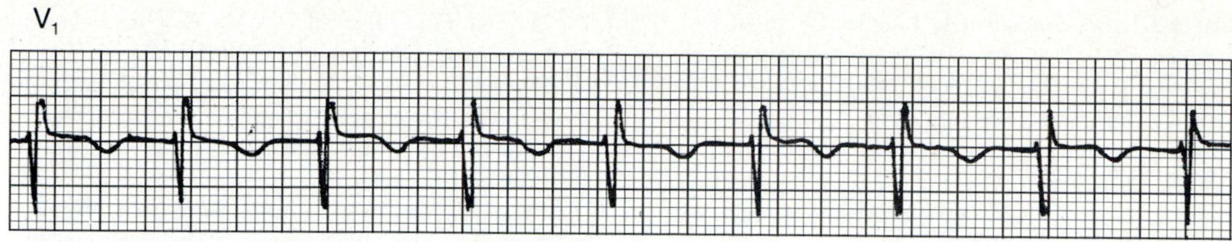

FIGURE 7-17 Accelerated idiojunctional rhythm.

Rate: 91 bpm
Rhythm: Regular
P waves: None visible
PR interval: None
QRS complex: 0.10 seconds. Note terminal R′ wave. In V_1, this may be indicative of RBBB. Inverted T waves.

Plan and Implementation

Patient goal. The patient will maintain adequate cardiac output during the arrhythmia and will maintain a serum digoxin level in therapeutic range.

Nursing interventions.

- Evaluate the significance of the arrhythmia. If AIJR is a result of acute inferior MI or postoperative open heart surgery, it is usually self-limiting and requires no treatment.
- If digitalis toxicity is present, assess the serum digoxin level and hold the digitalis as ordered by the physician.
- Document the arrhythmia. There is no need to notify the physician immediately if the patient is asymptomatic and AIJR is an expected part of the clinical picture. Nonetheless, the physician is notified at the earliest convenience.
- Evaluate the patient's response to measures taken, if any, to treat the arrhythmia.
- Evaluate progression of the arrhythmia and continue to evaluate the patient's response to it.

Evaluation

The patient remains hemodynamically stable as evidenced by the following:

- Strong peripheral pulses.
- No change in blood pressure.
- No complaints of light-headedness or dizziness.
- A serum digoxin level within therapeutic range.

Medical Treatment

Treatment is directed at the underlying cause. The arrhythmia usually requires no treatment unless it is a result of digitalis toxicity, in which case withdrawal of digitalis is indicated.

REFERENCES

1. Goldman MJ. *Principles of Clinical Electrocardiography*. 12th ed. Los Altos, CA: Lange Medical Publications, 1986.
2. Fowler NO. *Cardiac Diagnosis and Treatment*. 3rd ed. Philadelphia: Harper and Row, 1980.
3. Kernicki JG, Weiler KM. *Electrocardiography For Nurses: Physiological Correlates*. New York: John Wiley & Sons, 1981.
4. Schamroth L. *The Disorders of Cardiac Rhythm*. Vol. I. London: Blackwell Scientific Publications, 1981.
5. Marriott HJL, Bradley SM. Main-stem extrasystoles. *Circ.*, 1957, 16: 544.
6. Marriott HJL. *Practical Electrocardiography*. 8th ed. Baltimore: Williams & Wilkins, 1988.
7. Bleifer SB, Bleifer DJ, Hansmann DR, Sheppard JJ, Karpman HL. Diagnosis of occult arrhythmias by Holter electrocardiography. *Prog. Cardiovasc. Dis.*, May-Jun., 1974, 16(6): 569-99.
8. Marriott HJL, Conover M. *Advanced Concepts in Arrhythmias*. 2nd ed. St. Louis: The C.V. Mosby Co., 1989.
9. Garson A, Gillette PC. Junctional ectopic tachycardia in children: electrocardiography, electrophysiologic and pharmacologic response. *Am. J. Cardiol.*, Aug., 1979, 44(2): 298-302.
10. Gillette PC. Supraventricular arrhythmias in children. *J. Am. Coll. Cardiol.*, Jun., 1985, 5(6): 122B-129B.
11. Garson A, Gillette PC, McNamara DG. Supraventricular tachycardia in children: clinical features, response to treatment and long term follow-up in 217 patients. *J. Ped.*, 1981, 98: 875-82.
12. Roberts N, Moss J, Edelman E, Hartman K. Cardiac arrhythmias in children. Part I. Tachyarrhythmias. *J. Cardiovasc. Pulm. Tech.*, Aug.-Sept., 1980, 8(5): 53-60.
13. Garson A. The six most common acute cardiac dysrhythmias in children. Part II. *Appl. Cardiol.*, Jun.-Jul., 1984, 12(4): 13-23.
14. Grant JW, Serwer GA, Armstrong BE, Oldhom HN, Anderson P. Junctional tachycardia in infants and children after open heart surgery for congenital heart disease. *Am. J. Cardiol.*, May, 1987, 59(12): 1216-18.
15. Bär FW, Brugada P, Dassen WRM, Wellens HJJ. Differential diagnosis of tachycardia with narrow QRS complex (shorter than 0.12 sec.). *Am. J. Cardiol.*, 1984, 54(6): 555-60.
16. Clarke JM, Shelton JR, Hamer J, Taylor S, Venning GR. The rhythm of the normal heart. *Lancet*, Sept. 4, 1976, pp. 508-12.
17. Southall DP, Johnston F, Shinebourne EN, Johnston PGB. 24-hour electrocardiographic study of heart rate and rhythm patterns in population of healthy children. *Br. Heart J.*, 1981, 45: 281-91.
18. Scott O, Williams GJ, Fiddler GI. Results of 24-hour ambulatory monitoring in 130 healthy boys aged 10-13 years. *Br. Heart J.*, 1980, 44: 304-8.
19. Brodsky M, Wu D, Denis P, Kanakis C, Rosen KM. Arrhythmias documented by 24-hour continuous electrocardiographic monitoring in 50 male medical students without apparent heart disease. *Am. J. Cardiol.*, Mar., 1977, 39: 390-5.
20. Talan DA, Bauernfeind RA, Ashley WW, Kanakis C, Rosen KM. Twenty-four hour continuous ECG recordings in long distance runners. *Chest*, Jul., 1982, 82(1): 19-24.

21. Sobotka PA, Mayer JH, Bauernfeind RA, Kanakis C, Rosen KM. Arrhythmias documented by 24-hour continuous ambulatory electrocardiographic monitoring in young women without apparent heart disease. *Am. Heart J.*, Jun., 1981, 101(6): 753-9.
22. Fleg JL, Kennedy HL. Cardiac arrhythmias in a healthy elderly population. *Chest,* Mar., 1982, 81(3): 302-7.
23. Goldberger AL, Goldberger E. *Clinical Electrocardiography*. 4th ed. St Louis: The CV Mosby Co., 1990.
24. Jacquet L, Ziady G, Stein K, Griffith B, Armitage J, Hardesty R, Kormas R. Cardiac rhythm disturbances early after orthotopic heart transplantation: prevalence and clinical importance of the observed abnormalities. *J. Am. Coll. Cardiol.*, Oct., 1990, 16(4): 832-7.
25. Marriott HJL, Menendez MM. A-V dissociation revisited. *Prog. Cardiovasc. Dis.*, May, 1966, 8(6): 522-38.
26. Rosen MR, Fisch C, Hoffman BF, Danilo P, Lovelace DE, Knoebel SB. Can accelerated atrioventricular junctional escape rhythms be explained by delayed after-depolarizations? *Am. J. Cardiol.*, Jun., 1980, 45: 1272-84.
27. Kurer CC, Tanner CS, Norwood WI, Vetter VL. Perioperative arrhythmias after Fontan repair. *Circ.*, Nov., 1990, 82(5 Suppl.):IV 190-4.

SELF-ASSESSMENT

MULTIPLE CHOICE

Directions

For each of the questions below, select the correct answer(s) from the choices given. If more than one answer is correct, mark all that are correct.

Example

Examples of junctional arrhythmias include
 a. atrial fibrillation.
*b. junctional tachycardia.
*c. accelerated idiojunctional rhythm.
 d. ventricular tachycardia.

1. JPBs resemble APBs in the following respects:
   a. They are always preceded by a premature P′ wave.
   b. They are premature.
   c. Both their QRS complexes resemble those the sinus conducts.
   d. They are as common as APBs.

2. When a JPB is accompanied by a premature P′ wave, the P′ wave
   a. is negative on the inferior leads.
   b. is positive on the inferior leads.
   c. precedes or follows the QRS, or is not apparent.
   d. precedes the QRS complex.

3. Which of the following offers the best explanation for an echo beat?
   a. When a JPB does not produce retrograde atrial depolarization the sinus impulse is not disturbed, resulting in a sinus-conducted beat right after the JPB.
   b. JPBs usually occur in couplets. The second of the couplet is termed *echo beat* because it looks exactly like the first.
   c. When a JPB produces retrograde atrial depolarization the inverted P′ wave is known as the *echo beat* because it often occurs right after the JPB.
   d. When a P′ wave follows a JPB by a long enough interval, it may find the AV junction no longer refractory, enabling conduction to the ventricles with resultant ventricular depolarization.

4. Of the patients below, which one is in need of immediate attention?
   a. A 62-year-old female patient admitted with congestive heart failure is having occasional short runs of AIJR. Her digoxin level is in the toxic range. Vital signs are within normal limits and she is mildly dyspneic.
   b. A 14-year-old boy hospitalized after knee surgery has AV dissociation resulting from idiojunctional rhythm when he sleeps.
   c. A 2-day-old infant just went into junctional tachycardia at a rate of 240 bpm.
   d. A 42-year-old male patient, who has had an inferior MI, has a junctional escape rhythm at a rate of 58 bpm during slow phases of his sinus arrhythmia.

MATCHING

Directions

Match each arrhythmia in column A with its correct classification in column B.

Example

A	B
(B) 1. AT	A. Ventricular arrhythmia
(C) 2. JT	B. Atrial arrhythmia
(A) 3. VT	C. Junctional arrhythmia

A	B
( ) 5. Junctional tachycardia	A. Active or usurping
( ) 6. Junctional escape rhythm	B. Passive
( ) 7. Idiojunctional rhythm	
( ) 8. Junctional premature beat	

TRUE/FALSE

Directions

Determine whether each of the following statements is true or false and indicate with a *T* or *F*.

Example

(F) 1. AIJR is a lethal arrhythmia.

( ) 9. JPBs produce a QRS complex that typically is distinctly different from the sinus-conducted QRS complexes.

( ) 10. When a JPB is followed by a P′ wave that is inverted in the inferior leads, it is said to have produced retrograde atrial depolarization.

( ) 11. JPBs often display slight aberration.

( ) 12. A medication that may be related to the development of AIJR is digoxin.

( ) 13. A clinical setting in which AIJR occurs is acute inferior wall MI.

( ) 14. *Junctional automatic tachycardia* and *paroxysmal AV nodal reentrant tachycardia* are synonymous terms.

( ) 15. Prudent nursing intervention for the patient with a junctional escape rhythm includes immediate administration of intravenous lidocaine.

( ) 16. Isorhythmic AV dissociation occurs when the atria and ventricles are beating independently at approximately the same rates.

( ) 17. For the patient in IJR, atropine may be indicated if symptoms of low perfusion are present.

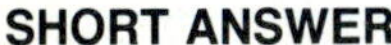

SHORT ANSWER

The following questions require short answers.

18. An 85-year-old male patient was admitted to your medical telemetry floor with a medical diagnosis of chronic obstructive pulmonary disease and bronchitis. After completing the admission assessment the attending nurse entered the following two nursing diagnoses on his care plan: impaired gas exchange and alteration in peripheral tissue perfusion. For the first 2 hours after admission, his heart rhythm was NSR with a rate of 84 to 88 bpm. Hearing the alarm sound at the central station, the nurse noted his patient was in IJR with a rate of 42 bpm on the monitor. What nursing measures are indicated in order of priority? Plan your interventions based on assessment findings.

***CASE:** At 0744 hours a 68-year-old male patient was admitted to the medical intensive care unit (MICU) after an "arrest" on the medical floor. The patient had been found apneic with a bradycardic rhythm and a rate of 20 to 30 bpm on the ECG. CPR was begun and the patient was given a stat dose of 5 ml epinephrine (1:10000 solution) IV. Within 2 minutes, he showed what appeared to be runs of ventricular tachycardia and sinus tachycardia at a rate of 150 bpm. In accordance with standard procedure a lidocaine infusion was begun after a lidocaine bolus of 50 mg was administered IV and the patient was transferred to the MICU. On arrival the patient was still intubated but was breathing on his own. The lidocaine drip was infusing at 2 mg/min. His MICU admission strip is presented here for your interpretation.*

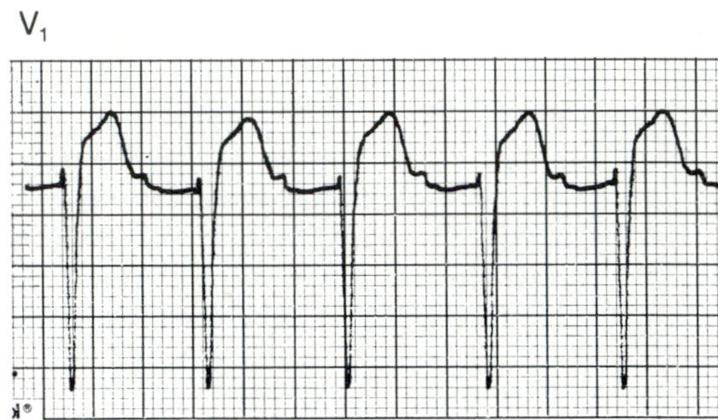

19. Analyze and interpret the rhythm below.
    At 0815 the physician ordered the patient be extubated. The family had requested that no resuscitative measures be taken because the patient was suffering from terminal metastatic cancer. The nurse extubated the patient. One-half hour after extubation the patient exhibited the rhythm below. On immediate examination, he was found to be apneic.
20. Analyze and interpret the arrhythmia and discuss probable contributing factors.

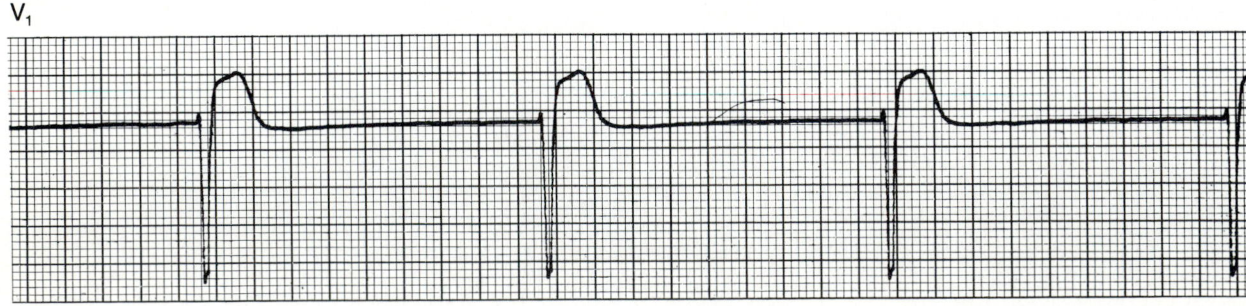

21. Assess this patient's arrhythmia.

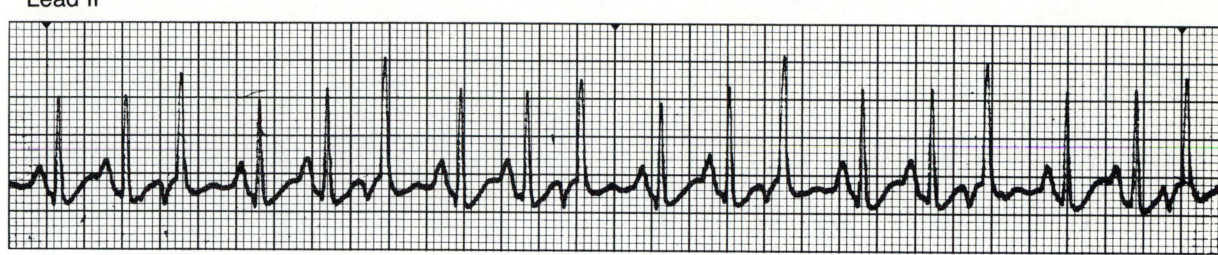

22. The patient with the arrhythmia below was admitted to the ICU after his acute inferior myocardial infarction. Analyze and interpret the arrhythmia. Would you expect such an arrhythmia with an inferior MI? Discuss the role of the coronary arteries in this patient's arrhythmia and MI. You may want to review the section on MI and coronary arteries in Chapter 1. Delineate nursing assessment and intervention measures.

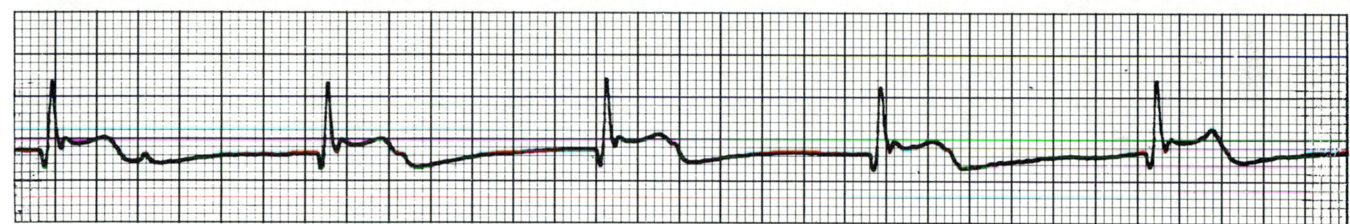

23. Analyze and interpret the arrhythmia below. Explain what is happening. List assessment measures and interventions in order of priority.

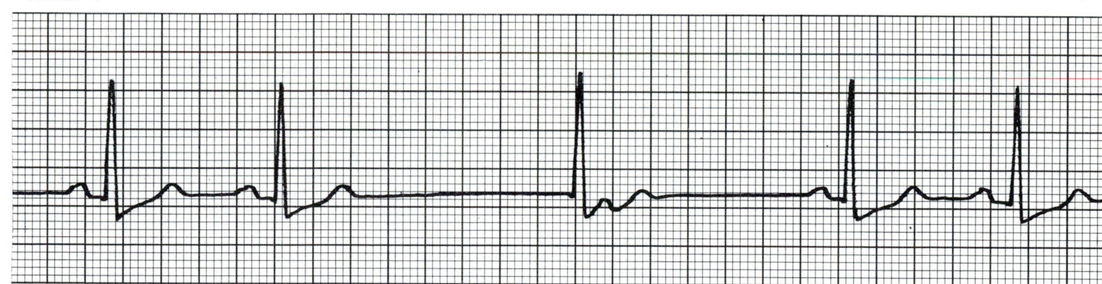

24. Analyze and interpret this arrhythmia.

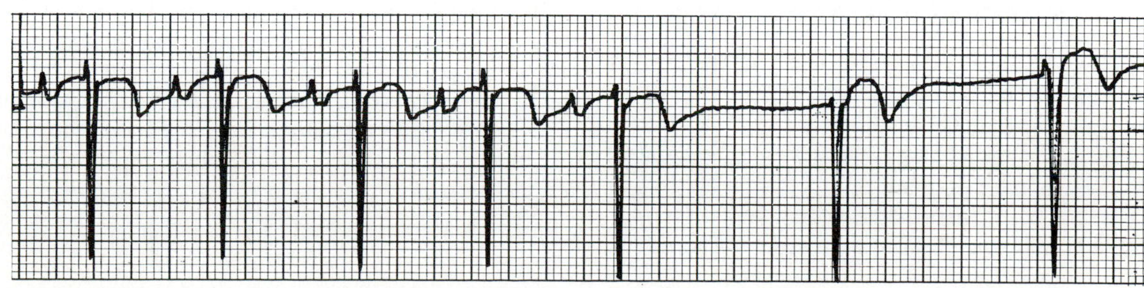

25. Analyze and interpret this arrhythmia.

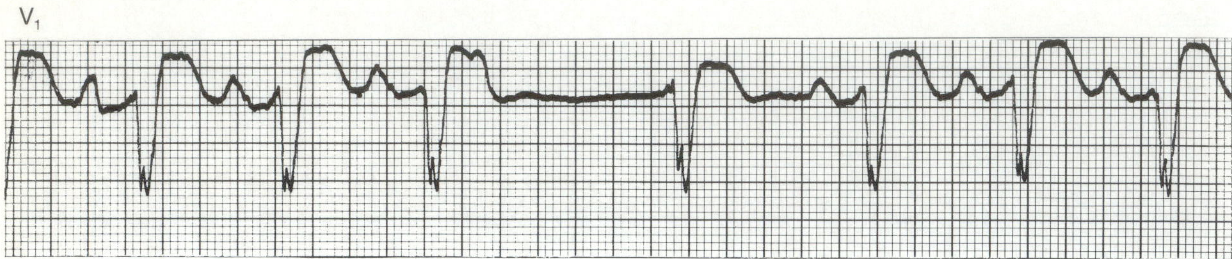

ANSWERS TO SELF-ASSESSMENT

1. b, c	5. A	9. F	14. F
2. a, c	6. B	10. T	15. F
3. d	7. B	11. T	16. T
4. c	8. A	12. T	17. T
		13. T	

18. Initial actions by the nurse would include immediately assessing the patient's response to this significant change in rhythm.
    Assess the following:
    1. Level of consciousness.
    2. Respiratory status.
    3. Blood pressure.
    4. Skin color.

The patient is found to be apneic, unconscious, with faint palpable pulses and a blood pressure of 66/30 mm Hg. His color was pale with cyanosis of the lips and nail beds. Immediate nursing interventions include the following:
1. Establish patent airway and initiate artificial respirations.
2. Call for help.
3. If ventilation does not improve the cardiac rhythm, atropine may be indicated. Usually, however, in situations of this nature, ventilatory assistance will result in resumption of NSR.
4. Notify the physician.
5. Stabilize the patient.
6. Alter plan of care to modify observation and assessment measures to prevent similar events.

19. *Rate:* 107 bpm
    Rhythm: Regular
    P wave: Normal, one precedes each QRS
    PR interval: 0.26 seconds, prolonged
    QRS complex: 0.09 seconds, normal rS configuration on V_1, elevated ST segment
    Interpretation: Sinus tachycardia with prolonged PR interval (first degree AV block, discussed in Chapter 9)

20. *Rate:* 33 bpm
    Rhythm: Regular
    P wave: Absent
    PR interval: None
    QRS complex: 0.09 seconds, normal rS complex on V_1, QRS looks just like those of sinus conduction
    Interpretation: Junctional escape rhythm at a rate of 33 bpm with apparent atrial asystole
    Discussion: The patient was not able to support his own airway, had a respiratory arrest and the resultant ECG manifestation. When a patent airway was established and ventilations provided with positive pressure/100% oxygen, his heart rate and rhythm returned to normal.
    Did you remember the lidocaine infusion that was left infusing? That is the likely reason this patient did not have any ventricular escape beats; the lidocaine suppressed ectopic ventricular activity.
    This situation actually occurred. It is presented here for purposes of discussion and to illustrate iatrogenic factors that may hasten death.

21. *Rate:* 170 bpm
    Rhythm: Irregular
    P wave: Some normal and upright, early ones are inverted on lead II and occur in a trigeminal pattern
    PR interval: 0.12 seconds with normal P waves; 0.08 to 0.09 seconds with inverted P waves
    QRS complex: 0.08 seconds; QRS complexes that are early show slight aberration: they are slightly taller, do not have the small initial q wave, and have smaller T waves
    Interpretation: Sinus tachycardia with trigeminal JPBs exhibiting retrograde atrial depolarization

22. *Rate:* 46 bpm
Rhythm: Regular
P wave: Present at a rate of 45 bpm (can you see them?) and regular; they do not bear a constant relationship to the QRS complex
PR interval: Not applicable since P waves are regular, QRS complexes are regular, and P waves do not bear a constant relationship to QRS complexes
QRS complex: 0.10 seconds, qR complex, elevated ST segment; QT interval 0.44 seconds
Interpretation: Idiojunctional rhythm, isorhythmic AV dissociation with atrial and junctional rates of 45 and 46 bpm respectively
Discussion: Since this patient has had an acute inferior MI, the coronary artery most often involved is the posterior descending branch, supplied in most patients by the right coronary artery. The right coronary artery also supplies the SA and AV nodes in most patients. Sinus bradycardia and AV blocks are very common with patients who have had inferior MIs. Marked sinus arrhythmia is also frequently exhibited by these patients.
Assessment: Immediately assess how well the patient is tolerating the arrhythmia by evaluating the sensorium, taking the blood pressure, inspecting the skin color, noting the skin temperature, and palpating peripheral pulses. If the patient is asymptomatic, no treatment is indicated. If the patient is hypotensive and showing other signs of low perfusion, atropine 0.5 mg may be indicated.

23. *Rate:* 50 bpm (based on 6-second estimation), 68 bpm for the sinus rhythm
Rhythm: Irregular
P wave: Normal in first two and last two complexes, but after the first two, there is a sinus pause (see the P wave in the ST segment of the third QRS complex?); a P wave does not precede the third QRS but does precede others and bears a constant relationship to the other QRS complexes
PR interval: 0.17 seconds on all but third complex
QRS complex: 0.08 seconds, depressed J point; QT interval 0.44 seconds
Interpretation: NSR at rate 68 bpm, sinus pause followed by a junctional escape beat and resumption of the sinus rhythm (The P wave in the ST segment of the junctional escape beat is upright on lead II, therefore not retrogradely conducted. It is probably a sinus P wave.)
Discussion: The sinus pause resulted in a junctional escape beat, a normal protective response by the junction in response to a decrease in heart rate.
Assessment: Assess the patient's tolerance of the arrhythmia by evaluating the sensorium, taking the blood pressure, assessing the peripheral pulses, measuring the pulse rate for a full minute, counting the number of sinus pauses per minute, and determining if the overall heart rate is affected. Review the medications the patient is taking and any other factors that may contribute to the development of a sinus pause.
Intervention: If the patient is symptomatic (i.e., if the sinus pauses are occurring with such frequency that the heart rate is significantly reduced and the patient has symptoms of inadequate cardiac output) correct the cause, if possible, by holding any medications that may be contributing to the arrhythmia until the physician is consulted. If you cannot eliminate a possible cause, notification of the physician is necessary and IV atropine may be indicated.

24. *Rate:* 88 bpm with abrupt slowing to 53 bpm
Rhythm: Irregular because of abrupt slowing
P wave: 0.10 to 0.11 seconds in duration, normal diphasic configuration for lead V_1; after first five P waves, no more P waves are detected
PR interval: 0.24 seconds (prolonged) in those beats preceded by a P wave
QRS complex: 0.06 seconds, normal rS configuration for V_1; beats not preceded by P waves have same configuration as those that are sinus conducted
Interpretation: NSR at rate of 88 bpm, prolonged PR interval (first degree AV block), abrupt sinus slowing resulting from apparent sinus arrest in excess of 2 seconds, junctional escape beats during sinus arrest
Discussion: Note on the last QRS complex, the initial r wave is different from the others and closely resembles the initial portion of the P waves. This is likely the result of a P wave, occurring just slightly earlier than the junctional escape.

25. *Rate:* 79 bpm with abrupt slowing, resulting in 6-second estimation of 60 bpm
Rhythm: Irregular
P wave: 0.14 to 0.16 seconds (wide) and tall; one precedes each QRS, except the QRS that occurs after the pause, and bears a constant relationship to those it precedes
PR interval: 0.26 seconds, prolonged in those QRS complexes preceded by a P wave
QRS complex: 0.16 to 0.18 seconds, prolonged because of intraventricular conduction defect (IVCD); all QRS complexes are the same configuration
Interpretation: Sinus rhythm with intraatrial conduction defect, IVCD, and nonconducted APB followed by a junctional escape beat
Discussion: This rhythm is disturbed by a pause. Since the most common causes of pauses are nonconducted APBs, search for a P wave hidden in the T wave of the preceding QRS complex. Do you see it there?

CHAPTER EIGHT

Ventricular Rhythm Disturbances

▶ GOAL

You will be able to distinguish lethal (or potentially lethal) from benign ventricular arrhythmias and use the nursing process in caring for patients with ventricular rhythm disturbances.

▶ OBJECTIVES

After studying this chapter and completing the self-assessment exercises, you should be able to:

1. Define sudden cardiac death (SCD) and relate the arrhythmias most often responsible for it and the type of patient most likely to be at higher risk.
2. List ten causes of ventricular premature beats (VPBs), recall common associated findings, and correlate the incidence of ventricular ectopy with age.
3. Describe and explain electrocardiographic features of and patterns of occurrence of VPBs.
4. Identify R-on-T and end-diastolic VPBs and appraise and contrast their significance.
5. Assess the patient with ventricular arrhythmias and evaluate the clinical significance of ventricular ectopy, deciding in which situations it may be an ominous sign.
6. Analyze the so-called warning arrhythmias.
7. Demonstrate ability to differentiate ventricular ectopy from supraventricular complexes conducted with aberration.
8. Determine nursing interventions for patients with ventricular arrhythmias and decide when prophylactic antiarrhythmic therapy is indicated.
9. Evaluate the patient's response to antiarrhythmic medications.
10. List several patient conditions in which ventricular tachycardia (VT) may be present and situations that might provoke its development.
11. Recognize VT, differentiate between monomorphic (uniform) and polymorphic (multiform) VT, and describe its electrocardiographic features.
12. Recall three electrocardiographic criteria supporting the diagnosis of VT versus supraventricular tachycardia with aberration.
13. Contrast nursing intervention measures for the patient in VT who is conscious with those for the patient who is unconscious.
14. Determine when electrical intervention is appropriate as an emergency nursing intervention and relate its significance to digitalis toxicity.
15. Identify and explain the ECG features of ventricular fibrillation (VF) and recall clinical situations in which VF is most likely to occur.
16. Establish priorities in assessing and planning emergency care for the patient in VF.
17. Recognize accelerated idioventricular rhythm (AIVR), differentiate it from VT, and contrast nursing interventions.
18. Demonstrate ability to recognize ventricular fusion and list three situations in which it may appear.
19. Recognize idioventricular rhythm (IVR), assess the patient who has the arrhythmia, and determine nursing intervention measures, explaining why lidocaine is contraindicated.
20. Recognize ventricular asystole and formulate a plan of emergency care for the asystolic patient.
21. Explain primary electromechanical dissociation (EMD), demonstrate ability to set priorities in assessing victims, and initiate appropriate emergency nursing interventions.
22. Define parasystole and differentiate it from other forms of ventricular ectopy.
23. Classify the arrhythmias studied as active (usurping) or passive (escape).

The ventricular arrhythmias are the most important of the cardiac rhythm disturbances because the ventricles are responsible for pumping blood to the body. If faulty ventricular depolarization results in little or no ventricular pumping, the result may be lethal. Yet, as will be seen in this chapter, ventricular arrhythmias are ubiquitous and may be benign or malignant (lethal).

Many cardiac and noncardiac stressors can contribute to

the neighborhood Jerry Van Amerongen

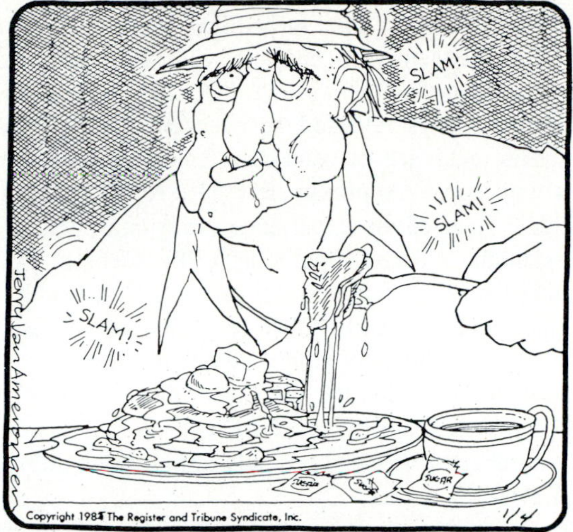

Half way through his "Hearty Man" breakfast, Dwayne thought he heard some of his smaller arteries slamming shut.

the development of ventricular rhythm disturbances. Noncardiac causes include disease, trauma, hypoxemia, excessive catecholamines, and stressors in healthy individuals. Among the cardiac etiologic factors are cardiovascular trauma and diseases of an organic and a structural nature.

SUDDEN CARDIAC DEATH

Some of the arrhythmias that will be discussed in this chapter are life-threatening and antecedent to sudden cardiac death (SCD) (death that occurs within 1 hour of symptom onset). Claiming 500,000 adult lives per year in this country, more than any other single entity, SCD accounts for about 50% of all deaths due to coronary heart disease (CHD).[1,2] For nearly half of these victims, death is the first symptom of CHD[3,4] and, although coronary atherosclerosis is present in most,[3,5-9] SCD is preceded by acute myocardial infarction in only 5% to 44% of cases.[3,5,10] SCD, most often the result of ventricular fibrillation,[11-13] may be secondary to myocardial ischemia.[14-17]

Ambulatory ECGs and cardiac electrophysiology studies suggest that the precipitating rhythm disturbance in the majority of SCD cases is one or more ventricular premature beats initiating a ventricular tachyarrhythmia that degenerates into ventricular fibrillation (VF).* Much less frequently, bradycardias have been documented before sudden death,† especially in the elderly.

Arrhythmias preceding adult cardiac arrests differ markedly from those of pediatric victims, in whom bradycardia is the most common antecedent arrhythmia. Some have documented that the most common progression of arrhythmias in pediatric cardiac arrests is from bradycardia to a ventricular arrhythmia.[25]

Pediatric patients at greatest risk of SCD are those with hypertrophic and dilated cardiomyopathies, congenital heart defects, acute myocarditis, aortic stenosis, mitral valve prolapse, previous surgery for congenital heart disease, complete heart block, Wolff-Parkinson-White (WPW) syndrome, long QT-interval syndrome, pulmonary

Heart Rate Variability

Many recent clinical studies have shown that the measurement of heart rate variability (HRV) is a valuable technique in clinical cardiology and that its import will increase in the future.

The physiologic framework of HRV has been attributed to the sympathovagal system, and the measurement of HRV reflects cardiac adaptation to changes in sympathovagal tone. Because the assessment of HRV is used as a measure of cardiac autonomic function and tone, it has emerged as an independent prognostic factor after acute myocardial infarction (MI).[28-32]

Methodology

There are a variety of recording techniques and methods for the measurement and numerical quantifications of HRV. This methodology falls primarily into two major categories: time indices and frequency domain indices.

Time indices can be expressed by the standard deviation of the RR interval[28,31,32] or by the mean of differences between consecutive RR intervals. These figures are calculated statistically from standard 24-hour ECG recordings. Many Holter system manufacturers have added the capability of assessing HRV to their systems.

The frequency domain indices determine the magnitude of individual components of the heart rate power spectrum and are expressed or quantified by power spectral variance analysis.[28,32] The spectral analysis of ECGs is performed on signal-averaged ECGs, which reveal cardiac late potentials and assess the synchrony and homogeneity of cardiac excitation.[29]

Prognostic significance

HRV is used to identify patients at high risk after acute MI. Recent clinical studies have demonstrated that reduced HRV carries an adverse prognosis in patients who have survived acute MI. Survivors of acute MI with low or reduced HRV have higher mortality than survivors with high HRV.[29,30]

HRV may be the single most important predictor of patients who are at high risk for SCD or malignant ventricular arrhythmias after myocardial infarction.[29,31] Recent research suggests that HRV, sympathovagal tone, and cardiac arrhythmias are linked.[29]

*6, 8, 9, 11, 18-24
†3, 8, 11, 12, 18, 19, 22

hypertension, and coronary artery abnormalities.[26,27]

Identification of people at risk for SCD may be accomplished by electrophysiology studies and determination of heart rate variability (see box on p. 191 for additional information on heart rate variability).

VENTRICULAR PREMATURE BEAT

Data Base: Problem Identification

Definitions, Etiology, and Mechanisms

Ventricular premature beats (VPBs) (also referred to as *premature ventricular complexes* [PVCs], *ventricular premature depolarizations* [VPDs], and *ventricular ectopic beats* [VEBs]) are the most common of the ectopic beats. (Review "The Premature Beat," Chapter 5.) Perhaps no other arrhythmia presents the prognostic dilemmas that VPBs do. On the one hand, they are a very common rhythm disorder; on the other hand, they are potentially lethal.

Their prognostic significance grew out of early experience in the acute care of myocardial infarction (MI) patients. In those early coronary care units, it was observed that ventricular fibrillation was often preceded by ventricular ectopy. Recent studies of SCD have supported this association. It has also been revealed that VPBs occur in most adults, healthy and diseased. Therefore the presence of VPBs is certainly not always a prodrome of disaster. Their prognostic importance is related to the clinical setting and the underlying type and severity of heart disease. For example, VPBs may be more ominous in acute MI than as an asymptomatic finding on a routine ambulatory electrocardiogram (ECG) in a stable patient.

VPBs are relatively rare in healthy children.[33,34] They occur more frequently in children with congenital heart disease[35] and Marfan's syndrome.[36] A study of healthy 10 to 13-year-old boys revealed an occasional VPB in only 26%.[37] The incidence of ventricular ectopy apparently increases with age.[38] Approximately 39% to 70% of young and middle-aged adults experience occasional VPBs,[38-43] whereas in the elderly population VPBs seem to be the rule rather than the exception. In studies[44,45] of healthy elderly individuals, nearly 80% experienced occasional VPBs, 49% exhibited complex ectopy (multifocal, couplets, and VT), and 12% displayed more than 30 per hour.[45] Thus the majority of adults with normal hearts has a small number of VPBs,[38] but only a minority exhibit frequent VPBs.

Coronary artery disease (CAD) is the most common cause of ventricular ectopy, and virtually all the other cardiac diseases may be associated with it to some degree. Although not an accurate predictor of disease, complex ventricular ectopy in many cases roughly parallels the severity of CAD[43] and the risk of sudden cardiac death.[3,46] The role of simple ventricular ectopy as a predictor of SCD is controversial.

There are many other causes and conditions correlated with the occurrence of VPBs. Mechanical stimulation from insertion of pacemaker wires and pulmonary artery catheters[47] and the situations presented in Table 8-1 are addi-

Table 8-1 Additional Etiologic Factors in Ventricular Ectopy[51-93]

Pharmacologic	Pathophysiologic	Physiologic
Adrenergic drugs	Acidosis	Before menstruation
Aerosols	Acute asthma	Emotional stress
Alcohol	After heart surgery	Exercise
Amphetamines	Afterload increase	Pregnancy
Caffeine*	Cardiomyopathies	
Carbon monoxide	Catecholamines	
Chloroform	Hypercalcemia	
Clofibrate	Hypocalcemia	
Cyclopropane	Hypokalemia	
Digitalis	Hypomagnesemia	
Dopamine	Hypoxia	
Isoproterenol	Impaired left ventricular function	
Lithium	Increased pulmonary wedge pressure	
Phenothiazines	Left ventricular hypertrophy	
Recombinant tissue plasminogen activator	Marfan's syndrome	
Solvents in typewriter correction fluid	Preload increase	
Theophylline	Reperfusion	
Thrombolytics		
Tobacco		
Tricyclic antidepressants		

*Equivocal.

tional etiologic factors associated with ventricular ectopy.

VPBs are thought to occur on the basis of two mechanisms, enhanced automaticity or reentry.[48,49] Immediately after coronary occlusion, they are likely due to reentry arising from the ischemic zone. This is also the most likely mechanism for SCD during this time.[49] Some studies have shown a tendency for VPBs to arise from the ventricle that is diseased.[50]

ECG Characteristics

A VPB occurs earlier in the cycle than the next expected QRS complex. Since its origin is within the ventricles, it is unable to traverse the rapid transit system of the ventricular conduction network, the bundle branches. Consequently, it makes its own path through the ventricles, causing ventricular depolarization sequentially rather than simultaneously, resulting in a QRS that is wider than normal. VPBs characteristically have a duration of 0.12 seconds or greater and their morphology is different from the other QRS complexes (see box on this page and Fig. 8-1). The shape and duration of the VPB depends on its source and the activation pathway it generates; it may resemble the sinus QRS if its origin is near the bifurcation of the His bundle or appear very bizarre and different when it originates lower in the ventricles[94] (Figs. 8-2 and 8-3).

Patterns of occurrence. Unlike APBs, VPBs usually exhibit full compensatory pauses. The reason for this is that the ectopic ventricular depolarization renders the AV junction refractory so that it cannot accept the next impulse arriving from the atria. This is known as a form of *concealed conduction* (Fig. 8-4). Sometimes, however, the VPB depolarizes the atria in retrograde fashion, resulting in a postectopic pause that is not compensatory (Fig. 8-5).

Features of Ventricular Premature Beats

- Premature QRS
- QRS different from sinus QRS
- 0.12 seconds or longer
- Not preceded by premature P′ wave
- Compensatory pause—usually

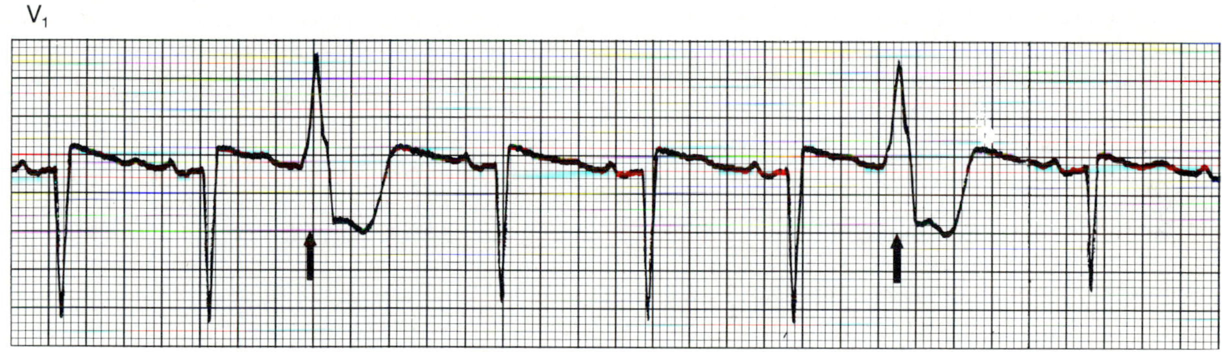

FIGURE 8-1 VPBs. Different from the other QRS complexes, VPBs are wider than normal *(arrows).*

Rate: 77 bpm
Rhythm: Irregular
P wave: Normal. One precedes each QRS complex except the VPB.
PR interval: 0.18 to 0.20 seconds
QRS complex: 0.07 seconds; VPB 0.18 seconds
Interpretation: NSR with two uniform VPBs

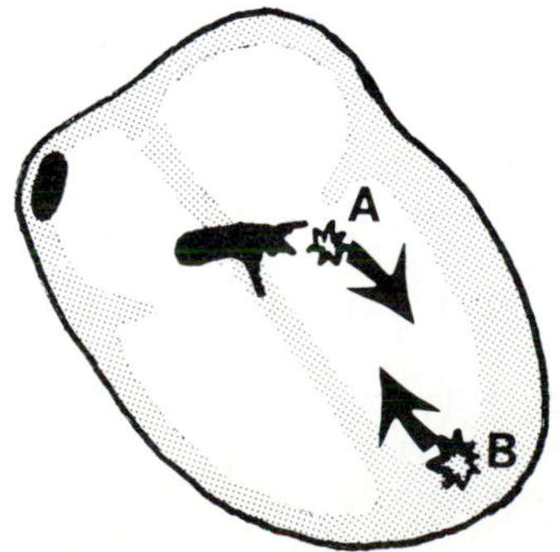

FIGURE 8-2 VPBs may be initiated anywhere in the ventricles. **A,** A VPB initiated high in the ventricles may closely resemble a sinus-conducted QRS complex because of close proximity to the bundle branch system (see Fig. 8-3). **B,** A VPB whose source is far from the intraventricular conduction system will appear much different from the sinus-conducted beats (see Fig. 8-1).

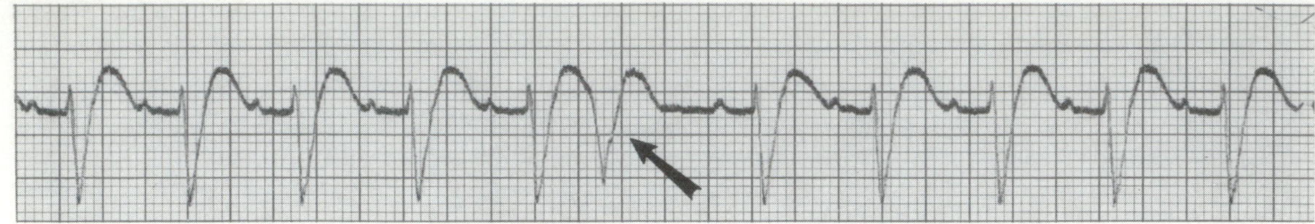

FIGURE 8-3 VPB closely resembles sinus-conducted QRS complexes *(arrow)*.

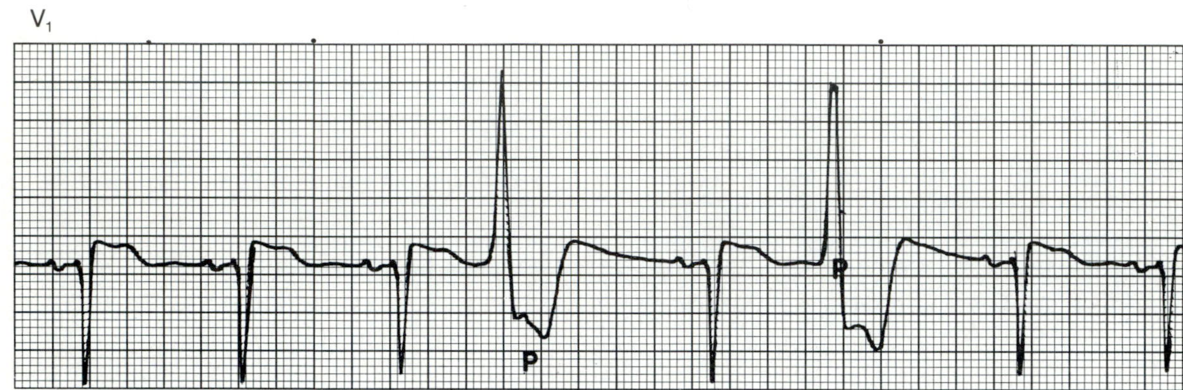

FIGURE 8-4 VPBs usually exhibit compensatory pauses. Undisturbed sinus rhythm prevails. The P waves obscured by the VPBs *(P)* do not produce QRS complexes, resulting in a compensatory pause after the VPB. Note after the first VPB, the sinus rate increases slightly. The second VPB completely obscures the P wave.

Rate: 73 to 79 bpm
Rhythm: Irregular
P wave: Normal
PR interval: 0.16 seconds
QRS complex: 0.10 to 0.11 seconds. VPBs 0.14 seconds. Sinus-conducted QRS complexes have elevated ST segments.
Interpretation: NSR with 2 VPBs

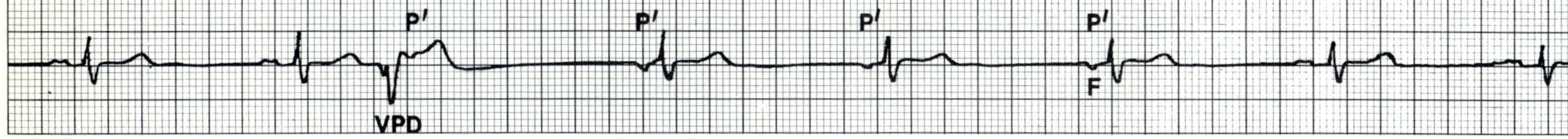

FIGURE 8-5 VPB producing a noncompensatory pause. VPB has resulted in retrograde atrial depolarization *(P′)* with subsequent atrial escape rhythm for three complexes before sinus rhythm resumes. Note fourth P′ wave is likely a fusion *(F)* of the sinus P wave and the P′ wave. It occurs "on schedule" for the escape rhythm and, if you measure the last two sinus P-P intervals, you will discover that it is the same as the P′-P interval.

Rate: 48 slowing to 45 bpm during atrial escape rhythm then increasing to 48 bpm with resumption of sinus rate
Rhythm: Irregular
P wave: Sinus P waves 0.10 to 0.12 seconds
PR interval: 0.19 to 0.20 seconds; 0.14 seconds during atrial escape rhythm
QRS complex: 0.10 seconds; VPB 0.13 seconds. Sinus-conducted QRS complexes exhibit a terminal s wave, abnormal for leads V_6 or MCL_6.
Interpretation: Sinus bradycardia with one VPB producing retrograde atrial depolarization resulting in an atrial escape rhythm lasting three complexes

The retrograde P′ and subsequent sinus P produce a P-P interval often longer than the P-P cycle of the basic rhythm.

Like APBs, VPBs may occur in bigeminal, trigeminal, or quadrigeminal patterns (Figs. 8-6 to 8-10); couplets or pairs (Figs. 8-11 and 8-12), and salvos (Fig. 8-13). A pattern of three VPBs in a salvo or triplet that is in rapid succession is a short run of ventricular tachycardia and may be uniform (monomorphic) or multiform (polymorphic) (Figs. 8-14 and 8-15). Interpolated VPBs are far more common than interpolated APBs and occur most commonly with slower sinus rates (Figs. 8-16 and 8-17). When a VPB is interpolated, the PR interval of the next sinus beat is usually longer, resulting in an R-R interval slightly longer than other R-R intervals. (It may be helpful at this point to review patterns of occurrence in Chapter 6.)

When a VPB occurs so early that it encroaches on the T wave of the preceding QRS complex, it is exhibiting the *R-on-T* phenomenon (Fig. 8-18). This is relatively uncom-

Text continues on p. 200.

V_1

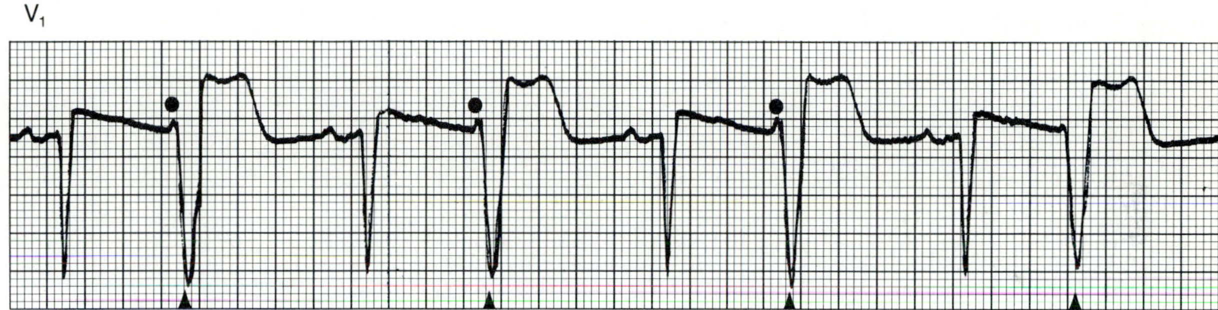

FIGURE 8-6 Ventricular bigeminy. Every second QRS complex is a VPB *(arrows).* Note what appears to be an initial r wave in some of the VPBs *(dots).* These are the beginnings of the regular occurring sinus P waves that are not disturbed by the VPBs.

Rate: 74 to 80 bpm
Rhythm: Irregular
P wave: Normal appearing (would need to confirm this on a 12-lead ECG. Is this a diphasic (+ −) P wave or just positive? It is difficult to ascertain from this tracing alone.)
PR interval: 0.20 seconds
QRS complex: 0.08 seconds; VPB 0.16 seconds
Interpretation: Ventricular bigeminy

V_1

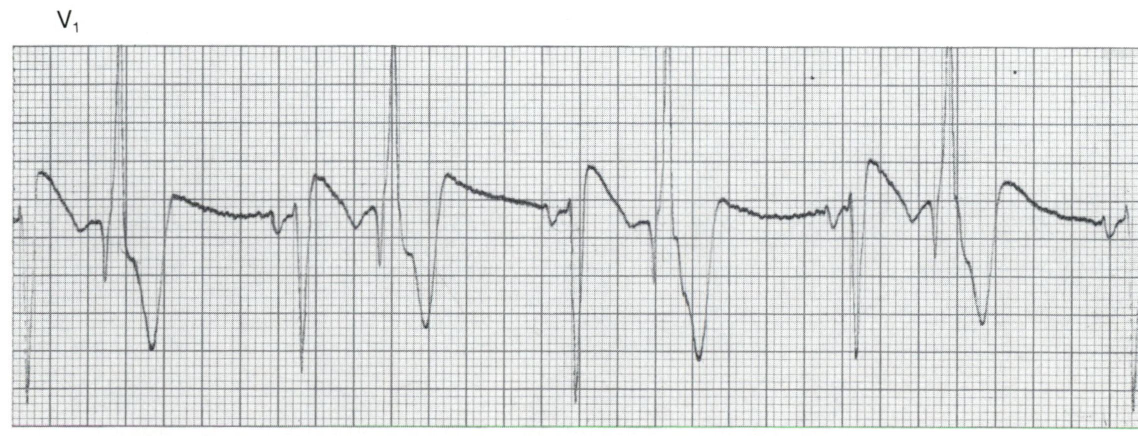

FIGURE 8-7 Ventricular bigeminy. Every other QRS complex is a VPB. VPBs have a qR configuration whereas the sinus-conducted QRS complexes have an rS morphology. Had the anomalous QRS complexes been initiated with a small, narrow r wave like the sinus-conducted beats, we would suspect RBBB aberration. Ventricular ectopy was confirmed by 12-lead ECG.

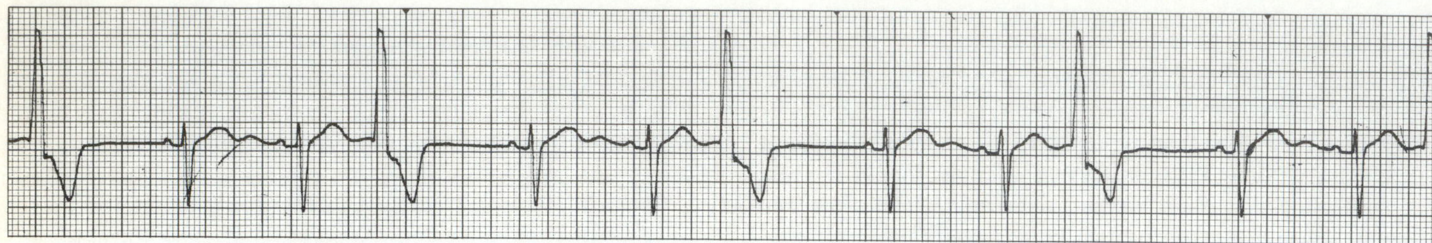

FIGURE 8-8 Ventricular trigeminy. Every third QRS complex is a VPB. Note compensatory pauses after VPBs.

Rate: 75 bpm
Rhythm: Irregular
P wave: Normal
PR interval: 0.14 seconds
QRS complex: 0.09 seconds. An rS complex on lead II is due to left axis deviation.
Interpretation: NSR with ventricular trigeminy

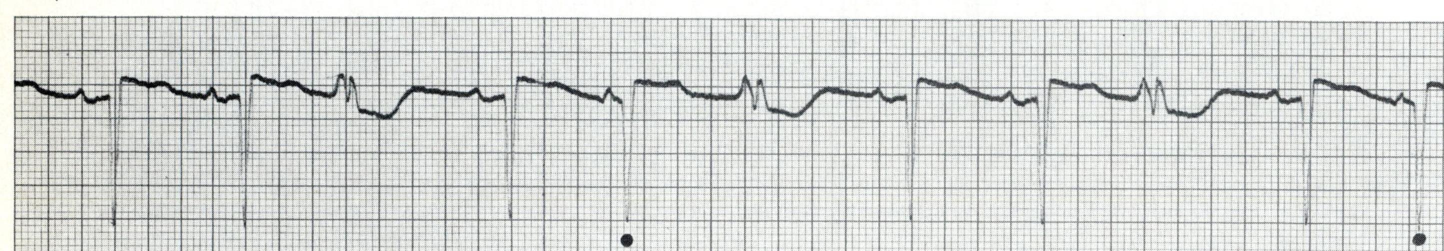

FIGURE 8-9 Ventricular trigeminy. Every third QRS complex is a VPB. Note compensatory pauses. There are also two JPBs *(dots)*. Note that the P′ waves preceding the JPBs are not premature and have a negative-positive diphasic appearance. Therefore they may be retrogradely conducted.

Rate: 75 bpm
Rhythm: Irregular
P wave: Appear normal. Verify with 12-lead ECG.
PR interval: 0.20 seconds
QRS complex: 0.07 to 0.08 seconds
Interpretation: NSR with ventricular trigeminy and two JPBS

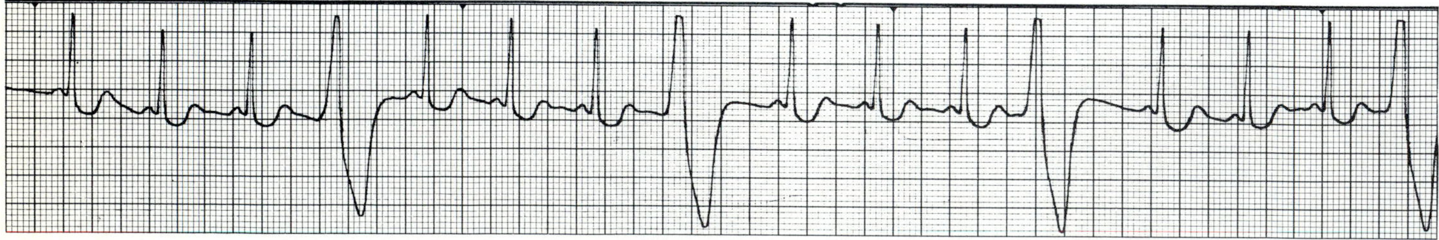

FIGURE 8-10 Ventricular quadrigeminy. Every fourth QRS complex is a VPB. This strip was taken from a healthy 36-year-old nurse while she was working in an intensive care unit.

Rate: 97 bpm
Rhythm: Irregular
P wave: Normal
PR interval: 0.12 seconds
QRS complex: 0.06 seconds; VPB 0.16 seconds
Interpretation: NSR with ventricular quadrigeminy

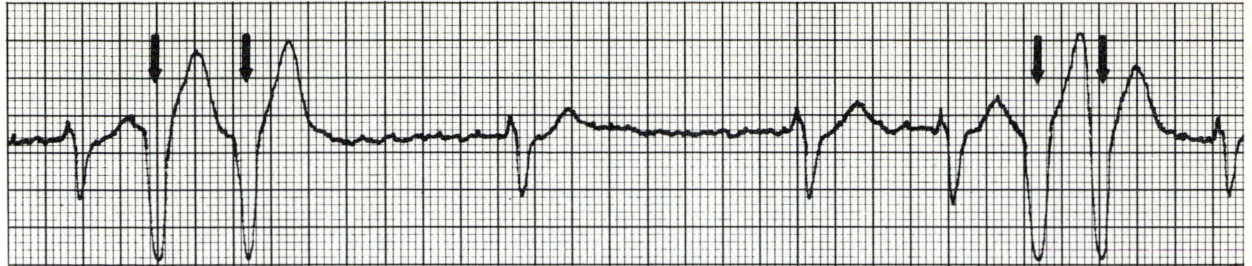

FIGURE 8-11 VPB couplet, pair, or salvo of two *(arrows).* The underlying rhythm is AF with a slow ventricular response. The tracing was taken during insertion of a pacing catheter into the right ventricle.

Rate: Approximately 60 bpm
Rhythm: Irregular
P wave: Chaotic appearing because of AF
PR interval: —
QRS complex: 0.14 to 0.16 seconds, IVCD
Interpretation: AF with slow ventricular response, two VPB couplets

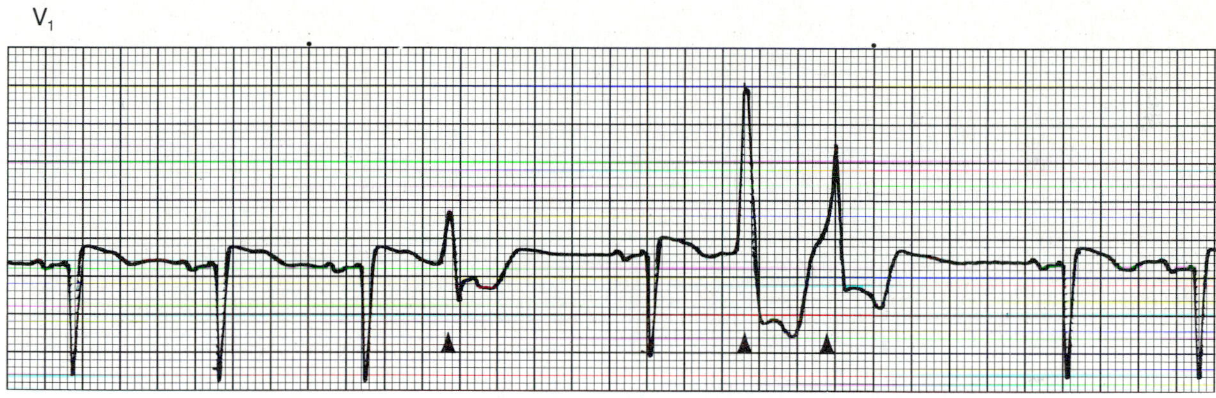

FIGURE 8-12 Single and paired VPBs. This strip shows VPBs *(arrows)* occurring singularly and in couplets or pairs.

Rate: 73 bpm
Rhythm: Irregular
P wave: 0.09 with + − diphasicity, normal for V_1
PR interval: 0.17 seconds
QRS complex: 0.10 seconds
Interpretation: NSR with VPBs occurring singularly and in pairs

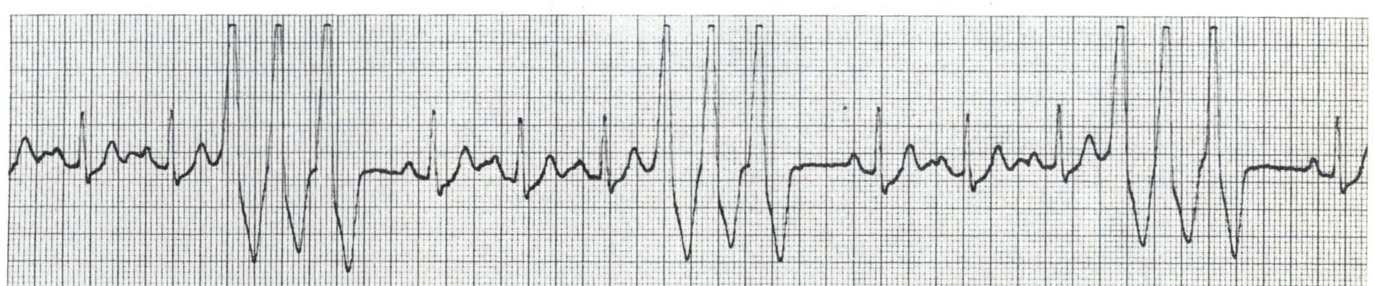

FIGURE 8-13 VPB triplets, salvos of three, or short bursts of VT. This is also an example of regular grouped beating as triplets occur after every three normal beats.

Rate: Approximately 120 bpm
Rhythm: Irregular (but regular grouped beating)
P wave: Normal
PR interval: 0.18 seconds
QRS complex: 0.10 seconds; depressed J point; VPB triplets
Interpretation: NSR with rate 91 bpm interrupted by frequent uniform VPB triplets at a rate of 176 bpm in a quadrigeminal pattern

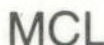

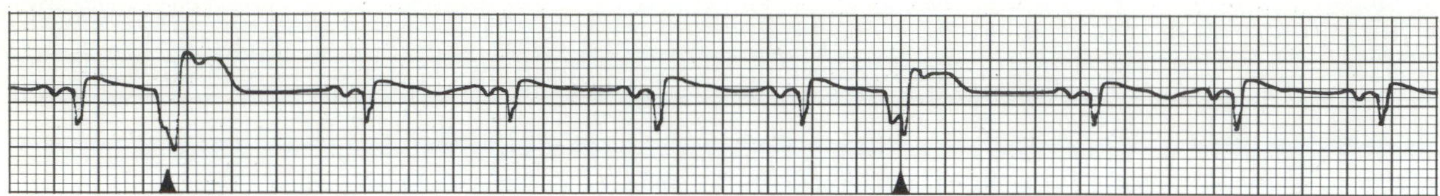

FIGURE 8-14 Uniform VPB. When VPBs *(arrows)* have similar morphologic characteristics, they are termed *uniform* or *monomorphic.*

Rate: 91 bpm
Rhythm: Irregular
P wave: Normal
PR interval: 0.14 to 0.16 seconds
QRS complex: 0.06 seconds
Interpretation: NSR with two monomorphic VPBs

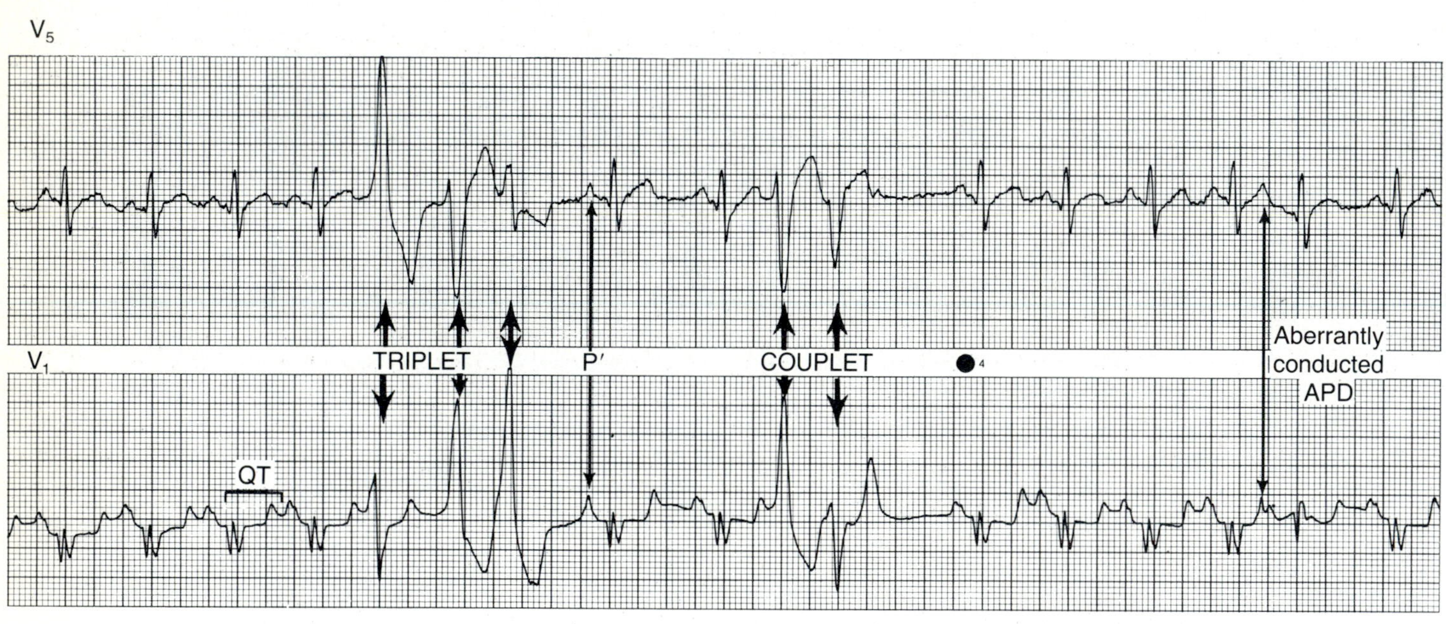

FIGURE 8-15 Multiformed or polymorphic VPBs. Simultaneous tracings in V_5 and V_1 exemplify how limited interpretation may be when only one lead is visualized. Note the VPB triplet in V_5 is clearly three different ventricular morphologies, whereas the same triplet visualized in V_1 appears as only two different morphologies. Likewise, the VPB couplet in V_1 is composed of two distinct morphologies that appear monomorphic in V_5.

Rate: Approximately 110 bpm
Rhythm: Irregular
P wave: Wide, notched, 0.12 seconds in duration
PR interval: 0.16 seconds
QRS complex: 0.12 seconds, prolonged, IVCD; QT interval 0.38 seconds, prolonged
Interpretation: Sinus Tachycardia (ST) at rate 100 bpm with IVCD and intraatrial conduction defect interrupted by triplet and couplet of polymorphic VPBs, prolonged QT interval, occasional APB

V_1

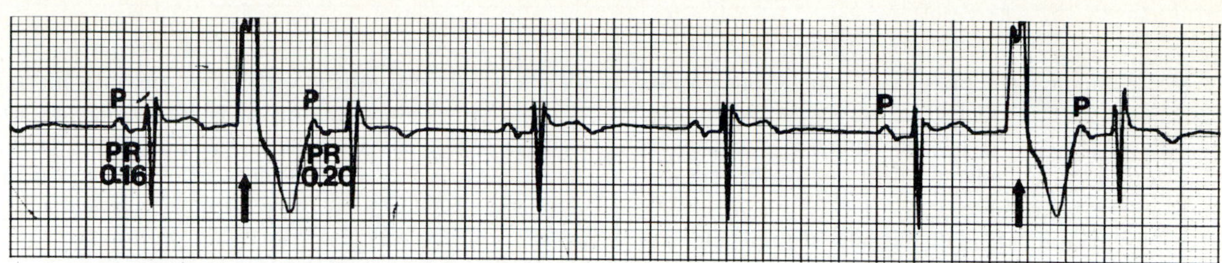

FIGURE 8-16 Interpolated VPBs. When a VPB is "sandwiched" between two sinus-conducted impulses, it is called *interpolated (arrows).* Note that sinus rhythm is not interrupted and the QRS conducted after the VPB is conducted with a longer PR interval (not unusual with interpolated VPBs).

Rate: 60 bpm
Rhythm: Irregular
P wave: 0.11 to 0.12 seconds
PR interval: 0.16 to 0.18 seconds
QRS complex: 0.10 seconds; VPB 0.14 seconds. Sinus-conducted QRSs have a terminal r wave, abnormal for V_1.
Interpretation: NSR with uniform, interpolated VPBs, rSr′ configuration in V_1

MCL_1

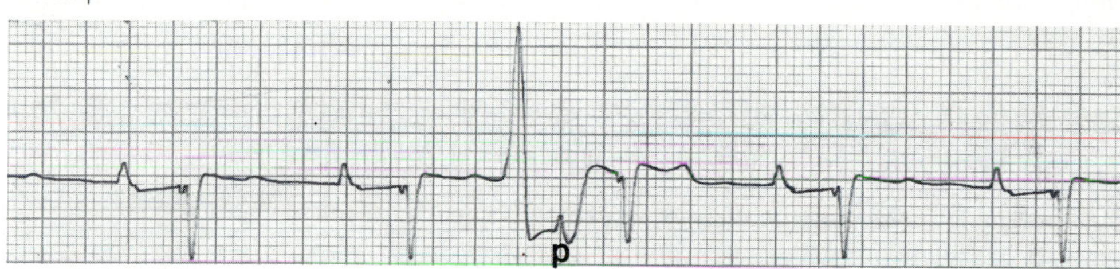

FIGURE 8-17 Interpolated VPB. Note the VPB does not interrupt sinus or the ventricular rhythm. The PR interval after the VPB is not prolonged beyond the others.

Rate: 60 bpm
Rhythm: Irregular
P wave: Peaked
PR interval: 0.26 to 0.28 seconds, prolonged
QRS complex: 0.10 seconds
Interpretation: NSR with prolonged PR interval and interpolated VPB

MCL_1

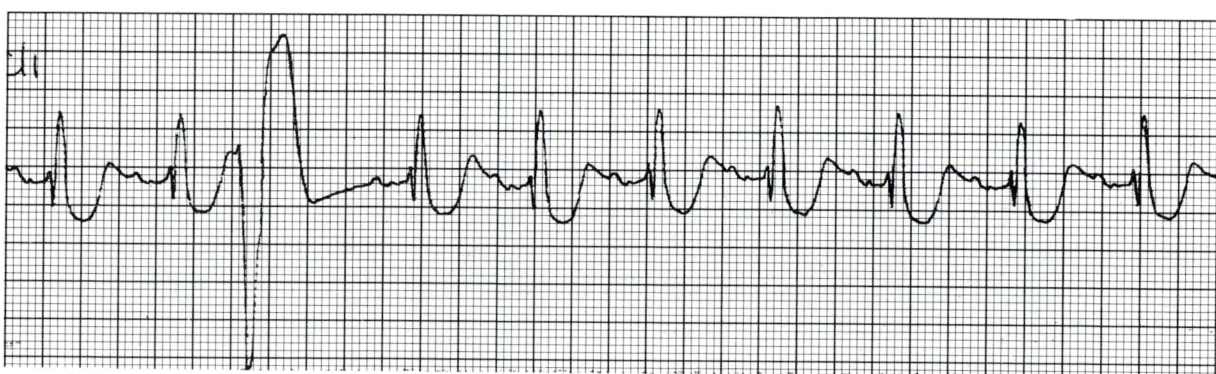

FIGURE 8-18 VPB exhibiting R-on-T phenomenon. Note VPB occurs on apex of the T wave of the preceding beat. (Also examine Figure 8-41 where an R-on-T VPB initiates VF.) R-on-T VPBs were once thought to be more dangerous than end-diastolic VPBs, but it is now realized that any VPB may be a harbinger of a fatal ventricular arrhythmia.

Rate: 94 bpm
Rhythm: Irregular
P wave: 0.12 seconds, wide
PR interval: 0.20 seconds
QRS complex: 0.12 seconds. Terminal R′ wave in MCL_1 is consistent with RBBB
Interpretation: NSR with one R-on-T VPB

mon.[95] In the middle-aged and elderly adult R-on-T VPBs occur in 1% to 2%,[45,96] and in normal young adults they occur in 0% to 4%.[41,42] (Also see Figure 8-19 that is included to serve as a reminder to always be on the look-out for equipment-related artifact.)

VPBs may also occur relatively late in the cycle, appearing earlier than the next expected QRS but late enough in the cycle to allow the P wave to appear. These late-in-cycle beats are known as *end-diastolic VPBs* (Figs. 8-20 and 8-21). In a study of 339 symptomatic cardiac patients with ventricular ectopy, Boudoulas et al[95] found that 5.6% of the VPBs were early (R-on-T), 26.8% were late in the cycle, and 67.6% were midcycle. Under the right physiologic conditions, lethal ventricular arrhythmias can be initiated by either early or late-in-cycle VPBs.[6,13,95,97-99]

Coupling interval. The distance (time) of the ventricular ectopic beat from the preceding QRS complex is referred to as the *coupling interval*. VPBs often exhibit fixed or constant coupling (see Figs. 8-1, 8-7, 8-8, 8-15, and 8-16) but also can display varying coupling intervals (see Fig. 8-4). Constant coupling intervals do not vary more than 0.08 seconds[100,101] (some authors extend this limit to 0.12 seconds[102]).

Rule of bigeminy.[100,101,103] The phenomenon of fixed coupling is especially apparent when bigeminal VPBs accompany a rhythm that is irregular, such as atrial fibrillation or sinus arrhythmia. These ventricular ectopic beats are precisely related to the preceding QRS, thought to be a product of reentry, and most likely occur after a relatively long pause. A pattern of bigeminy tends to perpetuate itself; the long pause that follows the VPB favors the development of another VPB. This phenomenon is known as *the rule of bigeminy*[100] (Fig. 8-22) and will be useful in the later discussion of aberration versus ectopy.

The box on this page summarizes features of VPBs.

Prognostic significance. The clinical setting in which VPBs occur is a critical variable in their significance, or the likelihood of promoting such life-threatening arrhythmias as ventricular tachycardia (VT) and fibrillation (VF). In the presence of CAD, VPBs are common and significant; over 60% of CAD patients have ventricular arrhythmias.[39] VPBs may be the first manifestation of latent CAD.[105] In the presence of overt heart disease, particularly angina, previous MI, and left ventricular hypertrophy, VPBs are associated with a considerably higher incidence of sudden death.[106] Those VPBs often noted before SCD include frequent polymorphic VPBs,[90,99] runs of VPBs, both early and late-in-cycle VPBs,[107] and couplets.[99] There is, however, **no specific antecedent arrhythmic pattern that has been consistently observed that can serve as a warning for SCD.**[7]

Ventricular ectopy in the presence of acute myocardial ischemia or infarction is far more significant than its occurrence in a healthy individual. It is believed that the threshold for VF is considerably reduced in people with organic heart disease as compared with patients without heart disease.[108,109] Immediately after MI, the incidence of VF, however, falls exponentially with time.[110] It has been shown that within 1 hour of acute MI, ventricular ar-

ECG Characteristics
Ventricular Premature Beats

Rate: Any
Rhythm: Irregular
P wave: VPBs not preceded by premature P′ waves
PR interval: Not present unless VPB is end-diastolic, then PR interval is < sinus-conducted PR.
QRS complex: 0.12 seconds or longer

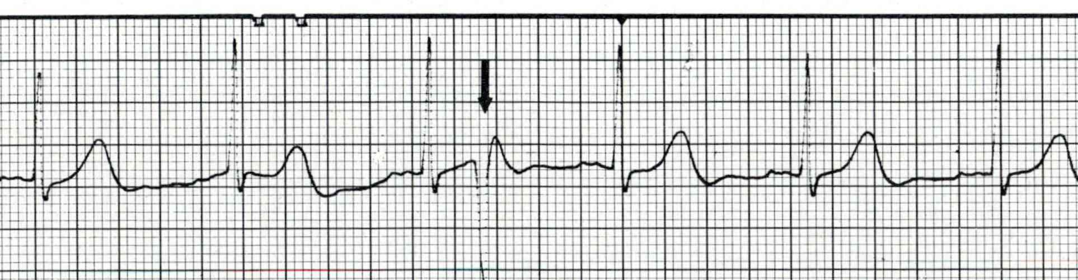

FIGURE 8-19 An R-on-T VPB *(arrow)?* No, this is simply artifact. Although this complex looks much like a premature beat, it is not. It is a peculiarity of a particular brand of monitoring equipment. It is included to stress the importance of knowing your equipment and familiarizing yourself with the artifacts it produces.

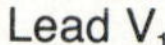

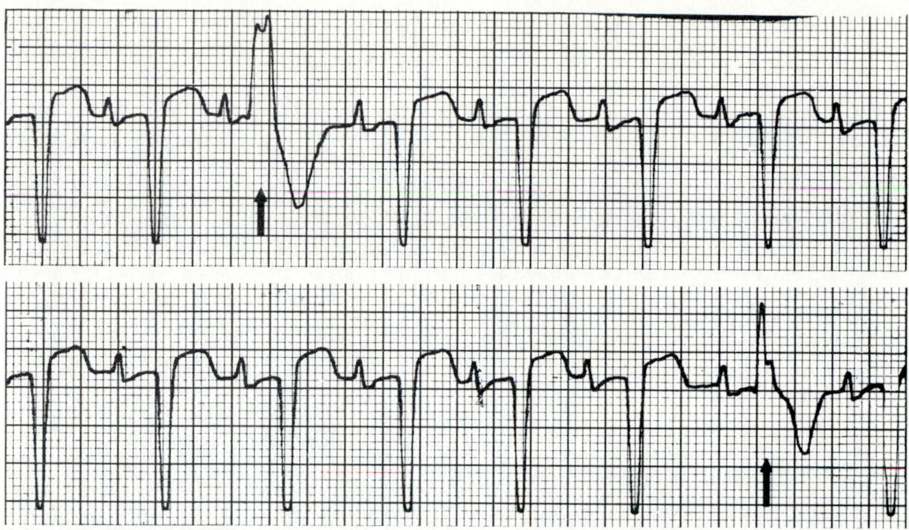

FIGURE 8-20 End-diastolic VPB. Top strip shows an early anomalous QRS complex *(arrow).* Note it is preceded by a P wave, but the P wave is not premature. The PR interval of all the other beats is 0.22 seconds, whereas the PR of the early QRS is 0.16 seconds. If this patient could conduct QRS complexes with a PR interval of 0.16 seconds, he would. The anomalous beat is early, yet late enough in diastole to have allowed the P wave to appear. Thus it is named *end-diastolic VPB.* The anomalous complex in the bottom strip *(arrow)* is likely a fusion beat—a sinus-conducted and end-diastolic VPB have occurred simultaneously, creating a combination complex. Remember the ECG is the algebraic sum of events. The positive VPB combined with the negative sinus-conducted QRS will create a complex that has both characteristics.

Rate: 100 bpm
Rhythm: Irregular
P wave: 0.12 seconds, wide, also tall
PR interval: 0.22 seconds, prolonged
QRS complex: 0.10 seconds; VPB 0.16 seconds
Interpretation: ST with end-diastolic VPBs and prolonged PR interval

MCL$_1$

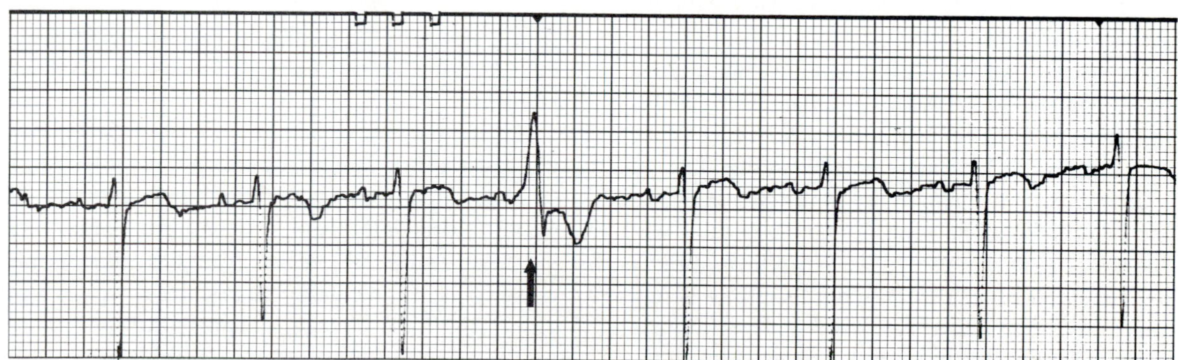

FIGURE 8-21 End-diastolic VPB. Note early QRS complex *(arrow)* is preceded by a P wave, but not an early P wave. The QRS is premature (earlier than the expected complex) but late enough in diastole to have allowed the P wave to appear. Do not confuse end-diastolic VPBs with aberrantly conducted APBs. Remember an APB has a premature P′ wave, whereas an end-diastolic VPB is preceded by the regularly occurring sinus P wave, which is not premature.

Rate: 79 bpm
Rhythm: Irregular
P wave: Normal
PR interval: 0.18 seconds
QRS complex: 0.09 seconds
Interpretation: NSR with one end-diastolic VPB

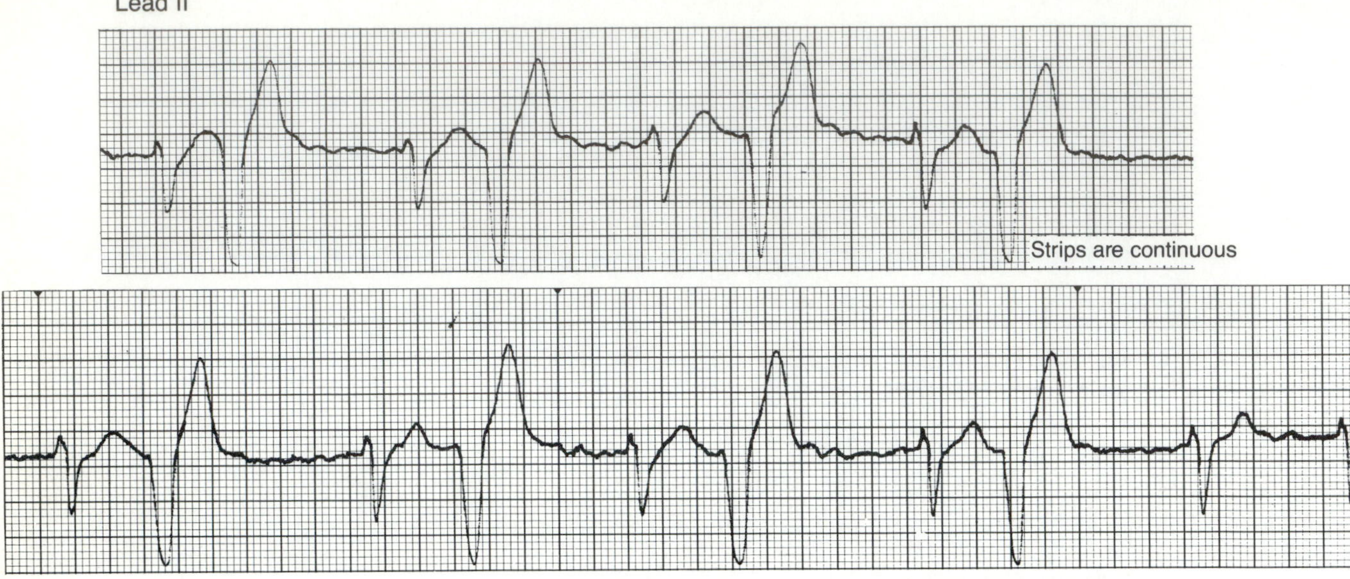

FIGURE 8-22 Ventricular bigeminy during AF with irregular ventricular response illustrating the rule of bigeminy.

rhythmias were present in nearly all the patients and 36% developed VF.[111] Since it takes the average patient over 3 hours to seek medical assistance,[112] overall in-hospital incidence of ventricular arrhythmias is approximately 84%,[113] with VF occurring in 2% to 11%.[113-119] (The incidence of VF has declined over the past several years and may be attributed to wide-spread use of beta blockers, better control of hypertension, and/or improved MI therapy, including the use of thrombolytics.) Interestingly, patients with acute MI who experience VF have a better prognosis than those who experience SCD as a primary arrhythmic event.[5,120] That is, when VF is not associated with MI, there is a tendency for recurrence.[5]

For many years, students of arrhythmology were taught to recognize what were known as *warning arrhythmias*-those that were reputed to be harbingers of VT or VF. Typically these warning arrhythmias included VPBs that occurred (1) in pairs, (2) in bigeminy, or (3) more than 5 times per minute; (4) exhibited the R on T phenomenon; or were (5) polymorphic or (6) in runs of VT. When these arrhythmias were detected, antiarrhythmic drug therapy was initiated. It is now recognized that these "warning arrhythmias" are a common phenomenon in acute MI rather than a warning.[113,114,121] In a group of acute MI patients not treated with antiarrhythmics, the incidence of warning arrhythmias is displayed in Table 8-2.

Roughly 60% of all hospitalized MI patients exhibit warning arrhythmias,[113,115] yet only 2% to 11% fibrillate.[18,72,113-116,118,121] Of those who fibrillate, only 50% to 60% exhibit warning arrhythmias before[18,113,121] and often those occur too close to the final event to institute therapy.[107] The remaining 40% to 50% of patients do not exhibit warning arrhythmias,[121,122] thus their clinical utility is dubious.

Table 8-2 Warning Arrhythmias in Acute Myocardial Infarction[113]

Type of warning arrhythmia	% of patients
R-on-T	10%
Bigeminal	13%
Multifocal	24%
Runs of VPBs	36%
>5/min	37%

To summarize, in the presence of an acute MI, the traditional warning arrhythmias are not reliable criteria for instituting prophylactic antiarrhythmic therapy.[113] Although-some[121] conclude there are no arrhythmias considered premonitory for VF, others recognize that simply an increase in heart rate and/or ventricular ectopy is a prodrome of VF.[8,11,14,19,107] To get an idea of the kinds of VPBs that are the culprits in initiating VF see Table 8-3.

Ventricular tachycardia is also considered a dangerous arrhythmia in the setting of acute MI and ischemia. Its incidence in the acute MI patient is 9% to 46%.[113,117,123-125] Yet as few as 4% of patients with VT exhibit warning arrhythmias in the 10 minutes preceding VT.[124] It has been concluded that there are no arrhythmias that can be considered premonitory for paroxysmal VT (PVT), since no positive correlation exists between PVT and the number or

Table 8-3 Ventricular Ectopy Initiating Ventricular Fibrillation[107,113,117,121]

VPBs initiating V	% of VF episodes
Closely coupled	45% to 69%
"Late"	35% to 45%
Deteriorated from VT	10% to 20%

Table 8-4 Ventricular Ectopy Initiating Ventricular Tachycardia[117,124,126]

VPBs initiating VT	% of VT episodes
Closely coupled	20%
"Late"	44% to 78%

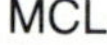

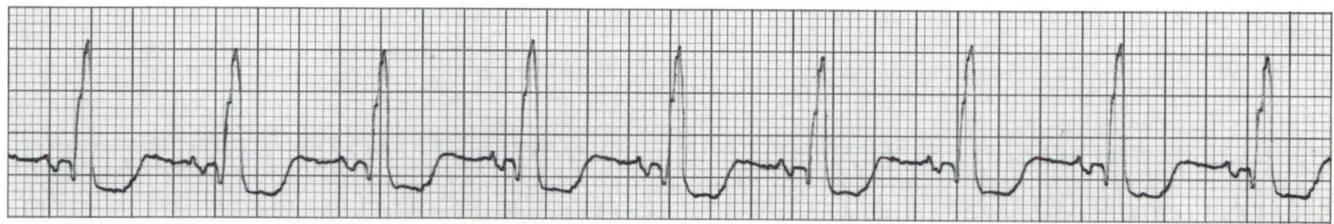

FIGURE 8-23 NSR with an intraventricular conduction defect (RBBB).

Rate: 83 bpm
Rhythm: Regular
P wave: Normal for MCL_1
PR interval: 0.12 seconds
QRS complex: 0.14 to 0.16 seconds (wide, terminal R wave is abnormal for MCL_1 or V_1 and is consistent with RBBB)

complexity of VPBs in the 10 minutes preceding it.[124] The kinds of VPBs responsible for initiating VT are presented in Table 8-4.

After the acute phase of MI, complex ventricular ectopy, such as couplets or runs, in the presence of left ventricular dysfunction seems to be an important risk factor for subsequent SCD.[127] Ruberman et al[128] report a high risk (25% probability) of SCD for post-MI patients who exhibit couplets, runs, or R-on-T VPBs. Their risk is five times that of patients who have no ventricular ectopy. Bigger et al[129] found the risk of an arrhythmic death begins to increase as soon as one VPB per hour is noted before discharge; the risk of SCD at 2 years is 3.6 times higher than in those patients who exhibited fewer than one VPB per hour. The presence of complex ventricular ectopy also seems to increase the risk for SCD in patients who have hypertrophic and dilated cardiomyopathy.[130] For those patients who are considered to be at high risk for SCD, there is no good evidence to support that treatment of their frequent VPBs prolongs their lives.

In summary, some important points deserve reemphasis.

- The significance of ventricular ectopy is related to the type and severity of the underlying heart disease.
- VPBs are ubiquitous, but they appear to be dangerous for those patients experiencing acute ischemia.
- For patients in the immediate post-MI period, the so-called warning arrhythmias are not good predictors of VT or VF, so do not wait for these arrhythmias to appear to begin prophylactic treatment. It only takes one VPB anywhere in the cycle to initiate VF.

Morphology. The morphologic structure of VPBs (their shape on the ECG) has earned prominent stature in electrocardiographic literature because differentiating ventricular ectopy from wide supraventricular complexes is often difficult.[131-134] Distinguishing the two is important because treatment differs.

A beginner in arrhythmology would have no difficulty diagnosing the rhythm in Fig. 8-23 as "normal sinus rhythm with an intraventricular conduction defect." The QRSs are wide, but each QRS is preceded by a P wave that bears a constant relationship to it. The rate is 83 bpm. We have no reason to suspect these QRS complexes are ventricular in origin because the rhythm fits the criteria for sinus rhythm.

Now look at Figure 8-24. The basic rhythm is normal sinus with an early complex interrupting the rhythm. The early QRS is wide and close examination reveals a P′ wave in the T wave of the preceding complex. This early complex is labeled as an aberrantly conducted APB. (It is conducted with a right bundle branch block (RBBB). Intraventricular conduction defects such as this are discussed in Chapter 9.) These two examples of wide complexes do not present major interpretive problems.

It is when the wide complexes occur rapidly or are not preceded by visible P′ waves that interpretation becomes

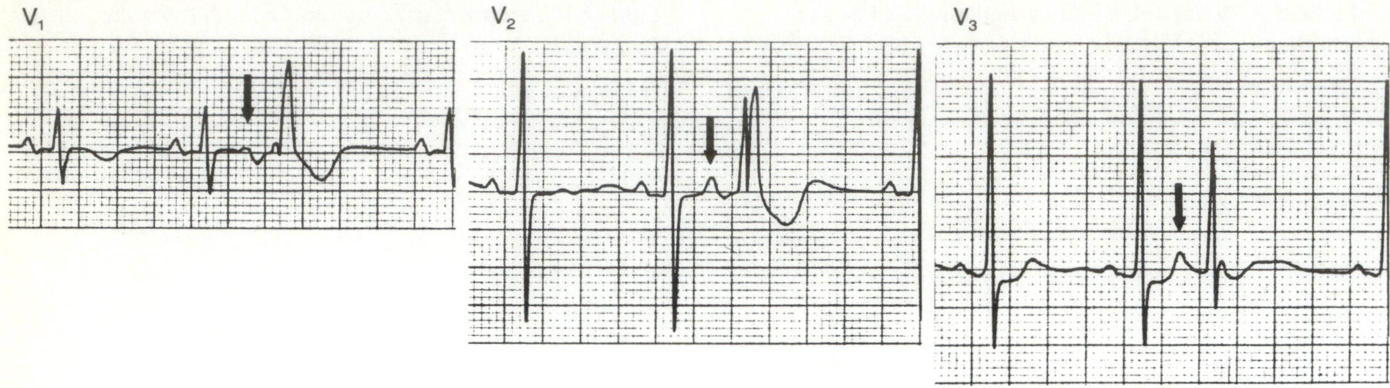

FIGURE 8-24 Three simultaneous tracings of an early wide beat. The anomalous QRS complex is wide and different from the other QRS complexes. The early QRS is preceded by an early P′ wave. Examination of the preceding T wave reveals a T wave that is different from the other normal T waves because it contains a P′ wave *(arrow)*.

Rate: 77 bpm
Rhythm: Irregular
P wave: Normal except for one APB
PR interval: 0.16 seconds
QRS complex: 0.09 seconds; aberrant QRS 0.14 seconds because of RBBB; best measured in V_1 or V_2
Interpretation: NSR, one APB conducted with RBBB aberration

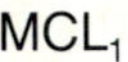

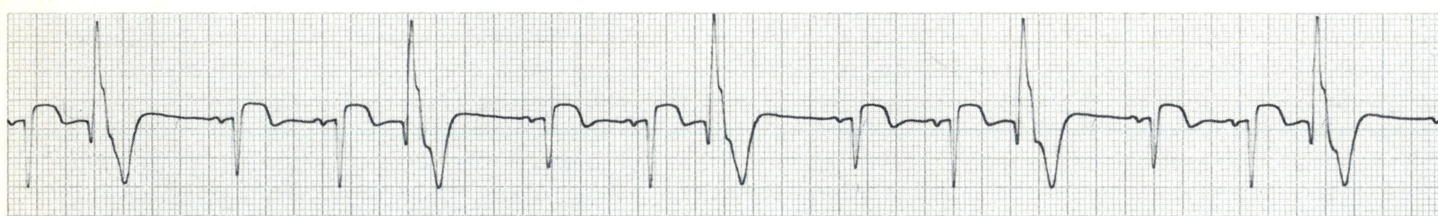

FIGURE 8-25 Ventricular trigeminy or trigeminal JPBs conducted with RBBB aberration? Every third complex is early and wide. Initial portions of both sinus-conducted and anomalous beats are similar (i.e., they both display initial negativity). The anomalous beats have a wide terminal R wave characteristic of RBBB. The beats display a compensatory pause after them, however. This kind of arrhythmia often poses a diagnostic dilemma. We believe these beats are ventricular in origin, but we advise using a 12-lead ECG to support the diagnosis.

Rate: 83 bpm
Rhythm: Irregular (but regular grouped beating)
P wave: Normal
PR interval: 0.15 seconds
QRS complex: 0.06 seconds; VPBs 0.14 seconds
Interpretation: NSR with ventricular trigeminy

problematic (Figs. 8-25 and 8-26). It is difficult to determine if these wide complexes are supraventricular with aberration or ventricular in origin. With no premature P′ waves to assist in the diagnosis, determination of the source of the wide complexes must be an educated guess based on research of morphologic characteristics of ventricular and aberrant supraventricular complexes. For example, sometimes on V_1 an anomalous beat displays a positive configuration with two points, dubbed *rabbit ears*. If the left rabbit ear of the QRS is taller than the right (Figs. 8-27 and 8-28), chances are it is ventricular in origin. If the right is taller (Fig. 8-16), the rabbit ears provide no diagnostic assistance.[131]

When wide, anomalous beats occur in the presence of atrial fibrillation (AF), differential diagnosis is often difficult (as it is in the presence of a tachycardia). In AF, helpful aids, such as premature P′ waves and compensatory pauses, are not present. Gulamhusein et al[134] studied patients with chronic AF who were treated with digitalis (none were digitalis toxic). Wide complexes were ana-

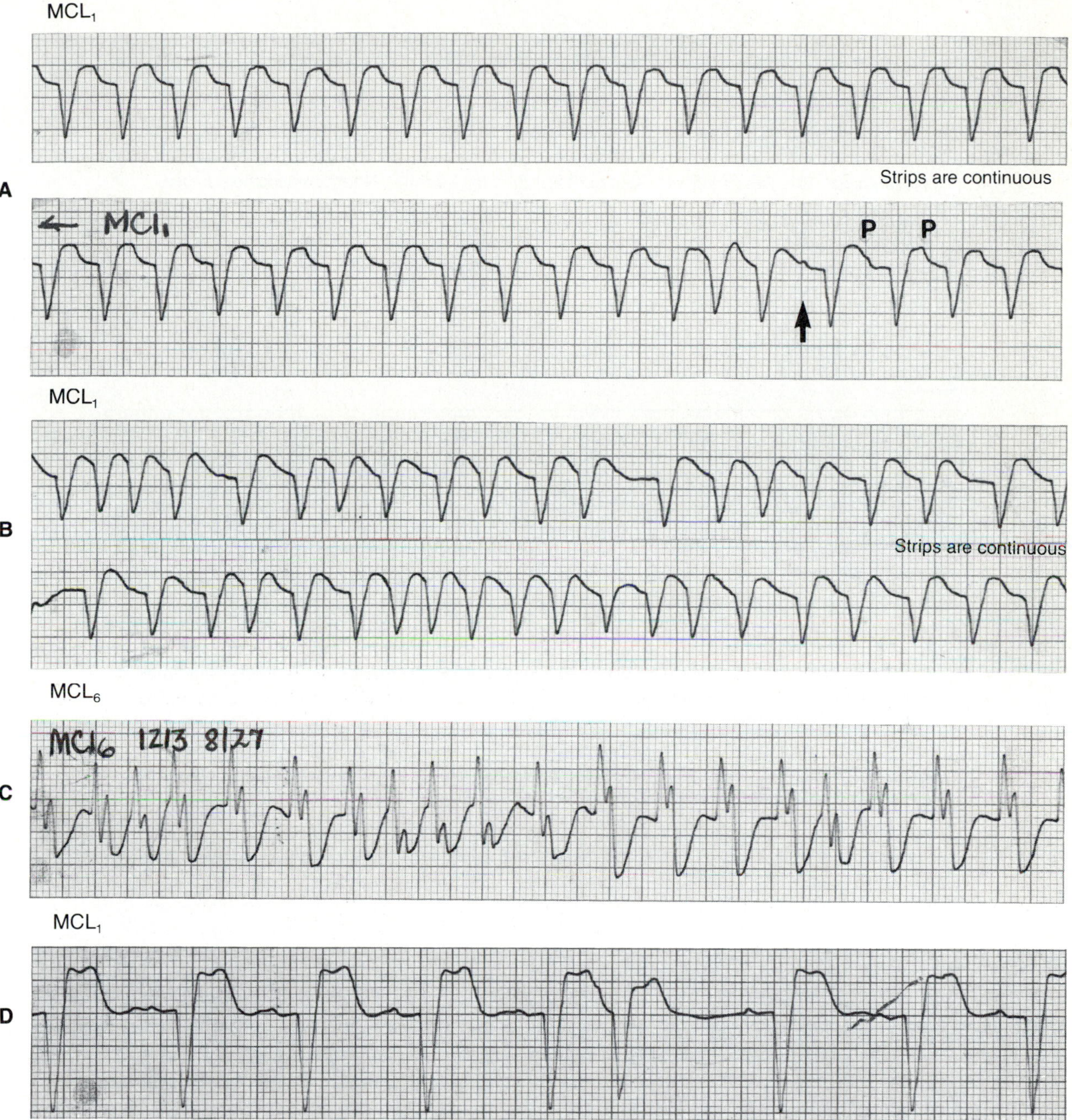

FIGURE 8-26 Wide-complex tachycardia.
A, Is the tachycardia supraventricular or ventricular in origin? The second strip in A offers diagnostic assistance when a pause in the rhythm *(arrow)* reveals a P wave allowing subsequent P wave identification *(P).* **B,** Minutes later the patient's rhythm becomes very irregular. The QRS complexes remain the same in morphology. Irregular ventricular rhythm and unidentifiable P waves suggest AF. **C,** Visualization of the rhythm on MCL$_6$. **D,** After digitalization. The QRS morphology is clearly an intraventricular conduction disturbance (LBBB).
Interpretations: **A,** SVT with LBBB. **B** and **C,** AF with LBBB. **D,** NSR with APBs and LBBB

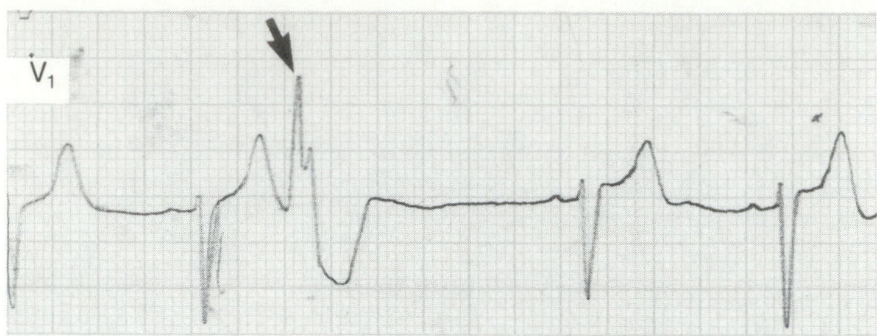

FIGURE 8-27 VPB illustrating left rabbit ear taller than right *(arrow)*. Note compensatory pause.

Rate: 71 bpm
Rhythm: Irregular
P wave: Normal
PR interval: 0.14 seconds
QRS complex: 0.09 seconds
Interpretation: NSR with VPB

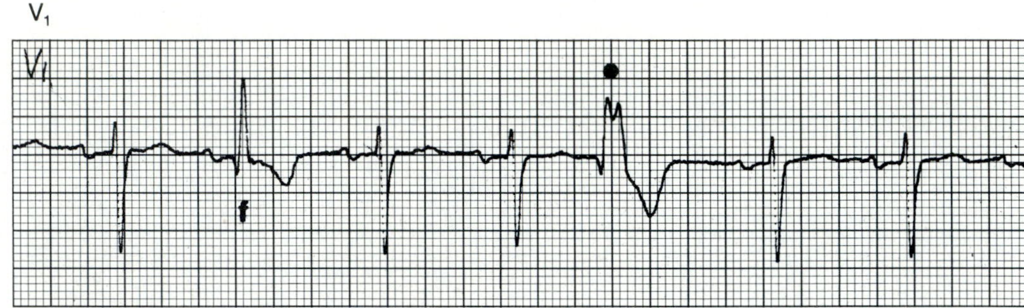

FIGURE 8-28 VPB *(dot)* resembles RBBB. Note compensatory pause, left rabbit ear taller than right. Another anomalous beat (f) is a fusion beat of the VPB and a sinus-conducted QRS complex. This patient was exhibiting VPBs with varying coupling intervals and many end-diastolic VPBs. Note PR interval of 0.18 seconds with all the normal complexes. The f beat is preceded by a P wave with a PR interval of 0.16 seconds. Note also that the initial 0.04 seconds of the QRS complexes of the anomalous beats is different from the sinus-conducted QRS complexes.

Rate: 86 bpm
Rhythm: Irregular
P wave: Normal
PR interval: 0.18 seconds
QRS complex: 0.10 seconds
Interpretation: NSR with VPBs displaying variable coupling intervals

lyzed with both intracardiac and electrocardiographic recordings. They found that 91% of the wide complexes were ventricular in origin, whereas only 9% were supraventricular impulses conducted with aberration. This high incidence of ventricular ectopy in the presence of atrial fibrillation may be related to digitalis or it may reflect coexistent underlying heart disease.

Of those wide beats that were found to be conducted with aberration, over 93% of them were conducted with RBBB showing a rSR′ in V_1 and a qRs complex in V_6, a pattern shown to be specific for RBBB aberration. Thus, when faced with the dilemma of differentiating a wide beat during AF, first realize that chances are high the beat is a VPB. Look at the beat in MCL_1 or V_1 and MCL_6 or V_6. If it is an rSR′ configuration in V_1 and a qRs in V_6, with the initial QRS vector (first 0.02-0.04 seconds of the QRS) identical to that of the normal beats, it is likely a supraventricular beat conducted with RBBB aberration.

Axis. The axis of the wide QRS may also provide some diagnostic help in the differential diagnosis of ectopy and aberration. The axes of ventricular ectopic beats may be directed to any of the four axis quandrants, including the superior right axis and the inferior right axis. It is rare for an aberrantly conducted beat to be directed to the superior right axis, and uncommon for it to be directed to the inferior right. Therefore, if frontal plane leads reveal the anomalous beat's axis to be −90 to −180 degrees, you can be reasonably confident the beat is ventricular in origin.

Fusion. At times, a ventricular ectopic beat activates

the ventricles simultaneously with or just milliseconds before the normal, supraventricular impulse does so. Late enough to have permitted appearance of the normal P wave and initiation of ventricular activation by the supraventricular impulse, the ventricular ectopic beat is not early enough to cancel depolarization of the ventricles by the supraventricular impulse. Consequently, the ventricles are depolarized by both ventricular and supraventricular impulses, with the resultant fusion beat resembling the beat initiating earliest activation. Thus the later the ventricular ectopic beat, the more the fusion beat resembles the sinus conducted QRS; the earlier the beat, the more it resembles the ventricular ectopic beat.

When an end-diastolic VPB occurs (after the regular sinus P wave but before the next scheduled QRS), the PR interval preceding the VPB will be shorter than the PR interval of the normal beats (Figs. 8-20 and 8-28). Be careful to diagnose fusion beats only when (1) there is evidence of end-diastolic ventricular ectopy, (2) the fusion beat combines morphologic characteristics of the VPB and sinus-conducted QRS, and (3) the PR interval preceding the fusion beat is the same or slightly shorter (but not more than 0.06 seconds shorter)[103] than the PR interval preceding the normal, sinus-conducted beats.

Fusion is a good criterion to support the diagnosis of ventricular ectopy. More criteria follow in Chapter 10.

Summary. ECG features of VPBs that favor the diagnosis of ventricular ectopy include:

- VPBs are more common.
- Taller left rabbit ear on V_1.
- Fusion.
- Superior right axis.

There are many more criteria used in differential diagnosis of wide QRS complexes; refer to references[103,132-134] and Chapters 9 and 10.

Applied Nursing Process

Clinical Assessment

- Detect:
  - An irregular pulse.
  - An irregularity in the ECG.
- Assess the patient and ECG.
  - Assessment of the patient with VPBs includes consideration of the clinical situation in which the VPBs are occurring. For example, in the presence of MI or myocardial ischemia they may be dangerous.
  - It is important to determine and document the frequency of VPBs in the patient's record:
    The number per minute; whether they are occurring consistently every minute.
    Their patterns of occurrence.
  - VPBs may occur more frequently or only at certain times during the day.
    Record time VPBs increase in frequency.
    Check for correlations with events such as meals, sleep, emotional excitement, exercise, hypoxemia, medication administration.
    Assess for symptoms such as light-headedness or palpitations.
  - VPBs may or may not produce strong peripheral pulses. Often their presence on the ECG is accompanied by a pulse deficit or a faint peripheral pulse. It is therefore important to assess perfusion in the presence of ventricular ectopy especially when they are frequent. For example, if a patient's heart rate is 60 per minute but she is having 20 VPBs per minute that do not produce peripheral pulses, her cardiac output will be significantly reduced. The VPBs will need to be terminated because of their adverse hemodynamic effects.
    Check blood pressure.
    Assess sensorium and question patient about symptoms such as light-headedness.
    Evaluate skin color, temperature.
  - Monitor serum electrolytes. (Is serum potassium within normal limits?)
  - Monitor oxygenation. (Is patient hypoxemic?)[66]
  - Review medications the patient is taking. (Are any arrhythmogenic, such as digoxin, aminophylline, isoproterenol, dopamine?)[66]
  - Question the patient about caffeine and other stimulant intake.
  - Observe for signs and symptoms of congestive heart failure.[66]
    Auscultate lungs for rales.
    Question the patient about shortness of breath.
    Inspect for distended neck veins.
    Assess for peripheral edema.
    Auscultate the heart for third heart sound (S_3).
  - Diagnose the arrhythmia. Detect an early wide QRS complex. Proceed with your diagnosis by using the algorithm in Figure 8-29. Chapter 10 provides detailed information needed for differentiating wide QRS complex beats.

❖ NURSING DIAGNOSIS

(1) Decreased cardiac output related to decreased ventricular filling. (2) Altered tissue perfusion: cerebral/peripheral/cardiopulmonary, related to decreased cardiac output. (3) Knowledge deficit regarding home management of ventricular ectopy.

❖ ECG DIAGNOSIS

Ventricular premature beats.

Plan and Implementation

Patient goal. The acutely ischemic (myocardial) patient will not develop ventricular ectopy.

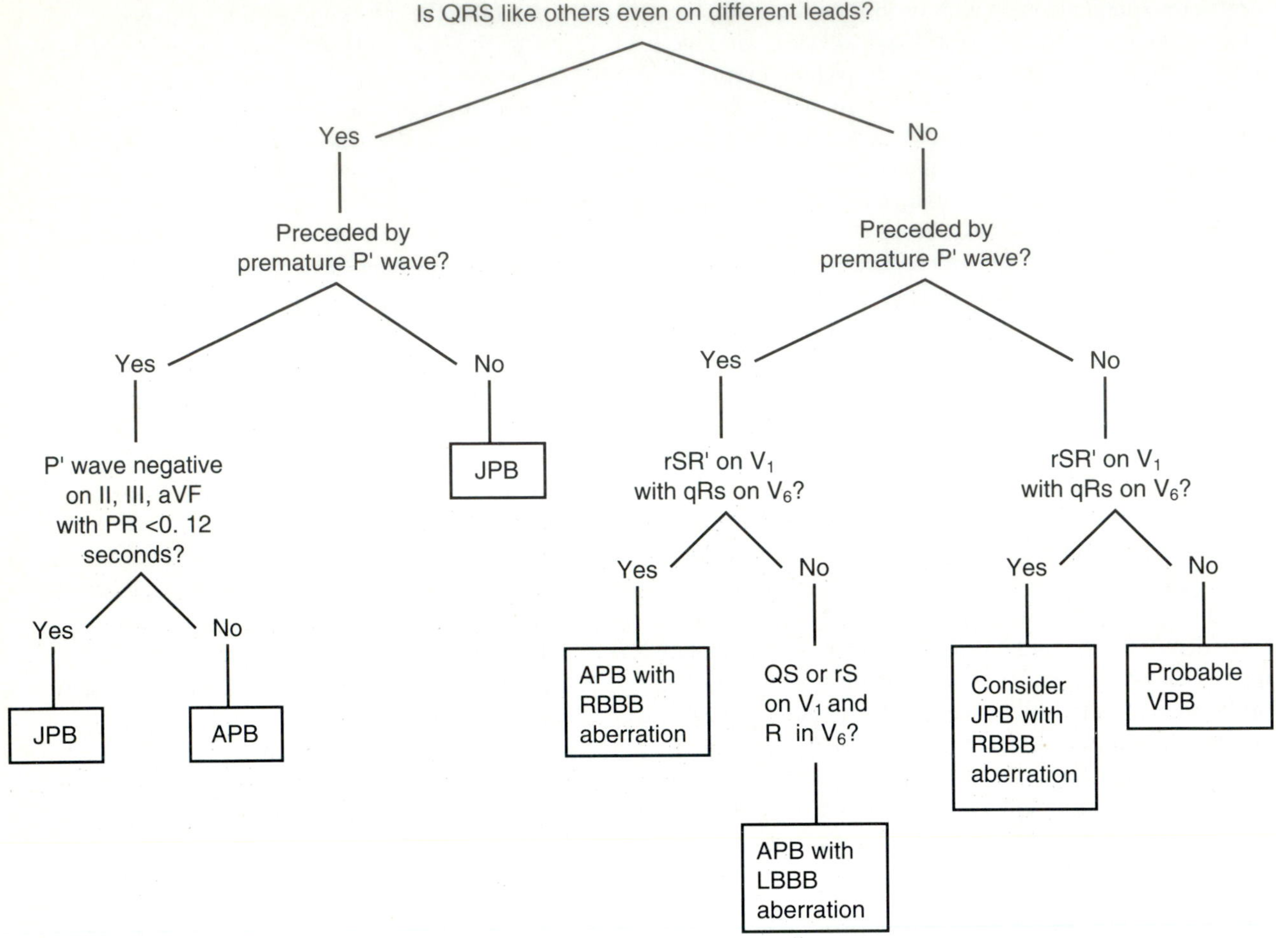

FIGURE 8-29 VPB algorithm.

The patient will not develop preventable, higher grade, dangerous, or malignant ventricular arrhythmias.

The patient will tolerate the ventricular ectopic activity with minimal symptoms and hemodynamic stability.

The patient will minimize or eliminate stressors/substances contributing to the ectopic beats.

The patient will relate appropriate information concerning important symptoms, antiarrhythmic drugs to be taken after discharge.

Nursing interventions.

- Keep emergency equipment and medications such as defibrillator, lidocaine, bretylium available.[66]
- Evaluate patient's tolerance of the arrhythmia.
- Start IV infusion as ordered to enable rapid medication administration, if necessary.
- Administer prophylactic antiarrhythmic therapy, if indicated (see box on p. 209).
- Administer oxygen PRN.
- Record the frequency of VPBs and notify the physician of significant increase in occurrence or change in the character of the ventricular ectopy.
- Record and document various patterns of occurrence such as multiform, bigeminy, couplets.
- Monitor patient on a lead that enables easy differentiation of wide QRS complexes: differentiate between VPB and supraventricular complex conducted with aberration. V_1 or MCL_1 would be a good choice. Also check the lead with the best P waves if they are not clear on V_1.[41]
- Take measures to correct hypokalemia, if present, especially in the presence of MI. Soon after MI, hypokalemia plays a significant role in ventricular ectopy.[72,135]
- Administer magnesium sulfate as ordered. In patients receiving long-term diuretic therapy and/or digitalis, hypomagnesemia is possible. Additionally, magnesium may be necessary to maintain intracellular potassium levels.[87]
- If the patient is experiencing emotional stress, intervene to maintain a restful environment.
- Discourage smoking.
- Eliminate sources of caffeine and other stimulants.
- Consult with physician regarding any medications that may be arrhythmogenic (see Table 8-1).
- Any nurse or paramedic administering antiarrhythmics

Prophylactic Antiarrhythmic Therapy.

In the presence of acute MI or myocardial ischemia, sudden increase in ventricular ectopy may warrant initiation of antiarrhythmic therapy such as lidocaine. If, however, prophylactic antiarrhythmic therapy is already being administered, consider either increasing dosage or changing drugs (e.g., to procainamide). Prophylactic antiarrhythmic therapy, initiated as soon after symptom onset as possible,[122,136] is advocated for selected patients. Although some[137] still recommend waiting for the so-called warning arrhythmias to appear before initiating prophylaxis, remember they are not particularly reliable predictors;[18,138-140] it takes only one VPB to initiate VT or VF. It must be stressed, however, that although prophylactic lidocaine is popular because of its ability to decrease the incidence of VF, routine use is controversial because of conflicting mortality reports and its implication in other serious arrhythmias.[139-144]

Since older patients (over 60 years) have been reported to have a lower incidence of primary VF after acute MI[12,14] and a higher incidence of adverse reactions to lidocaine,[140,145] prophylactic lidocaine may not be indicated for them, particularly outside the hospital.[145] Prophylactic lidocaine may also be contraindicated or reduced in dosage in the presence of second- or third-degree heart block, severe CHF, cardiogenic shock, sinus bradycardia with rates less than 50 bpm,[138] liver disease, or impaired hepatic perfusion.[115,138]

In the presence of AF or atrial flutter with fast ventricular responses, lidocaine's quinidine-like property of accelerating AV conduction in susceptible persons can lead to serious rate increases.[146,147] Consequently, some[146] believe the administration of lidocaine in the presence of atrial tachyarrhythmias with rapid ventricular response is relatively contraindicated, regardless of the presence of apparent ventricular ectopic beats, since the goal in therapy is to reduce the ventricular response. This enhancement of ventricular rate seems to be particularly true in patients receiving quinidine.[100] Fortunately, the occurrence of this phenomenon is relatively rare.

Alternatives to prophylactic lidocaine in the presence of acute MI include magnesium sulfate and beta blockers.[87,118,148]

must be fully cognizant of side effects, dosages, and contraindications of these agents.

- Implement medical orders; evaluate the patient's response to measures taken to treat the ventricular ectopy. For patients on the following drugs, adapt care plan accordingly. Refer to Chapter 11 for further drug information:
  - Procainamide. If QRS prolongs >25%, discontinue drug. Measure QRS during IV administration and every 8 hours during oral administration.
  - For any of the drugs that increase QT interval, measure QT every 4 to 8 hours and evaluate for lengthening. QT intervals longer than 0.5 seconds or a change in the QTc of >0.075 seconds have been associated with worsening ventricular arrhythmias. Drugs known to increase the QT interval include procainamide, quinidine, disopyramide, encainide.[148-150]
  - Watch for PR and QRS-interval prolongation for patients receiving flecainide and encainide.[150-153]
  - Note PR interval changes and QRS prolongation for patients receiving quinidine.[151,153]
  - Note heart rate changes for patients on acebutolol.[154]
  - For patients receiving drugs that may exert a negative inotropic effect such as mexiletine, disopyramide,[150] or flecainide,[151] evaluate hemodynamic response and appearance of signs and symptoms of congestive heart failure (CHF).
- Patient teaching is imperative for the patient who is receiving antiarrhythmics intravenously or orally, acutely ill or ready for discharge. The importance of dosage times, side effects, toxic reactions, and which symptoms require immediate attention is required information for any patient treated for ventricular arrhythmias.

Evaluation

- The patient maintains hemodynamic stability as evidenced by the following:
  - No change in blood pressure.
  - Lucid response without complaints of light-headedness.
  - Warm, dry skin without pallor or cyanosis.
- The patient with myocardial ischemia experiences relief of the ventricular ectopy.
- The patient with intractable ventricular ectopy stabilizes ventricular rhythm and remains comfortable as evidenced by denial of palpitations or other troublesome symptoms.
- The patient eliminates use of caffeine, nicotine, and other stimulants and describes ways to reduce other contributing stressors.

Medical Treatment

VPBs may or may not be treated pharmacologically, depending on the patient's clinical picture.[150-152,155-159] The prognosis of any electrocardiographic abnormality depends on that of the underlying disease process.

When treatment is necessary, drugs used may include the following:[106-108]

Class IA Antiarrhythmics
- Disopyramide
- Moricizine
- Procainamide
- Quinidine

Class IB Antiarrhythmics
- Lidocaine

Mexiletine
Phenytoin (in pediatric patients)
Tocainide
Class IC Antiarrhythmics
Encainide
Flecainide
Propafenone
Class II—Beta-Adrenergic Blockers
Acebutolol
Atenolol
Metoprolol
Propranolol
Timolol
Class IV—Calcium-Channel Blockers
Verapamil
Diltiazem

Medical management may include the periodic use of Holter monitoring to determine if ventricular ectopy is diminished or abolished. The treatment goal of symptomatic VPBs is the elimination of the symptoms.

VENTRICULAR TACHYCARDIA

Data Base: Problem Identification

Definitions, Etiology, and Mechanisms

Ventricular tachycardia (VT) is a common and significant rhythm disturbance. It may be life-threatening. Although it may be an isolated event, VT is more likely to be a chronic and recurrent problem. It is associated with many types of heart disease, but for most patients it is a major complication of acute MI and chronic ischemic heart disease, especially if associated with ventricular aneurysm formation.[160-163] It is also frequently associated with what is known as *prolonged QT interval syndrome,* a relatively rare disorder in which delayed ventricular repolarization is thought to play a role in its etiology.[164]

After orthotopic heart transplantation, VT is common.[165] VT may be a complication of cardiac catheterization[166] or seen in patients with disorders such as hypokalemia and hypomagnesemia,[87,162] anorexia nervosa,[167] mitral valve prolapse,[168] sarcoidosis,[169] aortic valve disease and after aortic balloon valvuloplasty,[170-172] rheumatic heart disease,[103] and hypertrophic and dilated cardiomyopathies.[81,160] Exercise, catecholamines,[103,173] antiarrhythmics (digoxin, procainamide, quinidine and others[162,174-176]), recombinant tissue plasminogen activator,[68,69] various anesthetics,[104] trazadone,[104] Mellaril,[54] and liquid protein diets[177] have all been associated with the occurrence of VT.

Occasionally this tachyarrhythmia is found in normal children and adults,[44,103,178] and it has been documented in all age groups, including infants.[179,180] Young adults with VT frequently have a history of cardiomyopathy, prolonged QT-interval syndrome, or mitral valve prolapse;[103,181] myocarditis and hypokalemia are also reported causes.[103] VT is quite uncommon in children who have not had intracardiac surgery,[182] but it may result from metabolic disturbances, antiarrhythmic drug toxicity,[182] cardiomyopathy,[183] or familial prolonged QT-interval syndrome.[34,184] It has also occurred rarely from intramyocardial tumor.[34,185]

In studies of SCD victims, VT deteriorating into VF was the rhythm present in the majority of cases.[6,11,19,22] When MI patients exhibit short runs of VT on a Holter monitor before discharge from the hospital, there is a higher incidence of subsequent SCD compared with those patients not exhibiting VT.[127-129]

What is the underlying mechanism in ventricular tachycardia and are there markers or indicators for its onset? These are questions that occupy a great deal of electrophysiologic research. It is known that there are two basic mechanisms: reentry and automaticity. Reentry is probably the responsible mechanism in VT as a late complication of MI and, therefore, the most commonly encountered.[160] Many things can facilitate the occurrence of ventricular tachycardia: ventricular ectopic activity, exercise, prolonged QT interval, drugs that influence the QT interval, catecholamines and catecholamine-like drugs such as isoproterenol, and severe digitalis toxicity.[160,187,188]

ECG Characteristics

Rate. Ventricular tachycardia is defined as three or more sequential, ventricular ectopic complexes, mostly regular and occurring at a rate greater than 100 bpm.[162] You will encounter in the literature varying rate definitions of VT from 120 to 140 bpm for the lower limit to 200 to 250 bpm for the higher limit. We have elected to use the lower limit of 100 bpm based on the traditional definition of a tachycardia (rate greater than 100 bpm).

QRS width. The duration of the QRS complex typically exceeds 0.12 seconds (Figs. 8-30 to 8-32). The criteria of rate and QRS width alone do not distinguish VT from a supraventricular tachycardia with aberration. Other electrocardiographic features that help to differentiate these two rhythms may be found in the box below and

Criteria Supporting VT

1. Superior right QRS axis
2. Fusion beats
3. AV dissociation
4. Monophasic R wave, qR, or RS in V_1
5. Taller left rabbit ear in V_1
6. rS, QS, or QR in V_6
7. Concordance in the precordial leads (QRS complexes are all positive or all negative in the six V leads) (Fig. 8-34)

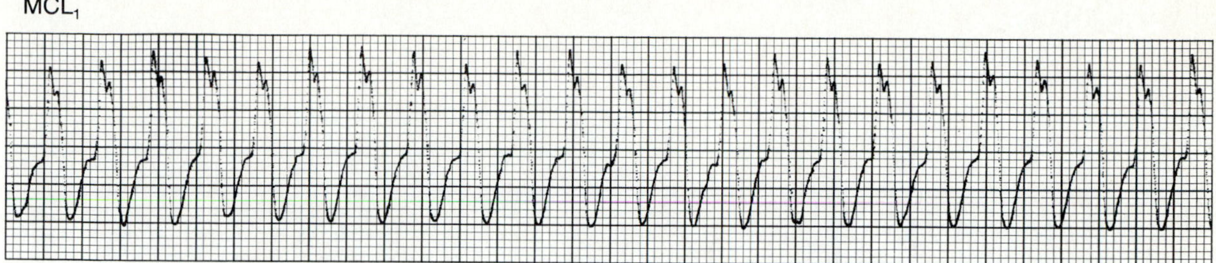

FIGURE 8-30 Ventricular tachycardia. Note wide complexes (0.12 to 0.14 seconds in duration) and left rabbit ear taller than right.

Rate: 214 bpm
Rhythm: Regular
P wave: Not identifiable
PR interval: —
QRS complex: 0.12 to 0.14 seconds
Interpretation: VT

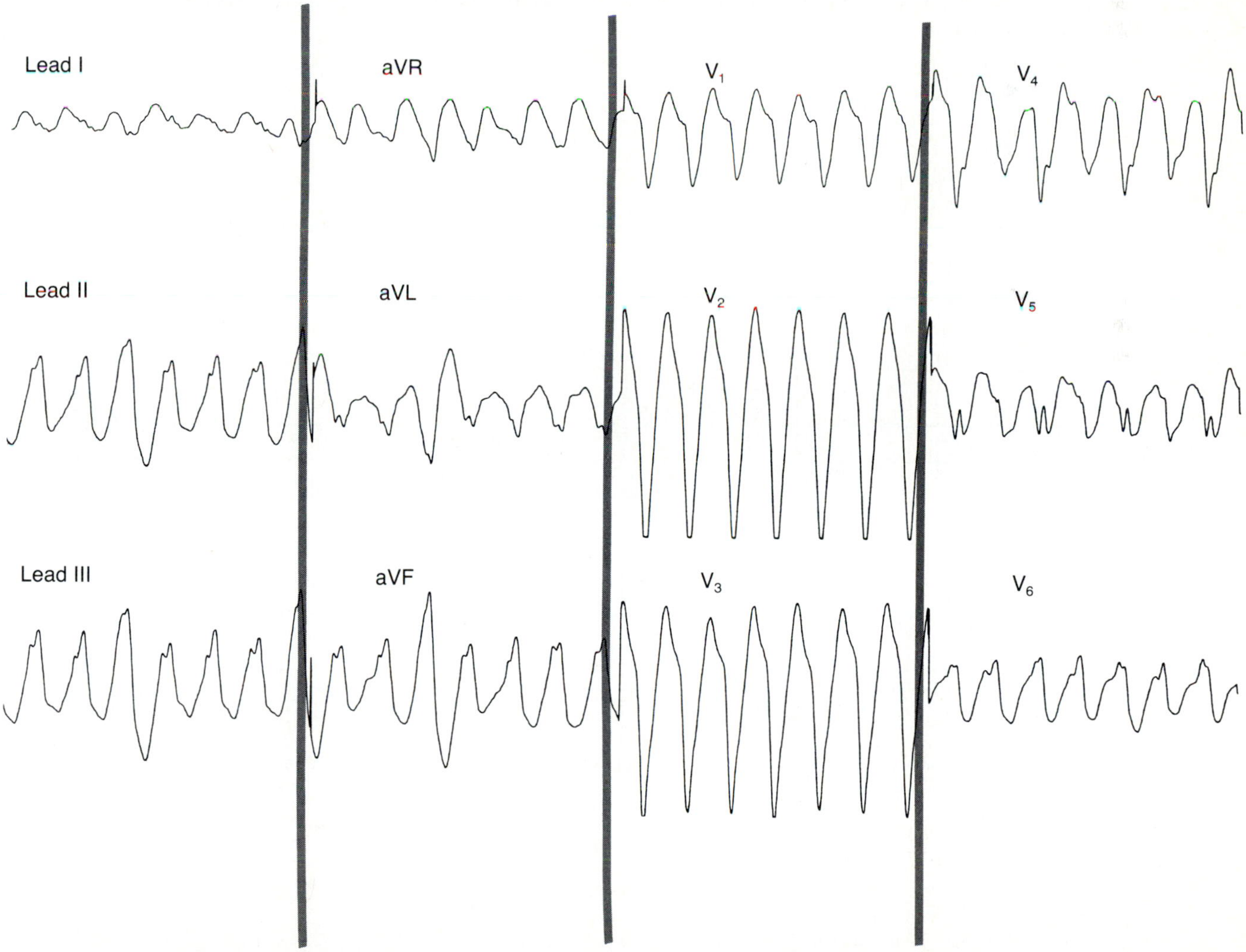

Lead I
aVR
V$_1$
V$_4$
Lead II
aVL
V$_2$
V$_5$
Lead III
aVF
V$_3$
V$_6$

FIGURE 8-31 Ventricular tachycardia recorded on a 12-lead ECG. QRS complexes are wide, 0.16 seconds. It is often difficult to ascertain the beginning and end of the QRS in wide complex tachycardias such as this. The rate is 167 bpm.

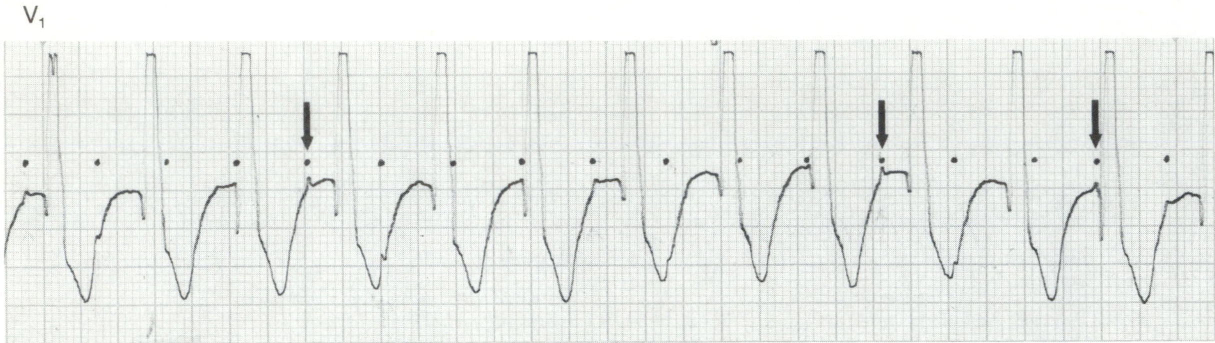

FIGURE 8-32 Ventricular tachycardia. Complexes are a wide qR pattern measuring 0.12 seconds. Independent atrial activity is identifiable *(dots).* To identify atrial activity, locate P waves *(arrows),* set your calipers to the P-P interval, then find obscured P waves. Note that atrial activity and ventricular activity are both independent (the atrial rhythm is regular at a rate of 150 bpm; the ventricular rhythm is regular at a rate of 115 to 120 bpm.). There is a P wave preceding each QRS, but it bears no constant relationship to the QRS complex.

Rate: Atrial: 150 bpm
Ventricular: 115 to 120 bpm
Rhythm: Atrial: Regular
Ventricular: Regular
P wave: Small, rapid. Atrial tachycardia. P waves bear no constant relation to QRSs.
PR interval: AV dissociation precludes PR interval measurement
QRS complex: 0.12 seconds
Interpretation: VT

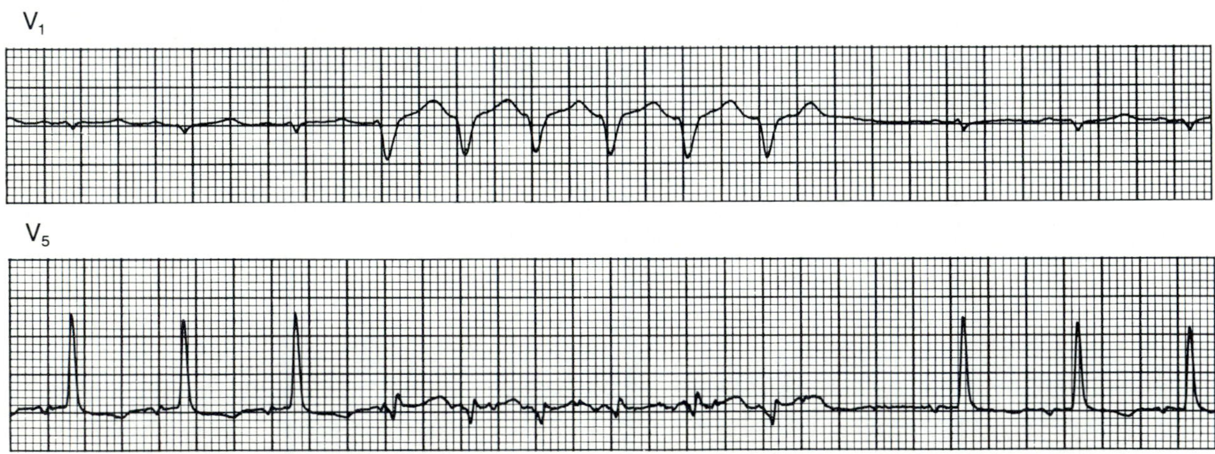

FIGURE 8-33 Nonsustained ventricular tachycardia. Simultaneous tracings of V_1 and V_5 show a short run of VT at a rate of 158 bpm.

Rate: 102 bpm increasing to 158 bpm
Rhythm: Regular rhythm interrupted by run of VT
P wave: Unusual morphology on V_5
PR interval: 0.16 to 0.18 seconds
QRS complex: 0.08 seconds. VT 0.11 to 0.12 seconds
Interpretation: ST interrupted by a 6-beat run of uniform VT

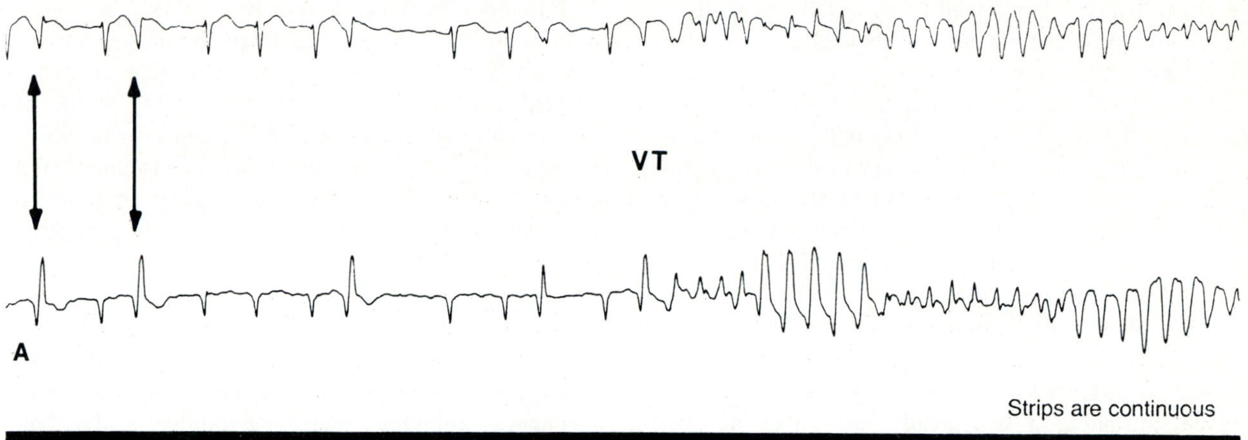

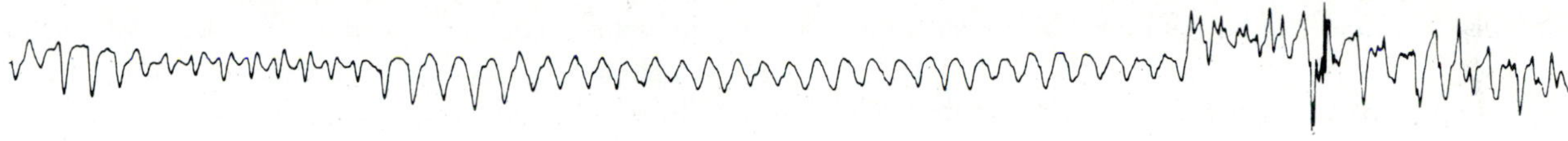

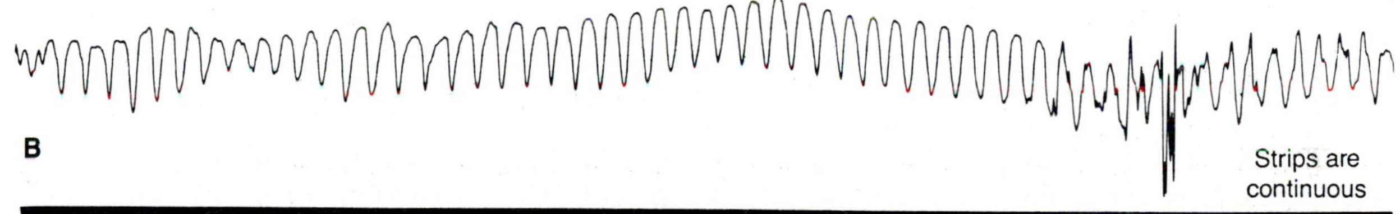

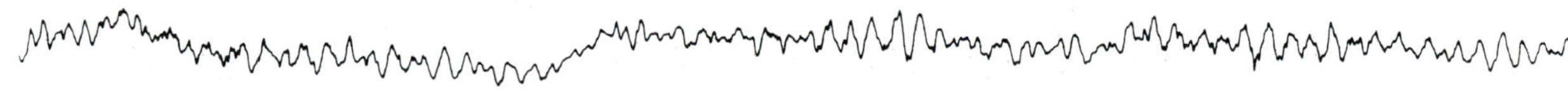

VF

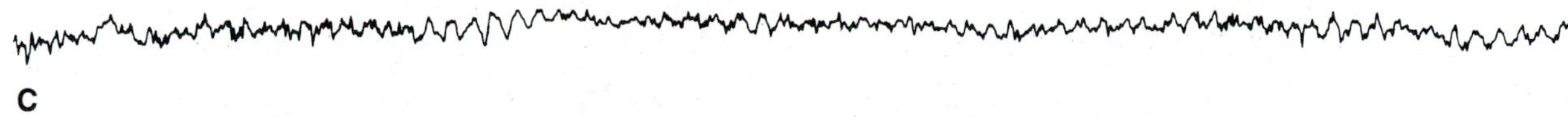

C

FIGURE 8-34 Ventricular tachycardia deteriorating into VF. Two tracings in each segment are simultaneous. Tracings are continuous. **A,** AF with frequent VPBs *(arrows)* going into a polymorphous VT (torsades de pointes). **B,** VT going into ventricular flutter and eventually deteriorating into VF in C. **C,** VF.

Chapter 10. Sometimes the origin of a tachycardia cannot be determined from surface electrocardiography and intracardiac recordings are performed to make the diagnosis.

The definition is simplistic but inadequate given the variation found in the rhythm's morphology, duration, and hemodynamic and electrical consequences. VT may be referred to as either *sustained* (duration greater than 30 seconds) or *nonsustained* (self-terminating in less than 30 seconds[162]) (Fig. 8-33). Although more likely to be well tolerated, nonsustained VT may cause serious hemodynamic compromise depending on its rate and the underlying heart disease and ventricular function.[162] Sustained VT may remain stable or deteriorate into VF (Fig. 8-34).

When VT is the rhythm preceding VF in SCD, it may be initiated by either a late-in-cycle or R-on-T VPB.[6,7,97] In this circumstance, it is typically faster than nonsustained VT with rates averaging 189 bpm and increasing to approximately 240 bpm before deteriorating into VF.[23] In Nikolic et al's review of monitored SCD cases, uniform VT with rates less than 200 bpm initiated VF in only 14% of the cases.[99]

Morphology. Morphology is another clue to the clinical import of VT. It may be monomorphic or polymorphic. Monomorphic (uniform) VTs most commonly occur in patients with chronic, ischemic heart disease who have had MIs complicated by ventricular aneurysm; they have also been observed in patients without underlying heart disease.[162] Uniform VT has variable rates and may be sustained or nonsustained (Figs. 8-30 to 8-33 and 8-35).

Polymorphic VTs. Polymorphic VTs (Figs. 8-34 and 8-36) are often very rapid and self-terminate, convert into a uniform and stable rhythm, or degenerate into VF. **Torsades de pointes** (French for twisting of the points) is a specifically recognized, rapid, and polymorphic tachyarrhythmia that is sustained or nonsustained, and not necessarily preceded by ventricular ectopy (Fig. 8-37). The rate can exceed 250 bpm, and it is often an irregular rhythm.[189]

Torsades de pointes is often, though not exclusively, associated with conditions producing a prolonged QT-interval. When it occurs, it is often observed during therapy with Class IA antiarrhythmic drugs, most commonly procainamide, quinidine, and disopyramide[6] and is believed to be the arrhythmia responsible for what is known as *quinidine syncope*[160] (syncopal episodes experienced by some individuals who take quinidine). It has also been reported with amiodarone therapy.[186] Electrolyte deficiencies in potassium, calcium, or magnesium may provoke the arrhythmia. Torsades de pointes has also been associated with coronary spasm, subarachnoid hemorrhage,[189] pneumoencephalography, intracranial trauma,[190] arsenic poisoning,[191] intracoronary papaverine,[192] terfanadine,[193] and psychotropic drugs.[194] Torsades de pointes is reported in up to 33% of monitored SCD as the arrhythmia preceding VF.[99]

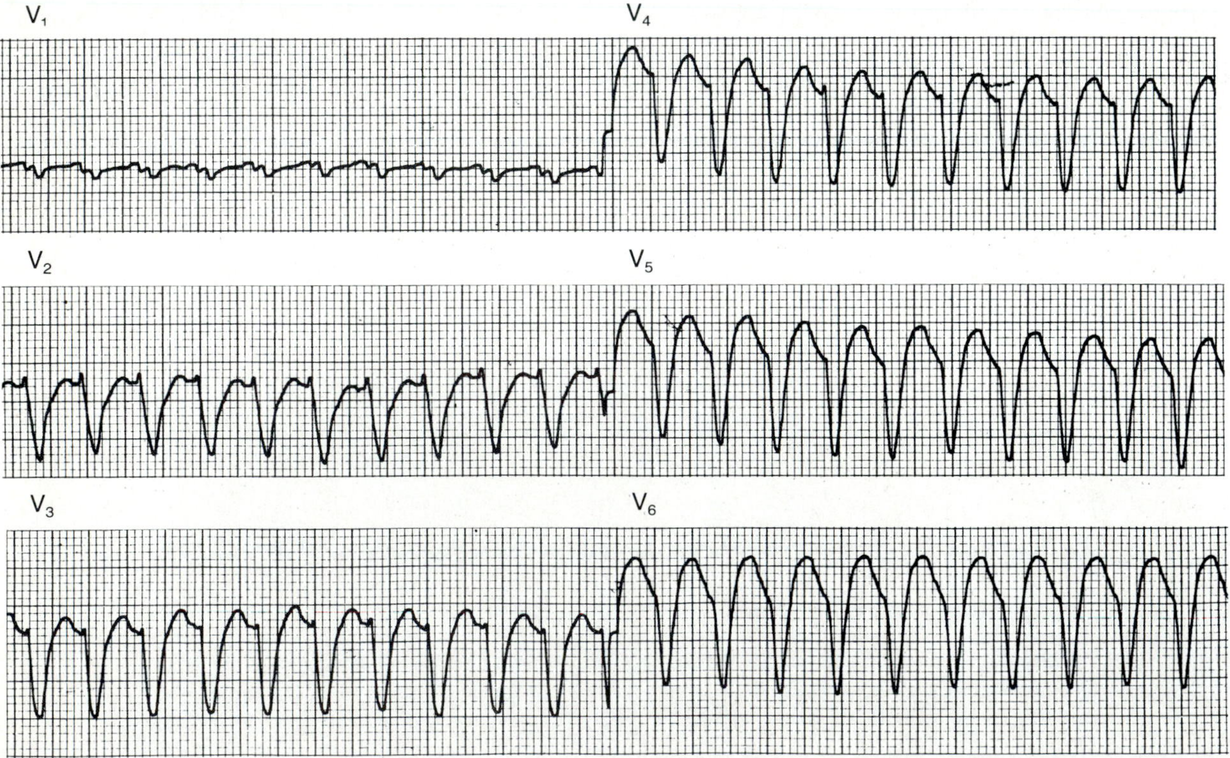

FIGURE 8-35 Monomorphic VT exhibiting concordance in the precordial leads. Note in all leads, the QRS complex is negative. When the V leads show either all positive or all negative QRS complexes, they are said to be concordant. When present, concordance supports the diagnosis of VT.

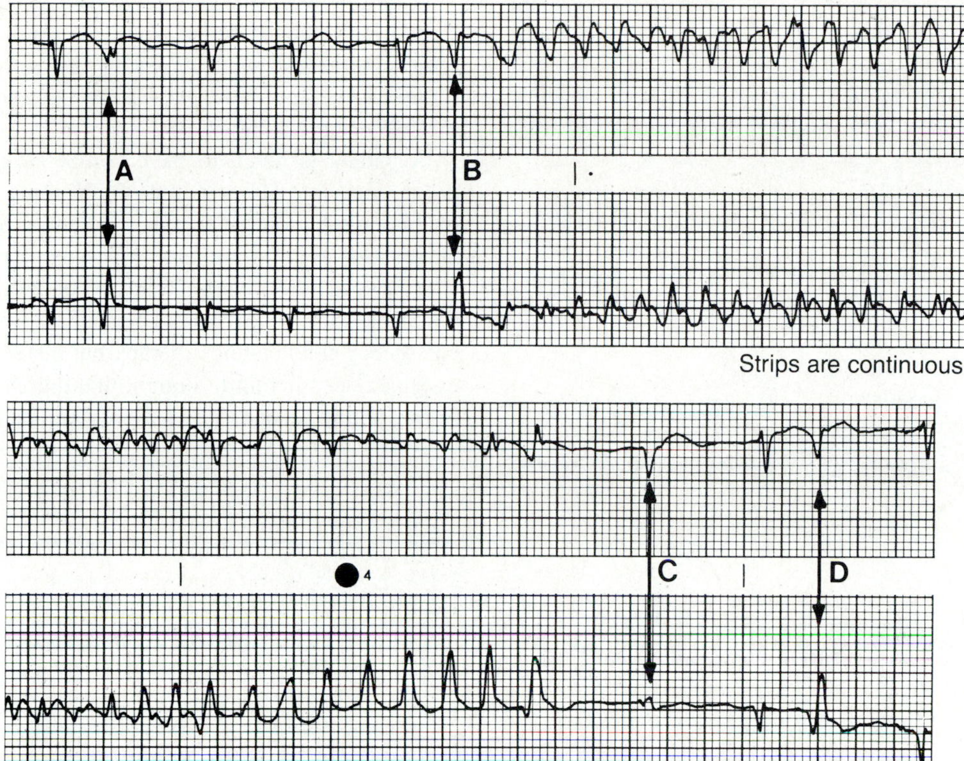

FIGURE 8-36 Polymorphic VT, nonsustained. Note in these two simultaneous tracings, the QRS complexes during the VT are of different morphologies. **A,** VPB. **B,** VPB initiating a 6-second run of polymorphic VT at a rate of approximately 320 bpm. **C,** After the VT spontaneously terminates, a ventricular ectopic beat is noted before the normally conducted QRS complex. **D,** VPB.

Rate: Approximately 120 bpm, then increases to 320 bpm, then approximately 120 bpm.
Rhythm: Irregular
P wave: Unidentifiable, AF
PR interval: —
QRS complex: 0.08 seconds; VT, VPBs 0.10 seconds and above
Interpretation: Uncontrolled AF interrupted by a 6-second run of polymorphic VT. Single VPBs precede and follow VT.

MCL$_1$

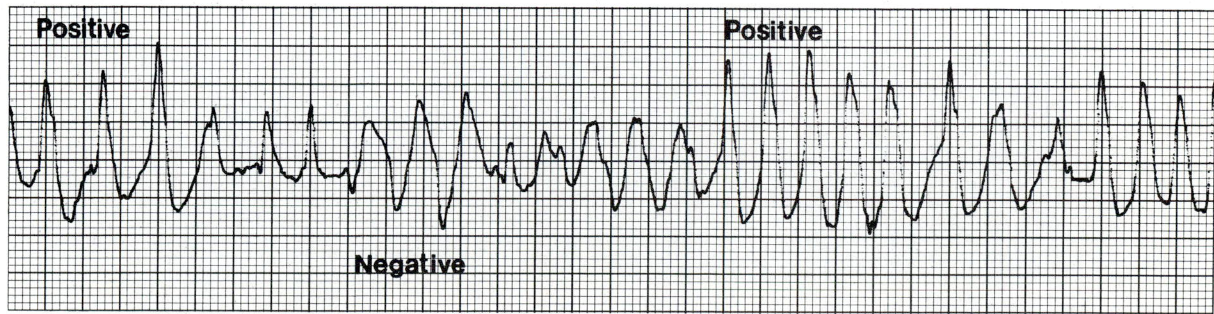

FIGURE 8-37 Torsades de pointes, a polymorphic VT, is characterized by alternating positive and negative QRS complexes.

Rate: 245 to 300 bpm
Rhythm: Irregular
P wave: Unidentifiable
PR interval: —
QRS complex: Wide, vary in morphology
Interpretation: Polymorphous VT (torsades de pointes)

It is most often initiated by late-in-cycle VPBs.[99]

See the box on this page for summary features of VT.

Ventricular flutter will be described here to avoid confusion with the use of this term. Ventricular flutter is a very rapid and coarse tachycardia in which the QRS complexes are not clearly defined. It may be thought of as a transitional or intermediary rhythm preceding VF (Fig. 8-38).

Summary.

Ventricular Tachycardia

- Three or more sequential ventricular ectopic complexes.
- Rate greater than 100 bpm (range generally 100 to 250 bpm).
- Rhythm generally regular.
- Sustained: >30 seconds.
- Nonsustained: <30 seconds.
- Prolonged QRS duration: ≥ 0.12 seconds (often >0.14 seconds).
- Can be uniform or polymorphic.

Torsades de Pointes

- Rate greater than 250 bpm.
- Polymorphic: QRS configuration continually changing.
- Often quite irregular.
- Nonsustained or sustained, can degenerate into VF.

Ventricular Flutter

- Rapid ventricular tachycardia with zigzag appearance (known as *sine wave*).
- QRS cannot be differentiated from T wave.
- When present, generally precedes VF.

Applied Nursing Process

Clinical Assessment

For the beginning practitioner, the sudden onset of VT in any patient must be immediately recognized, assessed, and regarded as a serious, potentially life-threatening arrhythmia. Note that recognition and assessment are emphasized first, before treatment. Although most patients with VT require immediate treatment, some do not. For those who require emergency management of the arrhythmia, the appropriate therapy must be quickly determined. Consider the following examples.

A patient is noted to have complex ventricular ectopy progressing into VT at a rate of 130 bpm. The recognition of this on the monitor signals a potential emergency to the nurse. However, immediate assessment reveals a patient who is conscious, complaining of palpitations, and has a blood pressure of 110/70. This patient would not require emergency countershock therapy but instead may require lidocaine. Keep in mind, though, that this rhythm could deteriorate within seconds into a more rapid tachycardia or VF.

ECG Characteristics
Ventricular Tachycardia

Rate: 100 to 250 bpm
Rhythm: Regular. May be slightly irregular. Polymorphic VT usually irregular.
P wave: May or may not be identifiable. May be retrograde atrial depolarization. AV dissociation may be present.
PR interval: Not relevant
QRS complex: 0.12 seconds or wider
Ventricular flutter QRS not differentiated from ST segment and T wave

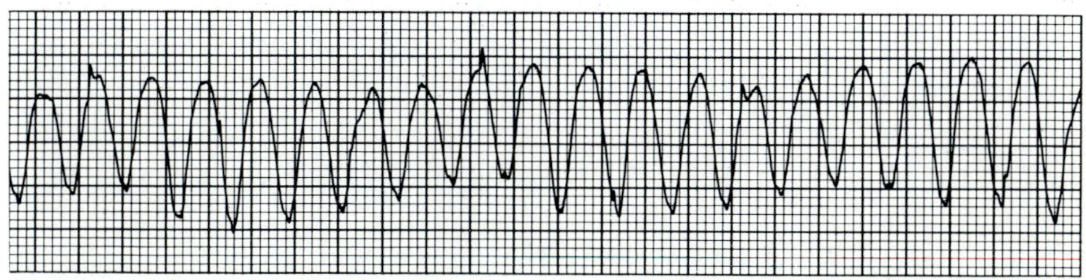

FIGURE 8-38 Ventricular flutter. VFl is diagnosed when the morphology of the QRS complexes cannot be ascertained. Is the complex negative or positive? The rhythm looks like a stretched-out spring.

Rate: 176 bpm
Rhythm: Regular
P wave: Unidentifiable
PR interval: —
QRS complex: Wide, cannot differentiate QRS complex from ST segment and T wave
Interpretation: VFl

Recognition of an unresponsive patient with VT, on the other hand, would warrant immediate electrical cardioversion before initiation of drug therapy. Rapid clinical assessment of a patient with a lethal arrhythmia, followed by the appropriate therapy, is imperative for successful management. Keep in mind that it is the patient being treated, not the arrhythmia seen on the oscilloscope.

- Detect:
  - A rapid pulse that is often thready (but not always) or no peripheral pulse.
  - A rapid, wide ventricular rhythm on the ECG.
- Assess patient and ECG.
  - Immediately assess level of consciousness: syncope or near-syncope, light-headedness, dizziness.
  - Measure blood pressure.
  - Palpate for peripheral pulses.
  - If the patient is conscious and stable, assess the following:

    Duration of rhythm.

    Character of arrhythmia (make certain it is not artifact such as scratching the positive electrode) (Fig. 8-39).

    Signs and symptoms that may indicate decreased myocardial perfusion such as chest discomfort and shortness of breath.

    Signs and symptoms that are consistent with decreased cardiac output such as pallor, cool and clammy skin, and altered mentation.

    Stat 12-lead ECG if there is opportunity to obtain one.

    Serum electrolytes: potassium, calcium, and magnesium.

    The clinical setting. Is the patient a candidate for VT (acute MI, history of wide-complex tachycardia, ventricular ectopic activity recorded on Holter, history of VF, syncope, other cardiac disorders, use of drug known to cause VT, hypokalemia, hypomagnesemia, hypocalcemia)? What is the underlying cardiac disorder (acute or chronic MI, mitral valve prolapse, ischemic heart disease, congestive cardiomyopathy, ventricular aneurysm, long QT syndrome)? Is there documented evidence of spontaneous VT on the ECG or Holter, or induced VT in the exercise or electrophysiology laboratory?
  - Always remember to ask the patient frequently how he/she feels. Useful information can be gained from doing this. Occasionally one encounters a patient who is unaware of the tachycardia, and this is significant for prognostic and future care planning reasons. VT with specific cause in children is usually symptomatic, but the idiopathic VT of childhood is generally asymptomatic; this may be due to the slower rate of this type of tachycardia.[182]
  - Diagnose the arrhythmia. Detect a regular wide QRS tachycardia and follow the algorithm in Fig. 8-40.

❖ NURSING DIAGNOSIS

(1) Decreased cardiac output related to tachycardia. (2) Altered tissue perfusion: cardiopulmonary/peripheral/cerebral, related to decreased cardiac output. (3) Pain (anginal), related to myocardial ischemia. (4) Knowledge deficit regarding management of ventricular tachycardia at home.

❖ ECG DIAGNOSIS:

Ventricular tachycardia.

Plan and Implementation

Patient goal. During VT, the patient's hemodynamic status will be maintained; the significance of the arrhythmia will be determined.

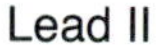

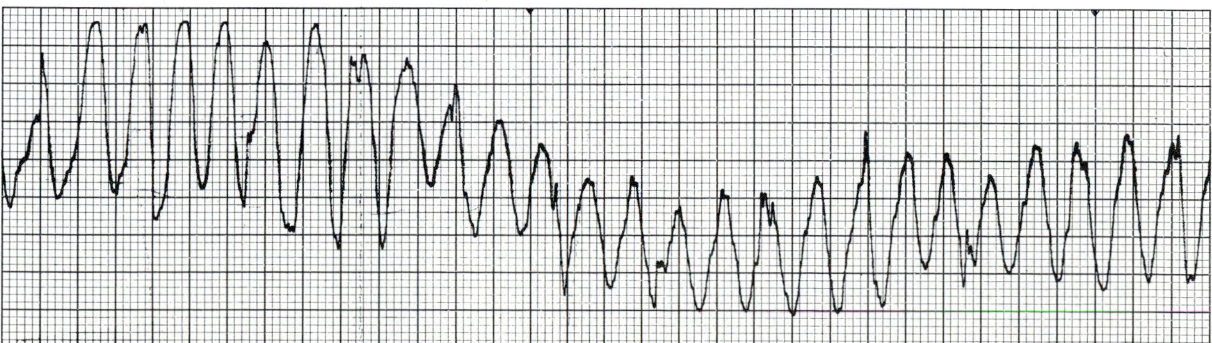

FIGURE 8-39 Ventricular flutter? No, just an itchy left leg electrode. This tracing was produced by scratching the electrode to relieve itching beneath it. It is included to stress the importance of treating the patient, not the monitor artifact.

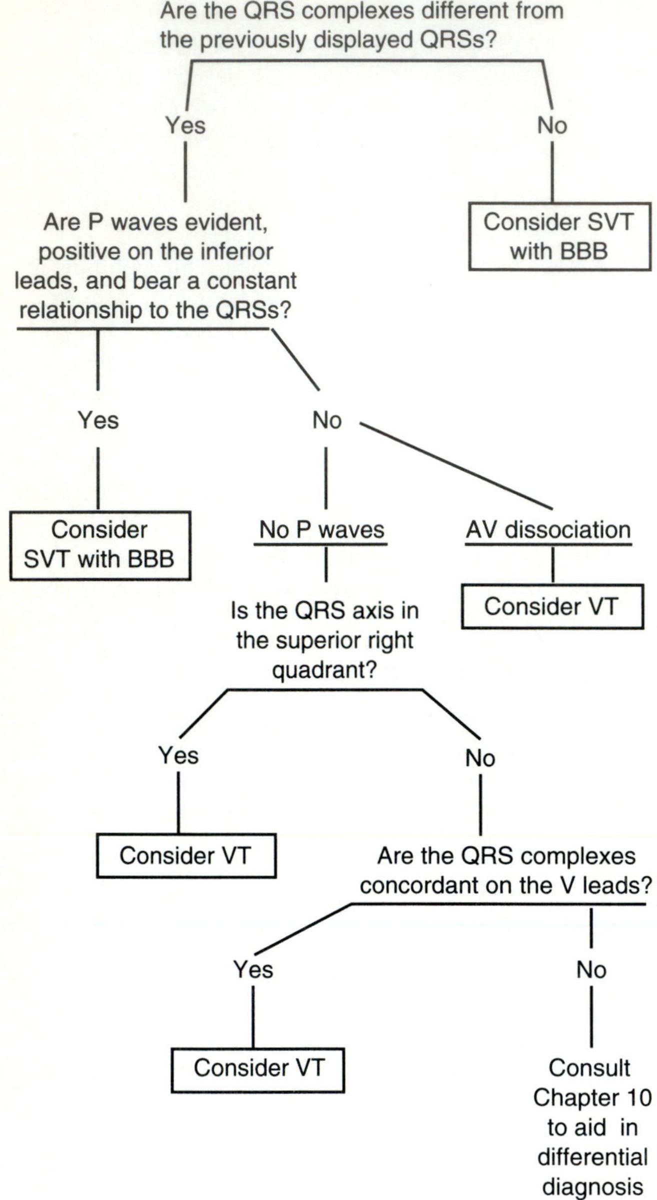

FIGURE 8-40 VT algorithm.

The patient will regain normal sinus rhythm in the easiest and safest way possible; the patient's arrhythmia will not deteriorate into VF.

Before discharge, the patient with chronic VT will relate appropriate information regarding drugs, diet, exercise, pacemaker management, automatic internal cardioverter/defibrillator (as indicated), and other self-care measures.

Nursing interventions.

- If the patient is unconscious, immediately consider the following interventions according to institutional policy and/or physician's orders, and your clinical judgment:
  - Precordial thump.
  - Electrical countershock.
  - CPR.
  - Antiarrhythmic drug therapy such as lidocaine, bretylium, or procainamide.
- Notify others of ***cardiac arrest***.
- Notify physician immediately.
- If the patient is near-syncopal:
  - Warn him or her of a precordial thump.
  - Cardiovert if thump is not effective.
- For those patients who require CPR, if you can intervene while the patient is still conscious, instruct the patient to cough hard every 1 to 3 seconds. Coughing forcefully produces hemodynamic events that are nearly identical to CPR. "Cough CPR" thus may be a useful adjunct in maintaining consciousness in the precious seconds immediately after a cardiac arrest not only for patients in VT but also for those in asystole, profound bradycardia with hypotension, and early VF.[195,196]
- If the patient is conscious:
  - Begin drug regimen (lidocaine, procainamide, quinidine, bretylium, or investigational agents according to institutional policy).
  - Sedate the patient if cardioversion is anticipated. Do not cardiovert someone who is awake.
  - Prepare for possible emergency pacemaker insertion for overdrive or underdrive pacing to abolish the arrhythmia.
- Remember that electrical cardioversion of patients who are digitalis toxic often elicits postcardioversion VPBs and possibly intractable VF or VT. This is not to say that these patients should not be countershocked; they should be if necessary. For these patients, VT has a high mortality rate. Treatment may include lidocaine, magnesium, or phenytoin. Future treatment will likely include antidigitalis antibodies. If the digitalis level is within therapeutic range, cardioversion does not appear to carry this risk.[198]
- Note the rate, duration, and morphology of the tachycardia and the beats that initiated or triggered the rhythm.
- For patients with torsades de pointes, proceed as described previously for the unconscious patient (except for the administration of procainamide, a class IA antiarrhythmic).
  - Treatment with isoproterenol, once normal rhythm has been restored, may be helpful in shortening the QT interval, if prolonged.[190] Its use is contraindicated in acute MI, angina pectoris, or hypertension. If given erroneously to a patient in VT that is not torsade de pointes, it may be fatal.[87]
  - If the patient is on any drugs that are known to cause this arrhythmia, such as the Class IA antiarrhythmics, hold subsequent doses until the physician has been notified.
  - Obtain serum potassium, magnesium, and calcium ac-

cording to hospital policy and administer magnesium and potassium supplements as ordered.
  - If the arrhythmia is associated with a prolonged QT interval, intravenous magnesium sulfate may be indicated, even if the patient's serum magnesium appears normal.[197]
  - Prepare for possible emergency pacemaker insertion. Pacing at a rate faster than the patient's rate is sometimes effective in shortening the QT interval.[190]
- Be fully informed of the dosage range, side effects, signs of toxicity, and electrocardiographic effects of the antiarrhythmic agents. Combination therapy (two or more drugs) for arrhythmia control has become fairly common.
- Routinely measure the PR interval and QRS width and calculate the QTc. Notify physician if a clinically significant change in QTc occurs in patients treated with antiarrhythmic drugs (a change of >0.075 seconds or a QTc value >0.50 seconds).[149]
- The patient with chronic, recurrent VT needs to be appropriately informed of the dosages and side effects of his/her antiarrhythmic drugs: procainamide, quinidine, calcium-channel blockers, beta blockers, digoxin, and investigational agents.
- Before discharge, reinforce the following points:
  - What symptoms warrant notifying the physician.
  - Outpatient clinic dates.
  - Exercise restrictions.
  - Driving restriction (if any).
- If indicated, arrange for the family to receive CPR training and instructions for use of the defibrillator in the home.
- If indicated, instruct the patient and family in other treatment modalities: arrhythmia surgery, magnet for radio frequency pacemakers, and internal cardioverter/defibrillator (ICD) (refer to Chapter 12).
- If indicated, instruct patient in use of transtelephonic and random (TAM II) ambulatory recorders.
- Obtain serum drug levels when ordered or indicated.
- Implement physician's orders; evaluate the effectiveness of measures taken to control the arrhythmia.

Evaluation

- The patient maintains/regains hemodynamic status during VT as evidenced by the following:
  - Maintenance of consciousness or immediate regaining of consciousness after arrhythmia terminated.
  - Maintenance of blood pressure or return of blood pressure with termination of the arrhythmia.
- The patient has stable cardiac rhythm as evidenced by normal sinus rhythm on the oscilloscope.
- If chronic VT, the patient understands the treatment regimen as evidenced by the ability to relate the appropriate information concerning care of the arrhythmia at home.

Important aspects in evaluating the patient with chronic, recurrent VT include all those aspects included in the preceding section, VPBs. The patient's physical response to antiarrhythmic drug therapy and understanding of it are very important because adverse physical and electrocardiographic effects are common. Ideally the patient has adapted to living with a chronic and life-threatening illness and complies with follow-up care.

Medical Treatment[160,173,199,200]

Pharmacologic

Because VT has many causes, successful drug therapy depends on the underlying disorder, the mechanism of the tachycardia, proper dosage, and the individual response to the drug. Failure of a pharmacologic regimen may be the result of toxic reactions necessitating discontinuance, insufficient dosage of an effective drug, or an ineffective drug. Antiarrhythmic drugs are classified by their effect on the action potential duration.

Class I. Traditionally used in the management of chronic, recurrent VT.

IA. Quinidine-like: procainamide, moricizine, quinidine, disopyramide.
Class IA drugs may be associated with the development of torsades de pointes.

IB. Lidocaine-like: lidocaine, phenytoin, mexiletine, tocainide.

IC. Flecainide, encainide, propafenone.

Class II. Beta-adrenergic blocking agents are used for VT associated with the following:

1. Transient, acute ischemia.
2. Catecholamine or exercise-induced VT.
3. Congenital long QT syndrome.
4. In combination with other antiarrhythmic drugs, particularly Class IA.

Class III. Sotalol, NAPA, bretylium, amiodarone.

Class IV. Calcium-channel blocking agents are traditionally used for the following:

1. Angina pectoris.
2. Unstable angina (from coronary spasm).
3. Supraventricular arrhythmias.

They are currently being investigated for use in ventricular tachyarrhythmias, especially in patients with VT who have no heart disease.

Nonpharmacologic

The following nonpharmacologic treatments may be used:

- Antitachycardia pacemakers.
- Implantable cardioverter defibrillator (ICD).
- Arrhythmia surgery and ablative therapy.
  - Endocardial resection with or without ventricular aneurysmectomy.
  - Encircling ventriculotomy.
  - Cryoablation.
  - Catheter ablation.
  - Epicardial and endocardial laser ablation.

VENTRICULAR FIBRILLATION

Data Base: Problem Identification

Definitions, Etiology, and Mechanisms

Ventricular fibrillation (VF) is the most common mechanism of SCD.[13] It is defined as chaotic asynchronous activation of cardiac tissue with numerous wavefronts of depolarization and repolarization resulting in multiple sites of reentrant activity.[201] The consequence is chaotic and ineffective mechanical activity with cessation of synchronous ventricular contraction.[201] The process can be initiated by reentry or rapid impulse formation.[13] Death ensues within minutes unless VF is terminated and a normal rhythm restored. Very rarely is VF self-terminating.[24,202,203]

VF is classified as either primary or secondary. Primary VF is of sudden onset in a patient without profound hypotension or cardiac failure. Secondary VF occurs as a terminal rhythm in patients with circulatory failure.[204] Primary VF is much easier to correct with electrical intervention, and our discussion is limited to it.

VF requires not only the presence of some excitable stimulus to initiate it and a critical mass of myocardium involved to sustain it but also nonuniformity of myocardial refractory period durations.[13,205] In other words, in order for the heart to fibrillate, something has to start it, enough of the myocardium has to be involved in the fibrillation, and electrical imbalance and instability are present.

VF is particularly common after acute MI or myocardial ischemia with the highest incidence immediately after insult.[115] Ischemia and infarction may reduce the threshold for VT or VF 30-fold.[108] The incidence of primary VF is 2% to 11%* to as high as 62.5%[111] within the first hour after symptom onset in acute MI. The mortality rate with primary VF may be as high as 47%.[116,206] In those who survive VF in the setting of acute MI, the prognosis resembles that of persons with similar infarctions who did not fibrillate.[5,207,208] In those episodes of VF resulting in SCD that are not associated with MI, however, the mortality rate is considerably higher.[5,120,207]

Other conditions that may facilitate the development of spontaneous VF include factors that provoke electrical instability of the myocardium such as:

- Prolonged QT interval†
- WPW syndrome[27]
- Electrocution and other electrical injuries[13]
- Cardiac catheterization
- Electrolyte imbalances:‡
  - Hypokalemia
  - Hypomagnesemia
- Metabolic acidosis[13]
- Hypothermia
- Drugs:[13,24,211-215]
  - Cocaine
  - Digitalis
  - Antiarrhythmic drugs, typically Class IA
  - Phenothiazines
  - Tricyclic antidepressants
- Inhalation of typewriter correction fluid[67]
- Cigarette smoking in the presence of myocardial ischemia[216-218]
- Exercise in the presence of myocardial ischemia[219]
- Autonomic nervous system imbalance:[13,191,205,220-222]
  - Beta-adrenergic stimulation
  - Vagal stimulation
  - High sympathetic tone combined with increasing parasympathetic tone
- Myocardial ischemia, reperfusion, and thrombolysis*
- Bradycardia[13]: A slow heart rate can have the following effects, all of which may enhance reentry:
  - Increase the duration of the relative refractory and vulnerability periods
  - Can increase the difference between the duration of action potential in the Purkinje and ventricular fibers
  - Can increase dispersion of refractoriness within the ventricular myocardium
- Emotional factors† including psychosocial stressors and intense activity of the central nervous system. Emotional arousal induces dramatic endocrine responses via the sympathetic-adrenal medullary system or the pituitary-adrenal cortical system. Emotional stress is a common precursor to SCD.
- Nonionic hyperosmolar angiography contrast medium[196]
- Other factors contributing to the pathogenesis of SCD include, but are not limited to, coronary artery disease, ventricular hypertrophy, cardiomyopathy, mitral valve prolapse, and conduction system pathology.[81,225-227]
- Myocardial scarring occurring in patients with previous MI and significant left ventricular dysfunction.[120]

In studies, victims of SCD (most often with documented VF) some similarities have been identified. The hearts of these people are significantly larger than those of control subjects,[228] they exhibit less heart rate variability,[229-230] and there is evidence in most of catecholamine excess.[220] SCD most commonly strikes men over the age of 50 who have coronary heart disease. Usually occurring during routine daily activities, most often in the morning, SCD is notorious for not providing any warning.[2,6,7,23] As can be surmised from the previous list, there are some puzzling and apparently contradictory contributing factors. There are likely subtle interactions that have not yet been fully recognized. What is known, however, is that many who fibrillate possess one or more of the above conditions. It is also recognized that a larger population possessing these same characteristics and conditions do not succumb to SCD.

*113-116, 118, 135, 145
†13, 17, 120, 209, 210
‡13, 72, 73, 86, 88, 89, 135

*13, 15-17, 49, 68, 120
†13, 205, 220, 221, 223, 224

"HEY, BACK OFF,
THIS WIRE JUST CAME
OFF!!"
Mindy Miller

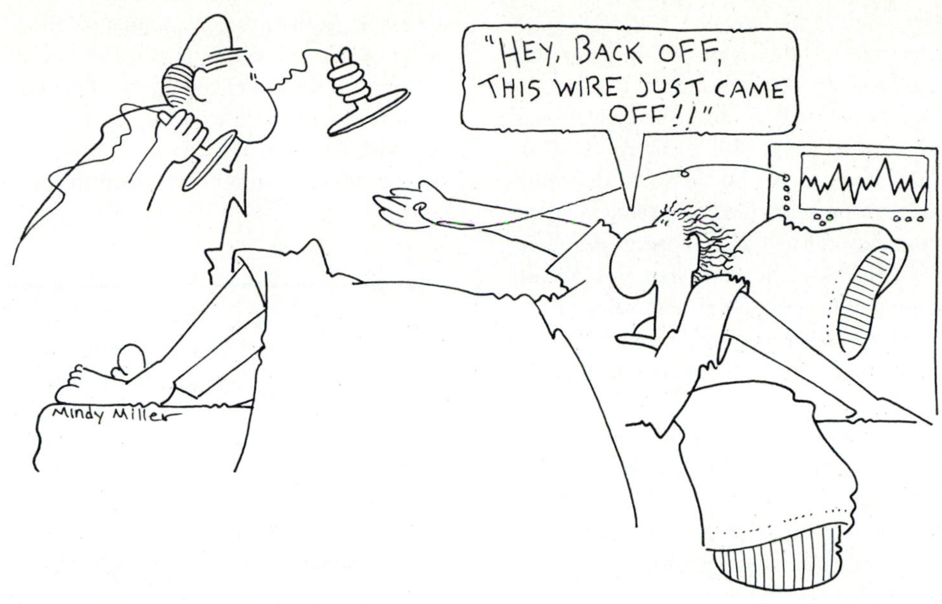

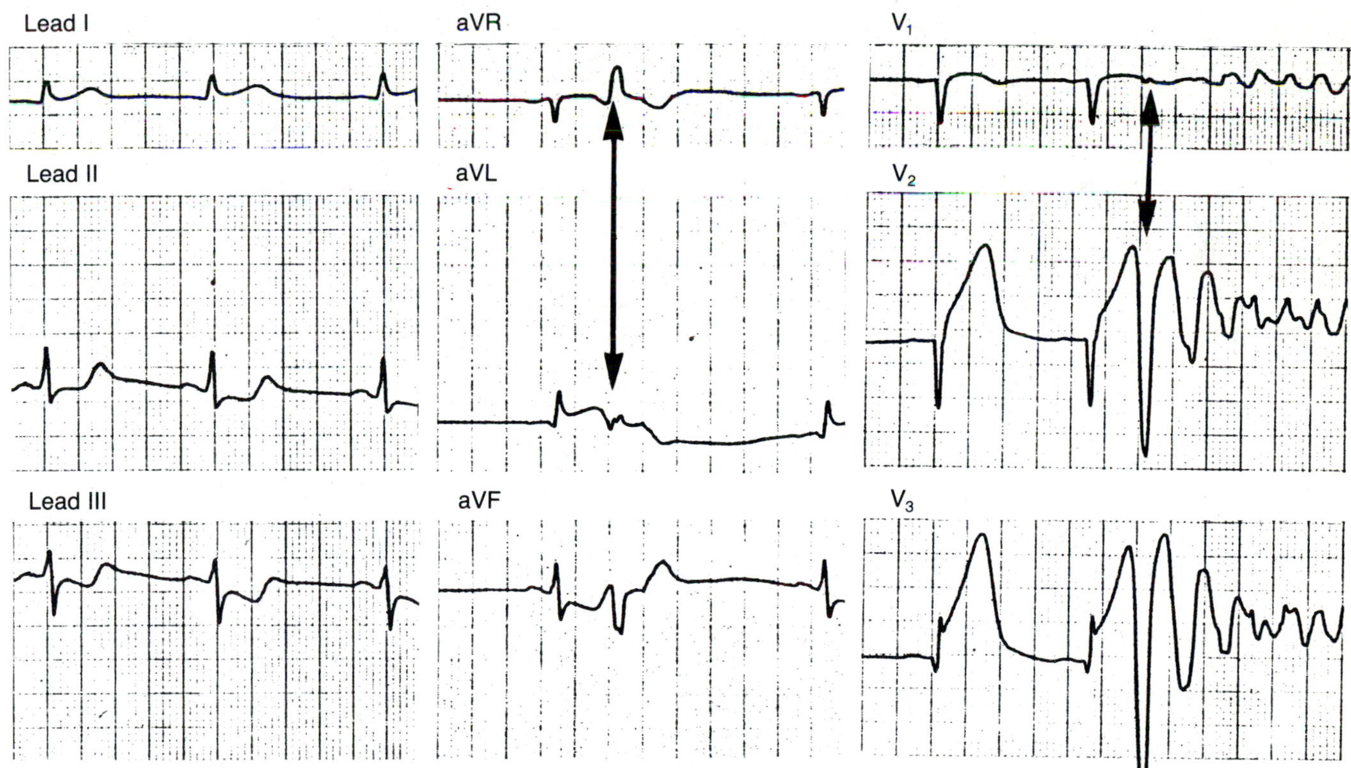

FIGURE 8-41 NSR to VF. During the recording of a 12-lead ECG, this patient, who experienced a recent anterolateral MI (note elevated ST segments in aVL, V_2, V_3), began exhibiting R-on-T VPBs *(arrow)* first detected during the simultaneous recording of aVR, aVL, and aVF. The next R-on-T VPB *(second arrow)* occurred during simultaneous recording of V_1, V_2, and V_3. Note how large the initiating VPB appears in leads V_2 and V_3, but it is nearly isoelectric in V_1. We hope this reinforces the recommendation to view arrhythmias on various leads. A unit should not have a policy of monitoring all patients on the same lead or on one lead.

ECG Characteristics

The rate of VF is rapid but too disorganized to count. The ECG pattern is irregular with no identifiable P waves or QRS complexes (Fig. 8-41). VF is described electrocardiographically as either fine (Fig. 8-42) or coarse (Fig. 8-43); the latter being much more amenable to defibrillation, probably because it represents the ECG early in arrest. Certain lead orientation may cause a VF to appear fine when, in fact, it is coarse[231] (Fig. 8-41, look at lead V_1). Should this situation be encountered, change the lead selector to a different lead. When VF persists for several minutes, it loses amplitude and becomes fine, reflecting degeneration of cellular function.[231]

VF can be initiated by either early or late-in-cycle VPBs, or it may be the end result of ventricular tachycardia (refer to previous discussions on SCD, VT, and VPBs initiating VF). Under rare circumstances, the origin of the excitable stimulus may be the atria. (Examples of situations in which this could happen include a patient who has accessory pathways, or conduction tissue that bypasses the AV node, as in WPW syndrome, the discussion of which is reserved for advanced study. This may also occur in situations where there is rapid AV nodal conduction coexisting with a long QT interval.[13]) Summary features for ventricular fibrillation are presented in the box below.

ECG Characteristics
Ventricular Fibrillation

Rate: Too fast to count
Rhythm: Grossly irregular
P wave: Not identifiable
PR interval: None
QRS complex: Not differentiated

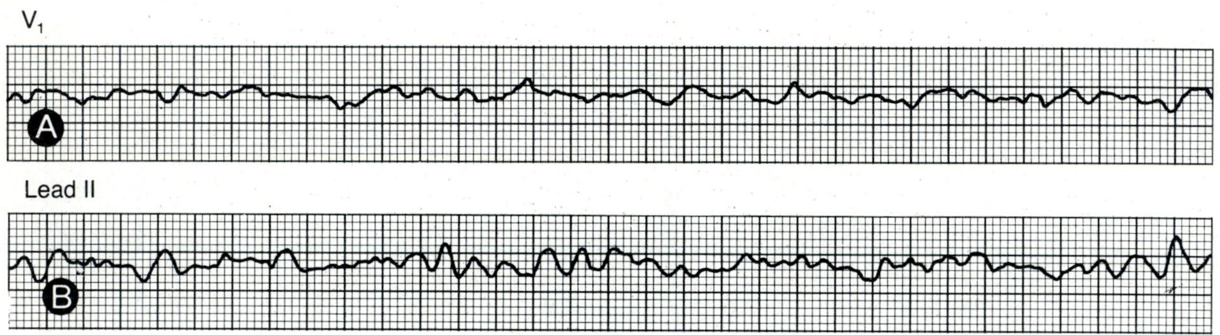

FIGURE 8-42 Two examples of fine VF.

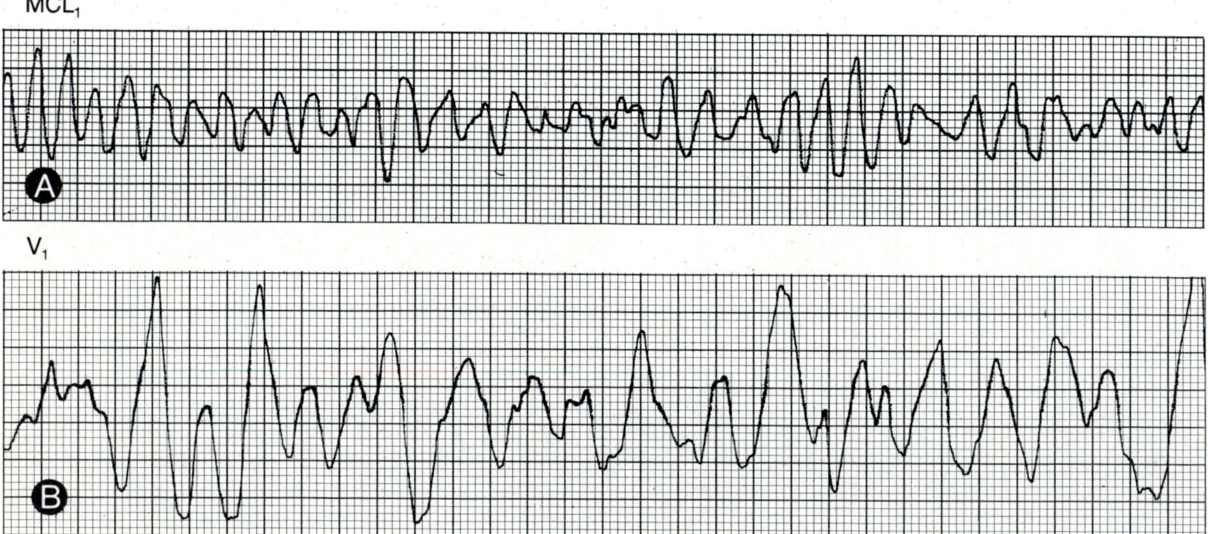

FIGURE 8-43 Two examples of coarse VF.

Applied Nursing Process

Clinical Assessment

- Detect:
  - Pulselessness, nonresponsiveness, apnea, or agonal respirations.
  - Chaotic ECG rhythm with no QRS complexes.
- Assess patient and ECG.

  The sudden onset of VF in any patient must be **immediately** recognized, assessed, and corrected. Prompt recognition and correction of the disturbance are imperative to prevent end-organ damage from prolonged circulatory collapse.
  - Identify VF on the monitor and make certain the rhythm is not artifact (Fig. 8-44) by confirming the ECG findings with the patient's clinical signs.
  - Establish pulselessness, apnea, and nonresponsiveness. On initial assessment, you may find the patient still semiconscious but deteriorating quickly.

❖ NURSING DIAGNOSIS

(1) Decreased cardiac output related to cessation of ventricular contraction. (2) Altered tissue perfusion: cerebral / cardiopulmonary / peripheral / renal / gastrointestinal, related to cessation of ventricular contraction. (3) Knowledge deficit regarding care of automatic implantable defibrillator/cardioverter at home.

❖ ECG DIAGNOSIS

Ventricular fibrillation.

Plan and Implementation

Patient goal. The patient will regain a pulse-producing rhythm before irreversible cellular damage has occurred.

The person with an implantable cardioverter/defibrillator will relate appropriate information concerning home care.

Nursing interventions.

- The presence of VF requires **immediate** conversion to a pulse-producing rhythm. If the VF is of recent onset (i.e., seconds) a precordial thump may, rarely, convert the rhythm. Usually, though, direct current (DC) countershock (see the box on p. 224) is required and is administered as soon as possible. The longer VF persists, the more resistant it is to electric shock.[201,232]
- As with VT, cough CPR may be used if the patient has not yet lost consciousness. Instruct the patient to "cough hard!" every 1 to 3 seconds.[195]
- Initiate CPR at once and continue for the duration of pulselessness.
- Notify others of **cardiac arrest.**
- Assess acid-base balance; correction of an imbalance makes successful resuscitation more likely.
- Administer medications to promote defibrillation and/or prevent recurrence of VF (see box on p. 224).
- Implement physician's orders; evaluate the effectiveness of measures taken to prevent recurrence of VF.
- If indicated, teach the patient and family home management for an implantable cardioverter/defibrillator (see Chapter 13).

Evaluation

- The patient has a return of a pulse-producing rhythm providing adequate tissue perfusion as evidenced by the following:
  - Palpable peripheral pulses.
  - Return of blood pressure.
  - Absence of pallor, cyanosis.
  - Warm, dry skin.
  - Return of consciousness.
- The patient with ICD relates appropriate information concerning care of ICD at home as evidenced by ability to state factors specific to individualized patient teaching plan.

Medical Treatment

In addition to those measures described in the preceding section, additional approaches may provide prophylaxis for VF. Intravenous nitroglycerin, provided hypotension is controlled, is thought to prevent VF in the presence of acute MI.[242] Other prophylactic measures include those that are used in the treatment of VT.

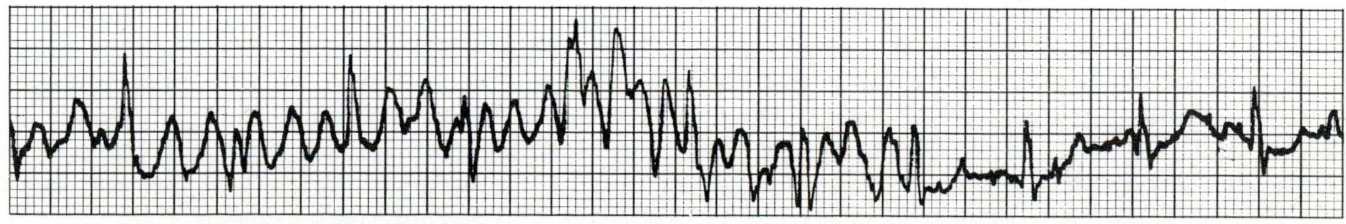

FIGURE 8-44 This tracing appears to be VF converting to ST. It is actually artifact produced by tapping the positive electrode.

Defibrillation

Countershock

Countershock accomplishes defibrillation by cardiac depolarization. The sinus node, or another pacemaker with higher automaticity, is then able to assume dominance with a well-ordered depolarization-repolarization sequence.[201]

Countershock is accomplished by delivering an electric shock 200 to 400 joules to the precordium. Repeated shocks at the same setting result in more energy delivered than the sum of the energy administered. When higher energies are used, the myocardium and subjacent tissues may sustain serious damage[233] and postconversion arrhythmias such as prolonged periods of asystole, third-degree AV block, and malignant ventricular arrhythmias.[201] Repeated shocks with high energy may result in resumption of VF because of progressive myocardial deterioration.[234] In the presence of digitalis toxicity, high energy defibrillation is extremely dangerous, the mechanism of which is not entirely clear.[201]

Variables complicating the threshold for defibrillation include the underlying condition of the myocardium, electrolyte and acid-base imbalance, and the degree of hypoxemia or hypothermia,[235] and the duration of VF.[232]

In children, 2 w-s/kg body weight has been recommended for a starting energy dose in defibrillation.[235] Refer to Chapter 12 for further details.

When a patient with an implanted pacemaker requires defibrillation, make certain the paddles are not overlying the battery pack or leads. Newer pulse generators have greatly improved resistance to the effects of external defibrillation, but damage can occur if the anterior paddles are placed directly over the generator or lead. Anterior paddles should be placed at least 5 inches from the generator and lead system, with confirmation of pacer function after defibrillation.[236]

Pharmacologic adjuncts to defibrillation

Bretylium tosylate has been found to be a helpful adjunct in the treatment of sustained VF refractory to lidocaine, other drugs, or multiple DC shocks[237,238] and should be used if DC countershock is not successful. Bretylium often renders the heart susceptible to defibrillation. It has also been credited with the ability to achieve chemical ventricular defibrillation.[239]

Administration of epinephrine often makes the VF more amenable to DC shock, especially if the VF is fine.[201] The routine use of epinephrine in the presence of VF is controversial, however. Since plasma levels of catecholamines in cardiac arrest are much higher than what is required to stimulate cardiac activity, some advocate the use of atropine if defibrillation has failed in the victim who is neither acidotic nor hypoxemic.[240]

Studies have shown that when prophylactic lidocaine is used immediately after symptom onset in MI, incidence of VF is less than 1%, ten times less than the incidence of VF when the warning arrhythmias are used as criteria for therapy initiation.[122,241] Magnesium sulfate may also be a useful adjunct in the prophylaxis of VF in susceptible individuals.[87,148]

ACCELERATED IDIOVENTRICULAR RHYTHM

Data Base: Problem Identification

Definitions, Etiology, and Mechanisms

In Chapter 1, subsidiary pacemakers were discussed. It was explained that pacemaker cells in the sinus (SA) node were normally in command of the heart's rhythm because the inherent rate of automatic depolarization in the SA node was faster than inherent rates of other pacemaker cells. If, for some reason the SA node fails to deliver an impulse, the next higher pacemaker would assume control. In most cases this would be the AV junction, whose inherent rate of diastolic depolarization is 40 to 70 bpm. The lowest of the subsidiary pacemakers are the pacemaker cells located in the ventricles. These possess an inherent rate of diastolic depolarization in the range of 10 to 40 bpm. When these subsidiary pacemakers are allowed to control the rhythm, the result is a slow rate (between 10 and 40 bpm) with wide, bizarre QRS complexes (that look like VPBs but are not premature). This rhythm is labeled *idioventricular rhythm* (IVR). Sometimes an IVR assumes control of the heart's rhythm but the rate at which it does so is faster than the inherent rate of the ventricle, 10 to 40 bpm, yet slower than tachycardia.[243] This is known as *accelerated idioventricular rhythm* (AIVR).

The term *accelerated idioventricular rhythm,* suggested by Marriott and Menendez,[244] describes the characteristics of the arrhythmia: an IVR that is accelerated beyond the inherent rate of the ventricles (10 to 40) yet below the "tachycardia" limit of VT. So the rate range established for AIVR is above 40 and less than 100 (although in practice the lower limit is more often 50).

The mechanism responsible for AIVR is probably the development of rapid phase 4 depolarization and discharge of normally latent pacemaker cells.[245] These pacemaker cells in the ventricles reach threshold and depolarize provided there is opportunity; either the basic sinus rhythm is decreased or the idioventricular pacemaker is enhanced[101,103] allowing the escape of, or usurpation by, the

AIVR. This discussion is limited to the escape type of AIVR.

The idioventricular pacemaker is depolarized by each conducted sinus impulse and only reaches threshold spontaneously when the interval between sinus beats is long enough. That is why the first beat of an AIVR is late in diastole with a long coupling interval.[246] AIVR is analogous to a ventricular triggered demand pacemaker[246] with a rate set similar to the sinus rate. Like the demand pacemaker, when the sinus rate decreases enough the pacemaker "kicks in".

Relatively common during the acute stages of MI, AIVR is believed to be a benign arrhythmia.[103,246-248] In this clinical setting, its incidence ranges from 9%[246] to 46%,[103,247] it occurs almost always within the first 48 hours[246] and most often during sleep. It was formerly believed that patients with inferior MIs were more likely to experience AIVR,[246-247] but it is now believed to occur as often with anterior infarctions.[103] Since AIVR usually does not compromise cardiac function,[246] does not progress to VT or VF,[246,247] and disappears spontaneously without treatment,[247] it is not considered a dangerous arrhythmia. Its resemblance to VT, however, tends to elicit what Marriott refers to as the *lidocaine reflex*. The arrhythmia usually bothers the caregivers more than it does the patient and it does not usually require treatment.

Other clinical settings in which AIVR has been documented include: digitalis toxicity,[246,249-250] myocardial reperfusion and thrombolysis,[68] pregnancy,[250] rheumatic heart disease, primary myocardial disease and hypertensive cardiac disease. It has been reported in people with no evidence of heart disease and is not unusual in the trained athlete, when its presence is a consequence of a low sinus rate.[243,249-251]

ECG Characteristics

AIVR is a type of IVR characterized by runs of between 4 and 30[247] wide, bizarre QRS complexes occurring at a rate similar to the prevailing sinus rate, seldom differing from it more than 5 bpm[246] (see box below, Figs. 8-45 and 8-46). The rate of the AIVR rarely exceeds 100 and is usually seen at rates between 60 and 90,[246] although some have been documented at rates as low as 40 and as high as 120 bpm.[58]

AIVR tends to occur when the basic rhythm slows, as it does in sinus arrhythmia. Since it starts near the end of diastole, the initiating beat has a long coupling interval.[246] Its appearance is often ushered in and out with fusion beats.[103,246] See Figs. 8-45 to 8-49 for examples of fusion beats and long initiating coupling intervals.

Ventricular fusion beats. An appropriate time to interject the concept of ventricular fusion beats is in a dis-

ECG Characteristics
Accelerated Idioventricular Rhythm

Rate: 40 to 100 bpm (usually 60 to 90 bpm, at times as high as 120 bpm)
Seldom differs from sinus rate by >5 bpm
Rhythm: Regular
P wave: Usually dissociated.
May be retrograde atrial depolarization.
PR Interval: Irrelevant
QRS Complex: 0.12 seconds or more

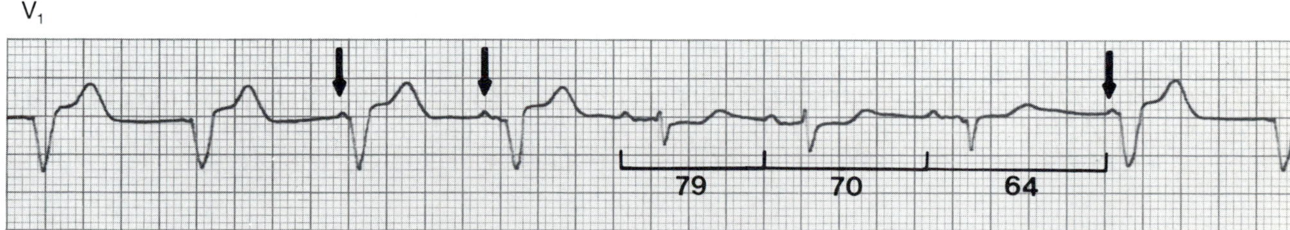

FIGURE 8-45 Accelerated idioventricular rhythm (AIVR). Note as sinus rate slows from 79 bpm to 64 bpm, the AIVR assumes control at a rate of 73 bpm. During the AIVR, the atria and ventricles are beating independently at similar rates. This is known as *isorhythmic AV dissociation.* Although a P wave occurs before some of the AIVR complexes *(arrows),* they are not conducting these impulses.

Rate: 71 to 78 bpm
Rhythm: Regular
P wave: Normal; dissociated from QRS during AIVR
PR interval: 0.20 seconds
QRS complex: 0.08 seconds; AIVR 0.12 seconds
Interpretation: AIVR

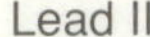

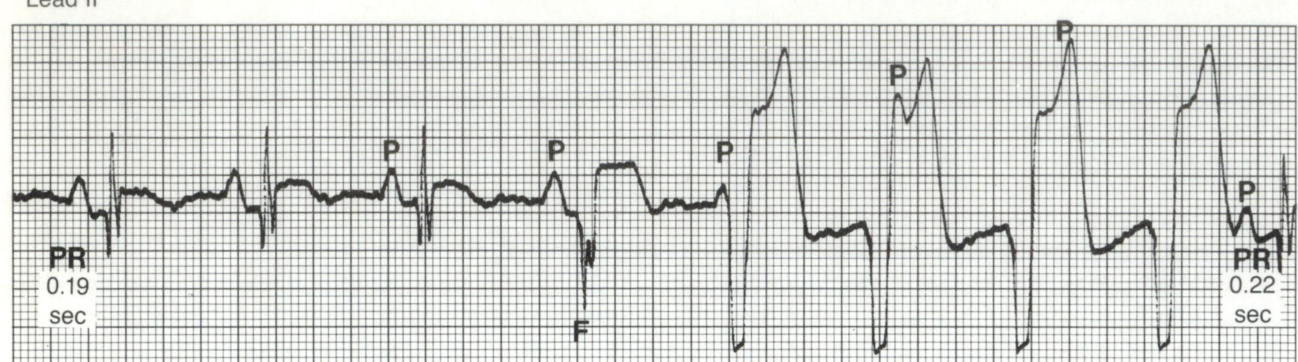

FIGURE 8-46 NSR to AIVR. The strip begins with NSR at a rate of 73 bpm. The fourth complex is a fusion beat *(F)*, which ushers in a short run of AIVR at a rate of 80 bpm. The sinus rate slowed from 73 to 67 bpm just before the AIVR assumed control. Note the independent atrial activity *(P)* that is dissociated from the AIVR. The last complex in the strip is called a *sinus capture;* the P wave was able to conduct a QRS complex because it found the ventricles recovered sufficiently, but it did so with a slightly longer PR interval.

Rate: 73 to 80 bpm
Rhythm: Irregular because of sinus capture
P wave: 0.13 seconds, wide, and tall
PR interval: 0.19 seconds; sinus capture has PR 0.22 seconds
QRS complex: 0.10 seconds
Interpretation: NSR with AIVR

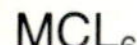

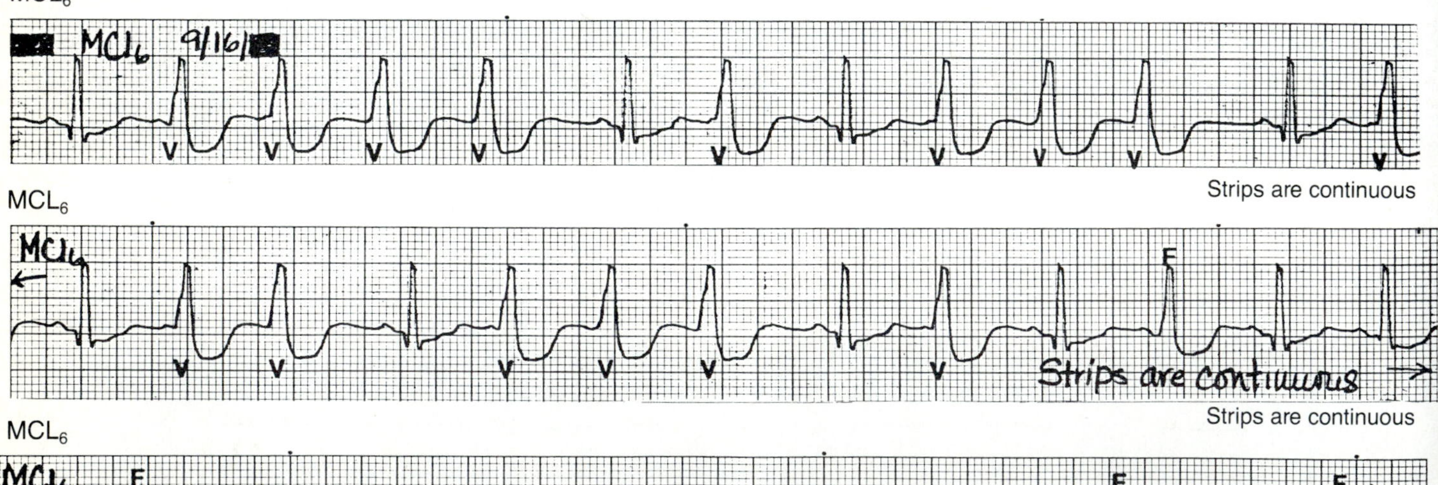

FIGURE 8-47 AIVR. Note the frequency with which this patient goes into and out of AIVR (marked *V*). In this example the AIVR rate is 107 while the sinus rate is 102 bpm. When rates of these two rhythms are so similar, fusion beats *(F)* are a common occurrence. Do we call this rhythm VT because the AIVR rate is over 100 bpm? This is one of those problems encountered when rate limits are set. No, this is not VT because the sinus and AIVR rates are so similar and because the R-R intervals initiating the runs of AIVR are similar to the R-R intervals of the sinus rhythm.

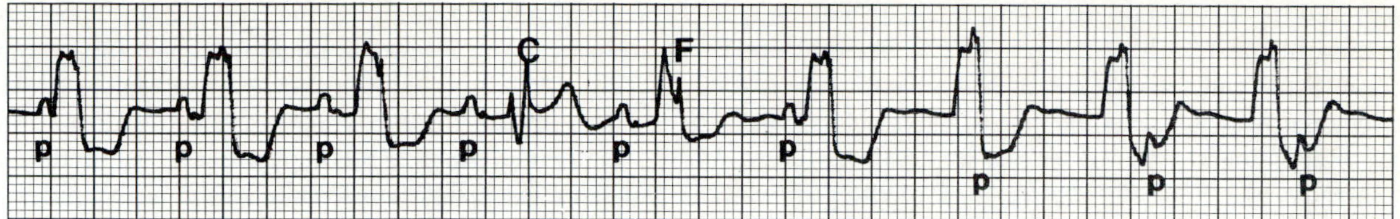

FIGURE 8-48 AIVR. At the start of this strip, AIVR is the prevailing rhythm at a rate of 88 bpm. The sinus rate, however, is slightly faster at 94 bpm allowing a sinus capture *(C)*. Here the sinus rate slows to 83 bpm allowing the AIVR to again assume control of the rhythm. Note fusion beat *(F)*.

Rate: 83 to 88 bpm
Rhythm: Regular
P wave: Normal; dissociated from ventricular rhythm during AIVR
PR interval: 0.21 seconds on the only sinus-conducted impulse *(C)*
QRS complex: 0.10 seconds capture beat; 0.14 seconds AIVR
Interpretation: AIVR

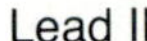

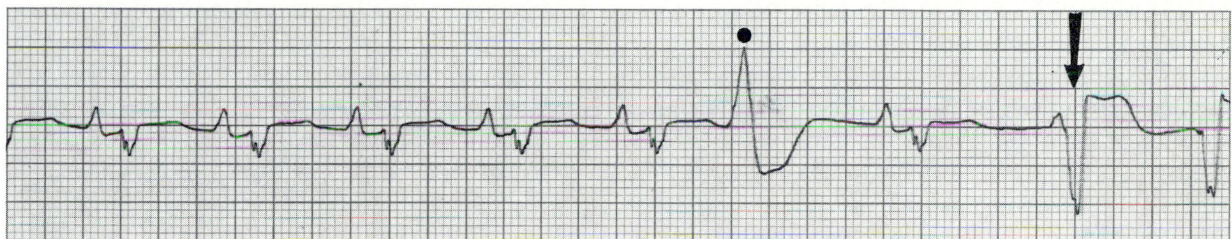

Strips are continuous

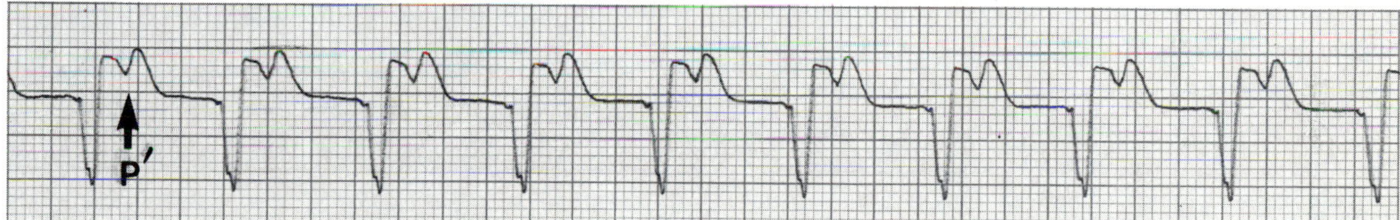

FIGURE 8-49 NSR into AIVR. This strip begins with NSR at a rate of 88 bpm. There is one VPB *(dot)* and another ventricular ectopic from a different focus that occurs in the end of diastole when the sinus rate slows to 67 bpm *(arrow)* initiating AIVR. This AIVR is producing retrograde atrial depolarization with each beat *(P′)*. Note negative dip in the ST segments of the AIVR on the bottom strip. This dip is not present in the initiating complex *(arrow)*.

Rate: Varies from 88 to 67 to 90 bpm. Such irregular rhythms should be counted for full minute.
Rhythm: Irregular
P wave: Slightly tall and peaked
PR interval: 0.18 seconds
QRS complex: 0.08 to 0.10 seconds. Negative on lead II because of left axis deviation. VPB present. AIVR 0.12 seconds.
Interpretation: NSR with one VPB. AIVR with retrograde atrial depolarization ensues with sinus slowing.

cussion of AIVR, since fusion is the rule rather than the exception in this setting.

In electrocardiography the term *fusion* refers to a complex that results when two impulses simultaneously activate parts of the same myocardial territory, whether atrial or ventricular.[252] (This discussion is limited to ventricular fusion complexes.) The resultant complex appears as a combination of two ventricular complexes. (Recall that the ECG is the algebraic sum of all the electrical events in the heart.) For example, if a sinus impulse arrives in the ventricles at the same instant a ventricular ectopic beat occurs, both beats will activate the ventricles, and the QRS complex representing the fusion beat on the ECG will be a combination of the two beats, bearing more resemblance to the beat that began activation first. In Fig. 8-46 the ventricular ectopic beat is predominantly negative. Combined with the predominantly positive sinus impulse, the complex written on the ECG will be the sum of the positive and negative forces.

Ventricular fusion beats can occur at any time it is likely that two impulses could activate the ventricles at the same time. End-diastolic VPBs, like AIVR, often occur just as the sinus impulse is arriving in the ventricles. Likewise, ventricular parasystole (discussed later in this chapter) may happen to deliver a ventricular ectopic at the same time a sinus impulse is activating the ventricles. Fusions may also occur in the midst of a ventricular tachycardia that does not conduct retrograde atrial impulses. In such a setting, fusion beats take the name of *Dressler*, the investigator who first described them in the presence of VT, elucidating that their presence is support for the diagnosis of VT when VT and supraventricular tachycardia with aberration require differential diagnosis.[253]

When a sinus complex and a ventricular ectopic beat are fused, the PR interval of the fusion beat may be the same or shorter than that of the sinus-conducted beat. When shorter, it will not be so by more than about 0.06 seconds.[254] The reason being that it takes virtually any ectopic impulse 0.06 seconds to reach the AV junction. Once the junction is depolarized, it cannot accept another impulse from above.[254]

As Marriott et al[254] admonish, fusion should be diagnosed only if you have cogent reason to believe the two impulses were due at that moment. There is a tendency to diagnose fusion when anomalous complexes are not readily explainable. Do not diagnose fusion unless proof exists of two impulses likely to activate the ventricles at the same time.

Other forms of fusion that may be encountered include the following:

- Atrial fusion (two foci activating the atria).
- Fusion occurring with ventricular pacemakers.
- Preexcitation (syndromes such as WPW syndrome).
- Junctional and ventricular ectopics fused.
- Ventricular ectopics from two foci producing fusion.

These examples of fusion complexes are beyond the scope of this book. The reader is encouraged, however, to study the various forms of fusion because they are often encountered and misdiagnosed.

Applied Nursing Process

Clinical Assessment

- Detect:
  - A run of ventricular beats at much the same rate as the previous sinus rhythm.
- Assess the patient and ECG.
  - When AIVR appears on the oscilloscope, most novice observers are prompt to diagnose it as VPBs or runs of VT. Close examination, however, reveals a resting or sleeping patient with a rate usually less than 100 bpm and an initiating QRS complex that is late in the cycle. Check the patient's tolerance of the arrhythmia by assessing the following:
    - Blood pressure.
    - Peripheral pulses.
    - Skin color and temperature.
    - Mentation. When awakening the patient, the rhythm will likely disappear with the increase in heart rate that accompanies wakefulness.
  - The first time the arrhythmia is displayed, awaken the patient to assess mentation. Subsequent similar episodes do not require repeated assessment if initial examination is negative.
  - The clinical situation in which the patient displays AIVR is an important consideration. AIVR noted during sleep in a patient who has recently experienced an acute MI is the clinical situation in which this rhythm is expected to occur. AIVR during an ambulance rescue of an apprehensive patient with chest pain, on the other hand, would be an example of an unusual clinical setting for this arrhythmia and should therefore alert the caregiver that the situation may not be so innocuous.
  - Diagnose the arrhythmia. Detect a run of regular, wide QRS beats that look like successive VPBs. Proceed with ECG diagnosis using the algorithm in Fig. 8-50.

❖ NURSING DIAGNOSIS

Decreased cardiac output related to ineffective ventricular contractions and/or loss of atrial contribution to cardiac output.

❖ ECG DIAGNOSIS

Accelerated idioventricular rhythm.

Plan and Implementation

Patient goal. The patient will remain hemodynamically stable and asymptomatic.

Nursing interventions.

- Document the rhythm.
- Awaken the patient (this will result in a rate increase sufficient to eradicate it in most cases).
- If patient is hemodynamically compromised, consider the following:
  - Atropine to increase the basic rate, if slow (remember atropine is not recommended immediately after acute MI).
  - AIVR may also respond to lidocaine, procainamide,[246] or other antiarrhythmic medications.
- Notify the physician of the presence of the arrhythmia and the patient's response to it.
- Reassure the patient that palpitations or mild symptoms

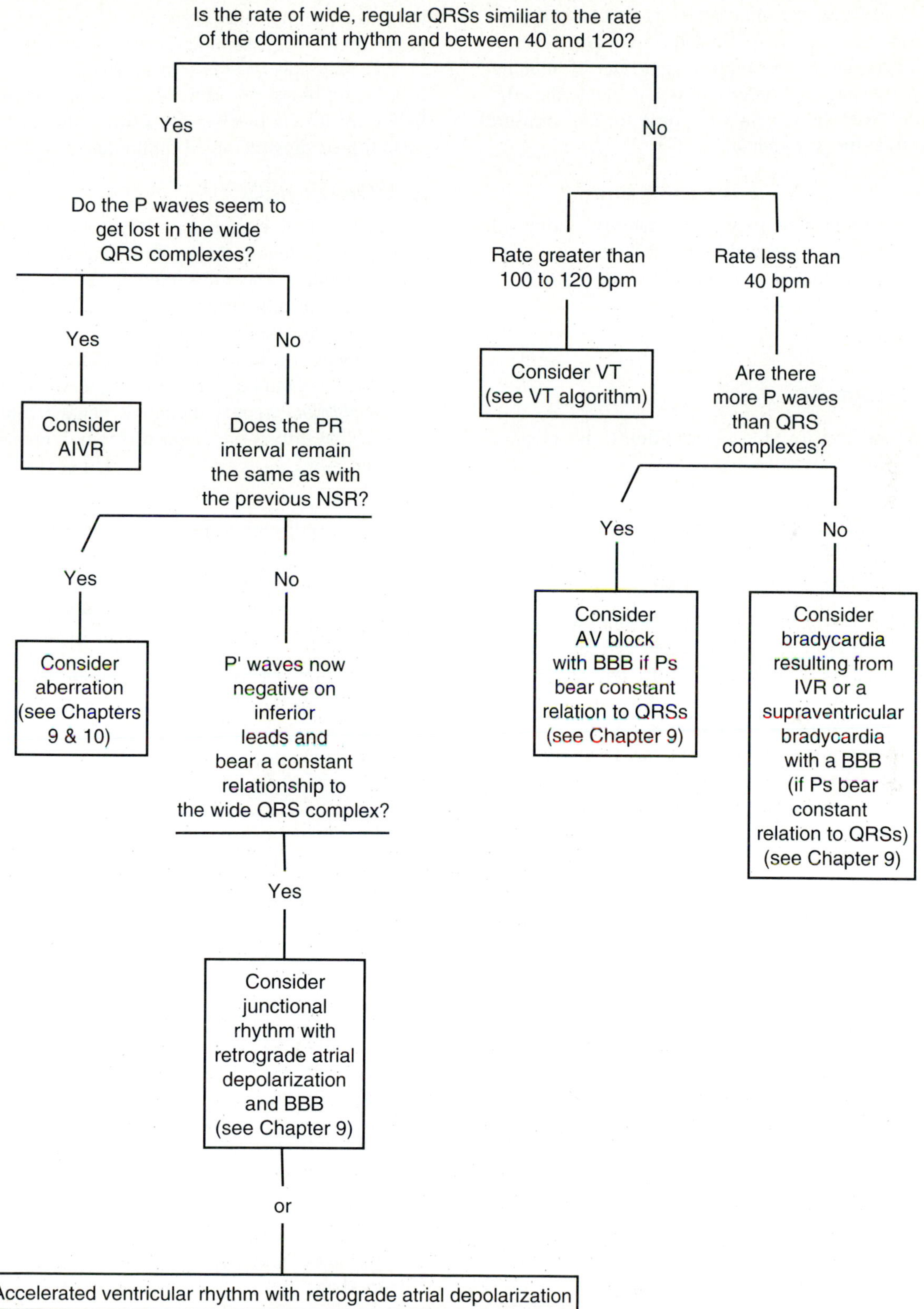

FIGURE 8-50 AIVR algorithm.

associated with the arrhythmia are not harmful.
- Continue to monitor the initiation of the arrhythmia for consistency of long coupling intervals. If coupling intervals shorten and rhythm is initiated by an early VPB, notify the physician of the change in character of initiation.
- Implement physician's orders, if any; evaluate the effectiveness of, and the patient's response to, any measures taken to treat the arrhythmia.

Evaluation

- The patient retains hemodynamic stability during episodes of AIVR as evidenced by the following:
  - Minimal or no change in blood pressure.
  - Palpable peripheral pulses.
  - Lucid response.

Medical Treatment

There is no medical treatment in addition to interventions above.

IDIOVENTRICULAR RHYTHM

Data Base: Problem Identification

Definitions, Etiology, and Mechanisms

Idioventricular rhythm (IVR), or ventricular escape rhythm, is not a primary electrical disturbance but occurs secondarily in response to a problem of either automaticity or conduction. IVR occurs when a higher supraventricular pacemaker, the SA node or AV junction, slows or fails or when supraventricular impulses are blocked somewhere beyond the AV node. Many conditions can depress automaticity or conduction, but the end result is the same. The wavefront of activation does not reach the ventricles, and ventricu ar depolarization would cease were it not for the lowest of the subsidiary pacemakers, the pacemaker cells in the ventricles, assuming control of the heart's rhythm.

IVR may appear as a transitional rhythm during complete heart block or artificial pacemaker malfunction or failure, or it may emerge and slow as the terminal agonal rhythm preceding electrical failure and death.

ECG Characteristics

The rate of IVR ranges from 10 to 40 bpm in a regular rhythm until rates reach very low ranges, when it may become irregular. The QRS complexes are wide, bizarre, and similar in appearance to VPBs. The atrial rate and rhythm may not be disturbed, or there may be concomitant atrial slowing or atrial asystole. A term used to describe IVR when it occurs as a terminal rhythm without pulses is *agonal rhythm*. Agonal rhythm is noted frequently when resuscitation efforts are stopped (see box below and Figs. 8-51 and 8-52).

ECG Characteristics
Idioventricular Rhythm

Rate: 40 bpm or less
Rhythm: Regular. With very slow rates, irregular.
P wave: May or may not be present. If present, dissociated from QRS complexes
PR interval: Irrelevant
QRS complex: 0.12 seconds or wider

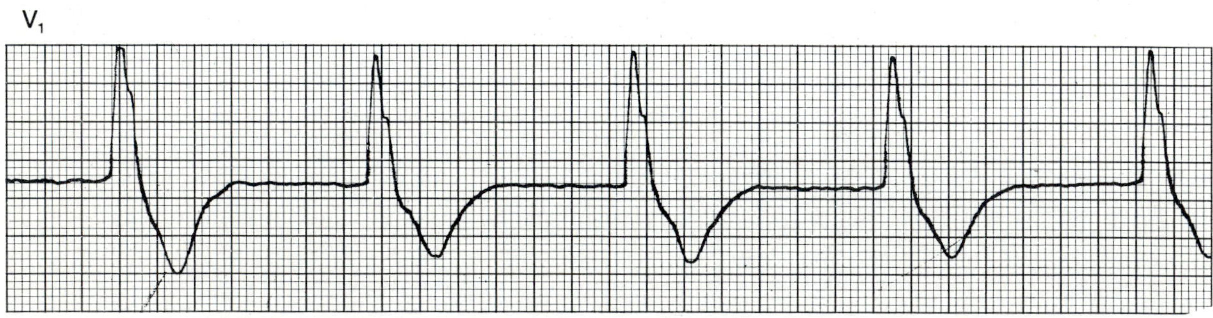

FIGURE 8-51 Idioventricular rhythm. Complexes are wide. There is no evidence of atrial activity.

Rate: 40 bpm
Rhythm: Regular
P wave: None identified
PR interval: —
QRS complex: 0.16 to 0.18 seconds
Interpretation: IVR

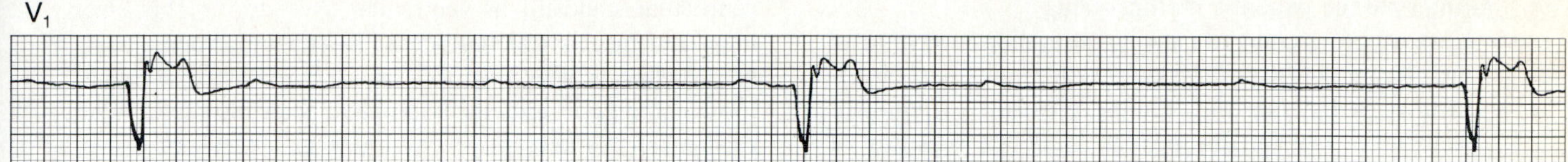

FIGURE 8-52 Idioventricular rhythm. Ventricular impulses are occurring at a rate of 15 bpm. Atria and ventricles are beating independently of one another, a condition referred to as *AV dissociation.*

Rate: Atrial: 40 bpm
Ventricular: 15 bpm
Rhythm: Atrial: Regular
Ventricular: Regular
P wave: Bear no relationship to QRS complexes
PR interval: Not relevant in AV dissociation
QRS complex: 0.14 to 0.16 seconds
Interpretation: IVR

Applied Nursing Process

Clinical Assessment

- Detect:
  - A possible decline in blood pressure.
  - Possibly weak or absent peripheral pulses.
  - Possibly symptoms of diminished cerebral perfusion.
  - Possibly a pulseless, apneic patient.
- Assess the patient and ECG.
  - Assess the patient for symptoms reflecting decreased cardiac output.

    Immediately determine if patient is conscious and breathing.

    Measure the blood pressure.

    Palpate peripheral pulses.

    Assess level of consciousness.

    Determine if syncope or near-syncope occurred.

    Question the patient about the presence of lightheadedness, dizziness.

❖ NURSING DIAGNOSIS

(1) Decreased cardiac output related to bradycardia and decreased stroke volume. (2) Altered tissue perfusion: cerebral/cardiopulmonary/peripheral, related to low cardiac output. (3) Knowledge deficit regarding temporary or permanent pacemaker therapy

❖ ECG DIAGNOSIS

Idioventricular Rhythm.

Plan and Implementation

Patient goal. The patient who is hemodynamically compromised will regain a perfusing rhythm before suffering irreversible cellular necrosis.

The patient's higher pacemaker failure will be identified and corrected.

The patient will relate appropriate information concerning temporary pacing and/or home management of permanent pacemaker.

Nursing interventions.

- If the patient is pulseless and apneic, initiate CPR at once. Initiation of cardiopulmonary resuscitation may be necessary if circulation is severely compromised from transitional heart block, artificial pacemaker failure, or Stokes-Adams attack.
- Notify others of **cardiac arrest.**
- Notify the physician immediately.
- Do not administer lidocaine. Because the complexes resemble VPBs, the inexperienced electrocardiographer might misinterpret the pattern and abolish the only means of depolarization the patient has left! If IVR appears after defibrillation or as a terminal rhythm during cardiac arrest, double check to be certain a lidocaine drip is not infusing.
- Give oxygen PRN.
- Start an IV infusion as ordered.
- If the IVR persists, an IV infusion of isoproterenol may be necessary. There is no firm consensus about whether atropine should be administered before isoproterenol is begun.
- Prepare for emergency temporary pacemaker insertion.
- Initiate external pacemaker as ordered.
- Observe for emergence of dangerous secondary tachyarrhythmias (generally VF) from profound hypotension and cardiac failure.
- If the patient with this rhythm is conscious and has adequate blood pressure, explain that measures are being taken to ensure a more stable heart rhythm. Explain the procedure for temporary pacemaker insertion and reassure the patient that little or no discomfort is usually experienced.
- For the stable patient in IVR who is hospitalized for elective pacemaker insertion, provide patient teaching concerning heart rate parameters, signs and symptoms of infection, and other self-care measures. (See Chapter 13 for further patient teaching details.)
- Implement physician's orders; evaluate measures taken

to improve the patient's rhythm status.

- If an isoproterenol infusion is sustaining a rhythm in the interim before pacemaker insertion, evaluate the effects of it by assessing for the presence of coronary ischemia. Question the patient about the presence of chest discomfort or shortness of breath.
- If a temporary pacemaker is inserted, evaluate its function and the patient's response to the increase in heart rate.

Evaluation

- The patient's arrhythmia is corrected (as in the patient who is hemodynamically unstable) or stabilized until temporary or permanent pacing is instituted. The patient maintains/regains hemodynamic stability as evidenced by the following:
  - Lucid response.
  - Palpable peripheral pulses.
  - A blood pressure sufficient to sustain life.
- The patient manages permanent pacemaker at home as evidenced by the following:
  - Ability to measure own pulse rate.
  - Ability to define heart rate ranges for optimum pacemaker function.
  - Using other self-care measures specific for him/her.

Medical Treatment

- Temporary ventricular pacemaker as an emergency measure and later a permanent ventricular pacemaker may be indicated.
- The underlying cause is corrected, if possible.

VENTRICULAR ASYSTOLE

Data Base: Problem Identification

Definitions, Etiology, and Mechanisms

Failure or progressive slowing of the idioventricular pacemaker rate to complete cessation of impulses results in ventricular standstill or ventricular asystole.[255] This electrical and mechanical quiescence is either transient, causing syncope or near-syncope, or a terminal cardiac event. It may emerge in untreated complete heart block, artificial pacemaker dysfunction or failure, or as a result of excessive vagal tone. It is a rare complication of exercise and hyperventilation and its occurrence in these settings is usually attributed to an exaggerated vasovagal reaction and preceded by a fall in blood pressure.[256-259] The problem in ventricular standstill is usually the failure of automatic discharge.[255] In the heart that is diseased, the idioventricular pacemakers or the regulatory mechanisms can be structurally or functionally altered.[255] As a terminal event, asystole follows IVR or VF in unsuccessful resuscitation attempts.

ECG Characteristics

Because there is no ventricular depolarization, there are no QRS complexes visible on the oscilloscope. If no atrial activity is present, the tracing is a simple flat line. If the atria are still depolarizing and contracting, the P waves may be regular and of normal size, irregular, or fibrillatory (see box below and Fig. 8-53).

> **ECG Characteristics**
> ***Ventricular Asystole***
>
> ***Rate:*** *Atrial:* Any
> *Ventricular:* 0
> ***Rhythm:*** *Atrial:* Any
> *Ventricular:* None
> ***P wave:*** None, abnormal, or normal
> ***PR interval:*** None
> ***QRS complex:*** None

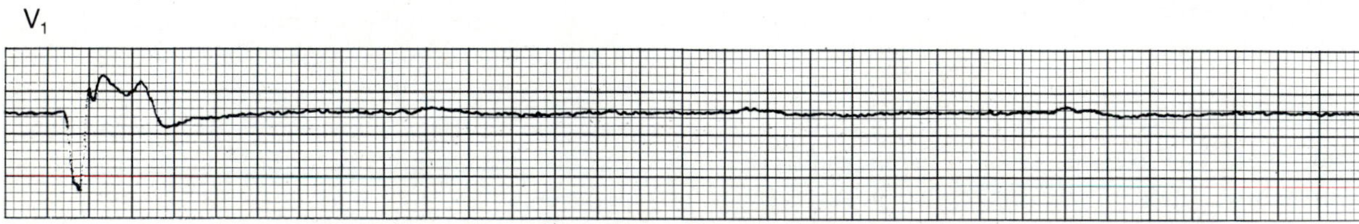

FIGURE 8-53 Ventricular asystole. After a ventricular complex, there is no more ventricular activity.

Rate: —
Rhythm: —
P wave: Evidence of very low voltage atrial activity
PR interval: —
QRS complex: None after initial beat on strip
Interpretation: Ventricular asystole

Applied Nursing Process

Clinical Assessment

- Detect:
  - Pulselessness, apnea or agonal respirations, declining or loss of consciousness.
  - A flat, or nearly flat, line on the ECG.
- Assess the patient and ECG.
  - The clinical assessment in ventricular standstill depends greatly on the underlying cause and the patient's prognosis. Whether it is a transient or terminal rhythm, it is a clinical emergency that requires **immediate** assessment of ventilation and perfusion.
  - If the arrhythmia appears suddenly, do the following immediately:

    Establish nonresponsiveness, apnea, pulselessness.

    Check monitor quickly to be certain that what you are seeing is not a mechanical malfunction such as a disconnected cable.

    Confirm asystole on at least two leads to be certain the arrhythmia is not fine ventricular fibrillation.[260]

❖ NURSING DIAGNOSIS

(1) Decreased cardiac output related to cessation of ventricular contraction. (2) Altered tissue perfusion: cerebral/cardiopulmonary/renal/gastrointestinal/peripheral, related to cessation of ventricular contraction. (3) Knowledge deficit regarding permanent pacemaker.

❖ ECG DIAGNOSIS

Ventricular asystole.

Plan and Implementation

Patient goal. The patient will regain hemodynamic stability by restoring normal sinus rhythm or receiving artificially paced rhythm; the patient will not experience prolonged hypoxemia and irreversible cellular necrosis.

Nursing interventions.

- If the patient is apneic and pulseless, initiate CPR at once.
- Cough CPR may be attempted if initiated before the patient becomes unconscious. Tell the patient to "cough hard!" every 1 to 3 seconds. Hard coughing produces hemodynamic changes that are similar to CPR.[190]
- Notify others of **cardiac arrest**.
- Notify the physician immediately.
- When asystole is of recent onset, a precordial thump may produce one or a series of ventricular depolarizations.
- If there is any doubt whether the arrhythmia is asystole or fine VF, treat as VF.[260]
- Emergency drugs that may be considered include epinephrine, atropine, sodium bicarbonate, and isoproterenol. Since plasma catecholamine concentrations are high in cardiac arrest, higher than what is normally required to stimulate cardiac activity, some recommend that atropine be administered before epinephrine. It is postulated that the heart may be held in asystole by an increase in vagal parasympathetic activity during the arrest.[240,261]
- If the asystole was transient and the patient did not experience loss of consciousness:
  - Assess vital signs and mentation frequently.
  - Hang an isoproterenol infusion at the bedside ready for infusion.
  - Assemble external pacing equipment and have it ready for immediate use.
  - Prepare for emergency temporary pacemaker insertion.
  - Explain to the patient that his/her heart rate dropped momentarily and you are taking measures to ensure it will not happen again.
  - Reassure the patient that little pain is experienced during external pacing and/or pacemaker insertion and that medication will be administered to promote comfort.
  - Make certain that a lidocaine infusion is not inadvertently left infusing in case the asystole is encountered as a secondary rhythm during a cardiac arrest.
- Implement physician's orders; evaluate the patient's response to measures taken to increase the heart rate.
  - If an external pacemaker is in use or a temporary pacemaker has been inserted, evaluate the patient's hemodynamic response to the increased rate.
  - Make sure the pacemaker is pacing properly.
  - If an isoproterenol infusion is being administered, evaluate the electrocardiographic response and resultant ischemic side effects by assessing the patient frequently for signs and symptoms of coronary ischemia.

Evaluation

- The patient exhibits a return to an adequate cardiac rhythm as evidenced by the following:
  - NSR, pulse-producing escape rhythm, or paced rhythm on the ECG.
  - Palpable peripheral pulses.
  - Lucid response.
  - Blood pressure sufficient to sustain perfusion.

Medical Treatment

Temporary transvenous ventricular pacing is indicated as an emergency measure followed by permanent ventricular pacing, if indicated. Correction of the underlying cause is corrected, if possible.

ELECTROMECHANICAL DISSOCIATION

Data Base: Problem Identification

Definitions, Etiology, and Mechanisms

A discussion of electromechanical dissociation (EMD) is included here for purposes of clarification and to avoid the misuse of the term. Like VF and asystole, EMD is a state of cardiovascular collapse. Unlike VF and asystole, EMD is not an arrhythmia. As the name implies, it is a condition in which electrical activity of the heart is not coupled with mechanical contraction. Thus EMD is distinctly different from VF and asystole with cardiovascular collapse resulting from mechanical, not electrical, failure. EMD is nearly always fatal, although there is a rare transient form that is associated with myocardial ischemia.[262] Whatever the form, EMD is an emergency that requires immediate attention.

With EMD, the heart ceases to contract effectively in the presence of either a normal ECG or a rhythm expected to produce a pulse. *Primary EMD,* as identified by Fozzard,[263] is observed in two clinical situations: (1) when the patient's heart rhythm is restored after prolonged cardiac arrest from any cause and (2) spontaneous occurrence in patients with ischemic cardiac disease.[262,264] The prevalence of primary EMD is difficult to determine because the patient does not exhibit prodromal symptoms or arrhythmias before sudden loss of consciousness. Carefully documented reports of primary EMD complicating acute MI indicate an incidence of 2.3%.[264]

There are many conditions that may mimic the clinical syndrome of EMD: (1) massive pulmonary embolus, (2) ball valve thrombus (in those with a prosthetic ball-type valve), causing obstructed inflow to the heart, (3) external or internal exsanguination, (4) cardiac rupture,[263] and (5) tension pneumothorax. Referred to by Fozzard[263] as *secondary EMD,* they differ importantly from primary EMD: the contractile ability of the heart is not impaired or is only secondarily affected. Although it is important to differentiate these syndromes from primary electromechanical dissociation because the treatments differ, some sources[260,265] do not differentiate them.

ECG Characteristics

In EMD there is **not** a characteristic QRS pattern. Careful observation of MI patients who have been victims of EMD has revealed a sinus rhythm at a normal rate with no palpable pulses or audible heart sounds. Subsequently, the ECG deteriorated to conduction block, IVR, or asystole.[264]

Applied Nursing Process
Clinical Assessment

- Detect:
  - Pulselessness, nonresponsiveness, apnea, or agonal respirations.
  - Normal ECG or a rhythm expected to produce a pulse.
- Assess the patient and ECG.
  - The hallmark of primary EMD is absence of pulses and heart sounds in the presence of a normal rhythm or a rhythm expected to produce a pulse. Immediate detection is unlikely unless the EMD is witnessed or the victim is being monitored hemodynamically. Loss of consciousness may go unnoticed until conduction delays, IVR, or asystole is detected on the monitor. A witnessed onset of EMD may reveal signs of circulatory collapse preceding loss of consciousness such as shortness of breath, chest pain, complaints of numbness or simply a "funny feeling," or blindness. **Immediately** assess the following:
    - Respiratory status.
    - Blood pressure and peripheral pulses.

Occasionally it is possible to rule out secondary EMD by assessment and knowing the patient's history before the catastrophe.

- Does the patient have an artificial ball valve? On rare occasions, a ball valve thrombus produces secondary EMD.
- Does the patient have an aortic aneurysm? Has the patient been involved in recent trauma? Could hemorrhage be causing the symptoms?
  - Assess for neck vein distension (presence of distension would tend to rule out hemorrhage unless pericardial tamponade or tension pneumothorax is also present).[260]
- Assess for signs of massive pulmonary embolism such as marked peripheral venous congestion.[263]
- Assess for pericardial tamponade in the postoperative cardiac surgery patient.
  - Assess color, sensorium, and urine output.
  - Inspect for jugular venous distension (presence of distension supports diagnosis).
  - Note presence of pulsus alternans and pulsus paradoxus.
  - Assess blood pressure parameters for arterial hypotension, equalization of right and left heart pressures, and increased left atrial or pulmonary artery diastolic pressures.
  - Auscultate lungs for muffled heart tones.
  - Inspect ECG for decreased amplitude of QRS complexes.
  - Note sudden decrease in amount of chest system drainage.
- Assess for sudden pericardial tamponade from a myocardial rupture (a rare occurrence).
  - Inspect for jugular venous distension (presence supports diagnosis).
  - Assess for signs of cardiovascular collapse.

❖ NURSING DIAGNOSIS

(1) Decreased cardiac output related to cessation of ventricular contraction. (2) Altered tissue perfusion: cerebral/cardiopulmonary/renal/gastrointestinal/peripheral, related to cardiovascular collapse.

❖ ECG DIAGNOSIS

Electromechanical dissociation accompanied by (ECG rhythm).

Plan and Implementation

Patient goal. The patient will regain adequate cardiac output.

Nursing interventions. EMD is an emergency that usually has a fatal outcome even with prudent and immediate intervention. Spontaneous primary EMD in patients with ischemic heart diseases requires **immediate** resuscitation regardless of the ECG pattern.

- Begin CPR.
- Alert others of **cardiac arrest.**
- Administer oxygen.
- Notify physician immediately.
- Manage acid-base balance based on arterial blood gas values.
- Administration of intravenous epinephrine or isoproterenol may help restore the electromechanical coupling. Atropine may be indicated if heart rate is slow.[260]
- When EMD occurs after prolonged cardiac arrest with restoration of adequate electrical activity, continue CPR until mechanical activity returns.

Secondary EMD also requires **immediate** treatment depending on the cause. It is beyond the scope of this book to address treatment protocols for these diverse conditions other than to offer minimal emergency actions to enable the caregiver to anticipate possible modes of therapy.

- Begin CPR.
- Notify others of **cardiac arrest.**
- Administer oxygen.
- Notify physician immediately.
- Following massive pulmonary embolism:
  - Prepare for emergency surgery.
  - Administer mechanical ventilations with 100% oxygen.
  - Obtain arterial blood gases as ordered.
- Try to alleviate the rare occurrence of a ball valve-thrombus by changing the patient's position.
- If cardiac tamponade is suspected:
  - Prepare for pericardiocentesis (unlikely to be successful in cardiac rupture).
  - Prepare for immediate thoracotomy if postoperative cardiac surgical patient (frequently successful).

Evaluation

- The patient's circulatory status is restored as evidenced by the following:
  - A return of consciousness.
  - Palpable pulses.
  - Blood pressure sufficient to sustain life.

Medical Treatment

- For primary EMD, CPR, along with other interventions as described previously, may help restore electromechanical coupling.
- The treatment for the various causes of secondary EMD is specific to the predisposing condition.

VENTRICULAR PARASYSTOLE

Data Base: Problem Identification

Definitions, Etiology, and Mechanisms

In its most basic form, ventricular parasystole is a fairly simple arrhythmia to understand. Its rather complex variations, such as parasystolic ventricular tachycardia, ventricular parasystole in combinations with other rhythms, and intermittent ventricular parasystole, are reserved for advanced study.

Recall that under normal conditions the dominant, controlling pacemaker in the heart, the SA node, has the highest inherent rate of automatic diastolic depolarization. In special circumstances with changes in myocardial automaticity, subsidiary pacemakers in the ventricles become capable of generating impulses independent of the SA node. Protecting the ectopic ventricular pacemaker from surrounding cells depolarizing it is known as either a persistent unidirectional *entrance block* or *interference*.[266] Thus the two rhythms are permitted to coexist (referred to as a *dual rhythm*), resulting in an ectopic ventricular pacemaker that emits a rhythm totally independent of the sinus rhythm, activating the ventricles whenever it finds them ready to receive an impulse. (Functionally and electrocardiographically, ventricular parasystole behaves just like an artificial fixed-rate ventricular pacemaker.) Sometimes, however, emission of the ectopic ventricular rhythm is prevented by what is called an *exit block*.[101]

Ventricular parasystole is not an uncommon disorder, but its true incidence is somewhat difficult to document since it is often misdiagnosed as frequent VPBs. It is easier to recognize and much more common than atrial or junctional parasystole.[252,267] It is thought that latent ventricular pacer cells under pathologic conditions may develop rapid phase 4 depolarization and discharge on a regular basis.[245] It is linked with coronary artery disease,[188,252,268] hypertensive cardiovascular disease, rheumatic heart disease, cor pulmonale, congenital heart disease, and cardiomyopathy. It is occasionally observed in the acute postmyocardial infarction population and in apparently healthy individuals. It is a relatively benign arrhythmia[269] and does not present a problem to many patients.

ECG Characteristics[101,103]

Often the first clue to the presence of ventricular parasystole is the appearance of monomorphic ventricular premature complexes with varying coupling intervals (recall that VPBs usually have fixed coupling intervals) (Figs. 8-54 and 8-55). This criterion by itself, however, does not confirm the diagnosis.

The second clue is mathematically related interectopic intervals. The interectopic interval is the interval from the beginning of one ectopic beat to the beginning of the next ectopic beat. Subsequent intervals between ectopic beats are the same as, or multiples of, the interectopic interval

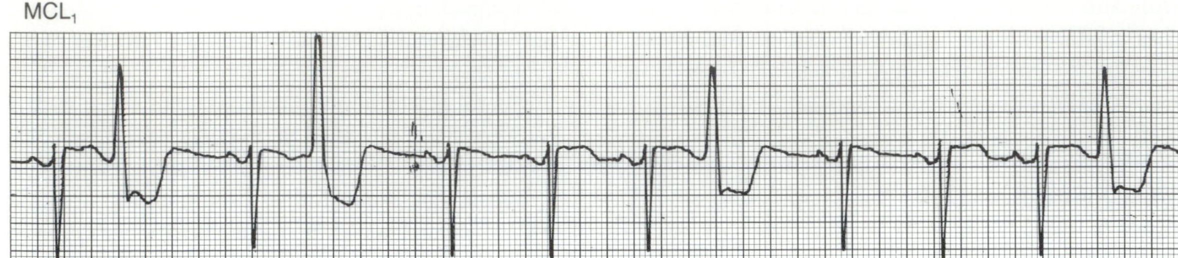

FIGURE 8-54 VPBs with fixed coupling intervals.

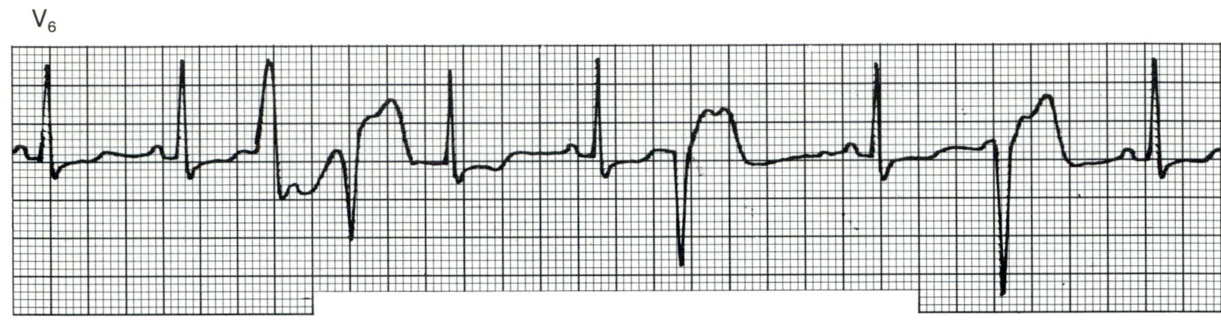

FIGURE 8-55 VPBs with varying coupling intervals.

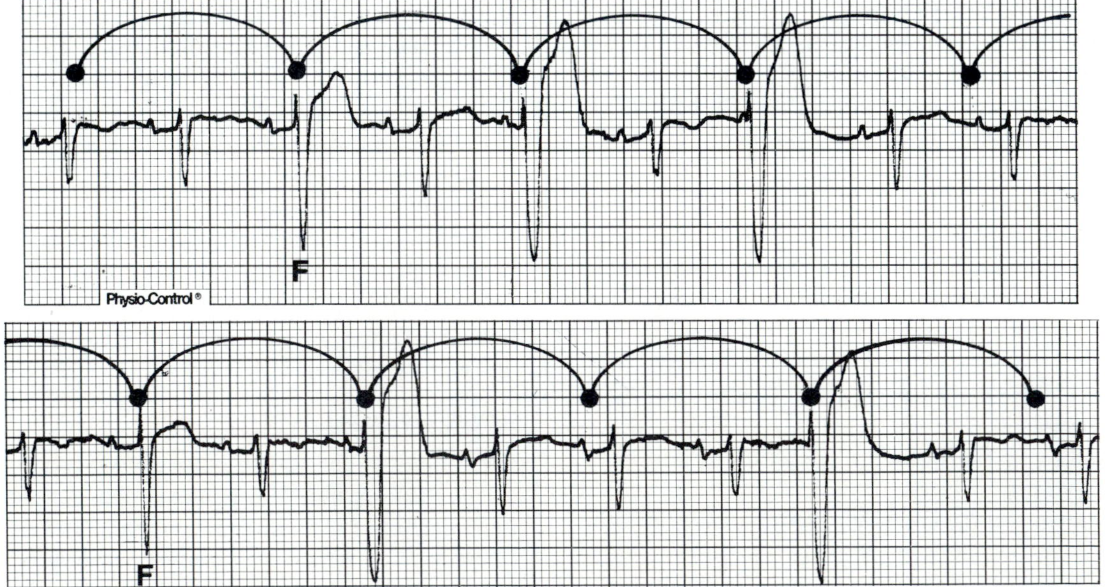

FIGURE 8-56 Ventricular parasystole. Ventricular ectopic beats occur at regular intervals. Interectopic intervals are mathematically related. Another characteristic is variable coupling intervals that often result in fusion beats *(F)*.

between two sequential beats (Fig. 8-56).

With dual rhythms competing for control of the ventricular rhythm, fusion complexes are common. The fusion beat is a combination of the ectopic ventricular beat and the sinus-conducted complex both activating the ventricles at the same time (see Fig. 8-56).

The rate of the parasystolic rhythm is often slow, usually between 38 and 60 bpm.[270] If the ectopic rate exceeds that of the sinus rate, the parasystolic rhythm will prevail and appear on the ECG as an IVR or AIVR. If the parasystolic rhythm is less than that of the sinus rate, the sinus rhythm will dominate and the parasystolic beats will appear whenever they can.

Table 8-5 and the box on this page provide useful summary features of ventricular parasystole.

Applied Nursing Process

Clinical Assessment

- Detect:
  - An irregular pulse.
  - Irregularities on the ECG caused by what look like VPBs.
- Assess the patient and ECG.
  - The clinical assessment is the same as for ventricular ectopy with attention to the possibility of pulse deficit. Palpate the peripheral pulses and determine pulse deficit by simultaneously listening to the apical pulse or watching the monitor.
  - Obtain the blood pressure and heart rate.
  - Assess skin temperature and color, level of consciousness.
  - Question the patient for the presence of symptoms such as palpitations.
  - Diagnose the arrhythmia. Detect what appear to be frequent monomorphic VPBs with varying coupling intervals. Proceed with the ECG diagnosis using the algorithm in Fig. 8-57.

Table 8-5 Comparison of VPBs with Ventricular Parasystole

Parasystole	VPBs
• Varying coupling intervals	• Fixed coupling usually
• Interectopic intervals mathematically related	• Interectopic intervals not related*
• Uniform	• Uniform or multiform

*Be careful analyzing VPBs that occur in a pattern, such as bigeminy, as they will appear to have the same interectopic intervals if the sinus rhythm is regular.

❖ NURSING DIAGNOSIS

(1) Decreased cardiac output related to decreased ventricular filling. (2) High risk for altered tissue perfusion: cerebral/peripheral/cardiopulmonary, related to decreased cardiac output. (3) Knowledge deficit regarding chronic nature and symptoms of arrhythmia.

❖ ECG DIAGNOSIS

Ventricular parasystole.

Plan and Implementation

Patient goal. The patient will remain hemodynamically stable; will relate appropriate information concerning the chronic nature and possible symptoms of the arrhythmia.

ECG Characteristics
Ventricular Parasystole

Rate: Parasystolic rate: 38 to 60 bpm
Underlying rate: Slow or normal
Rhythm: Parasystolic rhythm: regular
Underlying rhythm: regular or irregular
Overall rhythm: irregular
P wave: Any atrial rhythm may coexist
PR interval: PR interval of underlying rhythm not affected
QRS complex: Parasystolic: 0.12 seconds or wider, uniform
Underlying rhythm: Normal unless IVCD.

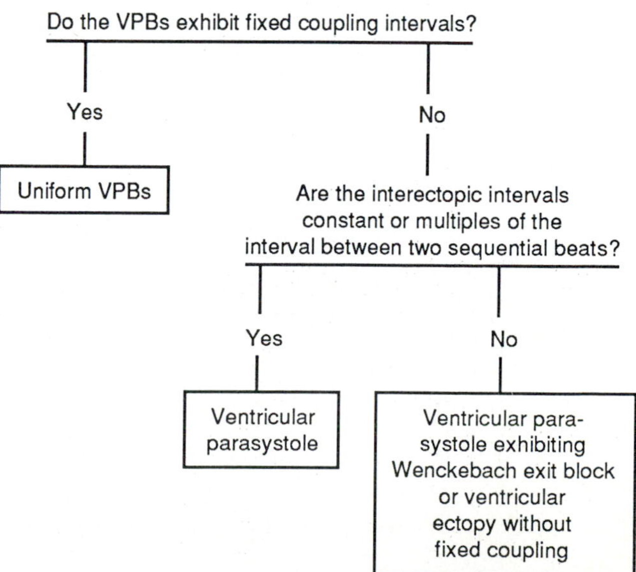

FIGURE 8-57 Ventricular parasystole algorithm.

Nursing interventions.

- Notify the physician of the presence of the arrhythmia, immediately if the patient is symptomatic.
- Implement physician's orders, if any.
- Save a very long sample of the rhythm strip to document the multiples of the interectopic intervals.
- If the patient experiences palpitations, teach about the nature of the arrhythmia to allay anxiety. Even if asymptomatic, patients should be taught about their arrhythmia.
- Teach patient the following:
  - The symptoms of poor perfusion.
  - How and when to take pulse.
  - To seek medical assistance if the pulse rate significantly drops and/or if symptoms of decreased perfusion develop.

Evaluation

- The patient's hemodynamic status remains unchanged as evidenced by the following:
  - No change in blood pressure.
  - Denial of discomfort.

Medical Treatment

Treatment may not be indicated.[271] If instituted, treatment depends on rate, symptoms, and underlying disease process. The rhythm is often found to be recalcitrant to antiarrhythmic therapy.

REFERENCES

1. Horowitz LN, Morganroth J. Can we prevent sudden cardiac death? *Am. J. Cardiol.*, Sept., 1982, 50: 535-8.
2. Kannel WB, Cupples A, D'Agostino RB. Sudden death risk in overt coronary heart disease: the Framingham Study. *Am. Heart J.*, Mar., 1987, 113(3): 799-804.
3. Hicks D. Medical grand rounds: sudden cardiac death. *J. Ark. Med. Soc.*, Oct., 1984, 85(5): 269-73.
4. Kannel WB, McGee DL, Schatzkin A. An epidemiological perspective of sudden death; 26-year follow-up in the Framingham Study. *Drugs*, 1984, 28(Suppl. 1): 1-16.
5. Sridharan MR, Checton J. Sudden cardiac death: identifying and managing the patient at risk. *Geriatrics*, Jan., 1985, 40(1): 63-9.
6. Panidis IP, Morganroth J. Holter monitoring and sudden cardiac death. *Cardiovasc. Rev. Rep.*, Mar., 1984, 5(3): 283; 287-90; 297-9; 303-4.
7. Roelandt J, Klootwijk P, Lubsen J. Prodromal and lethal arrhythmias in sixteen sudden death patients documented with longterm ambulatory electrocardiography. *Circ.*, Oct., 1983, 68(Suppl. III): 356.
8. Kempf FC, Josephson ME. Sudden cardiac death recorded on ambulatory electrocardiogram. *Circ.*, Oct, 1983, 68(Suppl. III): 355.
9. Rapaport E. Sudden cardiac death. *Am. J. Cardiol.*, Nov., 1988, 62: 3I-6I.
10. Brooks R, McGovern BA, Garan H, Ruskin JN. Current treatment of patients surviving out-of-hospital cardiac arrest. *JAMA*, Feb., 1991, 265(6): 762-8.
11. Olshausen KV, Witt T, Pop T, Treese N, Bethge K-P, Meyer J. Sudden cardiac death while wearing a Holter monitor. *Am. J. Cardiol.*, Feb., 1991, 67: 381-6.
12. Tresch DD, Thakur RK, Hoffmann RG, Aufderheide TP, Brooks HL. Comparison of outcome of paramedic-witnessed cardiac arrest in patients younger and older than 70 years. *Am. J. Cardiol.*, Feb., 1990, 65: 453-7.
13. Surawicz B. Ventricular fibrillation. *J. Am. Coll. Cardiol.*, Jun., 1985, 5(6): 43B-54B.
14. Northcote RJ, Ballantyne D. Ventricular fibrillation during ambulatory electrocardiography. *Am. Heart J.*, Dec., 1984, 108(6): 1560-2.
15. Hohnloser SH, Kasper W, Zehender M, Geibel A, Meinertz T, Just H. Silent myocardial ischemia as a predisposing factor for ventricular fibrillation. *Am. J. Cardiol.*, Feb., 1988, 61: 461-4.
16. Verheugt FWA, Brugada P. Sudden death after acute myocardial infarction: the forgotten thrombotic view. *Am. J. Cardiol.*, May, 1991, 67: 1130-4.
17. Marcus FI, Cobb LA, Edwards JE, Kuller L, Moss AJ, Bigger T Jr, Fleiss JL, Rolnitzky L, Serokman R. Mechanism of death and prevalence of myocardial ischemic symptoms in the terminal event after acute myocardial infarction. *Am. J. Cardiol.*, Jan., 1988, 61: 8-15.
18. Lie KI, Wellens HJ, Durrer D. Characteristics and predictability of primary ventricular fibrillation. *Eur. J. Cardiol.*, Apr., 1974, 1(4): 379-84.
19. Milner PG, Platia EV, Reid PR, Griffith SC. Holter monitor recordings at the time of sudden cardiac death. *Circ.*, Oct., 1983, 68(Suppl. III): 106.
20. Klein RC, Vera Z, Mason DT, DeMaria AN, Awan NA, Amsterdam EA. Ambulatory Holter monitor documentation of ventricular tachyarrhythmias as mechanism of sudden death in patients with coronary artery disease. *Clin. Res.*, Feb., 1979, 27(1): 7A.
21. Josephson ME, Horowitz LN, Spielman SR, Greenspan AM. Electrophysiologic and hemodynamic studies in patients resuscitated from cardiac arrest. *Am. J. Cardiol.*, Dec., 1980, 46(6): 948-55.
22. Panidis IP, Morganroth J. Sudden death in hospitalized patients: cardiac rhythm disturbances detected by ambulatory electrocardiographic monitoring. *J. Am. Coll. Cardiol.*, Nov., 1983, 2(5): 798-805.
23. Pratt CM, Francis MJ, Luck JC, Wyndham CR, Miller RR, Quinones MA. Analysis of ambulatory electrocardiograms in fifteen patients during spontaneous ventricular fibrillation with special reference to preceding arrhythmic events. *J. Am. Coll. Cardiol.*, Nov., 1983, 2(5): 789-97.
24. Denes P, Gabster A, Huang SK. Clinical, electrocardiographic and follow-up observations in patients having ventricular fibrillation during Holter monitoring. *Am. J. Cardiol.*, Jul., 1981, 48(1): 9-15.
25. Dorough D, Lyle T, Carrigan TA, Wright J. Arrhythmias precipitating pediatric cardiac arrest (abstract). *Heart & Lung*, May, 1987, 16(3): 335-6.
26. Denfield SW, Garson A Jr. Sudden death in children and young adults. *Pediatr. Clin. N. Am.*, Feb., 1990, 37(1): 215-31.
27. Klitzner TS. Sudden cardiac death in children. *Circ.*, Aug., 1990, 82(2): 629-32.
28. Hayano J, Sakakibara Y, Yamada A, Yamada M, Mukai S, Fujinami T, Yokoyama K, Watanabe Y, Takata K. Accuracy of assessment of cardiac vagal tone by heart rate variability in normal subjects. *Am. J. Cardiol.*, Jan., 1991, 67: 199-204.
29. Malik M, Camm AJ. Heart rate variability. *Clin. Cardiol.*, Aug., 1990, 13(8): 570-6.
30. Pipilis A, Flather M, Ormerod O, Sleight P. Heart rate variability in acute myocardial infarction and its association with infarct site and clinical course. *Am. J. Cardiol.*, May, 1991, 67: 1137-9.
31. Cripps TR, Malik M, Farrell TG, Camm AJ. Prognostic value of reduced heart rate variability after myocardial infarction: clinical evaluation of a new analysis method. *Br. Heart J.*, Jan., 1991, 65(1): 14-9.

32. Lombardi F, Sandrone G, Pernpruner S, Sala R, Garimoldi M, Cerutti S, Baselli G, Pagani M, Malliani A. Heart rate variability as an index of sympathovagal interaction after acute myocardial infarction. *Am. J. Cardiol.*, Dec., 1987, 60: 1239-45.
33. Southall DP, Johnston F, Shinebourne EA, Johnston PGB. 24-hour electrocardiographic study of heart rate and rhythm patterns in population of healthy children. *Br. Heart J.*, 1981, 45: 281-91.
34. Garson A Jr, Smith RT, Moak JP, Ross BA, McNamara DG. Ventricular arrhythmias and sudden death in children. *J. Am. Coll. Cardiol.*, Jun., 1985, 5(6): 130B-3B.
35. Dance D, Yates M. Nursing assessment and care of children with complications of congenital heart disease. *Heart & Lung,* May, 1985, 14(3): 209-17.
36. Chen S, Fagan LF, Nouri S, Donahoe JL. Ventricular dysrhythmias in children with Marfan's Syndrome. *Am. J. Dis. Child.*, Mar., 1985, 139: 273-6.
37. Scott O, Williams GJ, Fiddler GI. Results of 24 hour ambulatory monitoring of electrocardiogram in 130 healthy boys aged 10-13 years. *Br. Heart J.*, 1980, 44: 304-8.
38. Kostis JB, McCrone K, Moreyra AE, Gotzoyannis S, Aglitz NM, Natarajan N, Kuo PT. Premature ventricular complexes in the absence of identifiable heart disease. *Circ.*, Jun., 1981, 63(6): 1351-6.
39. Bleifer SB, Bleifer DJ, Hansmann DR, Sheppard JJ, Karpman HL. Diagnosis of occult arrhythmias by Holter electrocardiography. *Prog. Cardiovasc. Dis.* May/Jun., 1974, 16(6): 569-99.
40. Brodsky M, Wu D, Denes P, Kanakis C, Rosen KM. Arrhythmias documented by 24-hour continuous electrocardiographic monitoring in 50 male medical students without apparent heart disease. *Am. J. Cardiol.*, Mar. 5, 1977, 39: 390-5.
41. Sobotka PA, Mayer JH, Bauernfeind RA, Kanakis C, Rosen KM. Arrhythmias documented by 24-hour continuous ambulatory electrocardiographic monitoring in young women without apparent heart disease. *Am. Heart J.*, Jun., 1981, 101(6): 753-9.
42. Talan DA, Bauernfeind RA, Ashley WW, Kanakis C, Rosen KM. Twenty-four hour continuous ECG recordings in long distance runners. *Chest,* Jul., 1982, 82(1): 19-24.
43. Hinkle LE, Carver ST, Stevens M. The frequency of asymptomatic disturbances of cardiac rhythm and conduction in middle-aged men. *Am. J. Cardiol.*, Nov., 1969, 24: 629-50.
44. Wajngarten M, Grupi C, Bellotti GM, Da Luz PL, Azul LG, Pileggi F. Frequency and significance of cardiac rhythm disturbances in healthy elderly individuals. *J. Electrocardiol.*, Apr., 1990, 23(2): 171-6.
45. Fleg JL, Kennedy HL. Cardiac arrhythmias in a healthy elderly population. *Chest,* Mar., 1982, 81(3): 302-7.
46. Moss AJ, Davis HT, DeCamilla J, Bayer LW. Ventricular ectopic beats and their relation to sudden and nonsudden cardiac death after myocardial infarction. *Circ.*, Nov., 1979, 60(5): 998-1003.
47. Iberti TJ, Benjamin E, Gruppi L, Raskin JM. Ventricular arrhythmias during pulmonary artery catheterization in the intensive care unit. *Am. J. Med.*, Mar., 1985, 78(3): 451-4.
48. Chou T-C, Wenzke F. The importance of R on T phenomenon. *Am. Heart J.*, Aug., 1978, 96(2): 191-4.
49. Weiss JN, Nademanee K, Stevenson WG, Singh B. Ventricular arrhythmias in ischemic heart disease. *Ann. Intern Med.*, May, 1991, 114(9): 784-97.
50. Lewis S, Kanakis C, Rosen KM, Denes P. Significance of site of origin of premature ventricular contractions. *Am. Heart J.*, Feb., 1979, 97(2): 159-64.
51. LaRosa JC, Brown WV, Frommer PL, Levy RI. Clofibrate-induced ventricular arrhythmia. *Am. J. Cardiol.*, Feb., 1969, 23(2): 266-9.
52. Reinhardt CF, Azar A, Maxfield ME, Smith PE, Mullen LS. Cardiac arrhythmias and aerosol "sniffing." *Arch. Environ. Health,* Feb., 1971, 22: 265-79.
53. Surawicz B, Lasseter K. Effect of drugs on the electrocardiogram. *Prog. Cardiovasc. Dis.*, Jul., 1970, 13(1): 26-55.
54. Fowler NO, McCall D, Chou T-C, Holmes JC, Hanenson IB. Electrocardiographic changes and cardiac arrhythmias in patients receiving psychotropic drugs. *Am. J. Cardiol.*, Feb., 1976, 37: 223-30.
55. Tangedohl TN, Gau GT. Myocardial irritability associated with lithium carbonate therapy. *N. Engl. J. Med.*, Oct. 26, 1972, 287(17): 867-8.
56. Dreifus LS. The clinical significance of cardiac arrhythmias. *In* Dreifus LS, Likoff W (eds). *Mechanisms and Therapy of Cardiac Arrhythmias*. New York: Grune & Stratton, 1966.
57. Matoba R, Onishi S, Shimizu Y, Shikata I. Sudden death in methamphetamine abusers: a histological study of the heart. *Nippon Hoigaku Zasshi,* Apr., 1984, 38(2): 199-205.
58. Moss AJ, Akiyama T. Prognostic significance of ventricular premature beats. *In* Fisch C (ed). *Complex Electrocardiography 2*. Brest AN (ed). *Cardiovascular Clinics*. Philadelphia: FA Davis, 1974.
59. Sutherland DJ, McPherson DD, Renton KW, Spencer CA, Montague TJ. The effect of caffeine on cardiac rate, rhythm, and ventricular repolarization; analysis of 18 normal subjects and 18 patients with primary ventricular dysrhythmia. *Chest,* Mar., 1985, 87(3): 319-24.
60. Dietrich AM, Mortensen ME. Presentation and management of an acute caffeine overdose. *Pediatr. Emerg. Care,* Dec., 1990, 6(4): 296-8.
61. Chelsky LB, Cutler JE, Griffith K, Kron J, McClelland JH, McAnulty JH. Caffeine and ventricular arrhythmias. An electrophysiological approach. *JAMA,* Nov., 1990, 264(17): 2236-40.
62. Myers MG, Harris L. High dose caffeine and ventricular arrhythmias. *Can. J. Cardiol.* Apr., 1990, 6(3): 95-8.
63. Myers MG. Caffeine and cardiac arrhythmias. *Ann. Intern. Med.*, Jan., 1991, 114(2): 147-50.
64. Svedmyr N. Methylxanthines in asthma. *In* Morley J, Rainsford KO (eds). *Pharmacology of Asthma*. Boston: Birkhauser Verlag, 1983.
65. Sessler CN, Cohen MD. Cardiac arrhythmias during theophylline toxicity. A prospective continuous electrocardiographic study. *Chest,* Sept., 1990, 98(3): 672-8.
66. Vinsant M, Spence MI. *Commonsense Approach to Coronary Care*. 5th ed. St. Louis: The CV Mosby Co., 1989.
67. King GS, Smialek JE, Troutman WG. Sudden death in adolescents resulting from the inhalation of typewriter correction fluid. *JAMA,* Mar., 15, 1985, 253(11): 1604-6.
68. Lepley-Frey D. Dysrhythmias and blood pressure changes associated with thrombolysis. *Heart & Lung,* Jul., 1991, 20(4): 335-41.
69. Wilcox RG, Eastgate J, Harrison E, Skene AM. Ventricular arrhythmias during treatment with alteplase (recombinant tissue plasminogen activator) in suspected acute myocardial infarction. *Br. Heart J.*, Jan., 1991, 65(1): 4-8.
70. Sheps DS, Herbst MC, Hinderliter AL, Adams KF, Ekelund LG, O'Neil JJ, Goldstein GM, Bromberg PA, Dalton JL, Ballenger MN, et al. Production of arrhythmias by elevated carboxyhemoglobin in patients with coronary artery disease. *Ann. Intern. Med.*, Sept., 1990, 113(5): 343-51.
71. Arcebal AG, Lemberg L. Torsade de pointes (vignette). *Heart & Lung,* Nov./Dec., 1980, 9(6): 1096-1100.
72. Nordrehaug JE, Johannessen K-A, von der Lippe G. Serum potassium concentration as a risk factor of ventricular arrhythmias early in acute myocardial infarction. *Circ.*, Apr., 1985, 71(4): 645-9.
73. Podrid PJ. Potassium and ventricular arrhythmias. *Am. J. Cardiol.*, Mar., 1990, 65(10): 33E-44E.
74. Wessmann JP. Preventing ventricular dysrhythmias following myocardial infarction. *Dimens. Crit. Care Nurs.*, Jan./Feb., 1985, 4(1): 24-32.

75. Huikuri HV, Yli-Mayry S, Korhonen UR, Airaksine KE, Ikaheimo MJ, Linnaluoto MK, Takkunen JT. Prevalence and prognostic significance of complex ventricular arrhythmias after coronary arterial bypass graft surgery. *Int. J. Cardiol.*, Jun., 1990, 27(3): 333-9.
76. Houyel L, Vaksmann G, Fournier A, Davignon A. Ventricular arrhythmias after correction of ventricular septal defects: importance of surgical approach. *J. Am. Coll. Cardiol.*, Nov., 1990, 16(5): 1224-8.
77. Vaksmann G, Fournier A, Davignon A, Ducharme G, Houyel L, Fouron J-C. Frequency and prognosis of arrhythmias after operative "correction" of tetralogy of Fallot. *Am. J. Cardiol.*, Aug., 1990, 66: 346-9.
78. Pelliccia F, Cianfrocca C, Cristofani R, Romeo F, Reale A. Electrocardiographic findings in patients with hypertrophic cardiomyopathy. Relation to presenting features and prognosis. *J. Electrocardiol.*, Jul., 1990, 23(3): 213-22.
79. Chetty S, Mitha AS. Arrhythmias in idiopathic dilated cardiomyopathy. A preliminary study. *S. Afr. Med. J.*, Feb., 1990, 77(4): 190-3.
80. Pelliccio F, Gallo P, Cianfrocca C, d'Amati G, Bernucci P, Reale A. Relation of complex ventricular arrhythmias to presenting features and prognosis in dilated cardiomyopathy. *Int. J. Cardiol.*, Oct., 1990, 29(1): 47-54.
81. Chokshi SK, Nazari J, Mattioni T, Zheutlin T, Haffajee C, Kehoe R. Arrhythmias in idiopathic dilated cardiomyopathy. *Cardiovasc. Rev. Rep.*, Aug., 1990, pp 55-66.
82. McLenachan JM, Dargie HJ. A review of rhythm disorders in cardiac hypertrophy. *Am. J. Cardiol.*, Apr., 1990, 65(14): 42G-44G.
83. Siegel D, Cheitlin MD, Black DM, Seeley D, Hearst N, Hulley SB. Risk of ventricular arrhythmias in hypertensive men with left ventricular hypertrophy. *Am. J. Cardiol.*, Mar., 1990, 65(11): 742-7.
84. Aronow WS. Left ventricular hypertrophy. Significance in cardiac morbidity and mortality. *Postgrad. Med.*, Mar., 1990, 87(4): 147-50.
85. McLenachan JM, Dargie HJ. Ventricular arrhythmias in hypertensive left ventricular hypertrophy. Relationship to coronary artery disease, left ventricular dysfunction, and myocardial fibrosis. *Am. J. Hypertens.*, Oct., 1990, 3(10): 735-40.
86. Dyckner T. Serum magnesium in acute myocardial infarction; relation to arrhythmias. *Acta Med. Scand.*, 1980, 207(1-2): 59-66.
87. Tzivani D, Keren A. Suppression of ventricular arrhythmias by magnesium. *Am. J. Cardiol.*, Jun., 1990, 65: 1397-9.
88. Loeb HS, Pietras RJ, Gunnar RM, Tobin JR. Paroxysmal ventricular fibrillation in two patients with hypomagnesemia. *Circ.*, Feb., 1968, 37(2): 210-5.
89. Gottlieb SS, Baruch L, Kukin ML, Bernstein JL, Fisher ML, Packer M. Prognostic importance of the serum magnesium concentration in patients with congestive heart failure. *J. Am. Coll. Cardiol.*, Oct., 1990, 16(4): 827-31.
90. Freis ED. The cardiotoxicity of thiazide diuretics: review of the evidence. *J. Hypertens. Suppl.*, Jun., 1990, 8(2): S23-32.
91. Podrid PJ, Fuchs T, Candinas R. Role of the sympathetic nervous system in the genesis of ventricular arrhythmia. *Circ.*, Aug., 1990, 82(2 Suppl): I103-13.
92. Lesch M, Lewis E, Humphries JO, Ross RS. Paroxysmal ventricular tachycardia in the absence of organic heart disease. *Ann. Intern. Med.*, May, 1967, 66(5): 950-9.
93. Gorfinkel HJ, O'Driscoll RG. Control of paroxysmal ventricular tachycardia with oral contraceptives. *Chest*, Aug., 1973, 64(2): 279-80.
94. Watanabe Y, Dreifus LS. *Cardiac Arrhythmias; Electrophysiologic Basis for Clinical Interpretation*. New York: Grune & Stratton, 1977.
95. Boudalas H, Dervenagas S, Schaal SF, Lewis RP, Dalamangas G. Malignant premature ventricular beats in ambulatory patients. *Ann. Intern. Med.*, Nov., 1979, 91(5): 723-6.
96. Clarke JM, Shelton JR, Hamer J, Taylor S, Venning GR. The rhythm of the normal human heart. *Lancet*, Sept., 1976, 2: 508-12.
97. Campbell RW, Murray A, Julian DG. Ventricular arrhythmia in first 12 hours of acute myocardial infarction. Natural history study. *Br. Heart J.*, 1981, 40: 351-7.
98. Panidis IP, Morganroth J. Initiating events of sudden cardiac death. *In* Josephson ME (ed). *Sudden Cardiac Death*. Brest AN (ed) *Cardiovascular Clinics*, 15/3. Philadelphia: FA Davis, 1985.
99. Nikolic G, Bishop RL, Singh JB. Sudden death recorded during Holter monitoring. *Circ.*, Jul., 1982, 66(1): 218-25.
100. Langendorf R, Pick A, Winternitz M. Mechanisms of intermittent ventricular bigeminy. I. Appearance of ectopic beats dependent upon length of the ventricular cycle, the "Rule of Bigeminy." *Circ.*, Mar., 1955, 11: 422-30.
101. Schamroth L. *The Disorders of Cardiac Rhythm*. Vol. I. 2nd ed. London: Blackwell Scientific Publications, 1981.
102. Surawicz B, MacDonald MG. Ventricular ectopic beats with fixed and variable coupling: incidence, clinical significance and factors influencing the coupling interval. *Am. J. Cardiol.*, 1964, 13: 198.
103. Marriott HJL. *Practical Electrocardiography*. 8th ed. Baltimore: Williams & Wilkins, 1988.
104. Vitullo RN, Wharton JM, Allen NB, Pritchett EL. Trazodone-related exercise-induced nonsustained ventricular tachycardia. *Chest*, Jul., 1990, 98(1): 247-8.
105. Chiang BN, Perlman LV, Ostrander LD, Epstein FH. Relationship of premature systoles to coronary heart diseases and sudden death in the Tecumseh epidemiologic study. *Ann. Intern. Med.*, Jun., 1969, 70(6): 1159-66.
106. Alexander S, Desai DC, Hershberg PI. Clinical significance of ventricular premature beats in an outpatient population (abstract). *Am. J. Cardiol.*, Feb., 1972, 29: 250.
107. Adgey AAJ, Devlin JE, Webb SW, Mulholland HC. Initiation of ventricular fibrillation outside hospital in patients with acute ischaemic heart disease. *Br. Heart J.*, 1982, 47: 55-61.
108. Han J. Mechanisms of ventricular arrhythmias associated with acute myocardial infarction. *Am. J. Cardiol.*, Dec., 1969, 24(6): 800-13.
109. Han J. Ventricular vulnerability during acute coronary occlusion. *Am. J. Cardiol.*, Dec., 1969, 24(6): 857-64.
110. Adgey AAJ, Allen AD, Geddes JS, James RGG, Webb SW, Zaidi SA, Pantridge JF. Acute phase of myocardial infarction. *Lancet*, 1971, 2: 501.
111. Rose RM, Lewis AJ, Fewkes J, Clifton JF, Criley JM. Occurrence of arrhythmias during the first hour in acute M.I. (abstract). *Circ.*, Oct., 1974, 49,50(Suppl. III): 121.
112. Moss AJ, Goldstein S. The prehospital phase of acute myocardial infarction. *Circ.*, May, 1970, 41(5): 737-42.
113. Lie KI, Wellens HJJ, Downar E, Durrer D. Observations on patients with primary ventricular fibrillation complicating acute myocardial infarction. *Circ.*, Nov., 1975, 52: 755-9.
114. al Awadhi AH, Ravindran J, Abraham KA, Graham IM. The prevalence and outcome of ventricular arrhythmias in acute myocardial infarction. *Ir. J. Med. Sci.*, Apr., 1990, 159(4): 101-3.
115. Romhilt DW, Bloomfield SS, Chou T-C, Fowler NO. Unreliability of conventional electrocardiographic monitoring for arrhythmia detection in coronary care units. *Am. J. Cardiol.*, Apr., 1973, 31: 457-61.
116. Conley MG, McNeer JF, Lee KL, Wagner GS, Rosati RA. Cardiac arrest complicating acute myocardial infarction: predictability and prognosis. *Am. J. Cardiol.*, Jan., 1977, 39: 7-12.
117. Kuang-Hung T, Samant A, Desser KB, Benchimol A. R on T or R on P phenomenon? Relation to the genesis of ventricular tachycardia. *Am. J. Cardiol.*, Oct., 1979, 44: 632-7.
118. Antman EM, Braunwald E. Acute MI management in the 1990s. *Hosp. Practice*, Jul., 1990, pp 57-73.

119. Jensen GVH, Torp-Pedersen C, Kober L, Steensgaard-Hansen F, Rasmussen YH, Berning J, Skagen K, Pedersen A. Prognosis of late versus early ventricular fibrillation in acute myocardial infarction. *Am. J. Cardiol.*, Jul., 1990, 66: 10-15.
120. Bigger JT. Patients with malignant or potentially malignant ventricular arrhythmias: opportunities and limitations of drug therapy in prevention of sudden death. *J. Am. Coll. Cardiol.*, Jun., 1985, 5(6): 23B-6B.
121. El-Sherif N, Myerburg RJ, Scherlag BJ, Befeler B, Aranda JM, Castellanos A, Lazzara R. Electrocardiographic antecedents of primary ventricular fibrillation; value of the R-on-T phenomenon in myocardial infarction. *Br. Heart J.* Apr., 1976, 38(4): 415-22.
122. Wyman MG, Gore S. Lidocaine prophylaxis in myocardial infarction: a concept whose time has come. *Heart & Lung*, Jul., 1983, 12(4): 358-61.
123. Goldreyer BN, Wyman MG. The effects of first hour hospitalization in myocardial infarction (abstract). *Circ.*, Oct., 1974, 49-50(Suppl. III): 121.
124. De Soyza N, Meacham D, Murphy ML, Kane JJ, Doherty, JE, Bissett JK. Evaluation of warning arrhythmias before paroxysmal ventricular tachycardia during acute myocardial infarction in man. *Circ.*, Oct., 1979, 60(4): 814-8.
125. Chua TS, Koo CC, Tan AT, Ho CK. Mortality trends in the coronary care unit. *Ann. Acad. Med. Singapore*, Jan., 1990, 19(1): 3-8.
126. Roberts R, Ambos HD, Loh CW, Sobel BE. Initiation of repetitive ventricular depolarizations by relatively late premature complexes in patients with acute myocardial infarction. *Am. J. Cardiol.*, Apr., 1978, 41: 678-83.
127. Mukharji J, Rude R, Gustafson N, Poole K, Passamani E, Thomas LJ, Strauss HW, Muller JE, Roberts R, Raabe DS, Braunwald E, Willerson JT. Multicenter investigation of the limitation of infarct size (MILIS), Dallas, Texas. *J. Am. Coll. Cardiol. Abstracts*, Mar., 1983, 1(2): 585.
128. Ruberman W, Weinblatt AB, Goldberg JD, Frank CW, Chaudhary BS, Shapiro S. Ventricular premature complexes and sudden death after myocardial infarction. *Circ.*, Aug., 1981, 64(2): 297-305.
129. Bigger JT, Fleiss JL, Kleiger R, Miller VP, Rolnitzky LM. The multicenter post infarction research group: the relationship among ventricular arrhythmias, left ventricular dysfunction, and mortality in the two years after myocardial infarction. *Circ.*, 1984, 69: 250.
130. Armstrong WF, McHenry PL. Ambulatory electrocardiographic monitoring: can we predict sudden death? *J. Am. Coll. Cardiol.*, Jun., 1985, 5(6): 13B-6B.
131. Gozensky C, Thorne D. Rabbit ears: an aid in distinguishing ventricular ectopy from aberration. *Heart & Lung*, Jul./Aug., 1974, 3(4): 634-6.
132. Wellens HJJ, Bar FWHM, Lie KI. The value of the EKG in the differential diagnosis of a tachycardia with a widened QRS complex. *Am. J. Med.* Jan., 1978, 64: 27-33.
133. Akhtar M. Electrophysiologic bases for wide QRS complex tachycardias. *PACE*, Jan./Feb., 1983, 6: 81-97.
134. Gulamhusein S, Yee R, Ko PT, Klein GJ. Electrocardiographic criteria for differentiating aberrancy and ventricular extrasystoles in chronic atrial fibrillation: validation by intracardiac recordings. *J. Electrocardiol.*, 1985, 18(1): 41-50.
135. Nordrehaug JE, von der Lippe G. Hypokalemia and ventricular fibrillation in acute myocardial infarction. *Br. Heart J.*, 1983, 50: 525-9.
136. Barnaby PF, Barrett PA, Lvoff R. Routine prophylactic lidocaine in acute myocardial infarction. *Heart & Lung*, Jul., 1983, 12(4): 362-6.
137. AHA Medical/Scientific Statement. Special Report: ACC/AHA guidelines for the early management of patients with acute myocardial infarction. *Circ.*, Aug., 1990, 82(2): 664-73.
138. Romhilt DW. Lidocaine prophylaxis: An alternative to computerized arrhythmia monitoring. *Heart & Lung*, Nov./Dec., 1980, 9(6): 1007-8.
139. Dunn HM, McComb JM, Kinney CD, Campbell NPS, Shanks RG, MacKenzie G, Adgey AAJ. Prophylactic lidocaine in the early phase of suspected myocardial infarction. *Am. Heart J.*, 1985, 110(8): 353-62.
140. Lie KI. Lidocaine and prevention of ventricular fibrillation complicating acute myocardial infarction. *Int. J. Cardiol.*, Mar., 1985, 7(3): 321-5.
141. Hargarten K, Chapman PD, Stueven HA, Waite EM, Mateer JR, Haecker P, Aufderheide TP, Olson DW. Prehospital prophylactic lidocaine does not favorably affect outcome in patients with chest pain. *Ann. Emerg. Med.*, Nov., 1990, 19(11): 1274-9.
142. MacMahon S, Collins S, Peto R. Effects of prophylactic lidocaine in suspected acute myocardial infarction: an overview of results from the randomized controlled trials. *JAMA*, 1988, 260: 1910.
143. Zehender M, Kasper W, Just H. Lidocaine in the early phase of acute myocardial infarction: the controversy over prophylactic or selective use. *Clin. Cardiol.*, Aug., 1990, 13: 534-9.
144. Hine LK, Laird N, Hewitt P, Chalmers TC. Meta-analytic evidence against prophylactic use of lidocaine in acute myocardial infarction. *Arch. Intern Med.*, Dec., 1989, 149(12): 2694-8.
145. Lie KI, Wellens HJ, van Capelle FJ, Durrer D. Lidocaine in the prevention of primary V.F. *N. Engl. J. Med.*, Dec. 19, 1974, 291(25): 1324-6.
146. Marriott HJL, Bieza CF. Alarming ventricular acceleration after lidocaine administration. *Chest*, Jun., 1972, 61(7): 682-3.
147. Danahy DT, Aronow WS. Lidocaine-induced cardiac rate changes in atrial fibrillation and atrial flutter. *Am. Heart J.*, Apr., 1978, 95(4): 474-82.
148. Shechter M, Hod H, Marks N, Behar S, Kaplinsky E, Rabinowitz B. Beneficial effect of magnesium sulfate in acute myocardial infarction. *Am. J. Cardiol.*, Aug., 1990, 66: 271-4.
149. Morganroth J, Brozovich FV, McDonald JT, Jacobs RA. Variability of the QT measurement in healthy men, with implications for selection of an abnormal QT value to predict drug toxicity and proarrhythmia. *Am. J. Cardiol.*, Apr., 1991, 67: 774-6.
150. Heger JJ, Prystowsky EN, Zipes DP. New drugs for treatment of ventricular arrhythmias. *Heart & Lung*, May/Jun., 1981, 10(3): 475-83.
151. Salerno DM, Hodges M, Granrud G, Sharkey P. Comparison of flecainide with quinidine for suppression of chronic stable ventricular ectopic depolarization. *Ann. Intern. Med.*, Apr., 1983, 98(4): 455-60.
152. Anderson JL, Lutz JR, Allison SB. Electrophysiologic and antiarrhythmic effects of oral flecainide in patients with inducible ventricular tachycardia. *J. Am. Coll. Cardiol.*, Jul., 1983, 2(1): 105-14.
153. Oetgen WJ, Tibbits PA, Abt MEO, Goldstein RE. Clinical and electrophysiologic assessment of oral flecainide acetate for recurrent ventricular tachycardia: evidence for exacerbation of electrical instability. *Am. J. Cardiol.*, Oct., 1983, 52(7): 746-50.
154. Lui HK, Lee G, Dhurandhar R, Hungate EJ, Laddu A, Dietrich P, Mason DT. Reduction of ventricular ectopic beats with oral acebutolol: a double blind, randomized crossover study. *Am. Heart J.*, May, 1983, 105(5): 722-6.
155. Fisch C. Role of the electrocardiogram in identifying the patient at increased risk for sudden death. *J. Am. Coll. Cardiol.*, Jun., 1985, 5(6): 6B-8B.
156. Di Marco JP, Garan H, Ruskin JN. Quinidine for ventricular arrhythmias: value of electrophysiologic testing. *Am. J. Cardiol.*, Jan., 1983, 51(1): 90-5.
157. Winkle RA, Peters F, Kates RE, Harrison DC. Possible contribution of encainide metabolites to the long-term antiarrhythmic efficacy of encainide. *Am. J. Cardiol.*, Apr., 1983, 51(7): 1182-8.
158. Glasser SP, Clark PI, Laddu AR. Comparison of the antiarrhythmic effects of acebutolol and propranolol in the treatment of ventricular arrhythmias. *Am. J. Cardiol.*, Nov., 1983, 52(8): 992-5.

159. Pratt CM, Yepsen SC, Taylor AA, Mason DT, Miller RR, Quinones MA, Lewis RA. Ethmozine suppression of single and repetitive ventricular premature depolarizations during therapy: documentation of efficacy and long-term safety. *Am. Heart J.*, Jul., 1983, 106(1): 85-91.
160. Kienzle MG, Williams PD, Zygmont D, Doherty JU, Josephson ME. Antiarrhythmic drug therapy for sustained ventricular tachycardia. *Heart & Lung*, Nov., 1984, 13(6): 614-22.
161. Josephson ME, Kastor JA, Horowitz LN. Electrophysiologic management of recurrent ventricular tachycardia in acute and chronic ischemic heart disease. *In* Castellanos A (ed). *Cardiac Arrhythmias: Mechanisms and Management*. Brest AN (ed). *Cardiovascular Clinics*. Philadelphia: FA Davis, 1980.
162. Buxton AE, Josephson ME. Ventricular tachycardia-1983. *PACE*, Jan./Feb., 1984, 7(1-2): 96-108.
163. Hassapoyannes CA, Stuck LM, Hornung CA, Berbin MC, Flowers NC. Effect of left ventricular aneurysm on risk of sudden and nonsudden cardiac death. *Am. J. Cardiol.*, 1991, 67: 454-9.
164. Rosenthal ME, Oseran DS, Gang E, Peter T. Sudden cardiac death following acute myocardial infarction. *Am. Heart J.*, Apr., 1985, 109(4): 865-76.
165. Jacquet L, Ziady G, Stein K, Griffith B, Armitage J, Hardesty R, Kormos R. Cardiac rhythm disturbances early after orthotopic heart transplantation: prevalence and clinical importance of the observed abnormalities. *J. Amer. Coll. Cardiol.*, Oct., 1990, 16(4): 832-7.
166. Epstein AE, Davis KB, Kay GN, Plumb VJ, Rogers WJ. Significance of ventricular tachyarrhythmias complicating cardiac catheterization: a CASS Registry study. *Am. Heart J.*, Mar., 1990, 119(3 Pt 1): 494-502.
167. Isner JM, Roberts WC, Heymsfield SB, Yager J. Anorexia nervosa and sudden death. *Ann. Intern. Med.*, Jan., 1985, 102(1): 49-52.
168. Swartz MH, Teichholz LE, Donoso E. Mitral valve prolapse: a review of associated arrhythmias. *Am. J. Med.*, 1977, 62(3): 377-89.
169. Jain A, Starek PJ, Delany DL. Ventricular tachycardia and ventricular aneurysm due to unrecognized sarcoidosis. *Clin. Cardiol.*, Oct., 1990, 13(10): 738-40.
170. von Olshausen K, Witt T, Schmidt G, Meyer J. Ventricular tachycardia as a cause of sudden death in patients with aortic valve disease. *Am. J. Cardiol.*, May 1, 1987, 59(12): 1214-5.
171. Weesner KM. Ventricular arrhythmias after balloon aortic valvuloplasty. *Am. J. Cardiol.*, Dec. 15, 1990, 66: 1534-5.
172. Von Olshausen K, Witt T, Schmidt G, Meyer J. Ventricular tachycardia as a cause of sudden death in patients with aortic valve disease. *Am. J. Cardiol.*, May, 1987, 59: 1214-15.
173. Trippel DL, Gillette PC. Atenolol in children with ventricular arrhythmias. *Am. Heart J.*, Jun., 1990, 119(6): 1312-6.
174. Kudenchuk PJ, Kron J, Walance C, McAnulty JH. Spontaneous sustained ventricular tachyarrhythmias during treatment with type 1a antiarrhythmic agents. *Am. J. Cardiol.*, Feb. 15, 1990, 65(7): 446-52.
175. Hariman RJ, Hu DY, Gallastegui JL, Beckman KJ, Bauman JL. Long-term follow-up in patients with incessant ventricular tachycardia. *Am. J. Cardiol.*, Oct., 1990, 66(10): 831-6.
176. Rinkenberger RL, Prytowsky EN, Jackman WM, Naccarelli GV, Heger JJ, Zipes DP. Drug conversion of nonsustained ventricular tachycardia to sustained ventricular tachycardia during serial electrophysiologic studies. *Am. Heart J.* Feb., 1982, 103(2): 177-84.
177. Michiel RR, Sneider JS, Dickstein RA, et al. Sudden death in a patient on a liquid protein diet. *N. Engl. J. Med.*, May 4, 1978, 298(18): 1005-7.
178. Noh CI, Gillette PC, Case CL, Zeigler VL. Clinical and electrophysiological characteristics of ventricular tachycardias in children with normal hearts. *Am. Heart J.*, Dec., 1990, 120(6): 1326-33.
179. Lau KC, McGuire MA, Ross DL, Nunn GR, Knight WB, Uther JB. Incessant ventricular tachycardia in infancy. *J. Paediat. Child Health*, Apr., 1990, 26(2): 95-8.
180. Van Hare GF, Stanger P. Ventricular tachycardia and accelerated ventricular rhythm presenting in the first month of life. *Am. J. Cardiol.*, Jan. 1, 1991, 67: 42-5.
181. Morady F, Scheinman MM, Hess DS, Chen R, Stanger P. Clinical characteristics and results of electrophysiologic testing in young adults with ventricular tachycardia or ventricular fibrillation. *Am. Heart J.*, Dec., 1983, 106(6): 1306-14.
182. Gillette PC. Cardiac dysrhythmias in infants and children. *In* Engle MA (ed). *Pediatric Cardiovascular Disease*. Brest AN (ed). *Cardiovascular Clinics*, 11/2. Philadelphia: FA Davis, 1981.
183. Gillette PC. Ventricular arrhythmias. *In* Roberts NK, Gelband H (eds). *Cardiac Arrhythmias in the Neonate, Infant and Child*. New York: Appleton-Century-Crofts, 1977.
184. Garza LA, Vick RL, Nora JJ, McNamara DG. Heritable Q-T prolongation without deafness. *Circ.*, Jan., 1970, 41(1): 39-48.
185. Engle MA, Ebert PA, Redo SF. Recurrent ventricular tachycardia due to resectable cardiac tumor. *Circ.*, Nov., 1974, 50(5): 1052-7.
186. Keren A, Tzivoni D, Gottlieb S, Benhorin J, Stern S. Atypical ventricular tachycardia (Torsade de pointes) induced by amiodarone: arrhythmia previously induced by quinidine and disopyramide. *Chest*, 1982, 81: 384-6.
187. Schwartz AB, Scheinman MM. Ventricular tachycardia: newer insights. *Clin. Cardiol.*, Jul., 1983, 6: 307-11.
188. Rodriguez LM, Waleffe A, Brugada P, Dehareng A, Lezaun R, Sternick EB, Kulbertus HE. Exercise-induced sustained sympotomatic ventricular tachycardia: incidence, clinical, angiographic and electrophysiologic characteristics. *Eur. Heart J.*, Mar., 1990, 11(3): 225-32.
189. Lynch L. Torsade de pointes—a malignant arrhythmia. *Am. J. Nurs.*, Jul., 1986, 86(7): 826CC-7CC.
190. Tobias SL, Bookatz BJ, Diamond TH. Myocardial damage and electrocardiographic changes in acute cerebrovascular hemorrhage: a report of three cases and review. *Heart & Lung*, Sept., 1987, 16(5): 521-6.
191. Little RE, Kay GN, Cavender JB, Epstein AE, Plumb VJ. Torsade de pointes and T-U wave alternans associated with arsenic poisoning. *PACE*, Feb., 1990, 13(2): 164-70.
192. Talman CL, Winniford MD, Rossen JD, Simonetti I, Kienzle MG, Marcus ML. Polymorphous ventricular tachycardia: a side effect of intracoronary papaverine. *J. Am. Coll. Cardiol.*, Feb., 1990, 15(2): 275-8.
193. Monahan BP, Ferguson CL, Killeavy ES, Lloyd BK, Troy J, Cantilena LR Jr. Torsades de pointes occurring in association with terfenadine use. *JAMA*, Dec., 1990, 264(21): 2788-90.
194. Moore MT, Book MH. Sudden death in phenothiazine therapy: a clinicopathologic study of 12 cases. *Psychiatr. Q.*, 1970, 44: 389-402.
195. Schultz DD, Olivas GS. The use of cough cardiopulmonary resuscitation in clinical practice. *Heart & Lung*, May, 1986, 15(3): 273-80.
196. Marozsan I, Albared JL, Szatmary LJ. Life-threatening arrhythmias stopped by cough. *Cor Vasa.*, 1990, 32(5): 401-8.
197. *The Nurses' Handbook of Drug Alerts and Clinical Implications*. No. 1. New York: Am. J. Nurs., 1987.
198. Mann DL, Maisel AS, Atwood JE, Engler RL, LeWinter MM. Absence of cardioversion-induced ventricular arrhythmias in patients with therapeutic digitalis levels. *J. Am. Coll. Cardiol.*, Apr., 1985, 5(4): 882-90.
199. Smith A. Amiodarone: clinical considerations. *Focus Crit. Care*, 1984, 11(5): 30-7.
200. Teplitz L. Cryoablation for refractory ventricular dysrhythmias. *J. Cardiovasc. Nurs.*, Feb., 1990, 4(2): 63-9.
201. De Silva RA, Graboys TB, Podrid PJ, Lown B. Cardioversion and defibrillation. *Am. Heart J.*, Dec., 1980, 100(6): 881-95.
202. Interian A, Trohman RG, Castellanos A, Cox M, Zaman L, Myerburg RJ. Spontaneous conversion of ventricular fibrillation in cardiogenic shock from acute myocardial infarction. *Am. J. Cardiol.*, May 1, 1987, 59(12): 1200-1.

203. Kontny F, Dale J. Self-terminating idiopathic ventricular fibrillation presenting as syncope: a 40-year follow-up report. *J. Intern. Med.*, Mar., 1990, 227(3): 211-3.
204. Meltzer LE, Kitchell JB. The incidence of arrhythmias associated with acute myocardial infarction. *Prog. Cardiovasc. Dis.*, Jul., 1966, 9(1): 50-63.
205. Constant J. Preventing sudden death by raising the fibrillation threshold: a review-part 2. *Resident & Staff Physician*, Jun., 1991, 37(6): 29-32.
206. Wyman MG, Swan HJC, Rapaport E, Rockwell M. Arrhythmia deaths in 15,000 acute myocardial infarctions. *Circ.*, Oct., 1973, 48(4)(Suppl. IV): 40.
207. Schaffer WA, Cobb LA. Recurrent ventricular fibrillation and modes of death in survivors of out-of-hospital ventricular fibrillation. *N. Engl. J. Med.*, Aug. 7, 1975, 293(6): 259-62.
208. Tofler GH, Stone PH, Muller JE, Rutherford JD, Willich SN, Gustafson NF, Poole WK, Sobel BE, Willerson JT, Robertson T, Dassamani E, Braunwald E, and the MILIS Study Group. Prognosis after cardiac arrest due to ventricular tachycardia or ventricular fibrillation associated with acute myocardial infarction (the MILIS study). *Am. J. Cardiol.*, Oct. 1, 1987, 60(10): 755-61.
209. Vincent GM, Abildskov JA, Burgess MJ. Q-T interval syndromes. *Prog. Cardiovasc. Dis.*, May/Jun., 1974, 16(6): 523-34.
210. Johnson CT, Cowan M. Relationship between the prolonged QTc interval and ventricular fibrillation. *Heart & Lung*, Mar., 1986, 15(2): 141-50.
211. Billman GE. Mechanisms responsible for the cardiotoxic effects of cocaine. *FASEB-J.*, May, 1990, 4(8): 2469-75.
212. Loveys BJ. Physiologic effects of cocaine with particular reference to the cardiovascular system. *Heart & Lung*, Mar., 1987, 16(2): 175-80.
213. Goldberger AL, Goldberger E. *Clinical Electrocardiography*. 2nd ed. St. Louis: The CV Mosby Co., 1990.
214. Ruskin JN, McGovern B, Garan H, DiMarco JP, Kelly E. Antiarrhythmic drugs: a possible cause of out-of-hospital cardiac arrest. *N. Engl. J. Med.*, Nov. 24, 1983, 309(21): 1302-6.
215. Koster RW, Wellens HJJ. Quinidine-induced ventricular flutter and fibrillation without digitalis therapy. *Am. J. Cardiol.*, Oct., 1976, 38(4): 519-27.
216. Cryer PE, Haymond MW, Santiago JV, Shah SD. Norepinephrine and epinephrine release and adrenergic mediation of smoking associated hemodynamic and metabolic events. *N. Engl. J. Med.*, Sept. 9, 1976, 295(11): 573-7.
217. Bellet S, DeGuzman NT, Kostis JB, Roman L, Fleischmann D. The effect of inhalation of cigarette smoke on ventricular fibrillation threshold in normal dogs and dogs with acute myocardial infarction. *Am. Heart J.*, Jan., 1972, 83(1): 67-76.
218. Holbrook JH, Grundy SM, Hennekens CH, Kannel WB, Strong JP. Cigarette smoking and cardiovascular diseases. *Circ.*, Dec., 1984, 70(6): 1114A-7A.
219. Hoberg E, Schuler G, Kunze B, Obermoser AL, Hauer K, Mautner HP, Schlierf G, Kubler W. Silent myocardial ischemia as a potential link between lack of premonitoring symptoms and increased risk of cardiac arrest during physical stress. *Am. J. Cardiol.*, Mar. 1, 1990, 65(9): 583-9.
220. Eliot RS, Buell JC. Role of emotions and stress in the genesis of sudden death. *J. Am. Coll. Cardiol.*, Jun., 1985, 5(6): 95B-8B.
221. Skinner JE. Regulation of cardiac vulnerability by the cerebral defense system. *J. Am. Coll. Cardiol.*, Jun., 1985, 5(6): 88B-94B.
222. Amitzur G, Manoach M, Weinstock M. The influence of cardiac cholinergic activation on the induction and maintenance of ventricular fibrillation. *Basic Res. Cardiol.*, Nov.-Dec., 1984, 79(6): 690-7.
223. Verrier RL, Calvert A, Lown B. Effect of posterior hypothalmic stimulation on ventricular fibrillation threshold. *Am. J. Physiol.*, 1975, 228(3): 923-7.
224. Reich P, DeSilva RA, Lown B, Murawski BJ. Acute psychological disturbances preceding life-threatening ventricular arrhythmias. *JAMA*, Jul. 17, 1981, 246(3): 233-5.
225. James TN. Summary thoughts about sudden cardiac death. *J. Am. Coll. Cardiol.*, Jun., 1985, 5(6): 192B-8B.
226. Corrado D, Thiene G, Nava A, Rossi L, Pennelli N. Sudden death in young competitive athletes: clinicopathologic correlations in 22 cases. *Am. J. Med.*, Nov., 1990, 89:588-96.
227. Burke AP. Sports-related and non-sports-related sudden cardiac death in young adults. *Am. Heart J.*, 1991, 121: 568-75.
228. James TN. Morphologic substrate of sudden death. *J. Am. Coll. Cardiol.*, Jun., 1985, 5(6): 81B-2B.
229. Malik M, Farrell T, Camm AJ. Circadian rhythm of heart rate variability after acute myocardial infarction and its influence on the prognostic value of heart rate variability. *Am. J. Cardiol.*, Nov. 1, 1990, 66(15): 1049-54.
230. Cripps TR, Malik M, Farrell TG, Camm AJ. Prognostic value of reduced heart rate variability after myocardial infarction: clinical evaluation of a new analysis method. *Br. Heart J.*, Jan., 1991, 65(1): 14-9.
231. Jones DL, Klein GJ. Ventricular fibrillation: the importance of being coarse? *J. Electrocardiol.*, Oct., 1984, 17(4): 393-9.
232. Winkle RA, Mead RH, Ruder MA, Smith NA, Buch WS, Gaudiani VA. Effect of duration of ventricular fibrillation on defibrillation efficacy in humans. *Circ.*, May, 1990, 81(5): 1477-81.
233. Lown B, Crampton RS, DeSilva RA, Gascho J. The energy for ventricular defibrillation—too little or too much? Sounding Boards., *N. Engl. J. Med.*, Jun. 1, 1978, 298: 1252-3.
234. Peleska B. Cardiac arrhythmias following condenser discharges and their dependence upon strength of current and phase of cardiac cycle. *Circ. Res.*, Jul., 1963, 13(1): 21-32.
235. Gutgesell HP, Tacker WA, Geddes LA, Davis JS, Lie JT, McNamara DG. Energy dose for ventricular defibrillation of children. *Pediatrics*, Dec., 1976, 58(6): 898-901.
236. Frye SJ, Yacone LA. Cardiac pacing: a nursing perspective. *In* Hakki A-H (ed). *Ideal Cardiac Pacing*, Vol. 31 of *Major Problems in Clinical Surgery*. Philadelphia: WB Saunders, 1984.
237. Holder DA, Sniderman AD, Fraser G, Fallen EL. Experience with bretylium tosylate by a hospital cardiac arrest team. *Circ.*, Mar., 1977, 55(3): 541-4.
238. Heissenbuttel RH, Bigger JT Jr. Bretylium tosylate: a newly available antiarrhythmic drug for ventricular arrhythmias. *Ann. Intern. Med.*, Aug., 1979, 91(2): 229-38.
239. Sanna G, Arcidiacono R. Chemical ventricular defibrillation of the human heart with bretylium tosylate. *Am. J. Cardiol.*, Dec., 1973, 32(7): 982-7.
240. Little RA, Frayn KN, Randall PE, Stoner HB, Yates DW, Laing GS, Kumar S, Banks JM. Plasma catecholamines in patients with acute myocardial infarction and in cardiac arrest. *Q. J. Med.*, Feb., 1985, 54(214): 133-40.
241. Wyman MG, Hammersmith L. Comprehensive treatment plan for the prevention of primary ventricular fibrillation in acute myocardial infarction. *Am. J. Cardiol.* May, 1974, 33: 661-7.
242. Stockman MB, Verrier RL, Lown B. Effect of nitroglycerin on vulnerability of ventricular fibrillation during myocardial ischemia and reperfusion. *Am. J. Cardiol.*, Feb., 1979, 43: 233-8.
243. Gallagher JJ, Damato AN, Lau SH. Electrophysiologic studies during accelerated idioventricular rhythms. *Circ.*, Oct., 1971, 44(4): 671-7.
244. Marriott HJL, Menendez MM. A-V dissociation revisited. *Prog. Cardiovasc. Dis.*, May, 1966, 8(6): 522-38.
245. Bailey JC. The electrophysiologic basis for cardiac electrical activity: normal and abnormal. *Heart & Lung*, May/Jun., 1981, 10(3): 455-64.
246. Norris RM, Mercer CJ. Significance of idioventricular rhythms in acute myocardial infarction. *Prog. Cardiovasc. Dis.*, Mar/Apr., 1974, 16(5): 455-68.

247. Rothfeld EL, Zucker IR, Parsonnet V, Alinsonorin CA. Idioventricular rhythm in acute myocardial infarction. *Circ.*, Feb., 1968, 37(2): 203-9.
248. Rothfeld EL, Zucker IR, Leff WA, Parsonnet V. Idioventricular rhythm in acute myocardial infarction: a reappraisal. *Circ.*, Oct., 1970, 42(4)(Suppl. III): III: 193.
249. Massumi RA, Ali N. Accelerated isorhythmic ventricular rhythms. *Am. J. Cardiol.*, Aug., 1970, 26(2): 170-85.
250. Schamroth L. Idioventricular tachycardia. *J. Electrocardiol.*, 1968, 1(2): 205-12.
251. Zehender M, Meinertz T, Keul J, Just H. ECG variants and cardiac arrhythmias in athletes: clinical relevance and prognostic importance. *Am. Heart J.*, Jun., 1990, 1378-91.
252. Marriott HJL, Conover M. *Advanced Concepts in Arrhythmias*. 2nd ed. St. Louis: The CV Mosby Co., 1989.
253. Dressler W, Roesler H. The occurrence in paroxysmal ventricular tachycardia of ventricular complexes transitional in shape to sinoauricular beats. *Am. Heart J.*, Oct., 1952, 44(4): 485-93.
254. Marriott HJL, Schwartz NL, Bix HH. Ventricular fusion beats. *Circ.*, Nov., 1962, 26(5): 880-4.
255. Vasalle M. On the mechanisms underlying cardiac standstill: factors determining success or failure of escape pacemakers in the heart. *J. Am. Coll. Cardiol.*, Jun., 1985, 5(6): 35B-42B.
256. Tamura Y, Onodera O, Kodera K, Igarashi Y, Miida T, Aizawa Y, Izumi T, Shibata A, Takano S. Atrial standstill after treadmill exercise test and unique response to isoproterenol infusion in recurrent post exercise syncope. *Am. J. Cardiol.*, Feb. 15, 1990, 533-5.
257. Pederson WR, Janosik DL, Goldenberg IF, Stevens LL, Redd RM. Post-exercise asystolic arrest in a young man without organic heart disease: utility of head-up tilt testing in guiding therapy. *Am. Heart J.*, Aug., 1989, 118(2): 410-413.
258. Mark A. The Bezold-Jarisch relex revisited: clinical implications inhibitory relexes originating in the heart. *J. Am. Coll. Cardiol.*, 1983, 1: 90-102.
259. Buja G, Folino AF, Bittante M, Canciani B, Martini B, Miurelli M, Tognin D, Corrado D, Nava A. Asystole with syncope secondary to hyperventiltation in three young athletes. *PACE*, Mar., 1989, 12: 406-12.
260. American Heart Association. *Textbook of Advanced Cardiac Life Support*. Dallas: American Heart Association, 1987.
261. Brown DC, Lewis AJ, Criley JM. Asystole and its treatment: the possible role of the parasympathetic nervous system. *J. Am. Coll. Emerg. Physicians*, Nov., 1979, 8(11): 448-52.
262. Hurst JW, Logue RB, Walter PF. The clinical recognition and management of coronary atherosclerotic heart disease. *In* Hurst JW (ed). *The Heart; Arteries and Veins*. 4th ed. New York: McGraw-Hill, 1978, Chapter 62E.
263. Fozzard HA. Electromechanical dissociation and its possible role in sudden cardiac death. *J. Am. Coll. Cardiol.*, Jun., 1985, 5(6): 31B-4B.
264. Raizes G, Wagner GS, Hackel DB. Instantaneous nonarrhythmic cardiac death in acute myocardial infarction. *Am. J. Cardiol.*, Jan., 1977, 39(1): 1-6.
265. American Heart Association. Standards and guidelines for cardiopulmonary resuscitation and emergency cardiac care. *JAMA*, Jun. 6, 1986, 255(21): 2841-3044.
266. Kinoshita S, Konishi G, Kinohita Y. Protection of the ventricular parasystolic focus due to interference of sinus and parasystolic impulses in the ventricular-ectopic junction. *Cardiol.*, 1990, 77: 66-70.
267. Satullo G, Oreto G, Luzza F, Consolo A, Donato A. Sinus parasystole. *Am. Heart J.*, May, 1991, 121(5): 1507-12.
268. Andreoli KG, Fowkes VK, Zipes DP, Wallace AG (eds). *Comprehensive Cardiac Care*. 7th ed. St. Louis: The CV Mosby Co., 1991.
269. Baxter RH, McGuinness JB. Comparison of ventricular parasystole with other dysrhythmias after acute myocardial infarction. *Am. Heart J.*, Oct., 1974, 88(4): 443-8.
270. Watanabe, Y. Reassessment of parasystole. *Am. Heart J.* 1971, 81: 451.
271. Chung EKY. Parasystole. *Prog. Cardiovasc. Dis.*, 1968, 11: 64.

SELF-ASSESSMENT

MULTIPLE CHOICE
Directions

For each of the questions below, select the correct answer(s) from the choices given. If more than one answer is given, mark all that are correct.

Example

Ventricular rhythm disturbances are defined as arrhythmias originating in the
 a. atria.
 b. AV junction.
*c. ventricles.

Examples of ventricular rhythm disturbances include
*a. AIVR.
 b. AJR.
 c. PSVT.
*d. VT.

1. Which **one** statement below best defines sudden cardiac death (SCD)? SCD is defined as death
   a. resulting from rupture of the ventricular septum.
   b. occurring suddenly as a result of myocardial infarction.
   c. occurring within 24 hours of symptom onset.
   d. occurring within 1 hour of symptom onset.

2. SCD is most commonly due to which of the following arrhythmias?
   a. IVR.
   b. AIVR.
   c. VT.
   d. VF.
   e. Asystole.

3. Patients at higher risk for SCD include those who have
   a. coronary atherosclerosis.
   b. had SCD previously.
   c. acute myocardial ischemia.
   d. acute myocardial infarction.

4. The correlation of the incidence of VPBs with age is best described by which of the following statements?
   a. There is a linear relationship; with increasing age, the incidence of VPBs increases.
   b. There is an inverse relationship; with increasing age the incidence of VPBs decreases.
   c. There does not seem to be a relationship between age and the incidence of VPBs.
   d. VPBs occur only in elderly individuals with heart disease.

5. Ventricular ectopy is clinically significant
   a. whenever it occurs.
   b. when it results in compromise of cardiac output.
   c. in the presence of acute myocardial infarction.
   d. in the presence of myocardial ischemia.
   e. if it produces palpitations.

6. In evaluating a patient's response to antiarrhythmic drugs such as quinidine, procainamide, disopyramide, encainide, and amiodarone, it is necessary to regularly measure the
   a. blood pressure.
   b. peripheral pulse.
   c. ventricular rate.
   d. QT interval.

7. The following antiarrhythmic medication exerts a negative inotropic effect on the heart, a factor important in evaluating the patient's response:
   a. lidocaine.
   b. propranolol.
   c. procainamide.
   d. quinidine.

8. Which of the following is **not** a good criterion supporting the diagnosis of VT in the presence of a wide QRS tachycardia?
   a. An rSR′ QRS configuration.
   b. Concordance of the QRS complexes on all the precordial leads.
   c. Indeterminate QRS axis.
   d. QRS width >0.14 seconds without drug therapy.

9. Nursing intervention for the unconscious patient in VT depends on assessment findings. Which of the following is **not** indicated as initial intervention?
   a. CPR.
   b. Lidocaine.
   c. Cardioversion.
   d. Precordial thump.

10. Ventricular fibrillation is more likely to occur in the patient who has
    a. APBs.
    b. an acute myocardial infarction.
    c. hyperkalemia.
    d. chronic obstructive pulmonary disease.

MATCHING

Directions

Match each arrhythmia in column A with its correct classification in column B.

Examples

A	B
(C) 1. JPB	A. Ventricular arrhythmia
(B) 2. APB	B. Atrial arrhythmia
(A) 3. VPB	C. Junctional arrhythmia

A	B
( ) 11. VPB	A. Active or usurping
( ) 12. AIVR	B. Passive or escape
( ) 13. Primary VF	C. Either active or passive
( ) 14. IVR	
( ) 15. Torsades de pointes	

Directions

Match the patterns of occurrence of VPBs in column A with their definitions in column B. Choices in column B may be used more than once or not at all.

A	B
( ) 16. Bigeminy	A. Two VPBs in succession
( ) 17. Couplet	B. Every other beat is VPB
( ) 18. End-diastolic	C. Three VPBs in succession
( ) 19. Interpolated	D. Every third beat is VPB
( ) 20. Quadrigeminy	E. Three or more VPBs in rapid succession
( ) 21. R-on-T	F. Every fourth beat is VPB
( ) 22. Run of VT	G. VPB occurring in place of normal beat; results in compensatory pause
( ) 23. Salvo of two	H. VPB landing on T wave of preceding beat
( ) 24. Trigeminy	I. VPB occurring between two normal QRS complexes
( ) 25. Triplet	J. VPB occurring only slightly early, often allowing sinus P to show

Directions

Match the three arrhythmias in column A with characteristics in column B. Items in column B may be used more than once or not at all.

A	B
( ) 26. Rate usually 100 to 250 bpm	A. Torsades de pointes
( ) 27. Rate usually >250 bpm	B. Ventricular flutter
( ) 28. Always polymorphic	C. Ventricular tachycardia
( ) 29. May be uniform or polymorphic	
( ) 30. QRS complexes cannot be differentiated from T waves and are called sine waves	
( ) 31. Often irregular	

TRUE/FALSE

Directions

Determine whether each of the following statements is true or false and indicate with a *T* or *F*.

Example

(T) 1. Ventricular fibrillation is a lethal arrhythmia.

( ) 32. Uniform VPBs most often exhibit fixed coupling intervals.

( ) 33. EMD is defined as QRS complexes (electrical activity) not accompanied by mechanical activity (contraction).

( ) 34. The VPBs in ventricular parasystole often exhibit fixed coupling intervals.

( ) 35. Lidocaine is contraindicated in IVR.

( ) 36. In the presence of acute MI, prophylactic lidocaine should be administered as soon as one of the warning arrhythmias appears.

( ) 37. Ventricular fibrillation is a possibility when the digitalis-toxic patient is cardioverted.

( ) 38. Ventricular fibrillation is more likely to occur immediately after myocardial infarction than several hours after.

( ) 39. Multiformed VPBs are those that display three waves in the same complex, such as a qRSr′.

The remaining questions involve analysis of patient situations and assessment of rhythm strips. Responses required are short answer and essay.

CASE: *Mrs. M. is a 68-year-old patient on your telemetry unit. She was admitted 3 days ago with a medical diagnosis of congestive heart failure. Since you have just returned from a few days off, this is your first encounter with Mrs. M. You have made an initial brief assessment of vital signs: T 98.2; R 20; BP 128/78; AP 100.* ***A,*** *On the ECG, lead III reveals the pattern in this strip.* ***B,*** *Having difficulty assessing and diagnosing the rhythm, you switch to lead II.*

40. Can you determine the rhythm from strips **A** and **B?** Is there anything else can you do to assess the rhythm?

Lead III

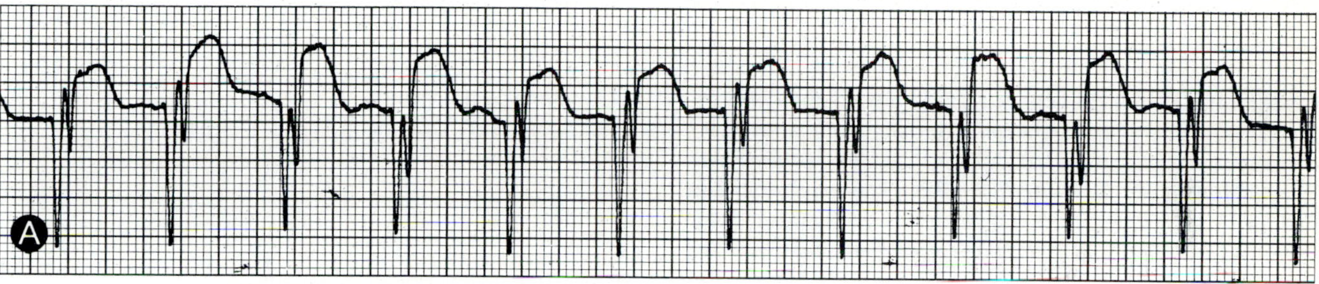

Lead II

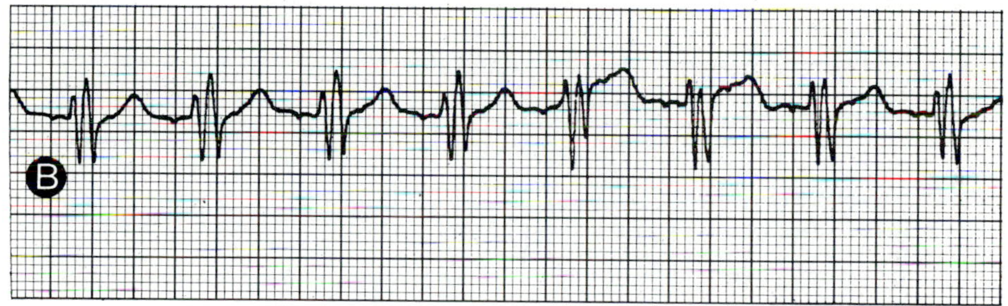

The rhythm strip below is the same pattern as viewed on V_1.

41. Proceed with your assessment and diagnosis of the arrhythmia.
42. What else will you include in your assessment?
43. What is the nursing diagnosis?
44. Delineate nursing interventions.
45. Relate some of the points to consider in evaluation of the patient after the above interventions.

V_1

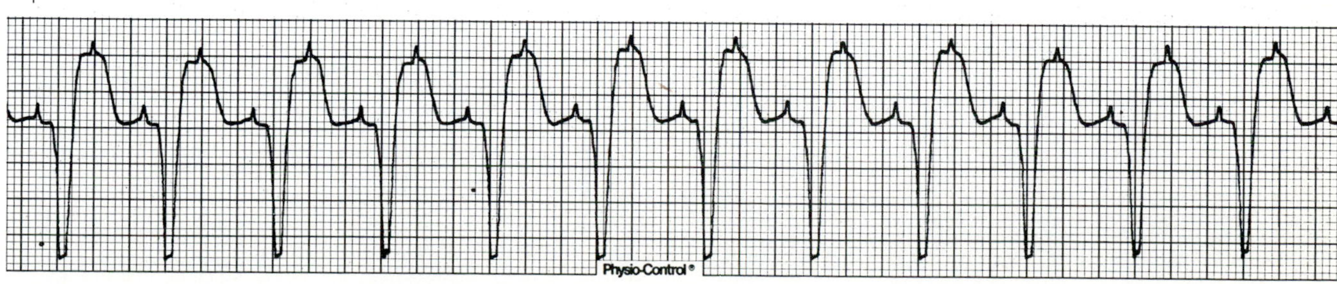

CASE: *Mr. S., a 79-year-old patient in the ICU, has been admitted for medical evaluation of syncopal episodes. His blood pressure is 156/90. His monitor strip is displayed here.*

46. Interpret and explain the rhythm. What nursing interventions related to the rhythm are indicated?

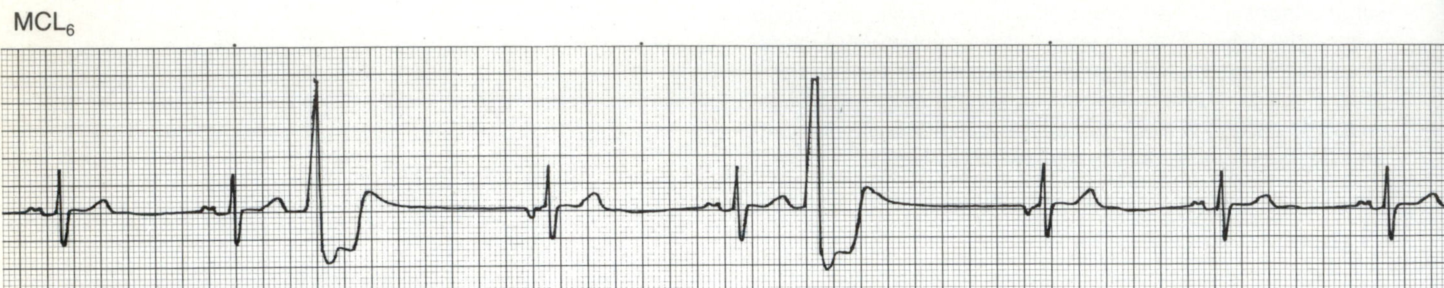

CASE: *Mr. G. is a 58-year-old client who summoned the ambulance when his severe retrosternal chest pain was not relieved by taking three nitroglycerin tablets sublingually. After attaching Mr. G. to the ECG, the following rhythm was displayed. The patient's blood pressure is 128/88, his skin is warm and moist with no signs of cyanosis, and he denies dyspnea.*

47. Interpret the rhythm.
48. Determine intervention in order of priority.

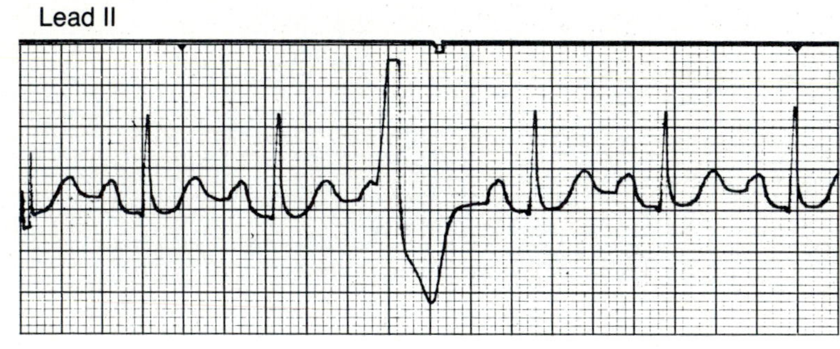

***CASE:** The following strips are two* different leads illustrating the same anomalous beat (arrow) *on leads III and aVL.*

49. Interpret the arrhythmia and determine nursing intervention.

Lead III

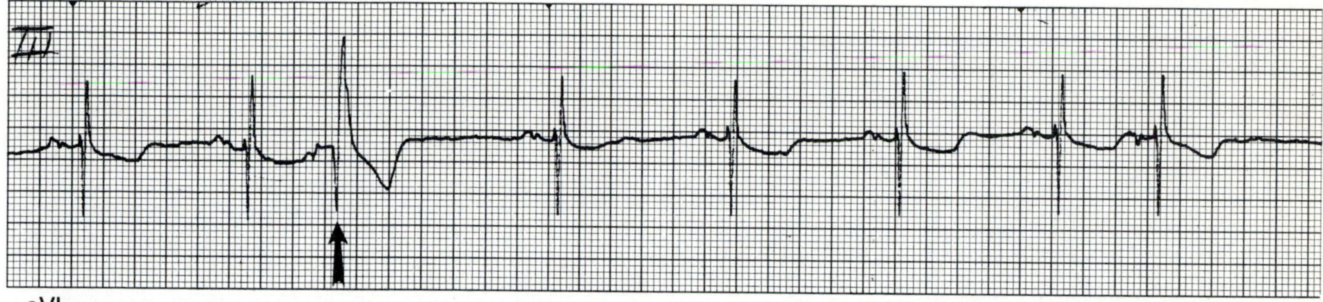

aVL

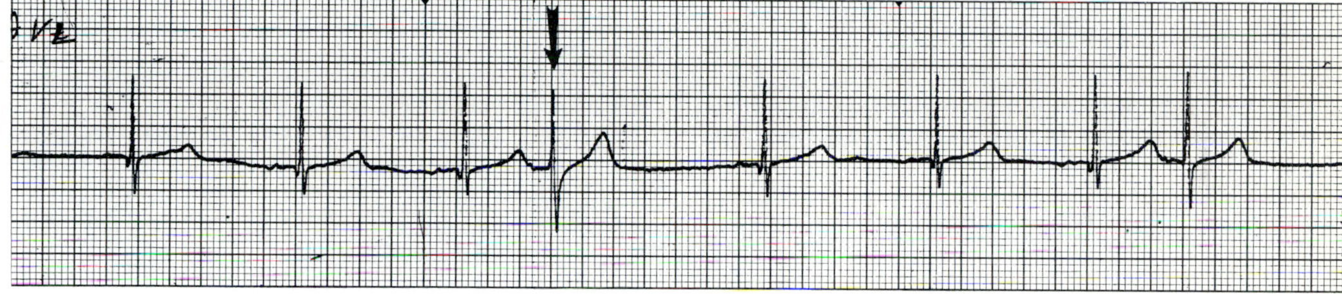

50. Interpret the rhythm strip below and write your interpretation as you would enter it in the patient's record.

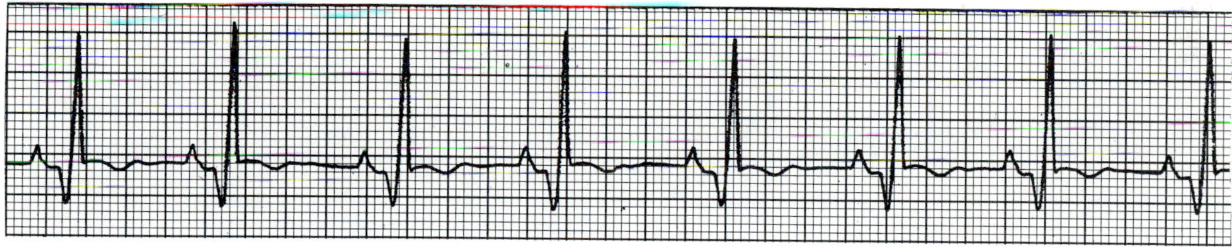

***CASE:** Ms. T. is a 42-year-old patient just admitted to the CCU with a medical diagnosis of probable acute MI. Moments after she arrived, she exhibited the rhythm displayed here.*

51. Assess the rhythm. What other assessments will you perform?
52. Emergency assessment reveals Ms. T. is not conscious. Formulate your plan of care and list your interventions by priority.

MCL_1

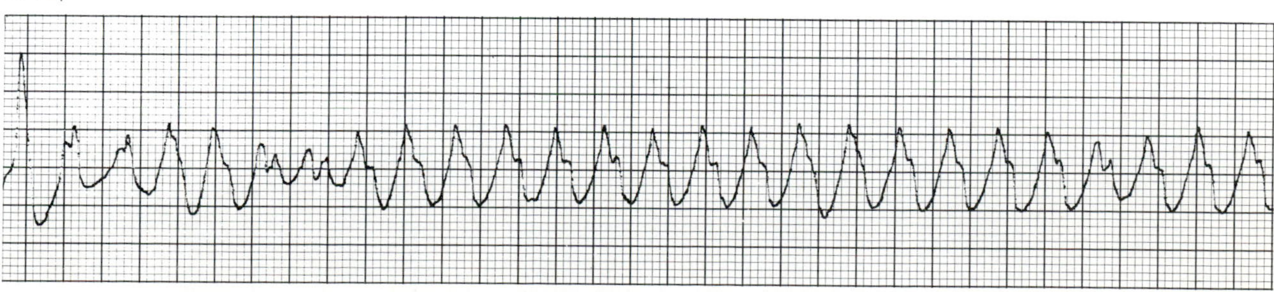

CASE: *Mr. L. is a 66-year-old client admitted to the CCU at 1000 hours with a medical diagnosis of acute MI. It is now 2330 hours and Mr. L is sleeping. He displays the rhythm below. Approximately 30 minutes ago he displayed the same arrhythmia at which time you awakened him to assess his response to the rhythm disturbance and found him to be asymptomatic. You also noted that as soon as you awakened him, the arrhythmia subsided.*

53. Interpret the rhythm.
54. Discuss your plan of care.

Lead II

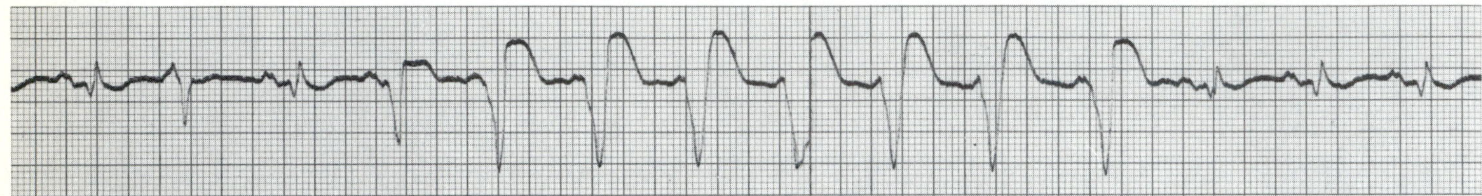

CASE: *Mr. K., a 38-year-old patient admitted to the telemetry unit for evaluation of chest pain, displays the rhythm below.*

55. Interpret the rhythm.
56. Explain why some of the QRS complexes are larger than others. In what other instances may this phenomenon be exhibited?
57. What factors will you consider in your initial care planning for this patient?
58. Discuss the arrhythmia in terms of its clinical significance.
59. List ten causes of ventricular ectopy.

Lead II

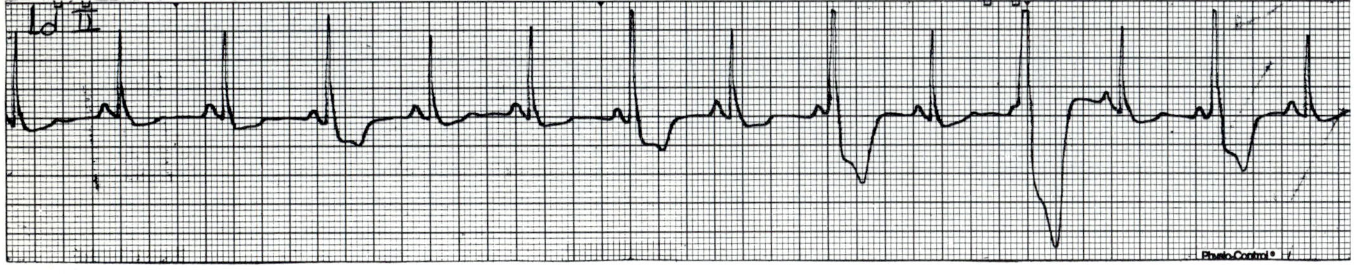

__CASE:__ Mr. M., 40, presented to the emergency room with complaints of chest pain, nausea, and weakness. As soon as he was connected to the ECG machine for his 12-lead ECG, he suddenly complained of worsening chest pain, began retching, and subsequently became semiconscious, pale with cool, clammy skin, and thready peripheral pulses with pulse deficit.

60. Interpret the rhythm. List two conditions in which this arrhythmia is likely to occur. List five situations that may provoke this arrhythmia.
61. Determine the QRS axis.
62. Does the morphology of the QRS complexes lend support to the diagnosis?
63. List immediate interventions in order of priority.
64. What can this rhythm deteriorate into?

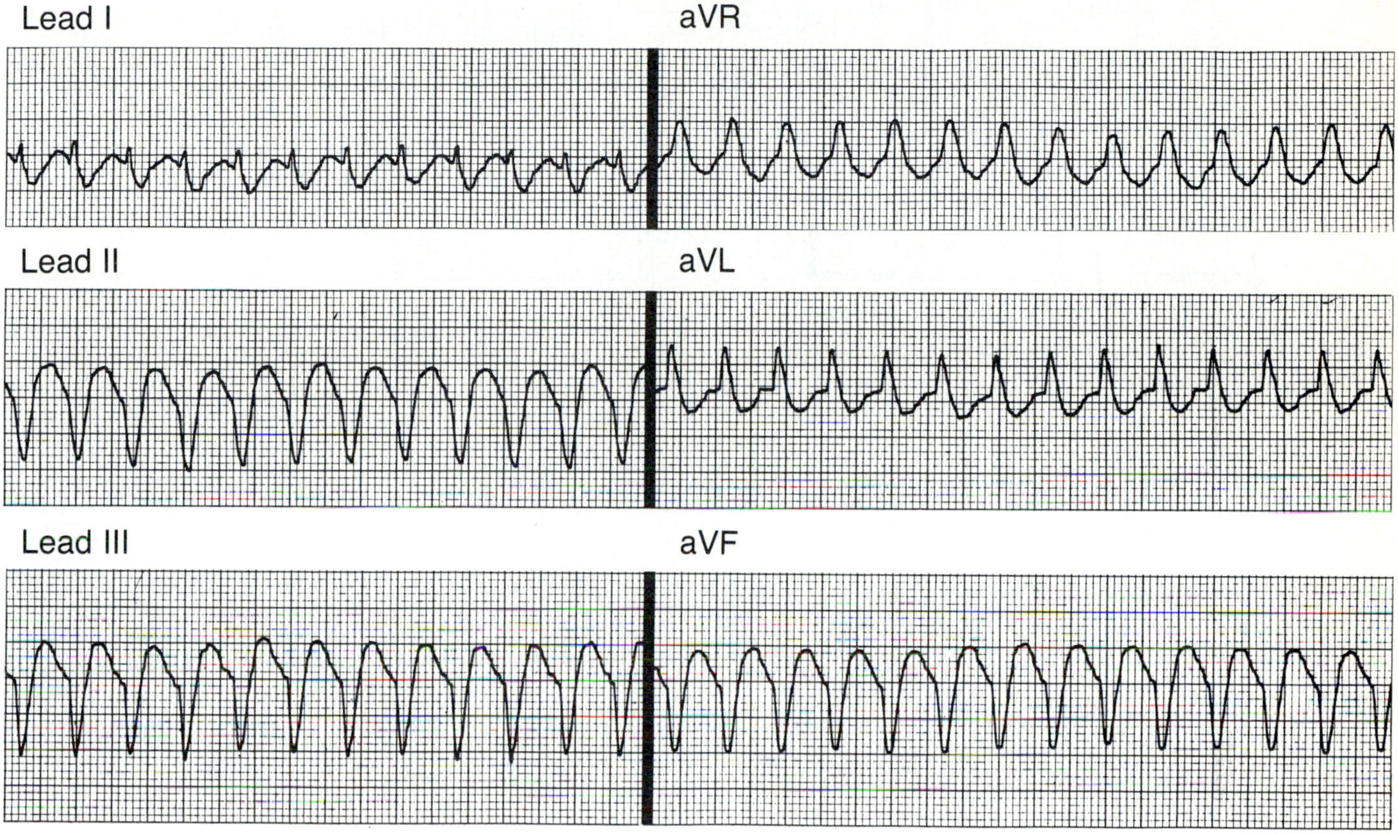

Lead I aVR

Lead II aVL

Lead III aVF

__CASE:__ Ms. P., 67, is hospitalized for evaluation and management of her angina pectoris. She recently began exhibiting anomalous beats. Leads V_1 and V_6 (not simultaneous) are presented here for your interpretation.

65. What is your interpretation of the rhythm?
66. Discuss nursing interventions.

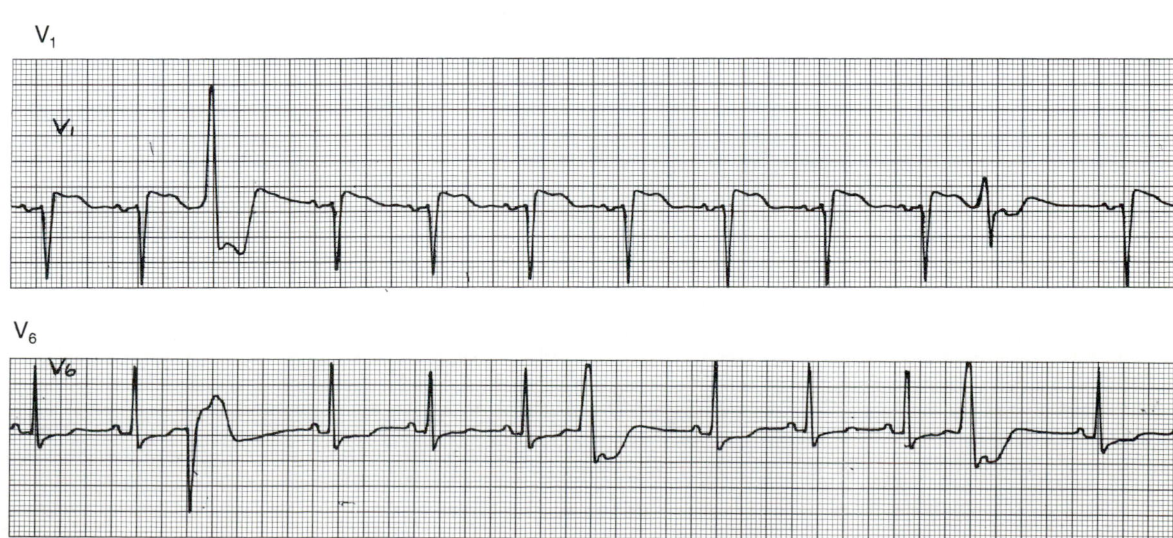

Presented below are rhythm strips. Analyze each.

67. Interpret the rhythm. Explain why there is a pause after the anomalous beat.

Lead II

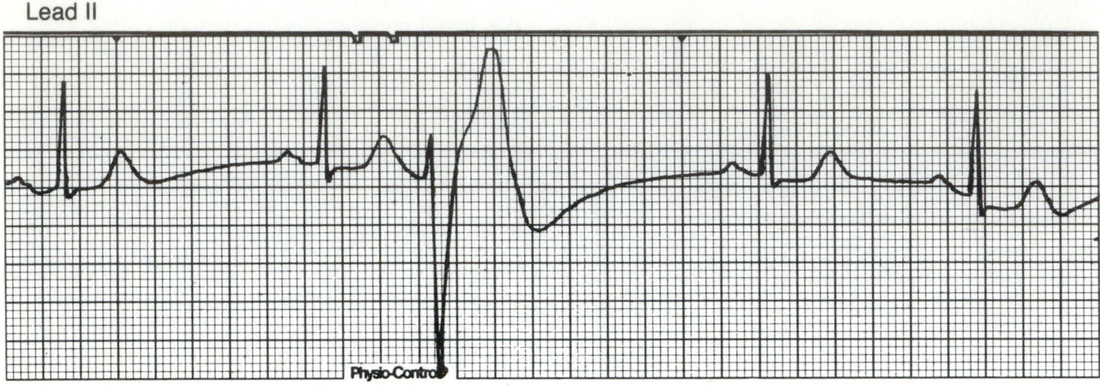

68. Analyze the rhythm.

V_1

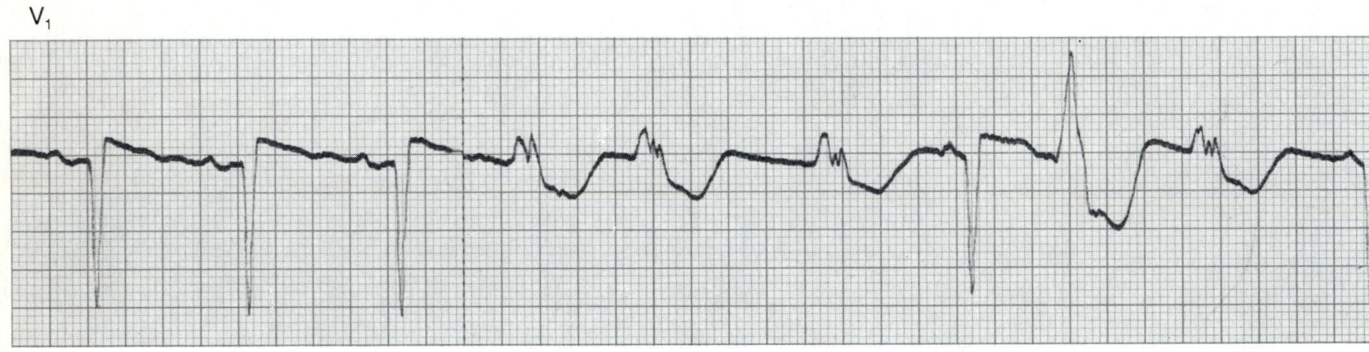

69. Analyze the rhythm. Discuss assessment and nursing intervention.

MCL_1

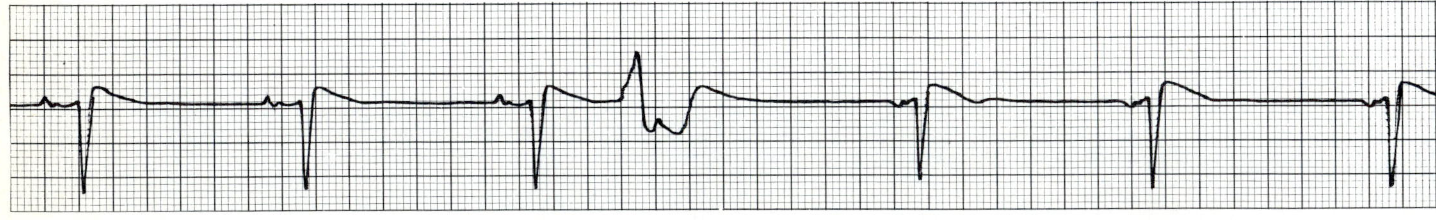

70. The patient with this rhythm was found nonresponsive, pulseless, and apneic. Analyze the rhythm. Discuss assessment and nursing intervention.

MCL_1

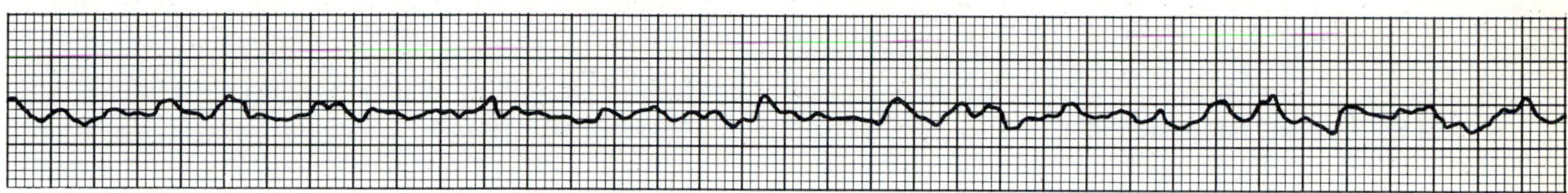

71. The two strips below are simultaneous tracings. Analyze the rhythm.

V_5

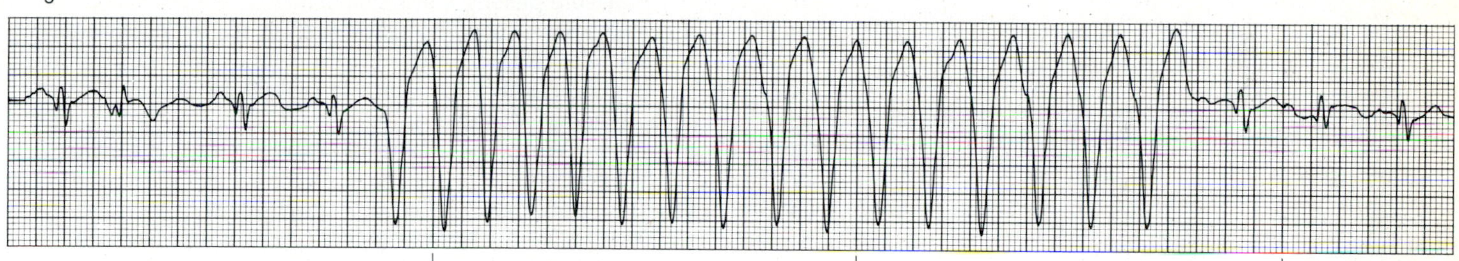

V_1

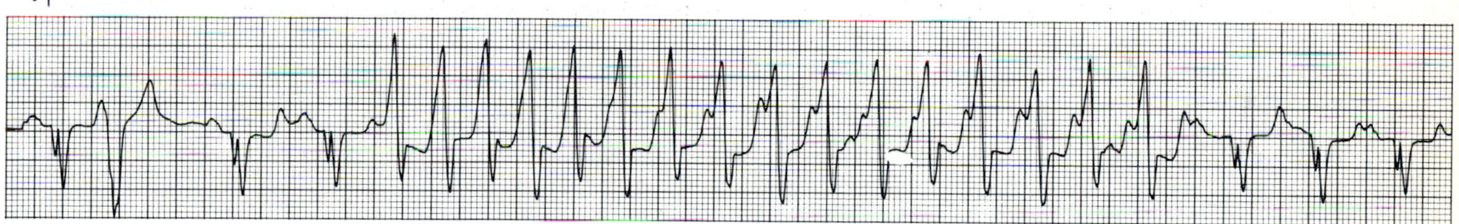

72. The patient with the rhythm below experienced a precipitous fall in blood pressure with the initiation of this arrhythmia. The patient was in the coronary care unit for evaluation of his chest pain.

MCL_1

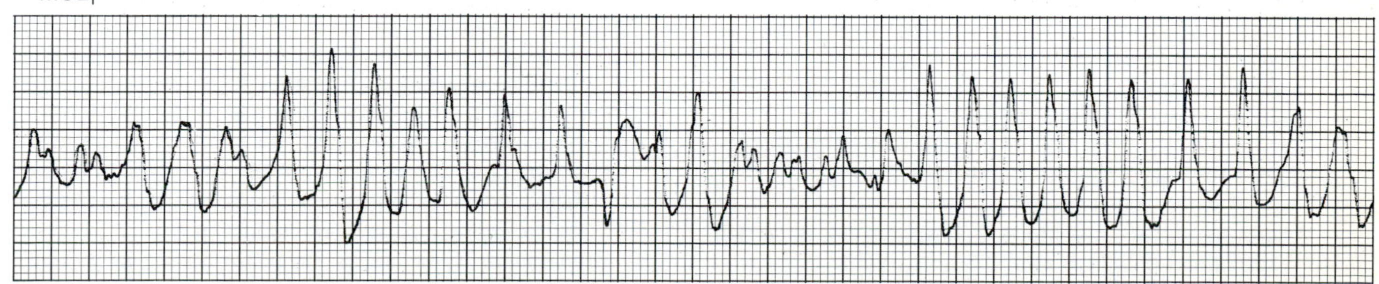

ANSWERS TO SELF-ASSESSMENT

1. d (choice b is one type of SCD. Recall that less than half of SCD victims have had an MI.)
2. c,d
3. a,b,c,d
4. a
5. b,c,d
6. d
7. b
8. a
9. b
10. b
11. A
12. B (C may also be correct, though less frequently)
13. A
14. B
15. A
16. B
17. A
18. J
19. I
20. F
21. H
22. C,E
23. A
24. D
25. C
26. C
27. A
28. A
29. C
30. B
31. A
32. T
33. T
34. F
35. T
36. F
37. T
38. T
39. F
40. From *A,* the only information that can be obtained is that the ventricular rhythm is regular and the complexes are wide. There is no consistent, identifiable atrial activity. The QRS complexes are wide at a rate of 100 bpm. It is necessary to differentiate between ventricular tachycardia and supraventricular tachycardia with an IVCD.

    In strip *B,* lead II, consistent atrial activity is evident preceding each QRS complex and bears a constant relation to it, indicating that the rhythm is probably supraventricular in origin. For confirmation, the rhythm requires analysis on still another lead.
41. Atrial activity is much clearer on this lead. Small, peaked P waves are identified not only preceding the QRS but in the ST-T wave area as well.

    Rate: Ventricular: 100 bpm
    Atrial: 200 bpm
    Rhythm: Ventricular: Regular
    Atrial: Regular
    P waves: Small, rate 200, regular
    PR interval: 0.11 seconds of the Ps preceding QRSs
    QRS complex: 0.12 to 0.13 seconds prolonged (IVCD); ST-T wave abnormalities
    Interpretation: AT with block, 2:1 conduction, atrial rate 200 bpm, ventricular rate 100 bpm, IVCD
42. As with any patient in, or approaching, tachycardia, assess blood pressure, peripheral pulses, sensorium. Since this rhythm is a classic digitalis toxicity arrhythmia, determine if the patient is on digitalis and obtain order for serum digoxin level. If indicated, assess for other signs of digitalis toxicity.
43. (1) Decreased cardiac output related to tachycardia (2) Decreased tissue perfusion related to decreased cardiac output.
44. Hold digoxin until serum level is obtained.
    Notify physician.
    Reassure patient, if symptomatic.
45. Your answer should include such things as the following:
    Evaluate rhythm for return to normal as digoxin level gradually decreases.
    Evaluate progress of other symptoms of digoxin toxicity, if present.
46. The basic rhythm is sinus bradycardia at a rate of approximately 48 bpm (see first two and last two complexes). Two uniform VPBs are each followed by a compensatory pause that is interrupted by atrial escape complex. Since the P wave measures 0.14 seconds, there is likely an intraatrial conduction defect present. Since the blood pressure is adequate, it is likely the rhythm is a sufficiently perfusing one. No intervention is indicated.
47. NSR with rate 95 bpm. One end-diastolic VPB. PR 0.18 seconds, QRS 0.08 seconds.
48. Interventions in order of priority: numbers 1 to 5 should be done nearly simultaneously and according to institutional policy.
    1. Reassure the patient.
    2. Administer oxygen.
    3. Start IV.
    4. Administer IV analgesic.
    5. Consider prophylactic lidocaine.
    6. Transport patient.
49. *Rate:* 54 to 60 bpm
    Rhythm: Irregular
    P wave: 0.11 to 0.12 seconds, wide, probable intraatrial conduction disturbance, APBs
    PR interval: 0.20 seconds
    QRS complex: 0.08 seconds
    Interpretation: Sinus bradycardia with rate 57 bpm. APBs, some of which are aberrantly conducted (in this example, best shown on lead III).
    Intervention: None unless the patient is showing signs and symptoms of an underlying disorder that may be related to the APBs, such as congestive heart failure.
50. Sinus rhythm with IVCD, regular rate 76 bpm. PR 0.14 seconds, QRS (qR) 0.12 seconds.

51. VT.
    Assess level of consciousness, presence of pulse and respirations.
52. Precordial thump.
    If no pulse begin CPR.
    Notify others of **cardiac arrest.**
    Cardiovert as soon as equipment available.
    Administer lidocaine, or other suitable antiarrhythmic medication according to institutional policies.
53. Sinus rhythm with AIVR and resultant AV dissociation. (Can you plot the P waves through the AIVR?)
54. Previous assessment attempts revealed that the arrhythmia subsided when the patient was awakened. There is probably no need to repeat that procedure if the patient's color is good and there are no other changes in his condition. AIVR is not unusual after MI and is, in most cases, an innocuous arrhythmia.
55. Basic rhythm is NSR with rate 82 to 85 bpm. Frequent end-diastolic VPBs result in frequent fusion beats (F).

Lead II

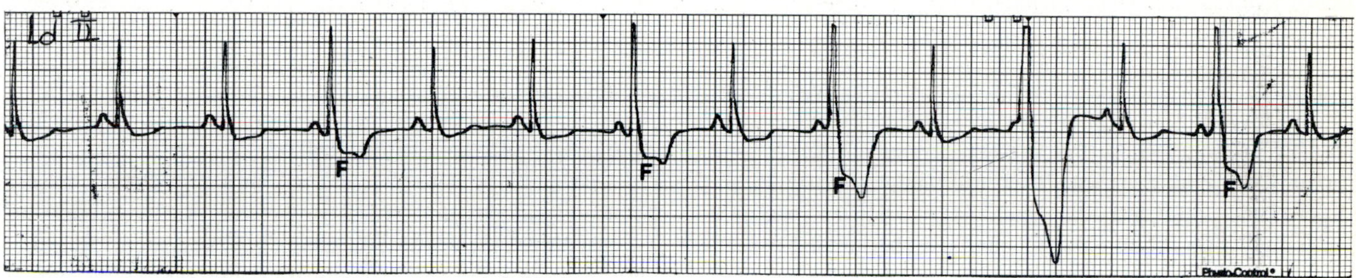

56. Fusion complexes *(F)* are wider because the sinus-conducted QRS is occurring at the same time as the VPB. The two QRS complexes are fused or combined. The larger the QRS complex, the greater the influence of the ectopic ventricular beat on the appearance of the QRS.
57. The possibility of ischemic heart disease.
58. VPBs are clinically significant in the presence of MI or ischemia. Late and early VPBs may initiate VT or VF.
59. See Table 8-1.
60. Probable VT.
    MI, coronary ischemia.
    Hypokalemia, hypomagnesemia, drug toxicity, prolonged QT interval syndrome, sympathomimetic amines.
61. Superior at approximately −90 degrees.
62. QRS is 0.12 seconds. Axis is superior. Need to assess V leads for more criteria.
63. Precordial thump. Administer lidocaine or comparable antiarrhythmic. Maintain airway patency.
64. VF.
65. NSR with polymorphic VPBs.
66. Consider prophylactic lidocaine. Notify physician of ventricular ectopy. Other interventions are based on assessment findings and might include oxygen therapy, allaying anxiety, etc.
67. Sinus bradycardia with VPB. Pause is compensatory (the sinus P in the VPB does not conduct a QRS complex).
68. NSR at rate 75 bpm, triplet of uniform VPBs followed by an end-diastolic JPB and couplet of polymorphic VPBs.
69. Sinus bradycardia with rate 43 bpm, prolonged PR interval of 0.22 seconds (first degree AV block, refer to Chapter 9), VPB followed by atrial escape rhythm at rate 41 bpm.
70. VF.
    Establish unresponsiveness and pulselessness.
    Defibrillate **immediately.**
    Continue CPR until defibrillator is available.
71. *Rate:* 94 bpm increasing to 202 bpm
    Rhythm: Irregular
    P wave: When present, is wide, 0.11 seconds
    PR interval: 0.18 to 0.28 seconds (PR longer with beats ending shorter cycles)
    QRS complex: 0.13 seconds, prolonged, IVCD; 16 beat run of monomorphic VT at slightly irregular rate 202 bpm
    Interpretation: Sinus rhythm with IVCD at rate 94 bpm. One VPB noted before rhythm interrupted by a run of monomorphic VT at rate 202 bpm. Initiating VPB different from singly occurring VPB.
72. *Rate:* 250 to 300 bpm
    Rhythm: Irregular
    P wave: None identifiable
    PR interval: —
    QRS complex: Wide, vary in morphology
    Interpretation: Polymorphic VT

CHAPTER NINE

Atrioventricular and Intraventricular Conduction Disturbances

▶ GOAL

You will be able to recognize significant atrioventricular (AV) and intraventricular conduction delays, determine which may be life threatening, and use the nursing process in caring for patients with these rhythm disturbances.

▶ OBJECTIVES

After studying this chapter and completing the self-assessment exercises, you should be able to do the following:

AV Blocks

1. Explain the conventional classification system for AV block.
2. Describe and recognize the ECG features of first, second, and third degree AV blocks, and determine nursing interventions based on assessment findings.
3. Compare and contrast the ECG features and treatments for Types I and II second degree AV blocks and differentiate one from the other on the ECG.
4. List two kinds of AV block that may occur in healthy individuals and explain their possible causes.
5. Offer two ECG diagnostic signs to assist in determining whether second degree AV block with 2:1 conduction is Type I or Type II.
6. Correlate the occurrence of Type I and Type II AV blocks with inferior and anterior myocardial infarctions (MI). State which of the two blocks may be a poorer prognostic sign and explain why.
7. Explain the etiology and clinical significance of first, second, and third degree AV blocks and compare assessment measures appropriate for each.

AV Dissociation

8. Define AV dissociation and relate it to third degree AV block. Identify three other arrhythmias in which AV dissociation is present.
9. Recognize AV dissociation on the ECG.

Intraventricular Conduction Delays

10. Explain the classification of intraventricular conduction delays and identify which may be found in healthy individuals and which may represent disease.
11. Appraise the clinical situation and determine which leads offer the most useful information in assessing patients with intraventricular conduction defects.
12. Contrast the ECG characteristics and clinical significance of right bundle branch block (RBBB) with left bundle branch block (LBBB). Recognize each on the ECG.
13. Explain how the electrical axis in left anterior hemiblock (LAH) differs from that in left posterior hemiblock (LPH) and choose the most appropriate lead to assess this.
14. Compare the clinical significance of hemiblocks with bundle branch blocks.
15. Explain the terms *monofascicular, bifascicular,* and *trifascicular blocks* and relate the clinical significance of each.

Ventricular Aberration

16. Describe the ECG characteristics of ventricular aberration and compare its clinical significance and treatment with ventricular ectopy.
17. Identify the most common form of ventricular aberration.
18. Recognize ventricular aberration on the monitor.
19. Discuss factors contributing to the development of ventricular aberration.

ATRIOVENTRICULAR BLOCKS

The anatomic structures of the AV conduction system consist of the AV node (AVN), bundle of His, bundle branches, and Purkinje fibers. Arrhythmias that result from a conduction delay or block within the AVN, bundle of His, or His-Purkinje system (HPS) are known as *AV blocks*. AV blocks (or conduction defects) have traditionally been classified by degrees: first, second, and third (complete). As a result of advances in cardiac electrophysiology with His bundle recordings, additional information concerning location and severity of AV block has been obtained, making this traditional classification deficient and impractical. However, we have elected to preserve the custom until a more desirable classification system prevails.

FIRST DEGREE AV BLOCK
Data Base: Problem Identification
Definitions, Etiology, and Mechanisms

First degree block is incomplete AV block due to slower than normal conduction through one or more sites of the AV conduction system (AVN, bundle of His, or HPS). Commonly the delay is located in the AVN[1,2] and results in a prolonged PR interval.

The causes of first degree AV block include increased vagal tone, acute inferior wall myocardial infarction (IWMI), myocarditis, subacute bacterial endocarditis (SBE), pharmacologic agents (e.g. digitalis, beta blockers, or calcium-channel blockers), and chronic heart disease of any kind. However, it is frequently a normal finding, especially in athletes. Holter studies have revealed its presence during sleep in healthy boys,[3,4] during sleep and

ECG Characteristics
First Degree AV Block

Rate: Any
Rhythm: Regular
P waves: Normal
PR interval: Above 0.20 seconds
QRS complex: Normal, unless IVCD present

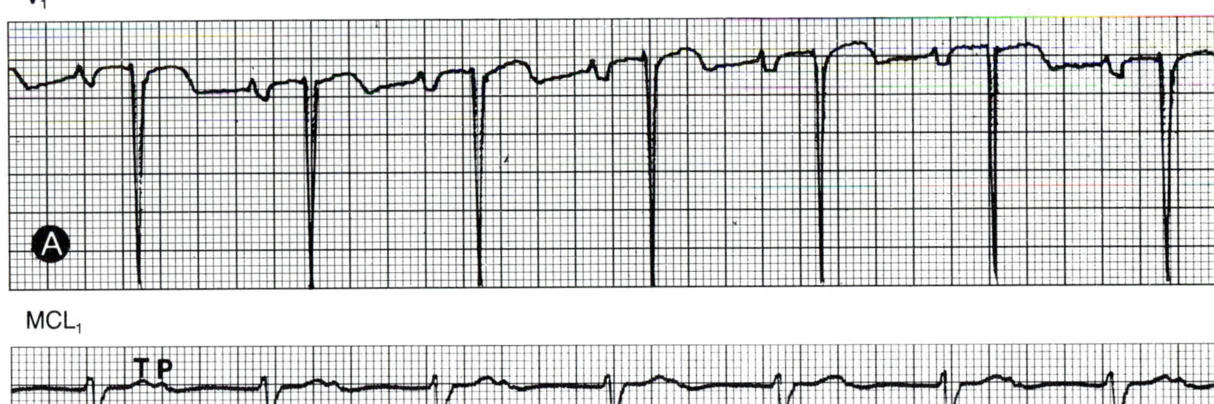

FIGURE 9-1 **A,** First degree AV block. **B,** First degree AV block with unusually long PR interval.

A.

Rate: 65 bpm
Rhythm: Regular
P wave: Normal; one precedes each QRS complex and bears a constant relation to it.
PR interval: 0.30 seconds, prolonged
QRS complex: 0.10 seconds, rS morphology normal on V_1
Interpretation: Sinus rhythm with first degree AV block

B.

Rate: 64 bpm
Rhythm: Regular
P wave: Normal; one precedes each QRS complex and bears a constant relation to it.
PR interval: 0.52 seconds, prolonged
QRS complex: 0.11 seconds, rS morphology normal on MCL_1
Interpretation: Sinus rhythm with first degree AV block.

wake periods in long-distance runners,[5] and in pilots and airmen.[6]

ECG Characteristics

First degree AV block is characterized by a PR interval of 0.21 seconds to as high as 0.60 seconds or more that does not change from beat to beat (see box on p. 257 and Fig. 9-1).

The PR interval is both age and rate dependent. In children under 14 years the normal PR interval is up to 0.18 seconds. The PR interval in adults with tachycardias should be no greater than 0.18 seconds. When the tachycardia exceeds 150 bpm, prolongation of the PR interval may occur because of the physiologic partial refractory period of the AV node.[7]

Applied Nursing Process

Clinical Assessment

- Detect:
  - A prolonged PR interval on the ECG.
- Assess the patient and ECG.
  - First degree AV block is usually only discovered by an ECG. However, in some individuals, the S_1 heart sound may become softer. When the PR interval is extremely long, the atria contract while the AV valves are closed, producing cannon waves in the jugular pulse.[8]

❖ NURSING DIAGNOSIS

Decreased cardiac output (rarely) related to loss of atrial contribution to cardiac output.

❖ ECG DIAGNOSIS

First degree AV block.

Plan and Implementation

Patient goal. The patient will be free from congestive heart failure and higher grades of block.

Nursing interventions.

- Document first degree AV block on the ECG and notify the physician if it is a new finding.
- Further nursing intervention is usually not required, since this arrhythmia is generally benign. However, if the PR interval becomes exceedingly prolonged, the atrial kick may be lost, resulting in decreased ventricular ejection. The diminished cardiac output could, in some cases, be sufficient to produce heart failure. Thus it is wise to keep such a possibility in mind and consider adapting the plan of care to include appropriate assessment measures.
- In the presence of an acute MI, observe and document any changes found to be present in the severity of the AV block.
- Inform the physician of the development of first degree block in digitalized patients. This may be an indication of impending digoxin toxicity.
- Be aware of the increased risk of higher grades of block when administering digitalis, beta blockers, or calcium-channel blockers to the patient with first degree AV block.[2]

Evaluation

The patient maintains hemodynamic stability and is free from advancing degrees of block as evidenced by the following:

- Stable blood pressure.
- No increase in the PR interval on the ECG and maintenance of 1:1 atrial-to-ventricular conduction.
- No signs of congestive heart failure.

Medical Treatment

No medical treatment is generally indicated.

SECOND DEGREE AV BLOCK

Second degree AV block exists when one or more atrial impulses fail to activate the ventricles. Two types of second degree block—Type I and Type II—were first identified on the basis of jugular pulse tracings by Wenckebach in the late nineteenth century in Vienna. In 1924, Mobitz utilized electrocardiography to identify the same AV conduction disturbances previously described by Wenckebach.[9,10] Present day terminology for Type I AV block is *Wenckebach* or *Mobitz I*. Type II AV block is referred to as *Mobitz II,* even though Wenckebach Type II might be more correct historically.

TYPE I SECOND DEGREE AV BLOCK

Data Base: Problem Identification

Definitions, Etiology, and Mechanisms

Type I AV block usually results from a conduction defect located within the AV node[1,8] and thus is sometimes referred to as *supra-Hisian*. It is characterized by progressive slowing and intermittent failure of AV conduction. Considered to be relatively benign, Type I second degree AV block generally does not progress to more advanced forms of AV block.[9,11]

Like first degree block, Type I second degree AV block is frequently associated with acute IWMI due to occlusion of the right coronary artery (RCA). With such an MI, the block is usually temporary, occurring within the first 24 to 48 hours. Type I AV block may also be seen with rheumatic fever or as a result of digitalis intoxication, beta blockers, or verapamil ingestion.[2,9,12] However, like first degree AV block, it may be a normal finding. It has been documented during sleep in healthy boys and athletes.[3-5]

Schamroth[7] suggests that AV block in athletes is a manifestation of increased vagal stimulation, and vagal stimulation has been shown specifically to induce Type I AV block.

ECG Characteristics

The classic form of Type I second degree AV block is differentiated from higher forms of AV block by characteristic ECG features. Most episodes, however, deviate somewhat from this classic pattern.[3,13,14]

Progressive lengthening of the PR interval.[9] In Type I AV block, what is known as the *Wenckebach phenomenon* is exhibited. The PR interval increases with each successive cycle until a QRS complex is dropped. This progressive lengthening of the PR interval occurs as each atrial impulse arrives earlier in the relative refractory period of the AV node. Increasing delay in the AVN eventually results in an atrial impulse that is unable to reach the ventricles in time to produce a beat. After the dropped QRS, the PR interval returns to normal (or near normal) and the sequence begins again (Fig. 9-2). The PR interval may become surprisingly prolonged with intervals up to 0.60 seconds not uncommon.

Grouped beating. Groups of beats occur in trios, couplets,[9] or other repetitive patterns of groups of beats. A common Wenckebach conduction ratio is 3:2 (three P waves to two QRS complexes) (Fig. 9-3), but other ratios producing larger groups (5:4, 6:5, and so on) are not unusual (see Fig. 9-2).

R-R interval shortening.[9,13] As the PR intervals lengthen in each group of beats, consecutive R-R intervals shorten (Fig. 9-4).

Longest cycle less than twice the shortest.[9,13] Measure the farthest distance between the QRS complexes (the last QRS in one group to the first QRS in the next group). This distance should be less than twice the shortest distance between QRS complexes. As illustrated in Figure 9-4, the longest R-R interval is the QRS that follows the longest PR interval and the first QRS after the dropped beat. This interval is not equal to twice the shortest cycle.

R-P/P-R reciprocity.[9] What is termed the *R-P interval* is the measurement from the beginning of the QRS to the beginning of the following P wave. As the PR interval lengthens, the R-P interval shortens; hence the reciprocal relationship.

Regular P-P interval.[15] The atrial rhythm is regular unless there is a sinus arrhythmia present (see box below).

Atypical Wenckebach variations include R-R interval lengthening, PR shortening, or concordant lengthening of RP and PR intervals.[14]

ECG Characteristics
Type I Second Degree AV Block

Rate: Usually within normal ranges
Rhythm: Atrial: Regular
Ventricular: Irregular (grouped beating)
P waves: Normal
PR interval: Progressive lengthening
QRS complex: Normal, unless IVCD present

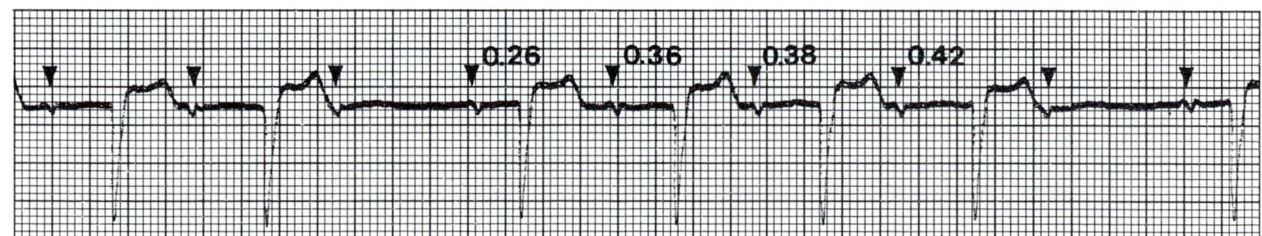

FIGURE 9-2 Second degree AV block, Type I.

Rate: Atrial: 79 bpm
Ventricular: 60 bpm
Rhythm: Atrial: Regular
Ventricular: Irregular
P wave: Normal; more P waves *(arrows)* than QRS complexes. Ps do not bear constant relation to QRSs.
PR interval: 0.26 to 0.42 seconds; progressively lengthens until QRS dropped
QRS complex: 0.10 seconds, elevated ST segment, one QRS complex dropped
Interpretation: Second degree AV block, Type I

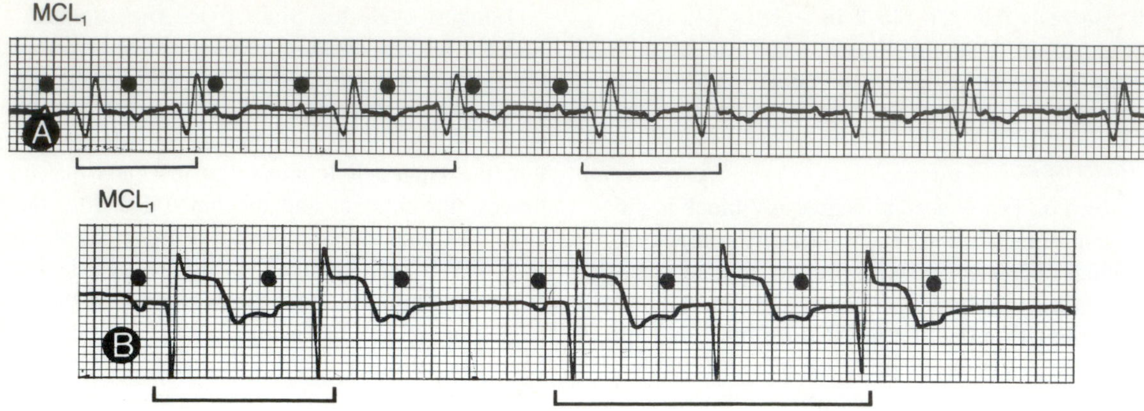

FIGURE 9-3 Two examples of grouped beating during Type I AV block. **A,** Note pairing *(brackets)* of QRS complexes, the result of a 3:2 conduction ratio (three P waves *[dots]* for each two QRS complexes) and **B,** the groups of two and three QRS complexes, the result of 3:2 and 4:2 conduction.

A.

Rate: Atrial: 130 bpm
Ventricular: 90 bpm
Rhythm: Atrial: Regular
Ventricular: Irregular
P wave: Normal, more P waves than QRS complexes; Ps bear no constant relation to QRSs
PR interval: 0.17 to 0.26 seconds, progressive lengthening until QRS dropped
QRS complex: 0.16 seconds, prolonged, rSR′ morphology in V_1 consistent with RBBB
Interpretation: Second degree AV block, Type I with 3:2 conduction, RBBB

B.

Rate: Atrial: 86 bpm
Ventricular: Approximately 60 bpm
Rhythm: Atrial: Regular
Ventricular: Irregular
P wave: Normal; more P waves than QRS complexes; Ps do not bear constant relation to QRSs
PR interval: 0.18 to 0.34 seconds, progressive lengthening until QRS dropped
QRS complex: 0.08 seconds; QR pattern on V_1 warrants further interpretation to rule out incomplete RBBB; elevated ST segment
Interpretation: Second degree AV block, Type I with 4:3 and 3:2 conduction

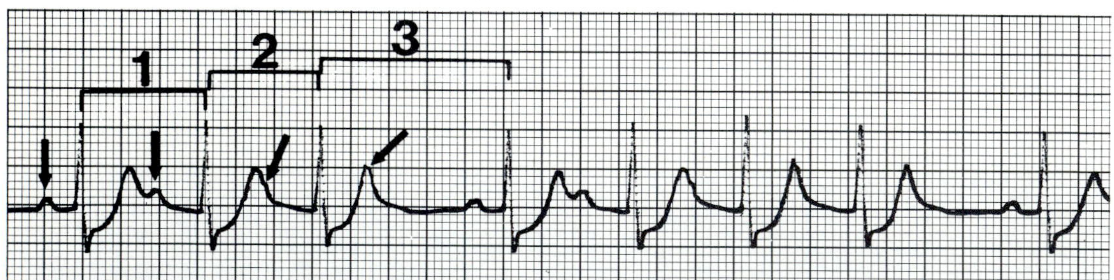

FIGURE 9-4 Second degree AV block, Type I. Note the R-R interval containing the dropped QRS complex *(3)* is less than twice the shortest R-R interval *(2)* P waves are marked with arrows.

Applied Nursing Process

Clinical Assessment

- Detect:
  - An irregular pulse.
  - An irregularity in the QRS complexes on the ECG manifested as groups of beats.
- Assess the patient and ECG.
  - Type I AV block will not usually cause symptoms unless the ventricular rate becomes exceedingly slow.
  - Carotid sinus massage (CSM) is often useful in identifying the site of block. Since CSM stimulates the vagus nerve, AVN block will increase if it already exists. Conversely, if the block is below the AVN, CSM should have no effect. If the AV block is the result of

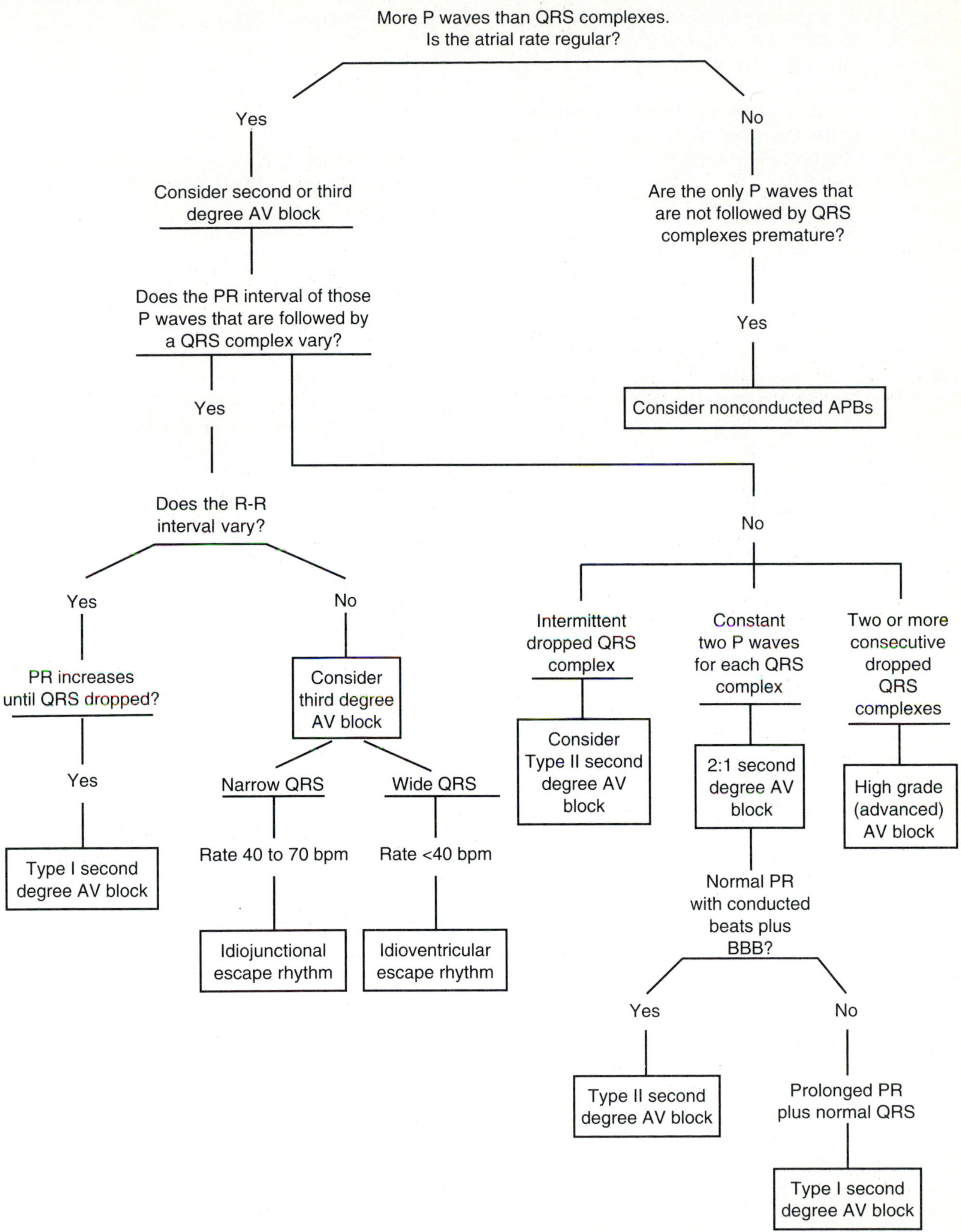

FIGURE 9-5 AV block algorithm.

an atrial rate that is too fast for AVN conduction, CSM may actually cause a decrease in block by slowing the sinus rate to allow 1:1 AV conduction.[1] (CSM as a nursing assessment measure may not be permitted in some institutions.)

- Assess how well the patient is tolerating the arrhythmia by checking the following (slow ventricular rates require more frequent assessments):
  Blood pressure.
  Skin color and temperature.
  Sensorium.
- Assess for possible causes of the arrhythmia such as:
  Increased vagal tone.
  IWMI.
  Digitalis toxicity.
- Diagnose the arrhythmia. Detect an atrial rate that is greater than the ventricular rate. The atrial rate must not be greater than 135 bpm. Use the algorithm in Fig. 9-5 for assistance in diagnosing second degree AV block.

❖ NURSING DIAGNOSIS

Decreased cardiac output related to bradycardia, if present.

❖ ECG DIAGNOSIS

Type I second degree AV block.

Plan and Implementation

Patient goal. The patient will remain hemodynamically stable, and the block will not progress.

The patient will regain NSR as the block subsides with time (as in the case of an IWMI) or when appropriate measures are taken to relieve etiologic factors such as digitalis toxicity.

Nursing interventions.

- Type I second degree AV block requires no intervention if the patient is asymptomatic and tolerates the arrhythmia. However, if intervention is necessary, it is based on the clinical findings and the clinical setting. For example, the healthy, young male athlete would not require intervention should the arrhythmia be detected during sleep. A patient who is digitalis toxic, on the other hand, would require interventions. These would include:
  - Notification of the physician.
  - Holding the digitalis.
  - Obtaining a serum digoxin level, as ordered.
- If the patient is symptomatic from a very slow ventricular rate, atropine or isoproterenol may be indicated. However, these medications are rarely required. With an acute MI, the best intervention is observation for the progression of block. Other interventions may be indicated such as:
  - An IV infusion, as ordered.
  - Oxygen PRN.
- Implement physician's orders and evaluate any measures taken to improve the block such as removal of digitalis from the treatment program.

Evaluation

- The patient's condition is stabilized as evidenced by:
  - Blood pressure within normal range.
  - A lucid response.
  - Warm and dry skin.
- The patient with an IWMI shows improvement as evidenced by:
  - Normal sinus rhythm on the ECG.

Medical Treatment

Although this arrhythmia is usually well tolerated, a temporary transvenous pacemaker may be indicated if the patient is symptomatic, if the ventricular response is less than 40 bpm, if congestive heart failure or ventricular arrhythmias exist, or for prophylaxis against progression to a higher grade of AV block (rare).[2]

Atropine or isoproterenol may be used as a means to improve AV conduction in the presence of excessive bradycardia or ventricular arrhythmias. Both drugs, however, increase myocardial oxygen consumption, which could be extremely detrimental in the patient with an acute MI.

TYPE II SECOND DEGREE AV BLOCK

Data Base: Problem Identification

Definitions, Etiology, and Mechanisms

Type II AV block is less common than Type I. The site of this abnormality in the His-Purkinje system is usually either within or distal to the bundle of His,[1] also called *infra-Hisian*. Type II involves blocking of both bundle branches—one bundle branch is blocked completely and the other blocks intermittently. The intermittent block of one branch causes intermittent dropping of QRS complexes. Because of the site of conduction defect, Type II AV block is more significant than Type I and may progress to complete AV block.[2,9]

Type II AV block is likely to be a chronic conduction disturbance.[15] When it is seen in the presence of an acute anteroseptal myocardial infarction (ASMI), it is usually associated with an irreversible defect in AV conduction.[11,16] Type II may also be seen with coronary artery disease or degenerative diseases of the His-Purkinje system.[17] Unlike Type I, Type II second degree AV block is generally not found in healthy individuals.

ECG Characteristics

The hallmark of Type II second degree AV block is the sudden dropping of a QRS complex. In contrast to Type I the PR interval in Type II AV block remains constant before and after the dropped QRS complex[18] and is usually within normal limits.[9] An important diagnostic criterion is the presence of two or more **consecutively** conducted P waves that have the same PR interval before the dropped beat.[9] In Type II, there is no R-P/P-R reciprocity. The PR remains constant even with changes in the R-P intervals[9] (Fig. 9-6).

> **ECG Characteristics**
> ***Type II Second Degree AV Block***
>
> ***Rate:*** *Atrial:* Within normal ranges
> *Ventricular:* May become very slow
> ***Rhythm:*** Irregular because of sudden dropping of QRS
> ***P waves:*** Constant P-P interval
> ***PR interval:*** Constant with two consecutively conducted P waves
> ***QRS complex:*** Sudden absence of QRS; often wide (0.12 seconds or more)

The QRS complex in Type II block may be normal, but it is frequently wide (0.12 seconds or more)[1,9,15,17] due to a bundle branch block, usually RBBB.[8] The P-P interval is constant.

Thus the distinguishing features of Type II second degree AV block are:

- Constant PR intervals.
- Constant P-P intervals.
- Sudden dropping of QRS complex.
- Normal or, more often, wide (0.12 seconds or more) QRS complex (see box on this page).

Applied Nursing Process

Clinical Assessment

- Detect:
  - An irregular pulse.
  - An irregularity in the ECG manifested by dropped QRS complexes.
  - The sudden onset of severe bradycardia (which could

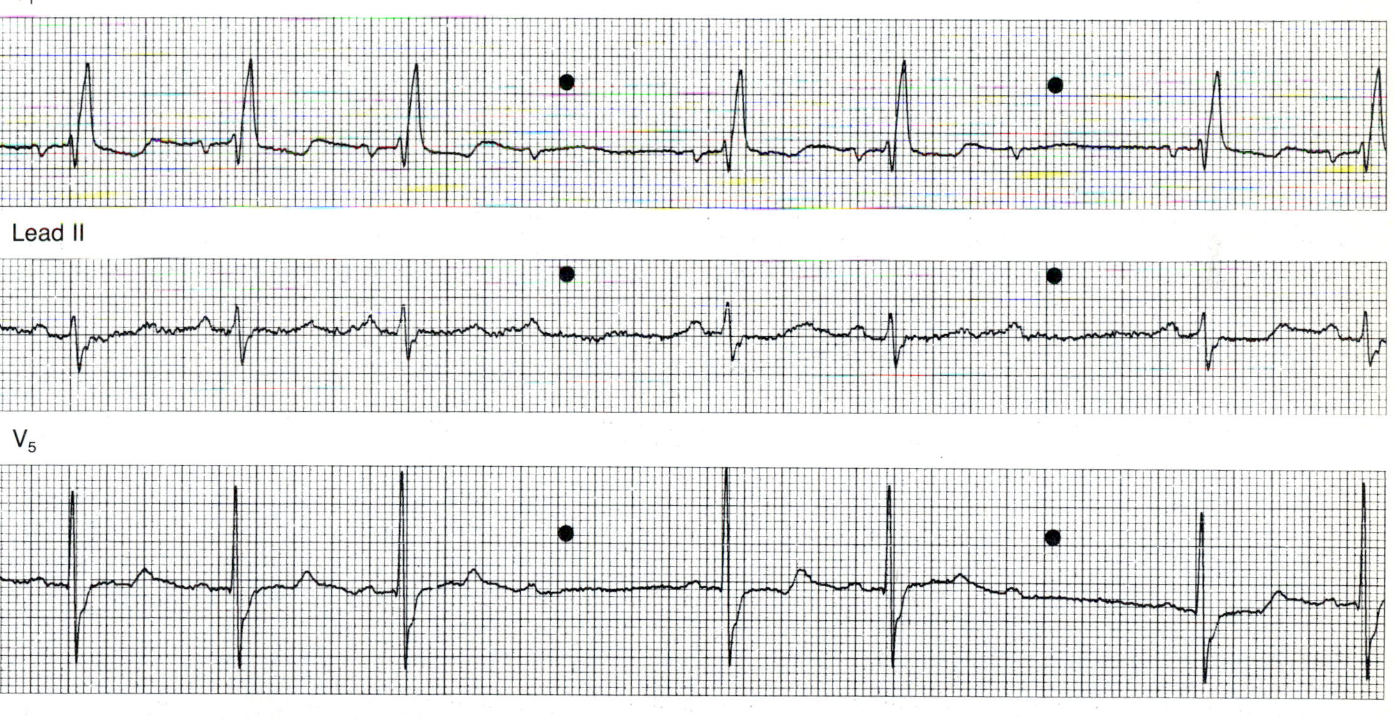

FIGURE 9-6 Second degree AV block, Type II. Note dropped QRS complex *(dot)* is preceded by constant PR intervals. There is an RBBB and also a left anterior hemiblock (see pp. 283-284).

Rate: Atrial: 68 bpm
Ventricular: Approximately 60 bpm
Rhythm: Atrial: Regular
Ventricular: Irregular
P wave: Normal; more P waves than QRS complexes; P precedes each QRS and bears a constant relation to it.
PR interval: 0.19 to 0.20 seconds, constant. Two P waves not followed by QRS complexes.
QRS complex: 0.13 seconds, rsR′ morphology in V_1 consistent with RBBB.
QT interval 0.48 seconds, prolonged
Interpretation: Type II second degree AV block with intermittent 2:1 conduction

be high grade AV block) with symptoms dependent on the degree of cardiac output reduction.

- Assess the patient and ECG.
  - See "Clinical Assessment," Type I AV Block.
  - The symptoms the patient experiences will be related to the ventricular rate. With little or no significant change in the heart rate, there will probably be few, if any, symptoms associated with the arrhythmia. However, if the ventricular rate is significantly slowed, the patient will likely become symptomatic.
  - Evaluate the patient's tolerance of the arrhythmia by assessing the following:
    Blood pressure.
    Peripheral pulses.
    Level of orientation.
    Skin color and temperature.
  - Diagnose the arrhythmia. Detect a sudden dropping of a QRS complex in the presence of a regular atrial rhythm (make certain it is not a nonconducted APB) and a constant PR interval with consecutively conducted P waves. Refer to the algorithm (see Fig. 9-5) for assistance in the differential diagnosis.
  - Continued observation of the patient's clinical tolerance of this arrhythmia is essential. Type II AV block may have the clinical effect of significantly reducing the ventricular rate.

❖ NURSING DIAGNOSIS

(1) Decreased cardiac output related to bradycardia. (2) Altered tissue perfusion: cerebral/cardiopulmonary/peripheral, related to reduced cardiac output. (3) Knowledge deficit concerning home management of permanent pacemaker.

❖ ECG DIAGNOSIS

Type II second degree AV block.

Plan and Implementation

Patient goal. The patient will remain stable and asymptomatic and will not exhibit significant hemodynamic changes resulting from a slowed ventricular rate.

Nursing interventions.

- On observing Type II block, notify the physician at once and prepare for an emergency temporary transvenous pacemaker insertion.
- Start IV infusion as ordered.
- Give oxygen PRN.
- Take the following measures to reduce metabolic expenditure and if the patient is symptomatic, promote cerebral perfusion:
  - Bed rest for the patient.
  - Lower the head of the bed to flat or low Fowler's position, if not contraindicated.
- If the patient is symptomatic from a slow ventricular rate, consider the following according to institutional policy and/or physician orders:
  - An IV isoproterenol infusion may be necessary to increase the ventricular rate. (The infusion should be prepared and ready as a precaution.)
  - External pacing (see Chapter 13).
- Implement physician's orders and evaluate measures taken to increase the ventricular rate.
  - For the patient who receives a pacemaker, monitor for proper functioning (see Chapter 13).
  - Monitor patients receiving IV isoproterenol for the following:
    Excessive heart rate elevation.
    Evidence of myocardial ischemia. (Isoproterenol increases myocardial oxygen consumption.)
    Ventricular ectopy. (By stimulating beta 1 receptors, isoproterenol enhances ventricular automaticity.)
    Hypokalemia, which may potentiate ventricular ectopy.

Evaluation

- The patient has a ventricular response within normal limits and sufficient cardiac output to maintain tissue perfusion as evidenced by the following:
  - Blood pressure within normal range.
  - Lucid response.
  - Warm, dry skin without pallor or cyanosis.
- The patient with a permanent pacemaker is capable of evaluating proper pacemaker function as evidenced by the following:
  - Ability to take own pulse.
  - Stating rate parameters consistent with proper pacemaker functioning.
  - Relating other information specific to individual patient problems.

Medical Treatment

Atropine is of minimal or no value in restoring AV conduction and may appear to increase the degree of AV block by increasing the sinus rate.[1,11] In such a situation the block is a result of the increased sinus rate rather than an increase in the pathology of the block itself. An isoproterenol infusion may be useful in accelerating the ventricular escape rhythm.

The presence of persistent Type II block in the presence of an anterior wall myocardial infarction (AWMI) is an indication for permanent pacing.[19] If Type II block is not persistent, there is no clear-cut indication for permanent pacing. Nevertheless, many physicians elect to implant permanent pacemakers in these circumstances to avoid the consequences of the development of third degree AV block. With IWMI, because few patients develop persistent, symptomatic AV blocks, few require permanent pacing. His-bundle electrocardiography and electrophysiology studies provide precise information on the location of the AV block, which may be indicated to validate the need for permanent pacing.

2:1 AV BLOCK

A 2:1 AV block may be a sequela of **either** Type I or Type II second degree AV block[18] and is characterized by block that increases without warning.

In the presence of 2:1 AV conduction the width of the QRS complex may be helpful in differentiating between Type I and Type II (Fig. 9-7). A narrow QRS complex is usually associated with Type I and a wide QRS with Type II. A search for evidence of Wenckebach block (Type I) on other rhythm strips may also be helpful in ruling out Type II.

HIGH GRADE AV BLOCK
Data Base: Problem Identification
Definitions, Etiology, and Mechanisms

High grade (advanced) AV block is more serious than previously described AV blocks, but it is not quite third degree (complete) AV block. It occurs when two or more consecutive atrial impulses do not reach the ventricles.[9] This AV block indicates instability in the conduction system and may lead to intermittent periods of ventricular asystole. The site of block is either the AVN or the HPS.[1]

ECG Characteristics

The ECG in high grade AV block reveals two or more consecutive dropped QRS complexes in association with constant PR intervals (Fig. 9-8). To indicate pathologic and not physiologic block, the atrial rate should be less than 135 bpm.[9] A normal QRS duration suggests the block is occurring at the AVN, whereas a wide QRS complex may be indicative of a block at or below the His bundle. The distinguishing features of this arrhythmia include:

- Two or more consecutive dropped QRS complexes.
- Constant PR intervals with conducted beats.

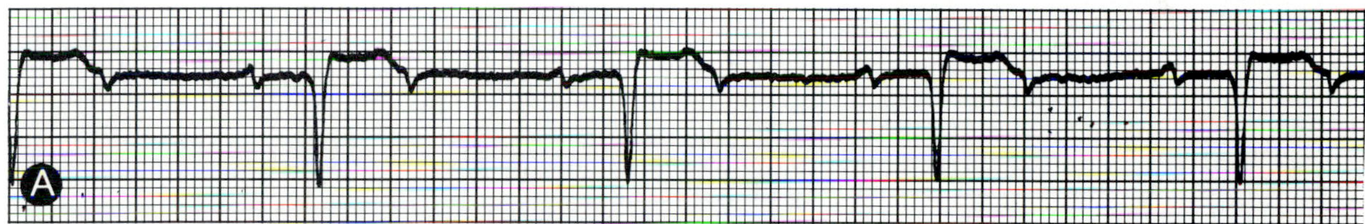

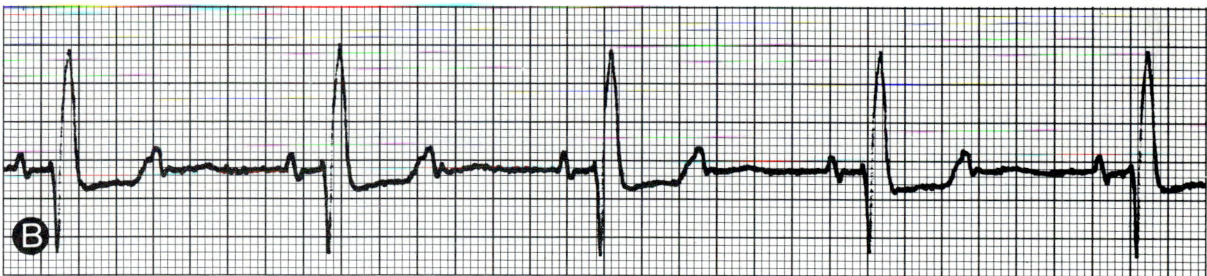

FIGURE 9-7 Two examples of 2:1 AV block.

A.

Rate: Atrial: 84 bpm
Ventricular: 42 bpm
Rhythm: Atrial: Regular
Ventricular: Regular
P wave: Normal; two P waves for every QRS complex
PR interval: 0.32 seconds, prolonged, for Ps preceding QRSs
QRS complex: 0.10 seconds, QS complex on MCL$_1$ (initial r wave absent); elevated ST segment
Interpretation: Type I second degree AV block with 2:1 conduction and RBBB (Because of the width of the QRS complex this arrhythmia probably originated from Type I AV block.)

B.

Rate: Atrial: 84 bpm
Ventricular: 42 bpm
Rhythm: Atrial: Regular
Ventricular: Regular
P wave: Normal; two P waves for every QRS
PR interval: 0.18 seconds for Ps preceding QRSs
QRS complex: 0.17 seconds, rSR′ in MCL$_1$ consistent with RBBB
Interpretation: Type II second degree AV block with 2:1 conduction and RBBB (Because of the width of the QRS complex this arrhythmia probably originated from Type II AV block.)

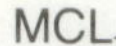

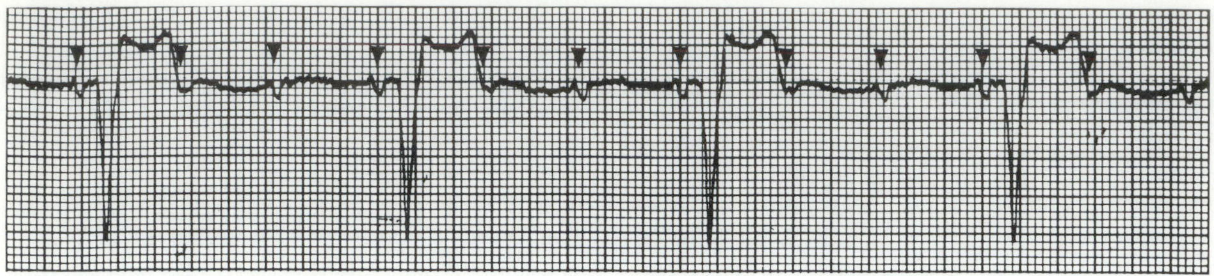

FIGURE 9-8 High grade AV block.

Rate: Atrial: 111 bpm
Ventricular: 37 bpm
Rhythm: Atrial: Regular
Ventricular: Regular
P wave: Normal; more Ps *(arrows)* than QRSs; Ps preceding QRSs bear constant relation to them.
PR interval: 0.16 seconds for Ps preceding QRSs
QRS complex: 0.12 seconds
Interpretation: High grade AV block with 3:1 conduction

ECG Characteristics
High Grade (Advanced) AV Block

Rate: *Atrial:* 135 bpm or less
Ventricular: 40 bpm or less
Rhythm: Regular or irregular
P waves: Regular
PR interval: Constant with conducted impulses
QRS complex: Normal or wide

- An atrial rate within normal limits, or no higher than 135 bpm (see box above).

Applied Nursing Process
Clinical Assessment

- Detect:
  - A slow pulse that may or may not be irregular.
  - A bradycardia on the ECG with more P waves than QRS complexes.
  - Probable symptoms of reduced cardiac output such as low blood pressure or pallor.
- Assess the patient and ECG.
  - High grade AV block will likely produce signs or symptoms associated with a slow ventricular rate. Assess the patient's response to the arrhythmia by determining the following:
    Blood pressure.
    Level of orientation.
    Skin color and temperature.
  - Assess for possible causes of high grade AV block such as drugs and ischemia.
  - Diagnose the arrhythmia. Detect more P waves than QRS complexes with a slow ventricular rate. Refer to Fig. 9-5.

❖ NURSING DIAGNOSIS

(1) Decreased cardiac output related to bradycardia. (2) Altered tissue perfusion: cerebral/cardiopulmonary/peripheral, related to reduced cardiac output. (3) Knowledge deficit regarding care of permanent pacemaker at home.

❖ ECG DIAGNOSIS

High grade AV block.

Plan and Implementation

Patient goal. The patient will remain hemodynamically stable and will not experience sudden or critical changes in cardiac output (e.g., syncope, hypotension, pallor, possible apnea).

The patient with a permanent pacemaker will relate the appropriate information concerning management of the pacemaker unit at home.

Nursing interventions.

- Monitor carefully for changes in the patient's tolerance of the arrhythmia. If there are lengthy periods of ventricular asystole, CPR will be necessary.
- Notify the physician immediately.
- Give oxygen PRN.
- Start IV infusion as ordered.
- Prepare an isoproterenol infusion and infuse if ordered or indicated.
- Prepare for emergency temporary pacemaker insertion.

- Initiate external pacing as ordered (see Chapter 13).
- Implement physician's orders and evaluate measures taken to increase the ventricular rate.

Evaluation

- The patient has a cardiac output sufficient to maintain adequate tissue perfusion as evidenced by the following:
  - Blood pressure within normal limits.
  - Clear sensorium.
  - Warm, dry skin without pallor or cyanosis.
- The patient's rhythm is restored with permanent artificial pacing or removal of the underlying cause.
- The patient manages the permanent pacemaker after discharge as evidenced by the following:
  - Ability to take own pulse.
  - Stating the pulse rate parameters indicative of proper pacemaker functioning.
  - Relating other information specific to the individual problem.

Medical Treatment

Permanent pacing is indicated if no reversible cause for the arrhythmia can be found (e.g., drugs).

THIRD DEGREE AV BLOCK

Data Base: Problem Identification

Definitions, Etiology, and Mechanisms

The total absence of AV conduction results in complete AV block. The block may occur at the AVN, but usually the lesion is located at the bundle of His or in both bundle branches.[1,20]

In adults the most frequent pathologic causes of complete AV block include acute MI, digitalis intoxication, and degenerative disease of the conduction system. In an IWMI, the block is located in the ischemic AVN and usually is transient. However, complete AV block complicating IWMI has been cited as a marker for poor prognosis.[22] In an AWMI, the site of block is below the bundle of His and may be irreversible.[9]

In newborn infants and children, third degree AV block is the most common cause of significant bradycardia. The abnormality is either congenital or acquired. Most congenital blocks occur in the AVN and therefore have a favorable prognosis because the intact escape pacemaker is junctional, under autonomic influence, and dependable. Surgical procedures are one cause of acquired heart block. This may occur when the surgical site is located in or adjacent to the conduction system. Surgically induced complete AV block is usually below the bundle of His and consequently has a poorer prognosis than the congenital form. The nonsurgical causes of acquired third degree AV block include infectious processes, idiopathic causes, and muscular diseases.[21]

ECG Characteristics

When complete AV block occurs, no atrial impulses are conducted to the ventricles. This block in conduction allows independent atrial and ventricular activity. The atria beat at their own rate, and the ventricles beat at a slower, regular rate usually less than 45 bpm. Complete AV block is one cause of AV dissociation (Fig. 9-9).

The control of the ventricles is by the escape mechanism of the AV junction or the ventricle.[9] When the pacemaker is in the area of the AVN the QRS will have a similar appearance to the sinus beat, be narrow, and provide a dependable rate[2,10] between 40 and 70 bpm. It may even respond to exercise.[1] When the AV junction is the pacemaker, the rhythm is called *idiojunctional* (IJR) (see Fig. 9-9).

A block below the bundle of His will produce a wide QRS complex and a slower, less stable rate (<40 bpm). A block within the bundle may produce a wide or narrow QRS complex[1,2,10,20] (Fig. 9-10). Such a rhythm is known as an *idioventricular rhythm* (IVR).

The distinguishing features of third degree (complete) AV block include:

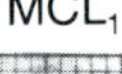

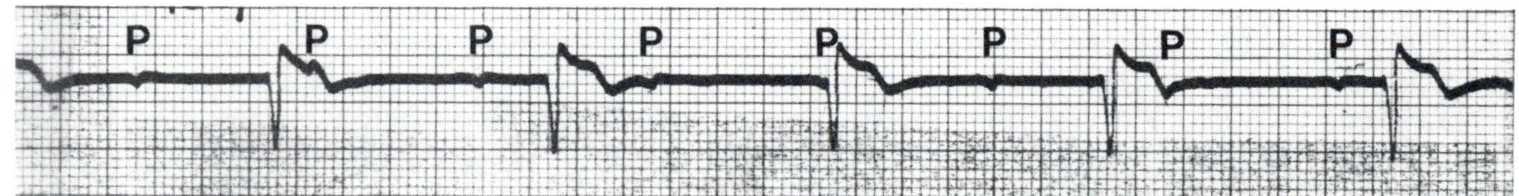

FIGURE 9-9 Third degree AV block.

Rate: Atrial: 81 bpm
Ventricular: 50 bpm
Rhythm: Atrial: Regular
Ventricular: Regular
P wave: Normal; more Ps than QRSs; Ps preceding QRSs bear no relation to QRSs (dissociated)
PR interval: (Not measured in AV dissociation)
QRS complex: 0.08 seconds; elevated ST segment
Interpretation: Third degree AV block with resultant AV dissociation and idiojunctional rhythm

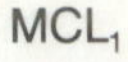

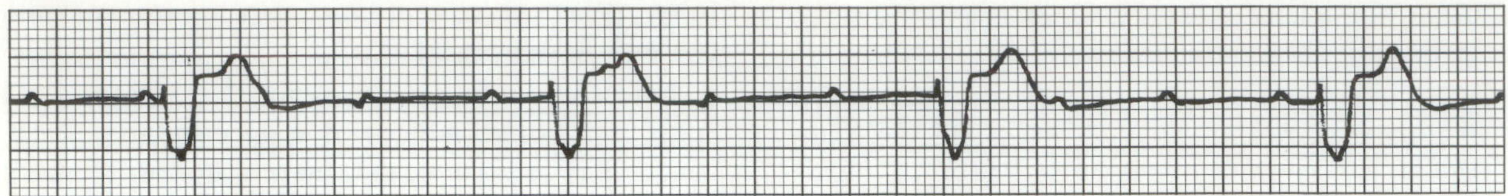

FIGURE 9-10 Third degree AV block.

Rate: Atrial: 125 bpm
Ventricular: 36 bpm
Rhythm: Atrial: Regular
Ventricular: Regular
P wave: Normal; more Ps than QRSs; Ps bear no relation to QRSs (dissociated)
PR interval: —
QRS complex: 0.17 seconds
Interpretation: Third degree AV block with resultant AV dissociation and idioventricular rhythm

- Slow ventricular rate (usually <45 bpm).
- Plenty of P waves with the atrial rate > the ventricular rate.
- AV dissociation (independent atrial activity and independent ventricular activity) (see box on this page).

Complete AV block may also occur in the presence of atrial fibrillation (AF) as a result of pathologic block or digitalis intoxication. The identifying feature is a **regular** ventricular response with the classic chaotic atrial activity[9] (Fig. 9-11). The rhythm controlling the ventricle in the situation of digitalis toxicity would be idiojunctional. The rhythm seen with a pathologic block may be either idiojunctional or idioventricular.

ECG Characteristics
Third Degree (Complete) AV Block

Rate: *Atrial:* Faster than ventricular
Ventricular: Usually <45 bpm
Rhythm: *Atrial:* Regular
Ventricular: Regular
P waves: Normal
PR interval: Appears to vary considerably because of AV dissociation; P waves bear no constant relation to QRS complexes
QRS complex: Narrow if junctional pacemaker with no BBB; wide if ventricular pacemaker

Applied Nursing Process
Clinical Assessment

- Detect:
  - A slow, regular pulse.
  - A slow rhythm on the ECG with the atrial rate higher than the ventricular rate; and with P waves bearing no constant relationship to the QRS complexes.
- Assess the patient and ECG.
  - The patient with third degree AV block will typically have clinical signs and symptoms associated with a slow heart rate. These may include fatigue, light-headedness, mental confusion, Stokes-Adams attacks, or congestive heart failure. Occasionally patients are asymptomatic.
  - Determine the patient's tolerance of the arrhythmia by assessing the following:
    Sensorium.
    Blood pressure.
    Skin color and temperature.
  - Assess for possible causes of the arrhythmia such as drug toxicity.
  - The other clinical signs of complete block are those found in AV dissociation (i.e., intermittent cannon waves and varying intensities of the S_1 heart sound).
  - Diagnose the arrhythmia. Detect a slow, regular ventricular rhythm with an atrial rate > the ventricular rate (See Fig. 9-5).

❖ NURSING DIAGNOSIS

(1) Decreased cardiac output related to bradycardia. (2) Altered tissue perfusion: cerebral/cardiopulmonary/peripheral, related to reduced cardiac output. (3) Knowledge deficit regarding care of permanent pacemaker.

❖ ECG DIAGNOSIS

Complete AV block.

Plan and Implementation

Patient goal. The patient will have a ventricular rate sufficient to maintain adequate blood pressure and perfusion.

The patient with a permanent pacemaker will relate important self-care measures before discharge.

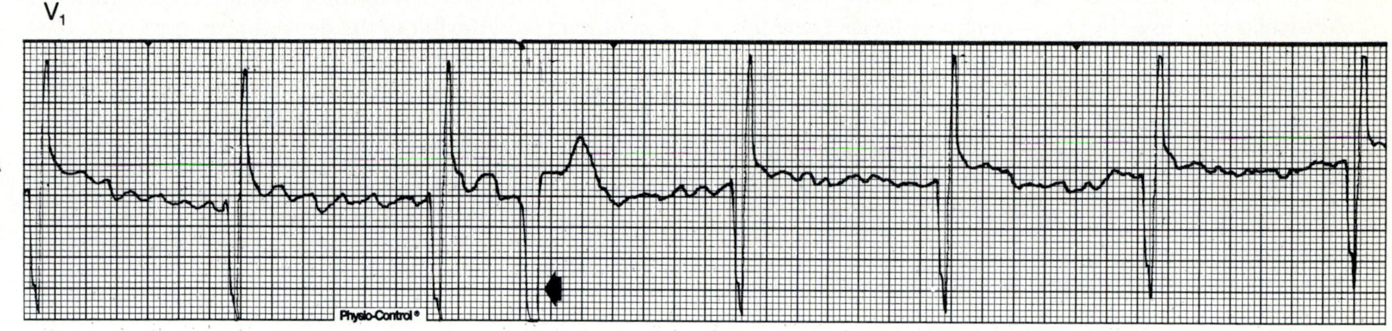

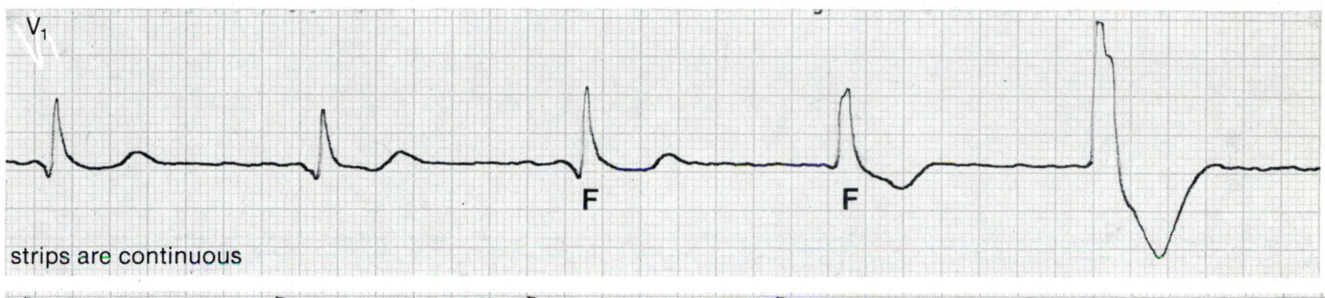

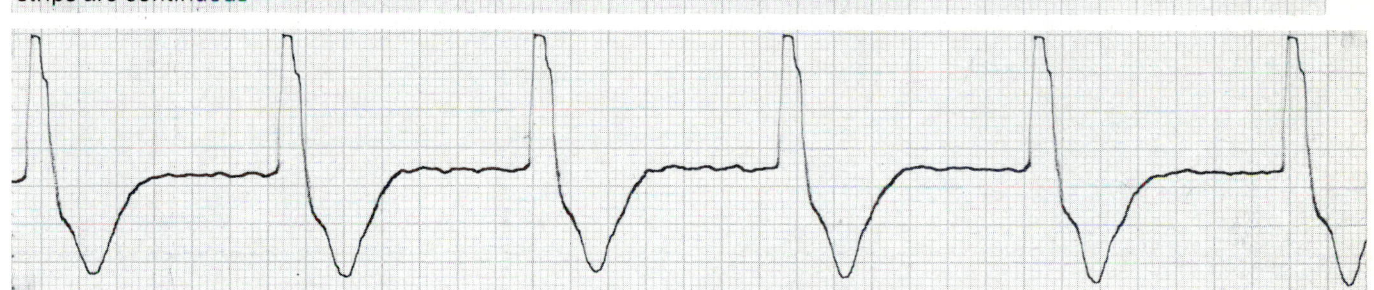

FIGURE 9-11 Two examples of AF with third degree AV block.

A.

Rate: Atrial: Chaotic, irregular
Ventricular: 45 bpm
Rhythm: Atrial: Irregular
Ventricular: Regular, except for one VPB *(arrow)*
P wave: "f" waves
PR interval: —
QRS complex: 0.14 seconds, rSR′ on V_1
Interpretation: AF with third degree AV block and probable idiojunctional rhythm with RBBB; one VPB.

B.

Rate: Atrial: Nonidentifiable P waves
Ventricular: 42 bpm accelerating to 45 bpm
Rhythm: Atrial: Irregular
Ventricular: Regular
P wave: "f" waves
PR interval: —
QRS complex: 0.10 to 0.12 seconds (first two QRSs), widening to 0.18 (bottom strip)
Interpretation: AF with third degree AV block. First two complexes are idiojunctional conducted with RBBB, displayed as qR complexes (initial r wave absent because of previous anteroseptal MI). The last complex on the top and all of them on the bottom strip represent an AIVR, usurping the IJR at a slightly faster rate of 45 bpm. The third and fourth complexes on the top strip are fusion beats *(F)*.

Nursing interventions.

- The urgency for nursing intervention primarily depends on the patient's clinical tolerance of the arrhythmia. A ventricular response of over 40 bpm may be adequate for systemic perfusion of the patient on bed rest.
- Continue to observe clinical tolerance of the arrhythmia by assessing sensorium and blood pressure at regular, frequent intervals and observe for change in the ventricular rate.
- Lower head of bed if congestive heart failure is not present.
- Although atropine is not typically effective in restoring AV conduction, it can be readily administered and may produce therapeutic results (Fig. 9-12).
- Prepare an isoproterenol infusion, administer as ordered, and titrate the infusion to the desired response.
  - Although isoproterenol probably will not restore AV conduction, by stimulating beta-1 receptors, it usually results in an increase in ventricular automaticity and, therefore, ventricular ectopy.
  - Use this drug with extreme caution in the presence of an acute MI as it increases myocardial oxygen consumption.
- Prepare for possible pacemaker insertion.

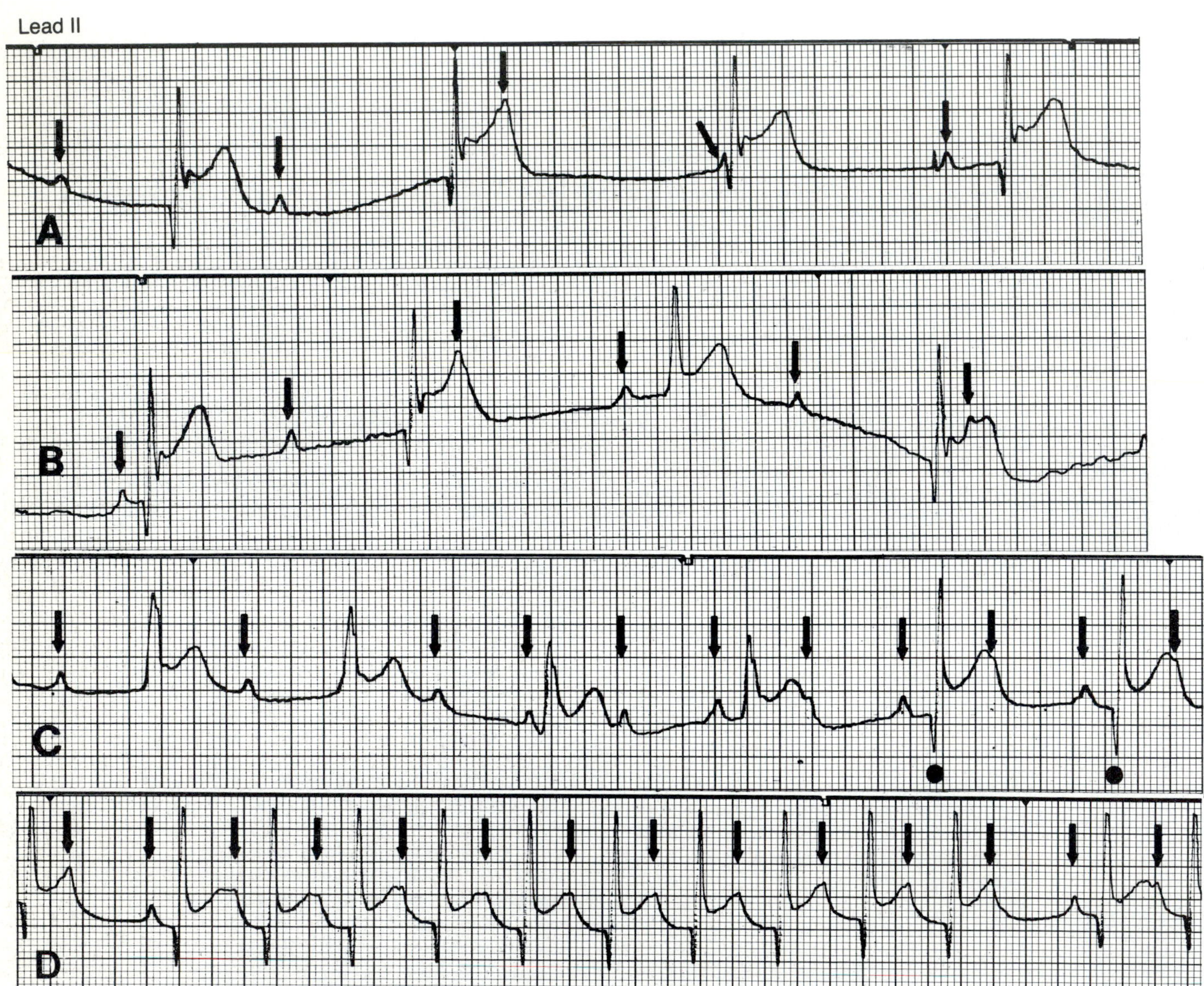

FIGURE 9-12 Third degree AV block. An unusual response to atropine.
A, Third degree AV block with atrial rate 44 bpm *(arrows)*, ventricular rate 35 bpm. **B,** Approximately 16 seconds after administration of IV atropine, atrial rate 58 bpm. **C,** Approximately 2½ minutes after atropine, atrial rate increases from 50 bpm to 108 bpm. AV conduction ratio is 2:1 at end of strip *(dots)*. **D,** Sinus tachycardia with atrial rate of 113 bpm. AV conduction is Type I, second degree block.

- Initiate external pacing as ordered (see Chapter 13).
- Implement physician's orders and evaluate any measures taken to increase the ventricular rate.
- Monitor patients receiving drugs to increase heart rate (i.e., atropine and isoproterenol) for the following:
  - Excessive rate elevation.
  - Evidence of myocardial ischemia.
  - Hypokalemia (may potentiate the propensity for isoproterenol to provoke ventricular ectopy).
- Monitor patients with AV block requiring temporary or permanent pacing for proper functioning of the pacemaker. Include regular assessments for signs and symptoms of infection, since the pacemaker insertion is a surgical procedure.

Evaluation

- The patient's ventricular response improves or remains adequate, and cardiac output is sufficient as evidenced by the following:
  - Blood pressure within normal limits.
  - Warm, dry skin without pallor or cyanosis.
  - A lucid response.
  - Absence of light-headedness or dizziness.
- The patient with a permanent pacemaker monitors proper pacemaker functioning as evidenced by the following:
  - The ability to measure own pulse.
  - Stating rate parameters consistent with proper pacemaker functioning.
  - Relating other information specific to the individual problem.

Medical Treatment

Patients with conduction defects distal to the bundle of His usually require permanent pacing.[1] Permanent pacemakers are also inserted in patients with symptomatic (i.e., dizziness, light-headedness, syncope, congestive heart failure, or ventricular arrhythmias) complete heart block.[2]

Patients with third degree AV block in the presence of an acute MI may benefit from an isoproterenol infusion to maintain an adequate ventricular rate (it will usually not be effective in restoring AV conduction). However, an infusion of this type is generally risky limited to emergency situations during pacemaker insertion because isoproterenol will increase the myocardial oxygen demand and worsen the MI. A temporary pacemaker is the treatment of choice followed by evaluation of the patient for permanent pacing.

AV DISSOCIATION

AV dissociation is not an arrhythmia. It is a phenomenon that accompanies various arrhythmias. We have included it in this chapter because it accompanies third degree AV block, but bear in mind that it is also present in several other arrhythmias as well.

Data Base: Problem Identification

Definitions, Etiology, and Mechanisms

AV dissociation is a common phenomenon that is manifested during a variety of cardiac arrhythmias. It occurs when the atria and ventricles fire at independent rates, and atrial activity does not result in ventricular activity,[15,23] altering the mechanical relationship between the atria and ventricles. Lost is the atrial kick of diastole that pumps additional blood into the ventricles, and for some patients, this has a deleterious effect on the cardiac output. *AV dissociation,* a nonspecific term described by Pick,[24,25] is "never a primary disturbance" but rather "the consequence of some other, more basic disorder." AV dissociation is a sign of an underlying process (see box below).

AV dissociation may be a normal finding, as in the athlete who develops a sinus bradycardia, which allows the AV junction to become the dominant pacemaker. It may also be seen in complete AV block, digitalis intoxication, acute MI, rheumatic fever, and after cardiac surgery. In the elderly, AV dissociation usually occurs as the result of degenerative cardiovascular disease.[26]

ECG Characteristics

AV dissociation can result from four basic disturbances.[10,24]

Slowing of the dominant pacemaker.* Slowing of the sinus rate below the inherent AV junctional rate allows the AV junction to assume the role of primary pacemaker. When this occurs, the atria are paced by the sinus node and the ventricles by the AV junction. AV dissociation that results from sinus or atrial slowing (e.g., sinus bradycardia or SA block) is known as *AV dissociation by default,* a frequently benign process (Fig. 9-13).

Increased automaticity of subsidiary pacemaker.* Examples of enhanced automaticity that create AV dissociation include accelerated idiojunctional rhythm (AIJR), junctional tachycardia (JT), accelerated idioventricular rhythm (AIVR), and ventricular tachycardia (VT). A common cause of enhanced automaticity of the AV junction is digitalis intoxication (Fig. 9-14). AIVR produces an AV dissociation seen most often in the presence of an acute MI and is generally considered benign (Fig.

*9, 10, 15, 23, 24, 26

Characteristics of AV Dissociation

- Not a primary disturbance.
- Independent atrial and ventricular rhythms.

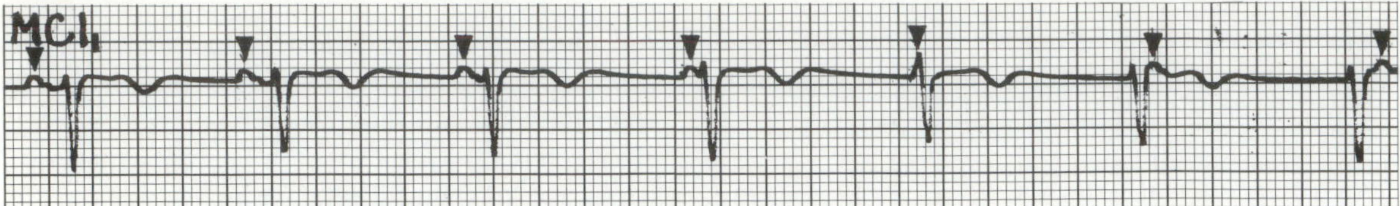

FIGURE 9-13 Isorhythmic AV dissociation by default. Note as the sinus rate slows, the AV junction becomes primary pacemaker.

Rate: Atrial: 63 slowing to 58 bpm
Ventricular: 63 bpm
Rhythm: Atrial: Regular
Ventricular: Regular
P wave: Normal; Ps *(arrows)* do not bear constant relation to QRSs (dissociated).
PR interval: 0.17 seconds at beginning of strip then AV dissociation ensues, so PR interval is not measured.
QRS complex: 0.09 seconds, rS in V_1 is normal.
Interpretation: Sinus rhythm to sinus bradycardia, resulting in a junctional rhythm by default and isorhythmic AV dissociation

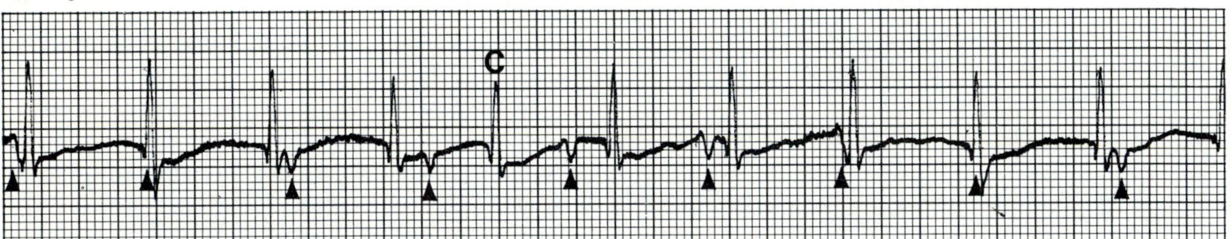

FIGURE 9-14 Enhanced automaticity of AV junction resulting in AV dissociation.

Rate: Atrial: 83 bpm
Ventricular: 94 bpm
Rhythm: Atrial: Regular
Ventricular: Regular except for fifth QRS complex *(C)* which represents a capture beat.
P wave: Normal; Ps *(arrows)* bear no relation to QRS complexes.
PR interval: Not measured in AV dissociation
QRS complex: 0.08 seconds
Interpretation: Accelerated idiojunctional rhythm with resultant isorhythmic AV dissociation with one capture beat

9-15). The takeover by a subsidiary pacemaker, referred to as *usurpation,* is nearly always abnormal because the subsidiary pacemaker dominates as a result of enhanced automaticity and excitability.

AV block.[9,10,15,23,24] In complete (third degree) AV block, no atrial impulses are transmitted to the ventricles; the atria and ventricles beat independently. Remember, complete AV block is just one cause of AV dissociation, but AV dissociation is not always complete AV block. This is an important point to remember to avoid the pitfall of diagnosing AV block based on the presence of AV dissociation (see Figs. 9-9 and 9-10).

Incomplete AV block may also favor AV dissociation. If the block causes the ventricular rate to fall below the inherent rate of a subsidiary pacemaker, the latter may take over.

Combinations and deviations.[9,10,23,24] Any of the previously mentioned ECG rhythm disturbances may occur in combinations to produce AV dissociation. Some of the mechanisms discussed previously may deviate from the descriptions. Fig. 9-16 illustrates AV dissociation in the presence of very slow atrial and ventricular rates. In this case the primary pacemaker slowed, the subsidiary junctional pacemaker failed, so the ventricles are paced by an

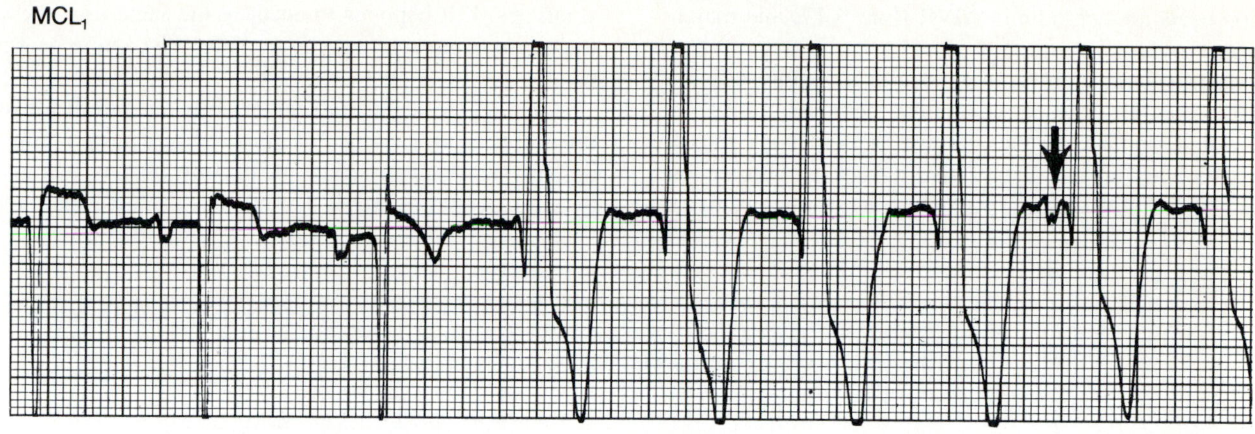

FIGURE 9-15 AV dissociation from increased automaticity.

Rate: Atrial: 68 slowing to 63 bpm
Ventricular: 68 increasing to 83 bpm
Rhythm: Atrial: Regular
Ventricular: Irregular because of sinus slowing and ventricular acceleration
P wave: Normal; Ps bear no relation to QRSs after first three beats. (Note P wave occurring before one of the AIVR complexes *[arrow]* does not conduct that impulse.)
PR interval: 0.24 seconds, first three beats
QRS complex: 0.08 seconds; 0.18 seconds during AIVR (note the monitor gain is too high, distorting the QRS)
Interpretation: Sinus rhythm with first degree AV block usurped by AIVR with resultant AV dissociation

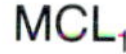

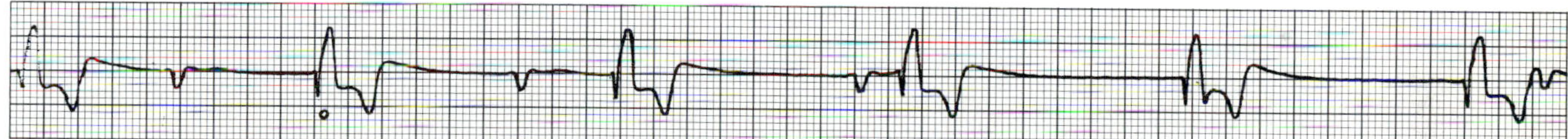

FIGURE 9-16 AV dissociation in the presence of a very slow atrial rate and idioventricular rhythm. Note that the atrial rate is less than the ventricular rate.

Rate: Atrial: 30 bpm
Ventricular: 35 bpm
Rhythm: Atrial: Regular
Ventricular: Regular
P wave: 0.12 seconds, prolonged. Ps bear no constant relation to QRSs (dissociated).
PR interval: Not applicable in AV dissociation
QRS complex: 0.15 seconds
Interpretation: Idioventricular rhythm with underlying sinus bradycardia and AV dissociation (The absence of an idiojunctional rhythm may indicate disease in the AV nodal area. The AV node should have been the backup pacemaker to take over at its escape rate.)

idioventricular rhythm. AV dissociation may be temporary (e.g., during sinus bradycardia or accelerated idioventricular rhythm) or permanent (e.g., complete AV block) (see box on this page).

Any of all of the following may be observed during AV dissociation:

Fusion beats. Ventricular fusion is common in AV dissociation (see Chapter 8). It occurs when the two independent impulses simultaneously activate the ventricles.

Four Basic Disturbances that can Result in AV Dissociation

1. Slowing of dominant cardiac pacemaker.
2. Increased automaticity of a subsidiary pacemaker—usurpation.
3. AV block.
4. Combinations of 1, 2, and 3.

Fusion beats are common in AIVR (Fig. 9-17) and may be seen as *Dressler beats* in VT.[23]

Capture beats. A capture beat is a supraventricular impulse that produces a ventricular complex during the dissociated rhythm. In the absence of AV block the supraventricular impulse may arrive during a nonrefractory period in the AV junction, allowing it to conduct to the ventricles. If it happens to occur at the same time the ventricles are being activated by an IVR, the capture beat may take on the ECG characteristics of a fusion beat.

Although occasionally seen in pairs, capture beats more often appear as a single "premature" beat interrupting the regular ventricular rhythm. A capture beat is recognized by a P wave preceding it that has a reasonable PR interval

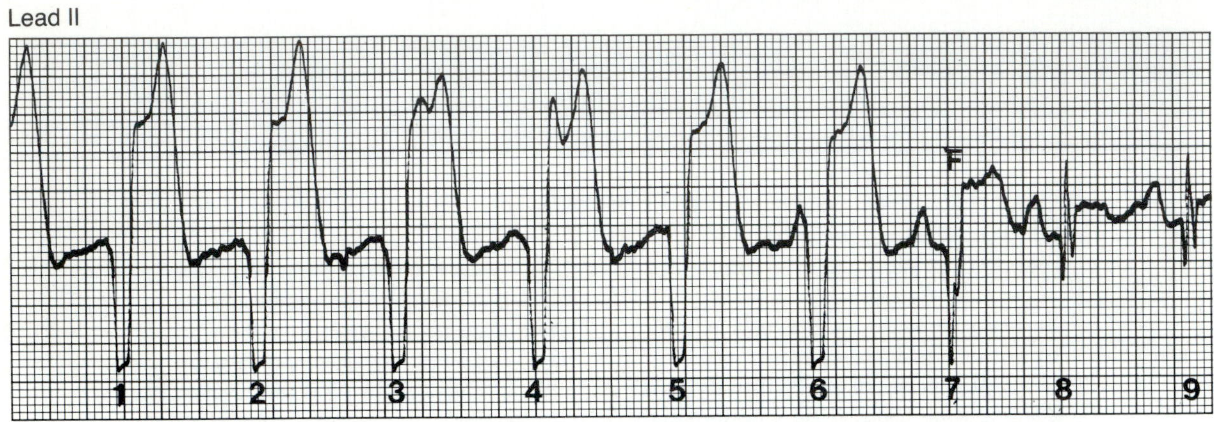

FIGURE 9-17 AV dissociation with fusion beat. Notice the change in appearance of the seventh QRS complex *(F)*. This represents a hybrid beat—it looks like a cross between the preceding and following QRSs. The fusion beat occurred as the two independent impulses simultanteously activated the myocardium. The PR interval on a fusion beat may be shorter than the normal sinus beat, but not by more than 0.06 seconds.

Rate: Atrial: 100 bpm for beats 7 to 9
Ventricular: 81 bpm for beats 1 to 6; 100 bpm for beats 7 to 9
P wave: Tall and wide. For beats 1 to 6, Ps are dissociated from QRSs.
PR interval: 0.20 seconds, beats 8 to 9; 0.16 seconds, beat 7
QRS complex: 0.15 seconds, beats 1 to 6; 0.10 seconds, beat 7 (fusion); 0.08 seconds, beats 8 to 9
Interpretation: AIVR with one fusion beat into sinus rhythm.

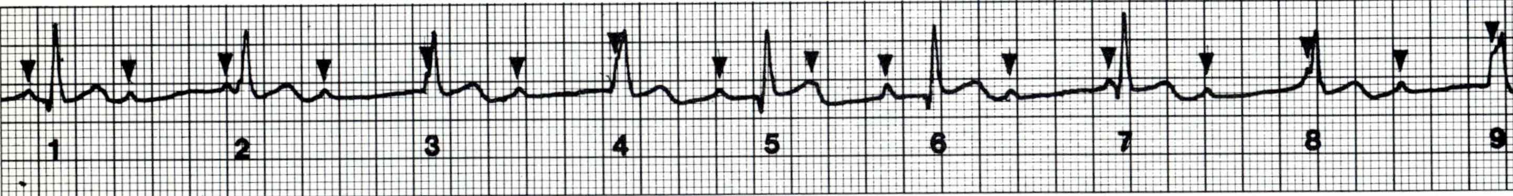

FIGURE 9-18 AV dissociation with capture beats and some degree of AV block. Note the regularity of the ventricular rhythm is interrupted by beats 5 and 6. Both of these beats are preceded by P waves with a PR interval of 0.23 seconds, resulting in normal conduction to the ventricles. Perhaps this patient could conduct 1:1 if the atrial rate were 79 bpm or less.

Rate: Atrial: 107 to 120 bpm *(arrows)*
Ventricular: 60 bpm
Rhythm: Atrial: Regular except for one APB that precedes beat 6
Ventricular: Irregular
P wave: Normal; more Ps than QRSs; Ps bear no constant relationship to QRSs except those preceding beats 5 and 6. Note occasional APB.
PR interval: 0.23 seconds for beats 5 to 6
QRS complex: 0.10 to 0.12 seconds
Interpretation: Sinus tachycardia with some degree of AV block, resulting in AV dissociation with an idiojunctional rhythm and two capture beats

capable of ventricular conduction (0.12 to 0.60 seconds). The appearance of the capture beat may or may not resemble the previous QRS complexes. When the ventricles are paced by the AV junction, the capture beat has the same QRS configuration (Fig. 9-18). When they are paced by an ectopic ventricular focus, the capture beat is narrower. Occasionally the capture beat occurs so prematurely that the QRS is wide from aberration.[9]

Isorhythmic AV dissociation. The term *isorhythmic AV dissociation* describes a unique AV dissociation during which the rates of the two independent pacemakers are virtually the same,[9] but the atrial and ventricular rhythms remain independent of each other. No consistent relationship between the P wave and QRS complex can be found (see Fig. 9-13). (Also refer to Chapter 8, Fig. 8-45.)

Applied Nursing Process

Clinical Assessment

- Detect:
  - A regular pulse.
  - P waves and QRS complexes that bear no relationship to one another with QRS complexes regular.
- Assess patient and ECG.
  - Assess the patient's tolerance of the arrhythmia by checking for signs and symptoms associated with alterations in hemodynamics from loss of the atrial kick (e.g., reduced cardiac output and congestive heart failure) such as:

    Blood pressure.
    Peripheral pulses.
    Mentation.
    Skin color and temperature.
    Lung sounds.
  - The diagnosis of AV dissociation may be aided by patient observation. In the presence of AV dissociation, irregularly occurring cannon waves may be noted in the jugular pulse.[9,27] Cannon waves (pulsations) occur as a result of atrial contraction being dissociated from ventricular diastole. In other words the atria are contracting against closed AV values.[9,28]
  - A second clinical sign in AV dissociation is discovered on auscultation of heart sounds. AV dissociation causes changing intensities of the first heart sound (S_1). As the PR interval shortens, the intensity of S_1 increases. As the atrial and ventricular activity becomes more "opposite," S_1 softens.[9]

❖ NURSING DIAGNOSIS

Decreased cardiac output related to loss of atrial contribution to cardiac output.

❖ ECG DIAGNOSIS

AV dissociation is never a diagnosis by itself. It is always due to another arrhythmia.

Plan and Implementation

Patient goal. The patient will remain hemodynamically stable for the duration of the arrhythmia and, if necessary, the cause of the AV dissociation will be corrected.

Nursing interventions.

- Notify the physician if the patient is symptomatic during episodes of AV dissociation.
- Assist in the identification of the primary cause of AV dissociation. If the patient has been taking digitalis, withholding further digitalis until a blood level is obtained may be indicated.
- Document ECG strips descriptive of the occurrence and duration of AV dissociation.
- Observe for any increasing frequency or symptomatology with AV dissociation.

Evaluation

The patient improves and tolerates the rhythm disturbance and is free from related symptoms as evidenced by the following:

- Stable blood pressure.
- Denial of light-headedness, dizziness, confusion, or shortness of breath.
- Warm, dry skin without pallor or cyanosis.

Medical Treatment

AV dissociation itself requires no treatment. However, the primary cause of the AV dissociation may necessitate treatment. An MI or chronic disease state producing advanced AV block and clinical symptoms (e.g., confusion, syncope, or dizziness) usually requires pacing therapy.

INTRAVENTRICULAR CONDUCTION DELAYS

Conduction delays that occur in the bundle of His or bundle branches are referred to as *intraventricular*. The most common and best recognized intraventricular conduction delays are those of the two bundle branches, commonly referred to as *bundle branch blocks*. Understand that the traditional term *block* connotes relative delay rather than structural blockade. Hemiblocks are another type of intraventricular conduction delay, resulting from delay in one of the fascicles, or divisions, of the left bundle branch.

In reviewing the anatomy of the common bundle and bundle branches, recall that the bundle branch system has two main divisions, both branching from the common bundle. The right bundle branch (RBB) travels down the right side of the interventricular septum, terminating in the right ventricular endocardial surface. The left bundle branch (LBB) separates into three major divisions: the anterior, posterior, and septal fascicles[25,29] (Fig. 9-19). The three fascicles are not discrete divisions but are parts of a sheet of Purkinje fibers.

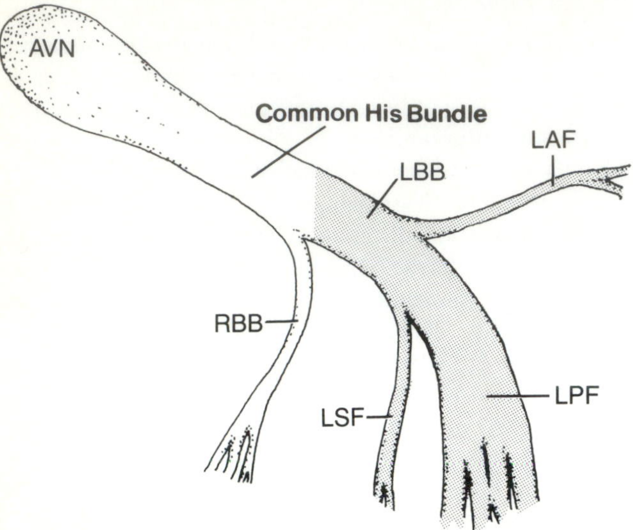

FIGURE 9-19 Schematic showing the divisions of the left bundle branch (shaded) as viewed on the frontal plane. RBB = Right bundle branch. LPF = Left posterior fascicle. LSF = Left septal fascicle. LAF = Left anterior fascicle.

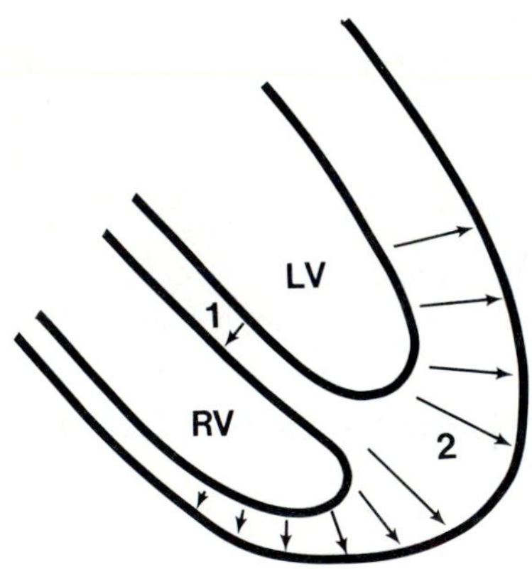

FIGURE 9-20 Schematic of ventricular depolarization. Septal depolarization—left to right (1). Ventricular depolarization—activation occurs simultaneously through both ventricles from endocardium to epicardium (2). The left ventricle (LV) provides the prominent force. RV = Right ventricle.

As you know, the order in which activation proceeds in the ventricles is important in generating the normal precordial ECG pattern. Initially, early septal activation from left to right produces the small r wave in V_1. To account for left-to-right septal activation, the traditional belief was that the impulse traveled down the LBB faster than it did the right and reached the left side of the septum first.[30,31] Recent electrophysiologic research indicates, however, that the speed of impulse transmission is essentially the same and that the slightly earlier activation of the left septum is likely due to the difference in pathway lengths. After septal depolarization, activation continues, involving the remaining ventricular muscle mass (left and right ventricles) and finally proceeds outward simultaneously through both ventricular walls from the endocardium to the epicardium. Owing to the greater left ventricular muscle mass, activation of the left ventricle is the prominent electrocardiographic force (Fig. 9-20). Chapter 1 provides a more detailed discussion of ventricular activation.

In bundle branch blocks the ventricles exhibit abnormal sequential activation. This results in the characteristically wide QRS complex of 0.12 seconds or more.

RIGHT BUNDLE BRANCH BLOCK

Data Base: Problem Identification

Definitions, Etiology, and Mechanisms

Recall that the RBB is much longer and thinner than the left. Because of its location and blood supply, the RBB is susceptible to a host of cardiac disorders. Because of this vulnerability, RBBB is observed frequently, sometimes in the absence of heart disease.[32] Its proximal segment is close to the aortic and tricuspid valves, making it vulnerable to degenerative or sclerotic valve changes. The AV nodal artery, a branch of the right coronary in most (90%) people,[29,33] supplies blood to this portion of the RBB. The middle segment, more commonly involved with coronary artery disease, derives its blood supply from the anterior descending branch of the left coronary artery. It is for this reason that patients with an anteroseptal MI may develop an RBBB.[29,33] The distal segment extends from the septum to the right ventricular endocardium and can be damaged by diseases of the right ventricle that cause dilation.

RBBB may appear transiently or nontransiently. As a transient arrhythmia, it is common, seen in aberrantly conducted APBs or supraventricular tachycardias. It has also been observed during Swan-Ganz catheter insertion.[34] The incidence of RBBB as a persistent arrhythmia is 2 to 3 per 1000 individuals with the incidence increasing in the elderly.[35]

ECG Characteristics

When the RBB does not allow normal impulse conduction, the normal relative activation sequence of the ventricles is disturbed. Unaffected by the RBBB, septal and left ventricular activation proceed normally, followed by the delayed right ventricular activation. The result is sequential rather than simultaneous depolarization (Fig. 9-21).

BBBs are best identified and differentiated from one another in leads V_1 and V_6.[30] V_1 lies over the right ventricle and V_6 lies over the left ventricle. The best ECG lead to identify RBBB is V_1 or MCL_1 whereas V_6 or MCL_6 may be used to confirm the diagnosis.

The classic pattern of RBBB includes the following:

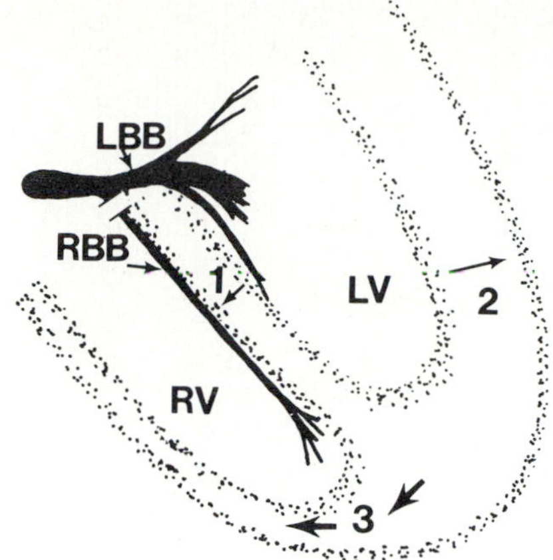

FIGURE 9-21 Schematic of right bundle branch block. RBBB delays right ventricular activation but does not alter septal or left ventricular activation. RBB = Right bundle branch. LBB = Left bundle branch. LV = Left ventricle. RV = Right ventricle.

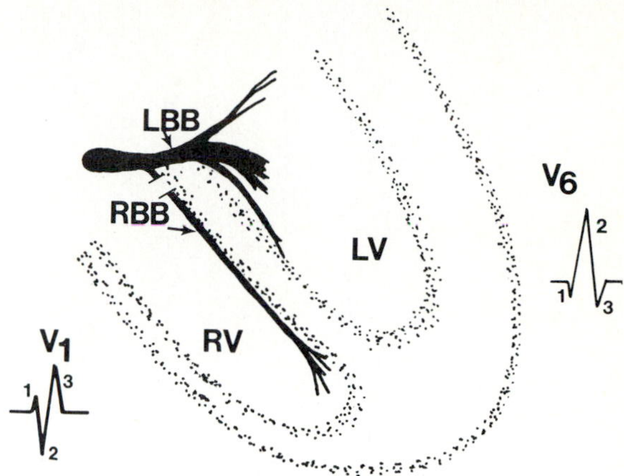

FIGURE 9-22 Schematic of triphasic QRS complex of RBBB in V_1 and V_6. RV = Right ventricle. LV = Left ventricle.

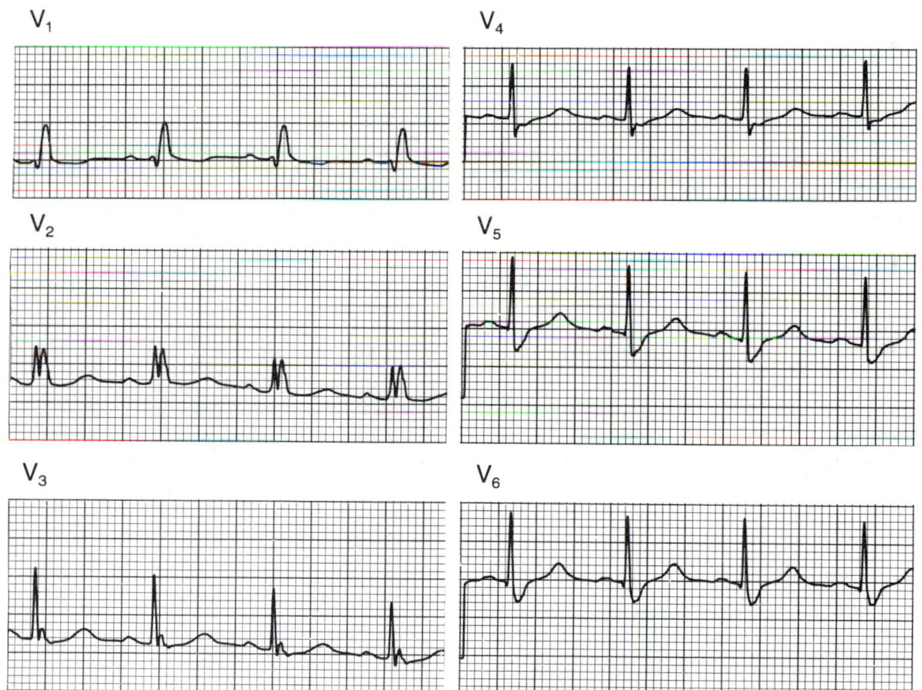

FIGURE 9-23 The precordial leads of an ECG showing RBBB with QRS complex prolonged to 0.12 seconds. Note triphasic QRS complex (rsR′) in V_1 with wide, terminal R′, and inverted T wave. In V_6, note the triphasic complex (qRs) with a wide, terminal s wave, and upright T wave.

Prolonged QRS complex (0.12 seconds or more).[9,10,17] Prolongation of the QRS complex to 0.12 seconds or more is due to the delay in conduction to the right ventricle.

Triphasic QRS complex.[9,10,17,30] In V_1 the initial r wave represents normal septal depolarization from left to right. The S wave represents activation of the left ventricle (away from the V_1 electrode). The RBBB creates an additional R′ wave as the impulse travels from the left ventricle through the interventricular septum to the right ventricle (toward V_1) writing an rSR′ complex (Figs. 9-22 and 9-23). Variations in the rSR′ configuration may occur and

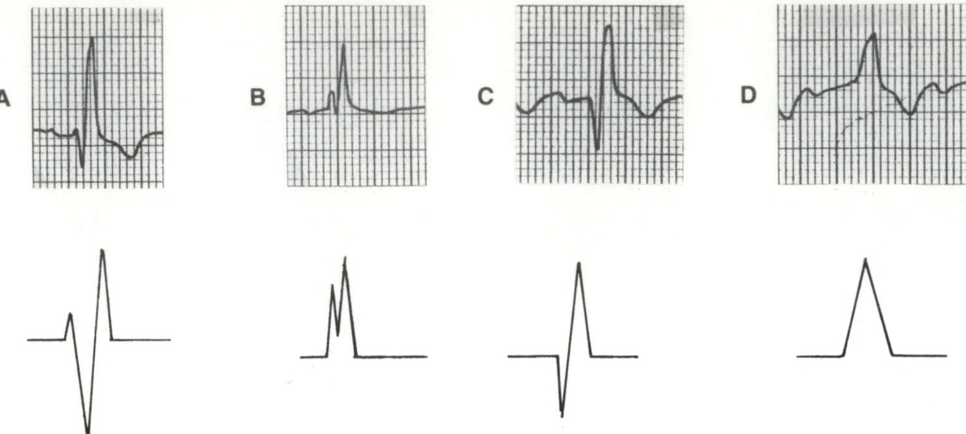

FIGURE 9-24 Variations in RBBB pattern in V_1. Note the feature that each variation has in common: a terminal R wave. **A,** rSR′, the most common form. **B,** R wave with two peaks. **C,** QR. Initial r wave missing because of previous septal infarction. **D,** R, the least common form.

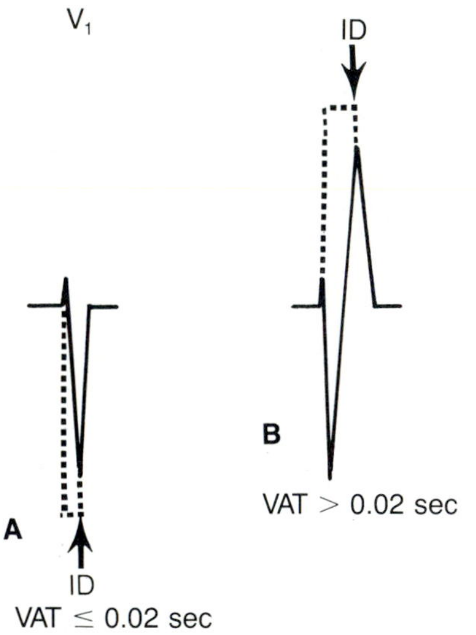

FIGURE 9-25 Schematic of intrinsicoid deflection (ID) and ventricular activation time (VAT) in normal QRS complex and in RBBB on lead V_1. Measure from the beginning of the initial r wave in V_1 (if it is present) to the maximum QRS deflection. **A,** Normal ID and VAT in V_1 occur within 0.02 seconds. **B,** In RBBB the ID and VAT are delayed beyond 0.02 seconds.

are illustrated in Fig. 9-24. Loss of the initial r wave may indicate septal infarction.

In V_6 the triphasic complex has a wide, terminal s wave (qRs). The initial q wave corresponds with normal left to right septal activation (away from the V_6 electrode). Left ventricular activation follows, resulting in an R wave. The s wave occurs as the impulse travels back towards the right ventricle (away from V_6). The change in appearance of the s wave ("slurring") is the characteristic feature of RBBB in V_6. The broad terminal s wave in V_6 and the terminal R′ wave of V_1 are the hallmarks of RBBB (see Figs. 9-22 and 9-23).

Prolonged ventricular activation time and intrinsicoid deflection in V_1.[9,30,31] Ventricular activation time (VAT) is defined as the time required for an impulse to travel from the ventricular endocardium to the epicardial surface and is measured on the ECG from the beginning of the QRS to its peak, the intrinsicoid deflection. Normal conduction produces a VAT within 0.02 seconds in V_1 and within 0.04 seconds in V_6. Since the right ventricle in RBBB has delayed activation, the lead overlying the right ventricle (V_1) will show this delayed activation with a prolonged VAT and delayed intrinsicoid deflection. The VAT and intrinsicoid deflection are within normal limits in V_6 in the presence of RBBB (Fig. 9-25).

T-wave changes. BBBs cause abnormal depolarization, resulting in abnormal repolarization. ECG changes seen in BBB are sometimes confused with myocardial ischemia or injury. For example, RBBB causes the T wave in V_1 to be inverted in a direction opposite to the positive terminal portion of the QRS complex. In V_6, this is evidenced by an upright T wave, opposite in direction to the terminal s wave. This T wave abnormality is secondary to the abnormal depolarization process of the RBBB.[9] Myocardial disease is suspected when, in the presence of RBBB, the T wave is in the same direction as the terminal component of the QRS complex.[10]

Other leads. V_1 and V_2 both "look at" the right ventricle and are very similar in QRS morphology. V_5, V_6, I, and aVL have similar QRS morphology because they all

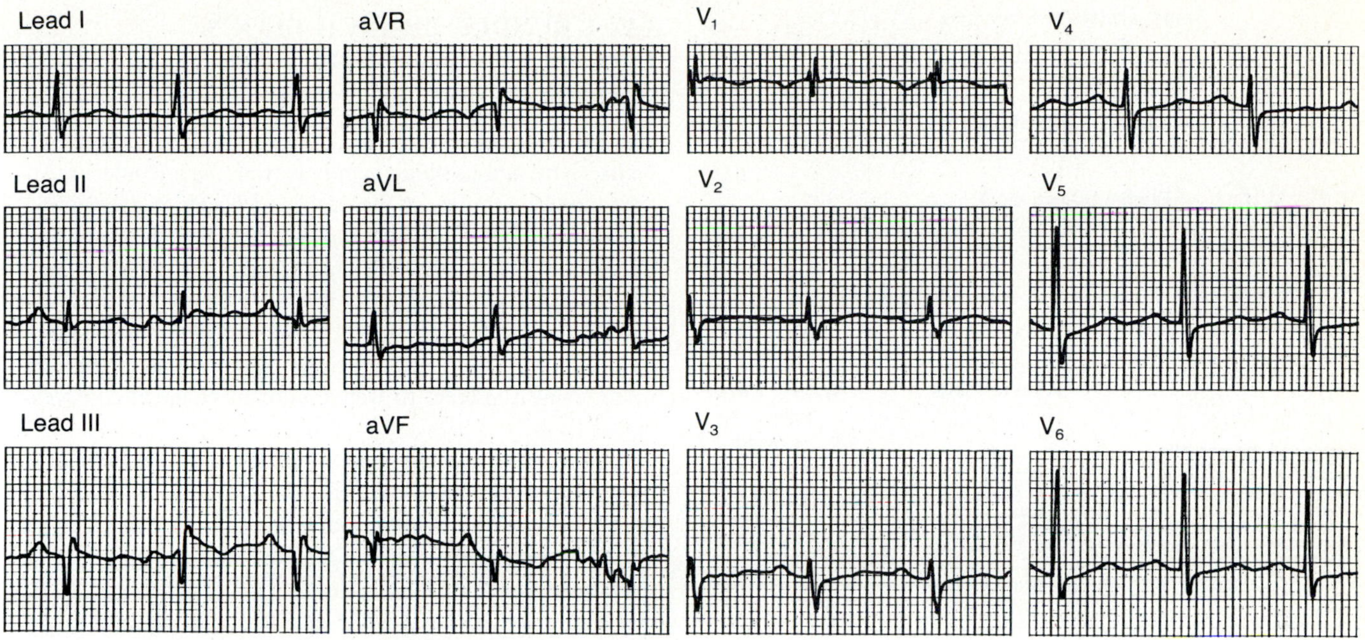

FIGURE 9-26 Incomplete RBBB. QRS morphology in V_1 shows rSR′. V_6 has terminal s wave. QRS duration is 0.08 seconds.

ECG Characteristics
Right Bundle Branch Block

- Prolonged duration of QRS complex—0.12 seconds or more.
- Triphasic QRS complex.
  V_1—rSR′.
  V_6—qRs.
- Wide terminal R′ wave in V_1.
- Wide terminal s wave in V_6.

"look at" the left ventricle from the anterolateral surface.

The box above summarizes the electrocardiographic characteristics of RBBB.

Incomplete RBBB.[9,10,17,30] Incomplete RBBB is diagnosed when the QRS morphology resembles that of an RBBB, but the duration is less than 0.12 seconds (Fig. 9-26). It occurs when there is delay in impulse conduction down the RBB, disturbing normally simultaneous ventricular activation. The left ventricle depolarizes slightly before the right ventricle. Incomplete RBBB is frequently seen in mitral stenosis and atrial septal defects. It may also be seen as a part of a juvenile pattern on an ECG.

Applied Nursing Process
Clinical Assessment

- Detect:
  - A wide QRS complex.
  - No significant clinical symptoms (usually).
- Assess the patient and ECG.
  - Check the patient's vital signs.
  - Diagnose the arrhythmia. Use the algorithm in Fig. 9-27 to assist you.

❖ NURSING DIAGNOSIS

Decreased cardiac output related to delayed right ventricular contraction.

❖ ECG DIAGNOSIS

Right bundle branch block.

Plan and Implementation

It is important to remember some facts about RBBB when planning patient care. It is a common intraventricular conduction delay noted on a routine ECG. In the presence of cardiovascular disease the prognosis is directly related to the nature and severity of the heart disease.[35] RBBB is sometimes found in normal healthy individuals and, in the absence of heart disease,[32,35] the prognosis is favorable.[36] When possible, your individualized plan of patient care should take into consideration the etiology of the RBBB, with goals identified accordingly.

Patient goal. The patient remains asymptomatic and

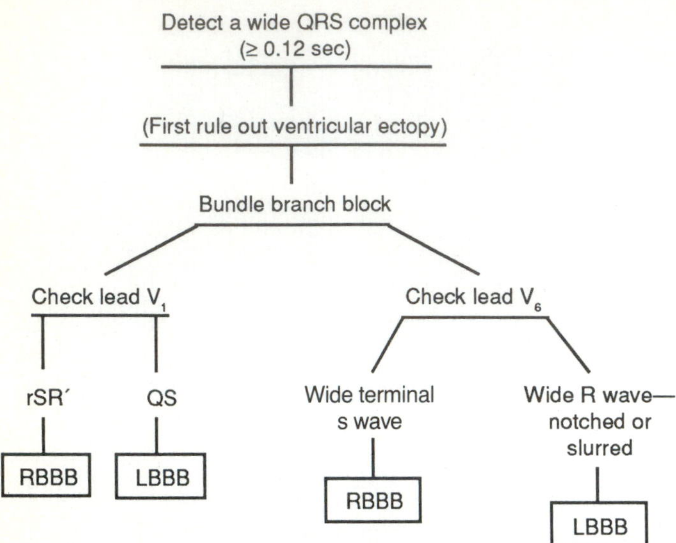

FIGURE 9-27 Bundle branch block algorithm.

will not develop additional conduction delays in the His-Purkinje system.

Nursing interventions.

- Use monitoring leads that allow for the identification of RBBB (MCL_1 and MCL_6 or V_1 and V_6).
- If your patient has had an acute anteroseptal or anterolateral MI (resulting from occlusion of the left anterior descending coronary artery), watch for the development of RBBB.[29,33] RBBB occurring acutely as a complication of an MI may be a poor prognostic sign if it represents a large loss in ventricular muscle mass.
- Observe for additional heart block that may dramatically impair impulse conduction (explained previously in this chapter).
- Identify changes in the RBBB pattern (e.g., intermittent episodes of RBBB).
- In addition to the patient's adaptive status, monitor for changes in the appearance of the ST segment or T wave.

Evaluation

The patient does not develop preventable, advanced degrees of heart block as evidenced by the following:

- The QRS axis within normal range.
- 1:1 AV conduction.

Medical Treatment

No pharmacologic intervention is needed. Electrical pacing is not generally indicated.

LEFT BUNDLE BRANCH BLOCK

Data Base: Problem Identification

Definitions, Etiology, and Mechanisms

The LBB is thick and broad compared with its counterpart on the right, and its blood supply is from the left anterior descending, circumflex, AV nodal, and posterior descending coronary arteries.[29,33] It was originally believed to have two major divisions (fascicles), but research has revealed variable anatomy with three identifiable fascicles.[25,29,38] Typically, block of the LBB occurs at its site of origin in the common bundle. This is because the initial segment may be narrow and is subject to ischemia or mechanical compression.[33,37,38]

Left bundle branch block (LBBB) is often indicative of significant organic heart disease.[31] Transient or permanent,[30] it is rare in healthy individuals.[39] The Framingham study[40] showed that, in the general adult population, the overall incidence of RBBB is slightly greater than LBBB, and both are associated with cardiovascular disease. In all age groups combined the incidence of both left and right bundle branch blocks is greater in men than in women. In addition, men who acquire LBBB are more likely to have or develop advanced cardiovascular abnormalities than are men who acquire RBBB. In another study the most frequent clinical cardiovascular event observed after the development of LBBB was sudden death without previous clinical evidence of ischemic heart disease. The 5-year incidence of sudden death as the first manifestation of heart disease was ten times greater in men with LBBB than in those men without it.[41] The prognosis of LBBB ultimately depends on the severity of the underlying heart disease.

Pathologies associated with LBBB include coronary artery disease, dilated cardiomyopathy, hypertension, and aortic insufficiency. It is recommended that the underlying cause of LBBB be determined.[42]

ECG Characteristics

LBBB totally alters the sequence of left ventricular activation, and septal excitation proceeds from right to left instead of left to right. The impulse activates the right ventricle after which it travels back across the septum to depolarize the left ventricle[10,31,39] (Fig. 9-28). The presence of LBBB invalidates ECG criteria for exercise stress testing, left ventricular hypertrophy, and MI. LBBB is best identified on lead V_6 (MCL_6). Leads V_1, I, and aVL may then be used to confirm the diagnosis.

The classic electrocardiographic pattern of LBBB includes the following:

Prolonged QRS complex (0.12 seconds or more).[10,30,31] QRS prolongation (0.12 seconds or more) sometimes beyond 0.20 seconds, is due to the delay in conduction to the comparatively bulky left ventricle. For this reason, LBBBs are usually wider than RBBBs.

Totally positive QRS complex in V_6.[10,30,31] In LBBB

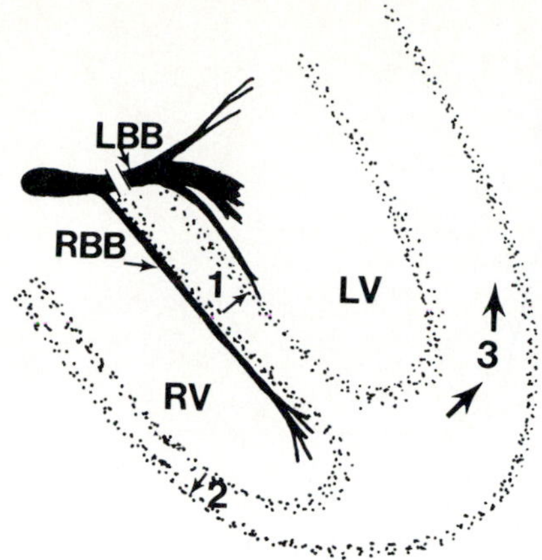

FIGURE 9-28 Schematic of LBBB that alters septal depolarization and delays left ventricular activation. LV = Left ventricle. RV = Right ventricle.

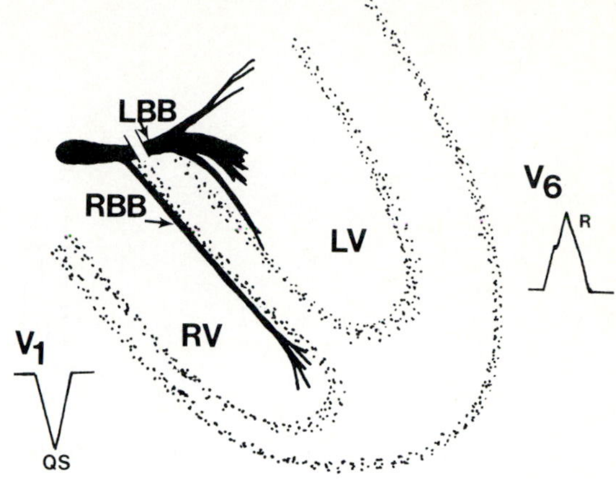

FIGURE 9-29 Schematic of LBBB morphology in leads V_1 and V_6. LV = Left ventricle. RV = Right ventricle.

the normal septal q wave is lost because the septum is activated from right to left. After the septal excitation, the right ventricle is activated, which may allow a slight downward deflection or notch to occur. The notch is not always so well defined, and its appearance may resemble a slurring of the R wave. The impulse continues toward the V_6 electrode as the left ventricle is activated (Figs. 9-29 and 9-30).

Predominantly negative QRS complex in V_1.[10,30,31] The QRS morphology in LBBB has two variations. The most common is a QS complex. The initial deflection is a small q wave (often obscured by subsequent negative deflections) representing right to left septal activation (away from the V_1 electrode). The right ventricle is activated, sometimes represented on the ECG by a small positive notching in the QRS complex. The impulse then travels to the left ventricle (away from V_1), producing a deep, wide S wave (see Figs. 9-29 and 9-30).[30,31]

The less common QRS appearance in LBBB is an rS configuration. The small r wave is not the result of septal depolarization but rather right ventricular depolarization. The left ventricle is subsequently activated sending the impulse away from the V_1 electrode (see Fig. 9-30).

Regardless of whether the complex is a QS or rS, downstroke in V_1 is typically slick and reaches its nadir, or deepest point, within 0.06 seconds.[66,67] The upstroke is often, but not always, notched or slurred (see Fig. 9-30).

Prolonged ventricular activation time and delay in intrinsicoid deflections.[10,30] In LBBB the left ventricle has delayed activation, resulting in a prolonged VAT and delayed intrinsicoid deflection in V_6 (>0.04 seconds) (Fig. 9-31).

T-wave changes. As in RBBB, abnormal repolarization also occurs in LBBB, resulting in T-wave changes. In

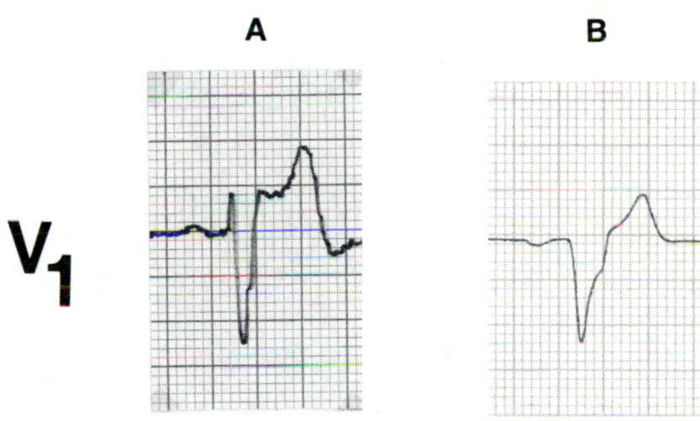

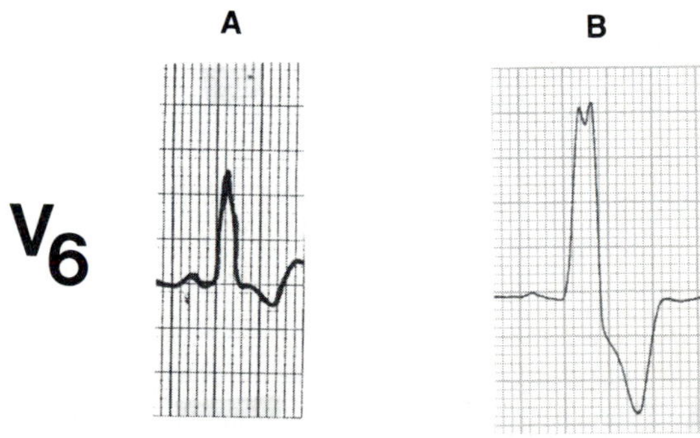

FIGURE 9-30 QRS morphology variations of LBBB in leads V_1 and V_6.

V_1: **A,** Initial r wave a result of right ventricular depolarization. **B,** QS complex, the most common form of LBBB. Note in both V_1 examples there is a slick downstroke of the S or Q wave and slurred or notched upstroke. The nadir, or most negative point of the QS or rS complex, is 0.06 seconds or less in LBBB. In both examples the nadir is reached in 0.06 seconds.

V_6: **A,** Slight slurring of R wave. **B,** Notching of R wave.

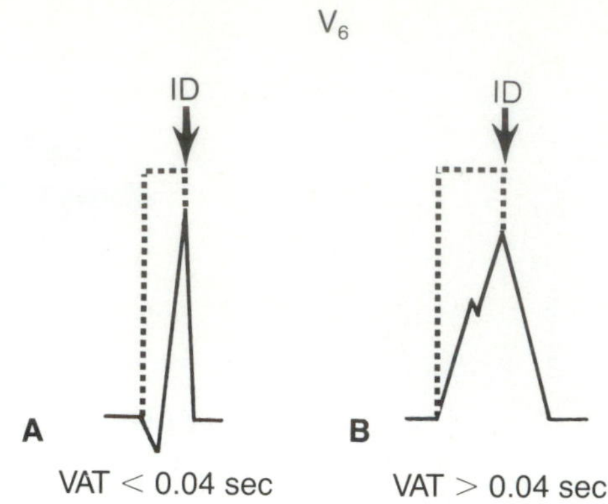

FIGURE 9-31 Schematic of ventricular activation time (VAT) and intrinsicoid deflection (ID) in normal QRS complex and in LBBB on lead V_6. **A,** Normal ID and VAT occur within 0.04 seconds in V_6. **B,** In LBBB the ID and VAT are delayed beyond 0.04 seconds.

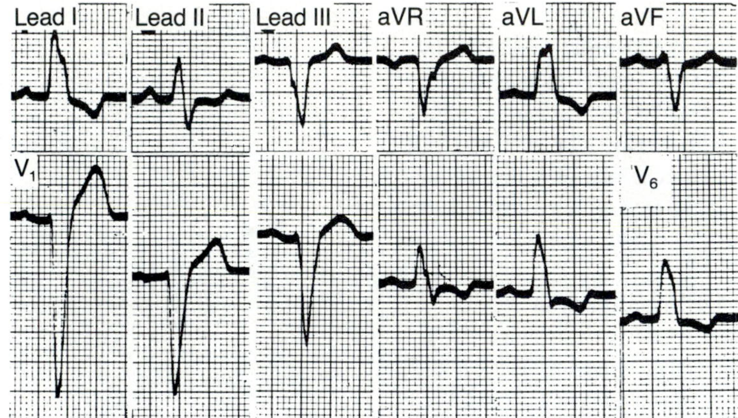

FIGURE 9-32 Left bundle branch block. Note wide QRS interval of 0.16 seconds with late intrinsicoid deflection in V_5 and V_6. Note alterations in ST segments.
V_1: rS with deep, wide S wave; upright T wave.
V_6: Wide R wave; inverted T wave.
Reproduced with permission from Marriott HJL. *Practical Electrocardiography.* 8th ed. Baltimore: Williams & Wilkins, 1988, p. 68.

V_6 the T wave is inverted, opposite in direction to the positive terminal portion of the QRS complex. The T wave is upright in V_1, since the terminal portion of the QRS is negative. The marked alterations in the ST segment and T wave that LBBB produces makes the ECG diagnosis of an acute anteroseptal MI difficult.

Other leads. Leads I, aVL, and V_5 should resemble the QRS complex in V_6 because they are all directed toward the left ventricle. The QRS morphology on V_2 is similar to that of V_1 (Fig. 9-32). The box on this page summarizes the ECG characteristics of LBBB.

ECG Characteristics
Left Bundle Branch Block

- Prolonged duration of QRS complex—0.12 seconds or more.
- Wide R wave in V_6 that may be slurred or notched.
- QS or rS in V_1 with slick downstroke, reaching nadir within 0.06 seconds.

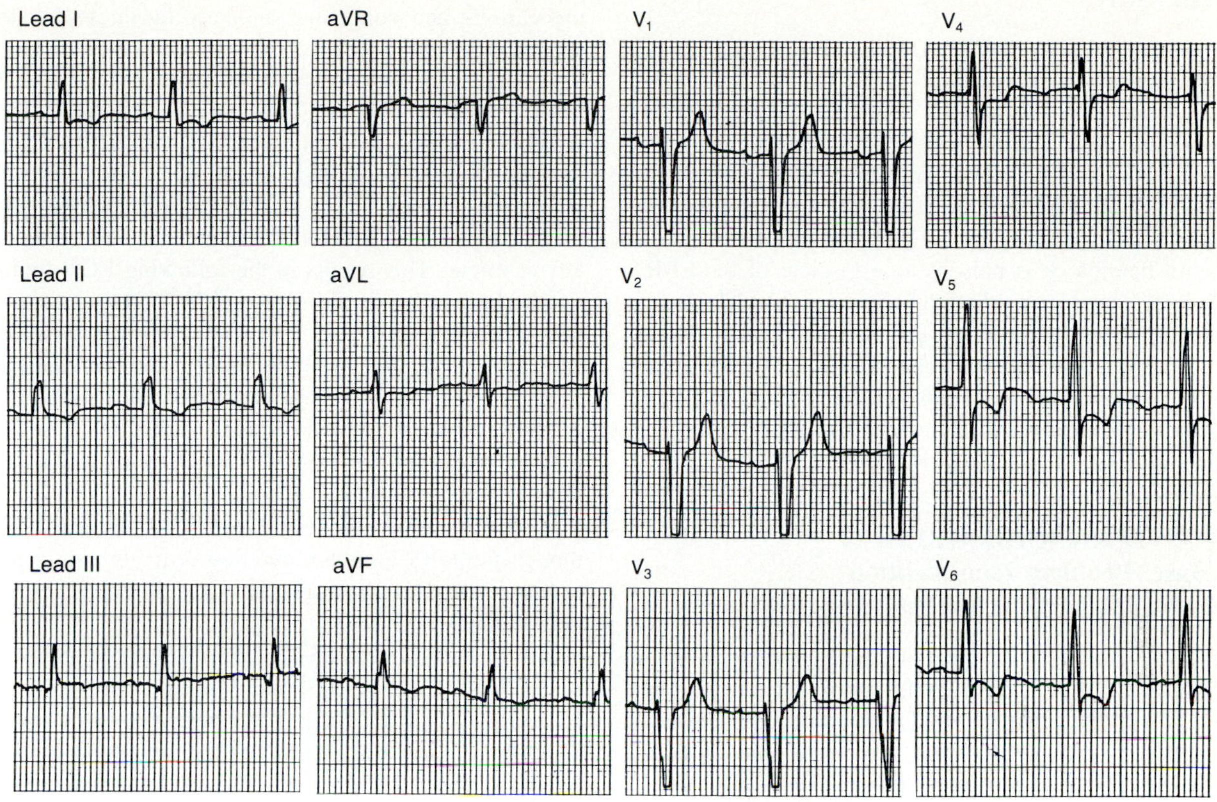

FIGURE 9-33 Incomplete LBBB. QRS morphology in V_1 is rS with a duration of slightly less than 0.12 seconds.

Incomplete left bundle branch block. The term *incomplete left bundle branch block* is used when the QRS morphology resembles LBBB but the QRS duration is normal (Fig. 9-33).

Applied Nursing Process

Clinical Assessment

The clinical assessment is the same as for RBBB.

❖ NURSING DIAGNOSIS

Decreased cardiac output related to slowed left ventricular contraction.

❖ ECG DIAGNOSIS

Left bundle branch block.

Plan and Implementation

Patient goal. The patient's rhythm will stabilize and not progress to a higher grade of block.

Nursing interventions.

- As in RBBB, monitor on leads that permit LBBB identification (MCL_1 and MCL_6; V_1 and V_6).
- In the presence of an acute anteroseptal or anterolateral MI,[43] observe for the development of LBBB, the emergence of which may indicate a poor prognosis if it represents a significant loss of ventricular muscle mass.
- Observe for the development of additional heart block that could have a deleterious effect on impulse conduction.
- Recall that during insertion of a Swan-Ganz catheter, RBBB may occur. Keep this in mind for the patient who has a preexisting LBBB. Although rare, simultaneous BBB is possible. Be prepared to alert the physician of the possibility of a RBBB to prevent a catastrophic event.
- Monitor changes in the appearance of the ST segment and T wave.

Evaluation

The patient remains free from additional conduction delays; is hemodynamically stable as evidenced by 1:1 AV conduction and no change in blood pressure.

Medical Treatment

Pharmacologic intervention is not indicated. The need for electrical pacing depends on individual clinical situations.

HEMIBLOCKS

The term *hemiblock* was popularized by Rosenbaum[44] as a result of studies suggesting that the LBB had only two main divisions, the left anterior (superior) and posterior (inferior) fascicles. Current research, however, indicates that the LBB is rarely, if ever, anatomically organized in this way.[29,38] Although *hemiblock* may be a misnomer, the terminology has not changed.

When a hemiblock is present, one fascicle of the LBB has a "block", or relative slowing of conduction. The term *left anterior hemiblock* (or *left anterior fascicular block*) refers to impaired or blocked conduction in the anterior fascicle. Likewise, the term *left posterior hemiblock* (or *left posterior fascicular block*) indicates conduction in the posterior fascicle is impaired or blocked.

LEFT ANTERIOR HEMIBLOCK
Data Base: Problem Identification
Definitions, Etiology, and Mechanisms

The anterior division of the LBB is thinner and longer than the posterior division.[44] Its blood supply is from the left anterior descending and AV nodal arteries. The anterior division lies in proximity to the left ventricular outflow tract, the anterior papillary muscle, and the aortic valve, increasing its vulnerability to disease.[29,37,44]

In patients over 50 years of age the most common cause of left anterior hemiblock (LAH) is anteroseptal or anterolateral MI.[44] Other causes include diffuse myocardial fibrosis, aortic valve disease, cardiomyopathies, atherosclerosis of the anterior descending coronary artery, hypertension, and Lev's disease. In the younger patient, myocarditis and congenital anomaly (atrial septal defect) are known to cause LAH.[44,45]

ECG Characteristics

A hemiblock is diagnosed by ECG alone. In LAH the initial impulse travels through the left posterior fascicle, activating the inferoposterior wall of the left ventricle. It then travels superiorly to activate the anterolateral wall of the left ventricle. This results in the following ECG findings:

Marked left axis deviation.[39,44,46] The shift in QRS axis to greater than −45 degrees is due to a delay in the activation of the upper anterior wall of the left ventricle. In LAH the impulse travels leftward and superiorly, instead of the normal left and downward vector (Fig. 9-34). (It may be be helpful to review "Axis Determination," Chapter 3.)

QRS duration of less than 0.12 seconds.[8,46] Although the QRS complex duration remains within normal limits, it tends to be longer than the individual's previous normal ECG.

qR in leads I and aVL.[47] The q wave represents initial activation of the posterior fascicle, with the impulse traveling away from the positive electrodes of I and aVL. The impulse then travels through the remainder of the ventricular network back toward the anterior fascicle (toward leads I and aVL), creating the upright R wave (Figs. 9-35 and 9-36).

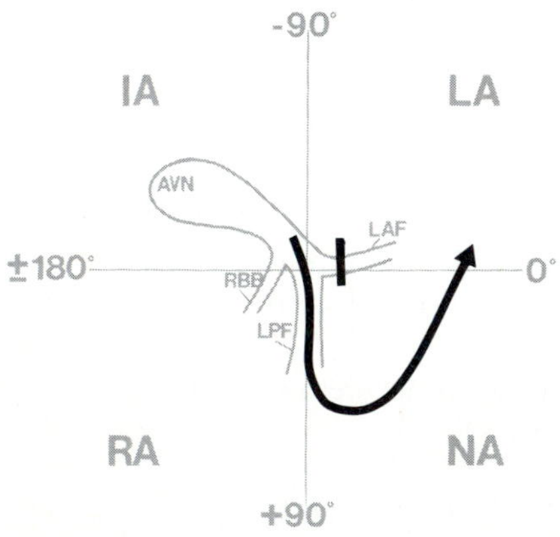

FIGURE 9-34 Schematic showing left anterior hemiblock (LAH). Recall that normal axis is downward and to the left, within the quadrant marked "NA." When the left anterior fascicle is blocked, the impulse travels down the left posterior fascicle. The mean vector is then directed up to the left axis quadrant, −45 to −90 degrees. IA = Indeterminate axis. LA = Left axis. NA = Normal axis. RA = right axis. RBB = Right bundle branch. LAF = Left anterior fascicle. LPF = Left posterior fascicle.

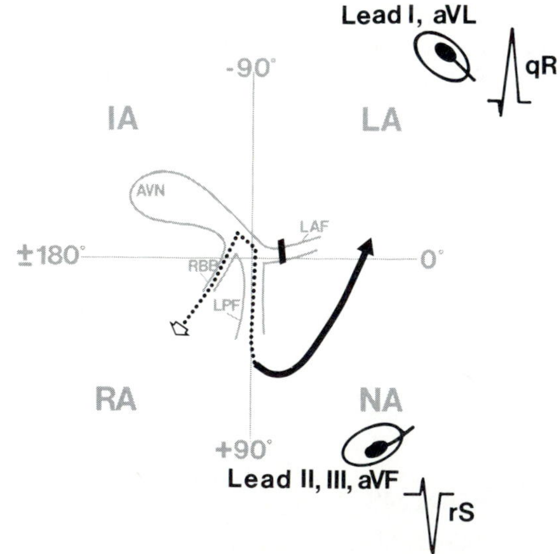

FIGURE 9-35 Schematic of QRS complex in left anterior hemiblock. Leads I and aVL: Initial impulse travels away from positive electrode of I and aVL. The impulse then travels back toward the positive electrode of I an aVL to complete ventricular activation.
Leads II, III, and aVF: Initial impulse travels toward the positive electrode of II, III, and aVF. The impulse then travels back away from the positive electrode of II, III, and aVF to complete ventricular activation.

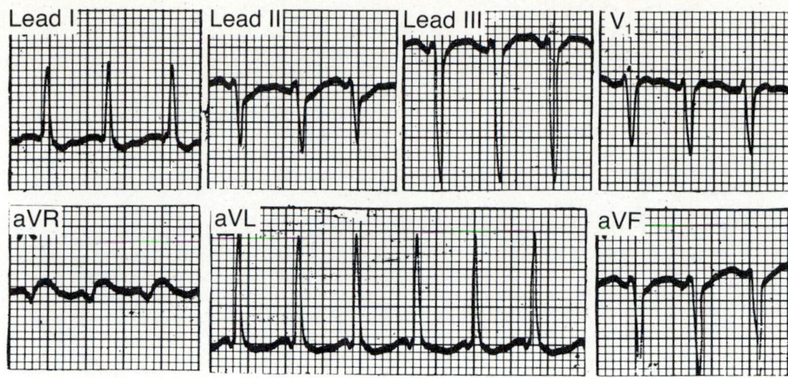

FIGURE 9-36 Left anterior hemiblock. Note left axis deviation, qR in lead I, rS in lead III, QRS duration of 0.08 seconds. Reproduced with permission from Marriott HJL. *Practical Electrocardiography*. 8th ed. Baltimore: Williams & Wilkins, 1988, p. 91.

ECG Characteristics
Left Anterior Hemiblock

- Marked left axis deviation greater than −45 degrees.
- QRS duration <0.12 seconds.
- qR in leads I and aVL.
- rS in leads II, III, and aVF.

rS in leads II, III, and aVF.[47] Recall leads II, III, and aVF have the positive electrode "looking" upward to the heart. In LAH, initial activation of the LBB is in the posterior fascicle. The activation is directed toward leads II, III, and aVF, and a positive r wave is recorded. As the impulse activates the remainder of the ventricular network, it travels back to the anterior fascicle (away from leads II, III, and aVF). The final activation is recorded as an S wave in leads II, III, and aVF (see Figs. 9-35 and 9-36).

The box above summarizes the ECG characteristics of LAH.

LEFT POSTERIOR HEMIBLOCK

Data Base: Problem Identification

Definitions, Etiology, and Mechanisms

The posterior fascicle (division) of the LBB is, by comparison, a sturdy one. Thicker and shorter than either the RBB or left anterior fascicle, it receives its blood supply from the AV nodal, posterior descending, and circumflex coronary arteries. Unlike the other fascicles, the posterior is situated in an area of the left ventricle that affords it protection from adverse conditions, such as disease and mechanical stress.[29] It is for these reasons—its size, multiple blood supply, and its protected location—that conduction delay in this fascicle is less likely and much less common than either the RBB or left anterior fascicle.

ECG Characteristics

LPH alters normal ventricular activation by delaying activation of the inferoposterior wall. The impulse first activates the anterolateral wall of the left ventricle and then travels downward to the inferioposterior wall. The following represent typical ECG changes exhibited with LPH.

Right axis deviation.[39,44] Shift in the QRS axis to approximately +120 degrees is due to the delay in activation of the inferoposterior left ventricular wall. The terminal activation is directed inferiorly and towards the right, causing right axis deviation (Fig. 9-37). (Refer again to Chapter 3, "Axis Determination.")

QRS duration.[8,46] Although the QRS complex duration remains within normal limits (less than 0.12 seconds), it tends to be longer than the individual's previous, normal ECG.

rS in leads I and aVL.[47] The QRS complex reflects an initial activation toward the positive pole of leads I and aVL, and then away from I and aVL as the remainder of the inferoposterior ventricular wall is activated (Figs. 9-38 and 9-39).

qR in leads II, III, and aVF.[47] Leads II, III, and aVF, with their positive poles located inferiorly on the body, view the initial activation traveling away from the positive electrode (thus the q wave). The terminal activation proceeds back toward the inferoposterior wall, resulting in the positive portion of the QRS complex (R wave) (see Figs. 9-38 and 9-39).

The box on 287 summarizes the ECG characteristics of LPH.

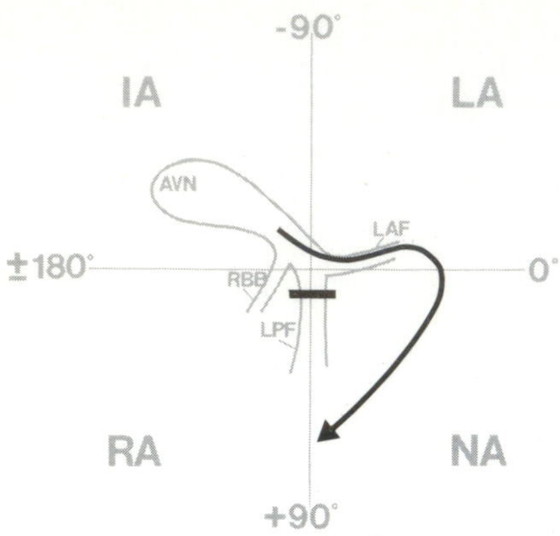

FIGURE 9-37 Schematic showing left posterior hemiblock (LPH). Normal axis is downward and to the left. When the impulse is unable to travel the posterior fascicle, it traverses the anterior fascicle. The mean vector force is then directed to the right axis quadrant, causing a right axis deviation 120 to 180 degrees. IA = Indeterminate axis. LA = Left axis. NA = Normal axis. RA = Right axis. RBB = Right bundle branch. LAF = Left anterior fascicle. LPF = Left posterior fascicle.

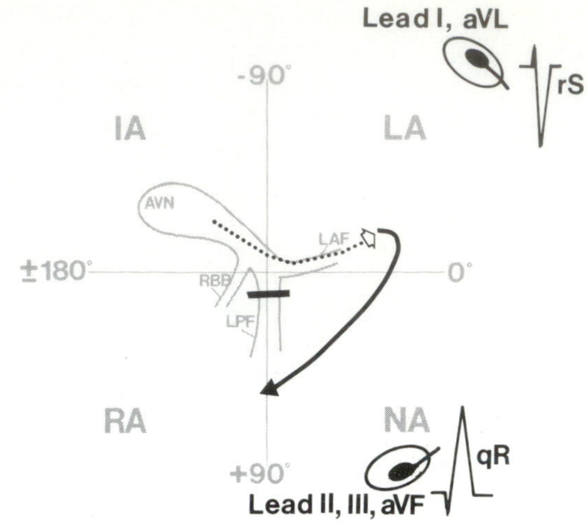

FIGURE 9-38 Schematic of QRS complex in left posterior hemiblock. Leads I and aVL: Initial impulse travels toward the positive electrode of I and aVL. The impulse then travels back away from the positive electrode of I and aVL to complete ventricular activation. Leads II, III, and aVF: Initial impulse travels away from the positive electrode of II, III, and aVF. The impulse then travels back toward the positive electrode of II, III, and aVF to complete ventricular activation.

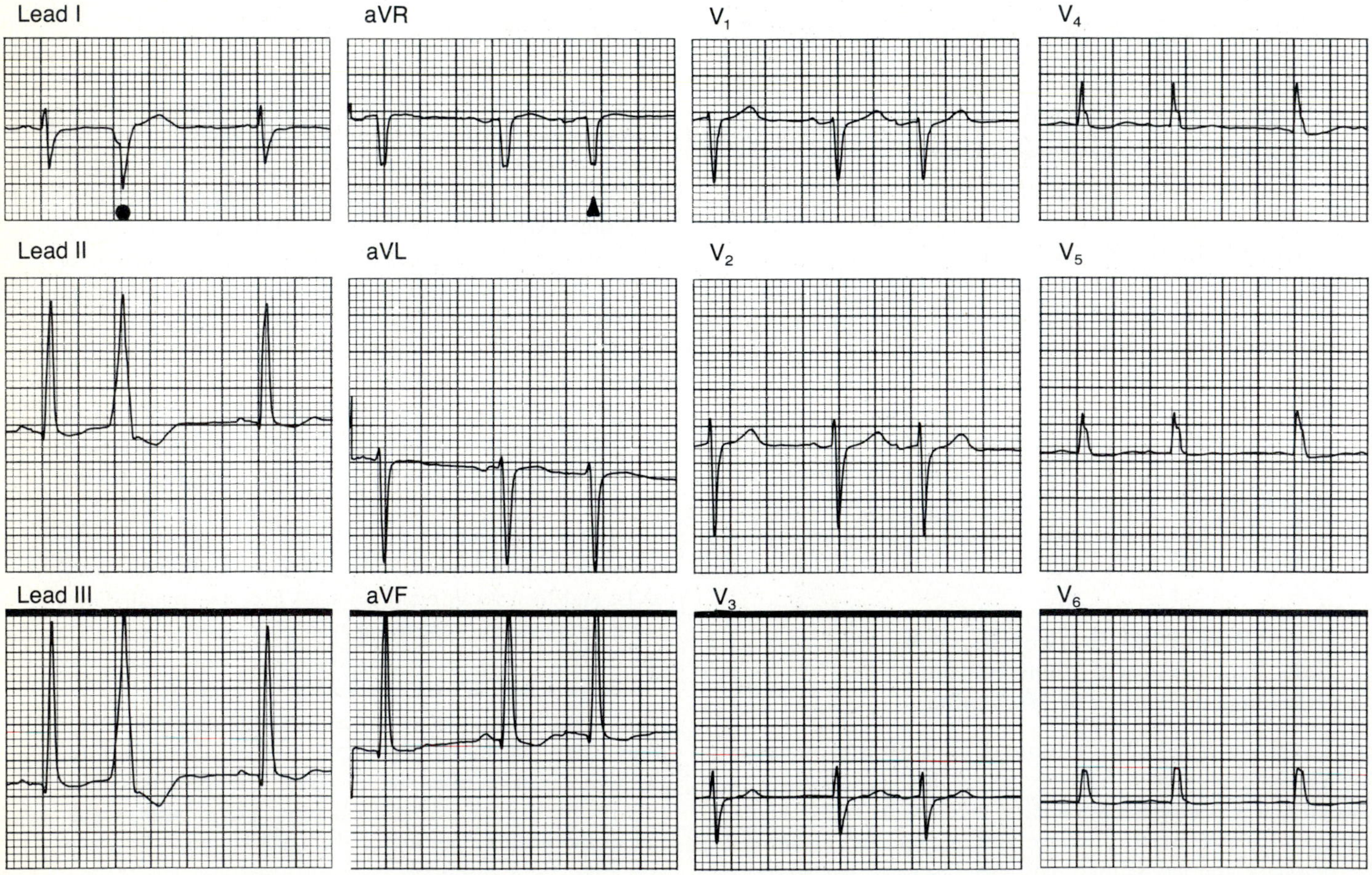

FIGURE 9-39 Left posterior hemiblock. VPB and APB marked with a dot and an arrow, respectively. Note right axis deviation, rS in lead I, qR in lead III, and QRS duration of 0.09 seconds.

Fascicular Blocks

As you know, the three major divisions, or fascicles, of the bundle branch network are the RBB, the left anterior fascicle of the LBB, and the left posterior fascicle of the LBB. To describe conduction delay that occurs in one of more of these fascicles, the terms *monofascicular, bifascicular,* and *trifascicular block* are used.

Monofascicular block. Monofascicular (or unifascicular) block involves conduction delay in only one fascicle, producing a RBBB, LAH, or LPH.

Bifascicular block. Bifascicular block involves a delay in impulse conduction in two of the three fascicles and produces three possible combinations.[17,47]

- RBBB with LAH. This combination is the most frequently seen, since these divisions share a common blood supply and point of origin (Fig. 9-40).
- RBBB with LPH.
- Complete LBBB. Both LAH and LPH are present.

Trifascicular block. Complete trifascicular block occurs when conduction is blocked in all three fascicles resulting in complete heart block.

Incomplete trifascicular block is a term that has been used when two of the three fascicles are blocked and the third shows evidence of incomplete block or delayed conduction. The tendency is to develop complete heart block; hence the empirical warning of first degree AV block with a wide QRS complex. Consider the following combinations.

- RBBB, LAH, and first or second degree AV block (Fig. 9-41).
- RBBB, LPH, and first or second degree AV block.
- Complete LBBB and first or second degree AV block.

ECG Characteristics
Left Posterior Hemiblock

- Right axis deviation of 120 degrees or greater.
- QRS duration <0.12 seconds.
- rS in leads I and aVL.
- qR in leads II, III, and aVF.

Applied Nursing Process
Clinical Assessment for LAH and LPH

- Detect:
  - A change in QRS axis. For example, if you are monitoring your patient on lead II and are noting a positive QRS complex, the sudden appearance of a negative QRS could indicate an LAH. Likewise, if you are monitoring on lead I, obtaining a positive QRS com-

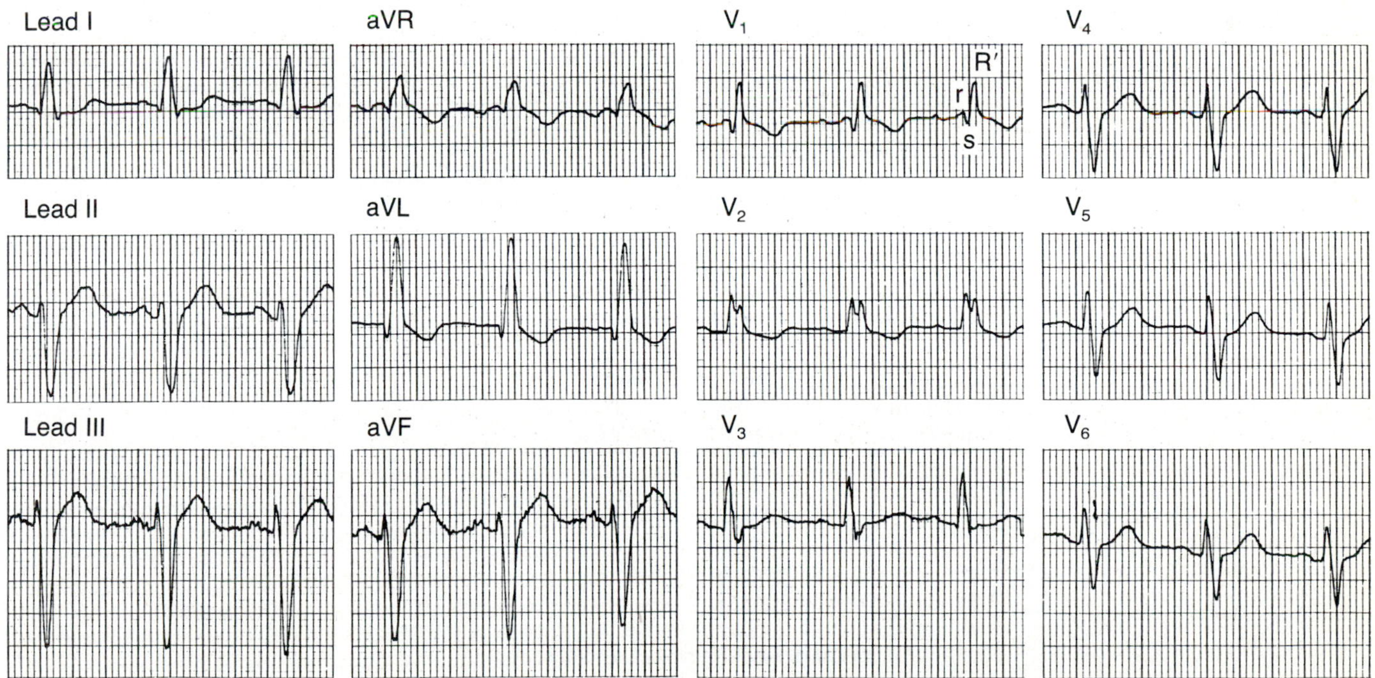

FIGURE 9-40 Bifascicular block, RBBB with LAH. Note rSR′ configuration in V_1 and a QRS duration of 0.14 seconds. There is also a left axis deviation, a qR in lead I, and rS in lead III.

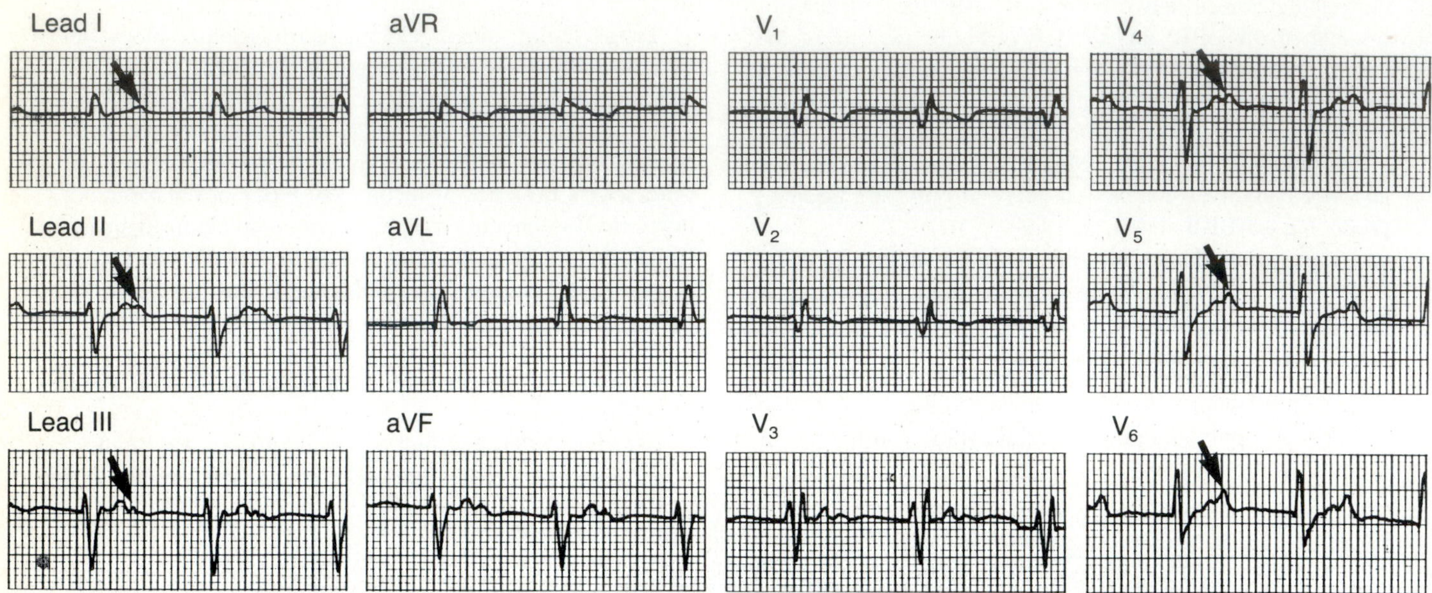

FIGURE 9-41 Incomplete trifascicular block (RBBB, LAH, and first degree AV block). RBBB: rSR′ configuration in V_1, wide terminal s wave in V_6, QRS duration of 0.12 seconds. LAH: Left axis deviation, qR in lead I, rS in lead III. First degree AV block: PR interval 0.44 seconds. P waves are marked *(arrows)*.

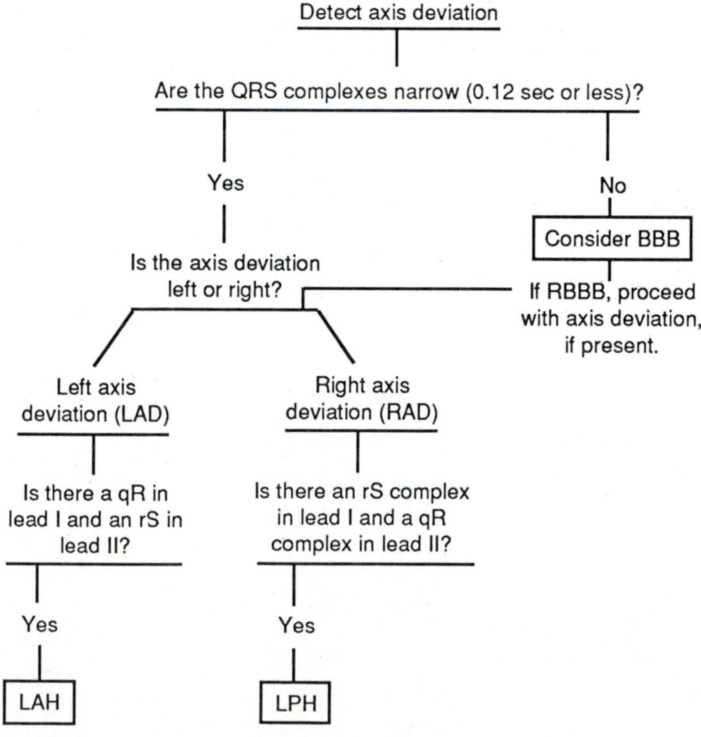

FIGURE 9-42 Hemiblock algorithm.

plex, and note a sudden change in the QRS to predominantly negative, this could indicate the presence of an LPH.
  - There is no clinical symptomatology that can predict the presence or absence of hemiblock.
- Assess the patient and ECG.
  - Assess vital signs.
  - Diagnose the arrhythmia using the algorithm in Figure 9-42.

❖ NURSING DIAGNOSIS

There is no alteration in cardiac output related to hemiblock.

❖ ECG DIAGNOSIS

Left anterior hemiblock or left posterior hemiblock.

Plan and Implementation

Patient goal. The patient will be free from a higher grade of AV or intraventricular block.

Nursing interventions.

- In the presence of an acute anteroseptal MI, observe for the development of fascicular block. If RBBB has been detected in MCL_1, monitor the frontal plane for the development of a hemiblock. Since LAH is more common, monitor one of the inferior leads, such as lead II, to detect a left axis deviation. Periodic checking of lead I for the development of a right axis deviation, indicating possible LPH, is recommended.
- Promptly notify the physician if any increase in fascicular block is observed (e.g., if the patient has an RBBB and suddenly develops a left axis deviation, or a prolongation of the PR interval).

Evaluation

The patient has no increase in block as evidenced by no change in the QRS morphology and 1 : 1 AV conduction.

Medical Treatment

Monofascicular block requires no special treatment. In the presence of a trifascicular block, prophylactic insertion of a temporary pacemaker is often indicated in the setting of an acute anterior MI. A permanent pacemaker may be required in the symptomatic individual.

VENTRICULAR ABERRATION

Data Base: Problem Identification

Definitions, Etiology, and Mechanisms

Ventricular aberration is defined as temporary, abnormal intraventricular conduction of a supraventricular impulse resulting in a wide QRS complex. The width is a result of incomplete recovery of the conducting tissue[48] with subsequent delay in depolarization. Because of this change in normal QRS complex morphology, aberration resembles ventricular ectopy and therefore causes arrhythmia identification dilemmas in many cardiac monitoring units.

Absolute identification of a supraventricular impulse with aberration versus ventricular ectopy is sometimes impossible. However, distinguishing between supraventricular and ventricular origins is important in determining appropriate intervention. Aberrant conduction is of little concern in either prognosis or treatment,[49] whereas ventricular ectopy without treatment may result in life-threatening arrhythmias. A good rule to follow is to consider funny-looking beats (FLBs) to be ventricular until you are able to prove the existence of aberration. A review of ventricular arrhythmias (Chapter 8) may be useful at this point. Differential diagnosis of wide QRS complexes follows in Chapter 10.

In recalling the anatomy of the bundle branches, remember that the RBB is longer and thinner than the left. The RBB also has a slightly longer refractory period[50] (refractoriness refers to the responsiveness of the myocardial tissue to an impulse). In aberrant conduction most often it is the RBB that is refractory, and thus a RBBB pattern is common.[51-53]

Aberration may occur in the presence of a rapid rate. The rapidity of the supraventricular impulse may not allow even healthy individuals to conduct a narrow QRS complex.[52,54] The rate at which the QRS becomes wide (or aberrant) is called the *critical rate*.[52] This tachycardia-dependent aberration is referred to as *Phase 3 block* (see Chapter 1, "Action Potential"). Such wide QRS tachycardias are often difficult to differentiate from VT. Supraventricular tachycardias with RBBB aberration often display heart rates between 170 and 200 bpm,[10,55] whereas rates of VT are frequently between 130 and 170 bpm.[10,52,54,55] Unfortunately, rate differentiation is a poor criterion for differential diagnosis because there is much overlap in the rates of these two tachycardias.

In AF, differentiation of anomalous beats or FLBs can be troublesome. In a study by Marriott and Sandler, over 50% of their tracings of AF contained FLBs.[56] Although aberration occurs in AF, studies using His bundle recordings suggest that approximately 90% of FLBs during AF are ventricular in origin.[57] When aberration occurs in AF, it is often a manifestation of what is known as *Ashman's phenomenon*. Ashman's phenomenon describes aberration that occurs when a short ventricular cycle follows a relatively long cycle.[58] Recall when there is an increase in the R-R interval, the refractory period lengthens. That is, the slower the rate, the longer the recovery.[59] When a short R-R interval follows a relatively long one, one of the bundle branches may still be refractory, resulting in an aberrant beat (Fig. 9-43). The aberration may be maintained in several consecutive QRS com-

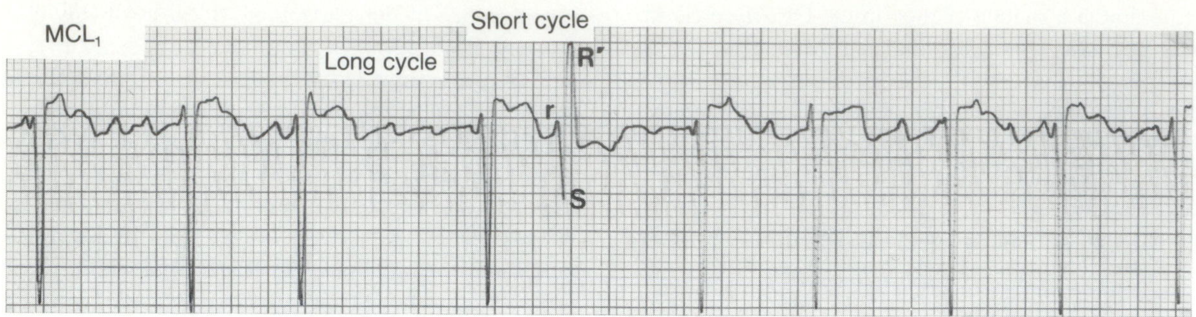

FIGURE 9-43 Ashman's phenomenon. An aberrant beat has RBBB morphology, rSR′. The aberrant beat occurs when a long cycle is followed by a relatively short cycle.

Rate: Atrial: Unable to determine
Ventricular: 90 bpm
Rhythm: Atrial: Irregular fib/flutter
Ventricular: Irregular
P wave: "f" waves
PR interval: —
QRS complex: Nonaberrant 0.08 seconds
Aberrant: 0.13 seconds
Interpretation: Atrial fib/flutter with intermittent RBBB aberration.

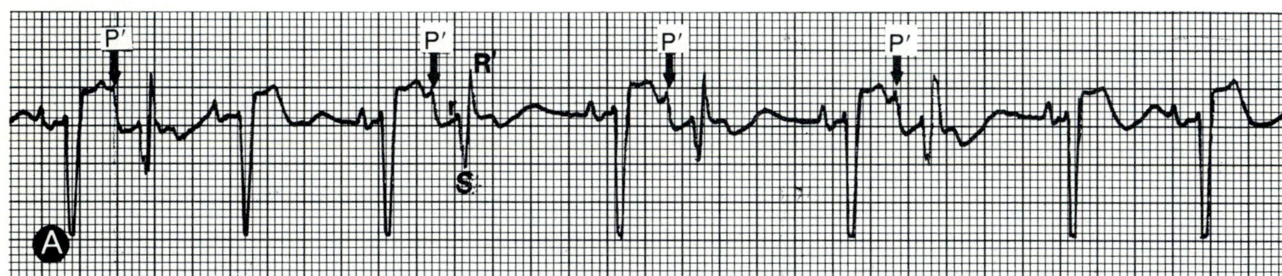

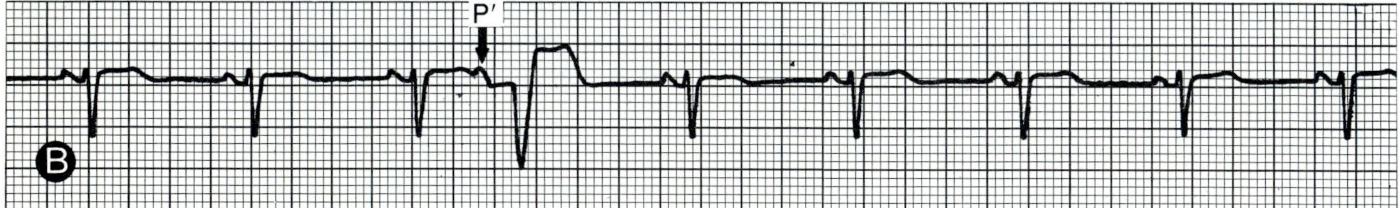

FIGURE 9-44 Two examples of sinus rhythm with aberrantly conducted APBs. **A,** Note the premature P′ waves *(arrows)* followed by a wide QRS with RBBB morphology. The PR interval is 0.14 seconds and the P′R interval is 0.16 seconds. **B,** Sinus rhythm with aberrantly conducted APB. Note the premature P′ wave followed by a wide QRS with LBBB morphology. The PR interval is 0.12 seconds and the P′R interval is 0.18 seconds.

plexes, until the supraventricular impulse occurs late enough in the cycle to permit recovery of both bundle branches.[48]

For similar reasons an atrial premature beat (APB) may find the conducting tissues of the bundle branch system refractory, resulting in a wide, aberrantly conducted QRS complex (Fig. 9-44). (Aberrantly conducted beats are also addressed in Chapters 6 and 10.)

Aberration may also occur when repolarization is prolonged.[52] Prolonged repolarization in turn lengthens the refractory period. The lengthening of the refractory period delays the responsiveness of the bundle branch and a wide QRS complex is recorded. This is referred to as *Phase 4 block* (see Chapter 1, "Action Potential"). This bradycardia-dependent BBB (also known as *reverse rate-related BBB*) is rare.[60,61]

ECG Characteristics

Several ECG features, when present, will aid in the diagnosis of aberration.

P waves.[17,52,62] The presence of a premature P′ wave preceding an abnormal premature QRS complex is strongly suggestive of aberrant conduction. The PR interval must be of reasonable length to permit AV conduction (see Fig. 9-44). The preceding ST segment and T wave of a wide premature QRS complex should always be inspected for a hidden P′ wave.

QRS morphology. In the absence of P waves, recognizing aberration is more difficult. Examining the morphologic characteristics of the anomalous QRS complex offers fairly reliable clues regarding its origin and at least enables us to make an educated guess (see pp. 203-207 and Chapter 10). Aberration usually has either a left or a right bundle branch block configuration. As previously stated, the RBBB configuration is more common and has the following QRS characteristics.[49,54-56,63]

- A triphasic configuration in V_1 (MCL_1). Approximately 70% of all aberrancy exhibits a triphasic QRS that may appear as rsR′, rSR′, or rsr′ on V_1 or MCL_1 (Fig. 9-45). In contrast, 92% of all ventricular ectopic beats demonstrate a monophasic or diphasic QRS complex on V_1 or MCL_1: R, qR, QR, or Rs. The remaining 30% of aberrant beats manifest as either a monophasic or diphasic QRS complex. It is this 30% that makes the differentiation between aberration and ventricular ectopy so difficult. To assist in differentiating the positive complex with two peaks in V_1, an approach identified by Gozensky and Thorne,[64] known as *rabbit ears,* may be helpful. If the left rabbit ear is taller than the right ear on V_1 or MCL_1, ventricular ectopy is favored. A taller right rabbit ear does not favor either ventricular ectopy or aberration. Remember, the rabbit ear criterion is applied only on V_1 or MCL_1.
- A triphasic QRS complex, qRs, in V_6 or MCL_6 (Fig. 9-46).
- Width of QRS less than 0.14 seconds.[55,62,65] In aberration the QRS complex is usually narrower than 0.14 seconds.

The box on this page summarizes the most common ECG characteristics of aberration.

Ashman's phenomenon. As previously described, Ashman's phenomenon may occur in the presence of AF. It is characterized by an aberrant QRS of a short cycle that was preceded by a long cycle, or from a very short cycle after an average length cycle.[58] Because the cycle length is short, the supraventricular impulse arrives while parts of the conduction system are still refractory. Since the RBB has the longest refractory period, the QRS most often resembles a RBBB (rSR′ on V_1 or MCI_1). Ashman's phenomenon is commonly found in the absence of heart disease.[62]

Initial vector. The initial vector (first 0.02 to 0.04 seconds of the QRS) of a supraventricular beat conducted with RBBB aberration is often identical to that of the sinus beat.[49] In RBBB aberration, initial activation is not affected. Thus on V_1, RBBB aberration frequently exhibits an identical initial vector. When the initial vector is also identical in leads V_6, I, II, and III, the likelihood of aber-

Most Common ECG Characteristics of Aberration

- Triphasic QRS configuration in V_1 and V_6 (MCL_1 and MCL_6).
- QRS complex <0.14 seconds.

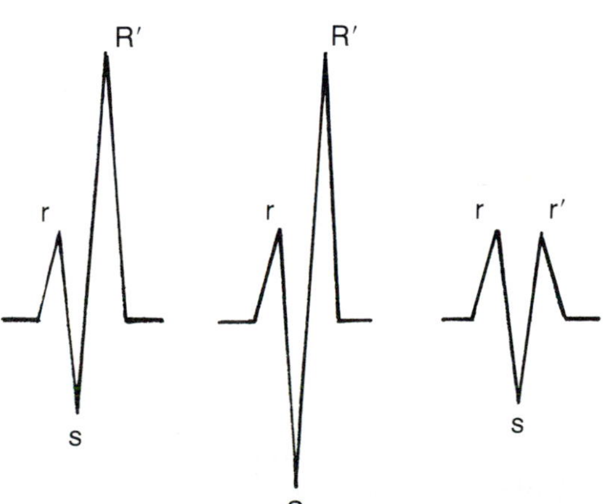

FIGURE 9-45 Schematic of most common forms of aberrant QRS morphology in V_1, RBBB type.

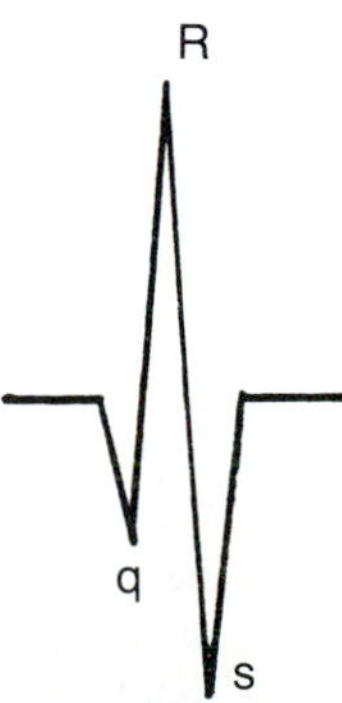

FIGURE 9-46 Schematic of common aberrant QRS morphology in V_6, RBBB type.

ration is further enhanced.[55] Although an identical initial vector supports aberration, it is not diagnostic and is only valuable with RBBB aberration. Ventricular ectopic and LBBB aberrant beats usually have abnormal septal activation and therefore display different initial vectors.[49,58]

Compensatory pause. The presence or absence of a compensatory pause is not very helpful. Premature supraventricular impulses do not usually display a full compensatory pause whereas ventricular premature beats (VPBs) generally are followed by a compensatory pause, with the exception of interpolated VPBs. Do not rely on the presence or absence of the pause to confirm a differential diagnosis, since it is only a supporting feature.

Fixed coupling intervals. The presence of fixed coupling intervals lends support to the diagnosis of ventricular ectopy, but it is not always a reliable criterion. For example, it is of no use with the single FLB, and some VPBs, as well as ventricular parasystole, exhibit variable coupling intervals. Although we can say that fixed coupling intervals favor the diagnosis of ventricular ectopy, we cannot say that variable coupling intervals indicates aberration.

Rhythm. Rhythm may be of some value in differential diagnosis. The R-R interval in VT is usually regular. When the rhythm is irregular in the presence of a rapid (above 220 bpm), wide-QRS tachycardia, consider AF with aberration[55] or Wolff-Parkinson-White syndrome (WPW is an AV "bypass" arrhythmia that may result in a supraventricular tachycardia with a wide QRS complex).

Chapters 8 and 10 offer additional criteria that may be used in the differential diagnosis of aberration versus ventricular ectopy.

Applied Nursing Process

Clinical Assessment

- Detect:
  - (Often) an irregularity in the pulse.
  - Intermittent wide QRS complexes.
- Assess the patient and ECG.
  - Evaluate the patient's clinical tolerance of the arrhythmia by assessing the following:
    - Blood pressure.
    - Peripheral pulses.
    - Sensorium.
    - Skin color and temperature.
    - Associated symptoms such as palpitations, lightheadedness, dizziness.
  - Differentiate aberration from ventricular ectopy. Certain clinical observations and interventions may assist in the differential diagnosis of aberration.
    - Vagal stimulation slows conduction of supraventricular impulses through the AV node and consequently decreases the ventricular rate. Vagal stimulation does not usually affect the rate of ventricular discharges, so it rarely, if ever, affects VT.[50,52] The absence of vagal slowing, however, does not confirm the presence of VT.
  - Two other previously described physical assessment findings may be considered in the differential diagnosis of aberration versus ventricular ectopy. They are of limited value, however, for they may be present in both ventricular and junctional tachycardias.[62]
    - Irregular and varying amplitude of cannon waves suggests the presence of AV dissociation (refer to "AV Dissociation").
    - Variation in amplitude of the first heart sound on auscultation lends support to the diagnosis of AV dissociation or VT.
  - Another auscultatory finding may be helpful. In RBBB (the most frequent form of aberration) it is common to find a splitting of the heart sounds resulting from the delay in activation of the right ventricle. Supraventricular tachycardia with aberration will have close splitting of the heart sounds whereas in VT, splitting of the first heart sound is significant.[28]

❖ NURSING DIAGNOSIS

Decreased cardiac output related to tachycardia (if present).

❖ ECG DIAGNOSIS

Supraventricular impulses (specify) conducted with ventricular aberration.

Plan and Implementation

Patient goal. The patient will remain asymptomatic and hemodynamically stable.

Nursing interventions.

- The nurse who is continuously monitoring the patient may encounter instances when independent decisions must be made concerning the initiation of prophylactic antiarrhythmic treatment protocols. To assist you in making the interpretations more confidently, here are some guidelines:
  - Obtain a long ECG strip recording to show the relationship of the FLBs to the preceding cycle.
  - Use MCL_1 or V_1 as the primary monitoring lead, and change to MCL_6 or V_6 for a different "look" at the FLB. Use multiple lead analysis whenever necessary.
  - Keep QRS morphology tables close to the central monitoring station and become well acquainted with them.
  - Look for P waves buried in the preceding ST segments and T waves.
  - Compare previous ECG strips with sinus beats, VPBs, and bundle branch blocks with the FLBs.
  - Finally, use other health team members when needed to confirm your diagnosis.
- Do not become monitor dependent. Apply your good observation and assessment skills to the individual patient.
- Administer pharmacologic agents as prescribed and evaluate the patient's response to them.

Evaluation

The patient is free from arrhythmia-related symptoms as evidenced by the following:

- Blood pressure within normal limits.
- Warm, dry skin.
- A lucid response.

Medical Treatment

Medical treatment is based on the diagnosis of the arrhythmia. If VT is diagnosed, lidocaine is usually indicated and, if unsuccessful, electrical cardioversion is performed.

To control the ventricular rate in supraventricular tachycardias with aberration, verapamil or esmolol is often effective. Later the patient may benefit from the administration of digitalis. Adequate digitalization must occur to establish therapeutic blood levels. Any patient who has been previously taking digitalis should have a serum level determined to check for the presence of toxicity prior to administering additional digitalis.

If there is uncertainty about the tachycardia diagnosis and the patient is symptomatic, electrical cardioversion is indicated.

REFERENCES

1. McVay MR. Atrioventricular block—a review. *S. Dakota Med.*, Jan., 1984, 37(1): 21-6.
2. Gomes JA, El-Sherif N. Atrioventricular block: mechanism, clinical presentation, and therapy. *Med. Clin. N. Am.*, Jul., 1984, 68(4): 955-67.
3. Scott O, Williams GJ, Fiddler GI. Results of 24-hour ambulatory monitoring of electrocardiograms in 131 healthy boys aged 10-13 years. *Br. Heart J.*, 1980, 44: 304-8.
4. Dickinson DF, Scott O. Ambulatory electrocardiographic monitoring in 100 healthy teenage boys. *Br. Heart J.*, Feb., 1984, 51: 179-83.
5. Talan DA, Bauernfeind RA, Ashley WW, Kanakis C, Rosen KM. Twenty-four hour continuous ECG recordings in long-distance runners. *Chest*, Jul., 1982, 82(1): 19-24.
6. Bexton RS, Camm AJ. First degree atrioventricular block. *Eur. Heart J.* 1984, 5(Suppl. A): 107-9.
7. Schamroth L. *The Disorders of Cardiac Rhythm*. Oxford: Blackwell Scientific Publications, 1971.
8. Braunwald E. *Heart Disease: A Textbook of Cardiovascular Medicine*. 3rd ed. Philadelphia: WB Saunders, 1988.
9. Marriott HJL. *Practical Electrocardiography*. 8th ed. Baltimore: Williams & Wilkins, 1988.
10. Conover MB. *Understanding Electrocardiography*. 5th ed. St. Louis: The CV Mosby Co., 1988.
11. Zipes DP. Second-degree atrioventricular block. *Circ.*, Sept., 1979, 60(3): 465-72.
12. Strasberg B, Amat-Y-Leon F, Dhingra R, Palileo E, Swiryn S, Bauernfeind R, Wyndham C, Rosen K. Natural history of chronic second-degree atrioventricular nodal block. *Circ.*, May, 1981, 63(5): 1043-9.
13. Denes P, Levy L, Pick A, Rosen KM. The incidence of typical and atypical A-V Wenckebach periodicity. *Am. Heart J.*, Jan., 1975, 89(1): 26-31.
14. Kupfer JM, Kligfield P. A generalized description of Wenckebach behavior with analysis of determinants of ventricular cycle-length variation during ambulatory electrocardiography. *Am. J. Cardiol.*, May, 1991, 67(5): 981-6.
15. Bailey JC. Atrioventricular dissociation. *Heart & Lung*, Jul.-Aug., 1981 10(4): 629-33.
16. Langendorf R, Pick A. Atrioventricular block, type II (Mobitz)—its nature and clinical significance. *Circ.*, Nov., 1968, 38(5): 819-21.
17. Sweetwood HM. *Clinical Electrocardiography for Nurses*. 2nd ed. Rockville, MD: Aspen Systems, 1988.
18. Barold SS, Friedberg HD. Second degree atrioventricular block: A matter of definition. *Am. J. Cardiol.* Feb., 1974, 33(2): 311-15.
19. Frye RL, Collins JJ, DeSanctis RW, Dodge HT, Dreifus LS, Fisch C. Guidelines for permanent cardiac pacemaker implantation, May 1984; a report of the Joint American College of Cardiology/American Heart Association Task Force on Assessment of Cardiovascular Procedures (Subcommittee on Pacemaker Implantation). *Circ.*, Aug., 1984, 70(2): 331A-9A.
20. Ohkawa S, Hackel DB, Ideker RE. Correlation of the width of the QRS complex with the pathologic anatomy of the cardiac conduction system in patients with chronic complete atrioventricular block. *Circ.*, Apr., 1981, 63(4): 938-47.
21. Gillette PC. Cardiac dysrhythmias in infants and children. *In* Engle MA (ed). *Cardiovascular Clinics: Pediatric Cardiovascular Disease*. Brest AN (ed). *Cardiovascular Clinics*, 11/2. Philadelphia: FA Davis, 1981.
22. Clemmensen P, et al. Complete atrioventricular block complicating inferior wall acute myocardial infarction treated with reperfusion therapy. *Am. J. Cardiol.*, Feb., 1991, 67(4): 225-30.
23. Marriott HJ, Menendez MM. A-V dissociation revisited. *Prog. Cardiovasc. Dis.*, May, 1966, 8(6): 522-38.
24. Pick A. AV dissociation. A proposal for a comprehensive classification and consistent terminology. *Am. Heart J.*, Aug., 1963, 66(2): 147-50.
25. Hecht HH, Kossmann CE, Childers RW, Langendorf R, Lev M, Rosen KM, Pruitt RD, Truex RC, Uhley HN, Watt TB. Atrioventricular and intraventricular conduction: revised nomenclature and concepts. *Am. J. Cardiol.*, Feb., 1973, 31(2): 232-44.
26. Marriott HJ, Schubart AF, Bradley SM. A-V dissociation: a reappraisal. *Am. J. Cardiol.*, Nov., 1958, 11(5): 586-605.
27. Marriott HJ, Conover MH. *Advanced Concepts in Arrhythmias*. 2nd ed. St. Louis: The CV Mosby Co., 1989.
28. Schrire V, Vogelpoel L. The clinical and electrocardiographic differentiation of supraventricular and ventricular tachycardias with regular rhythms. *Am. Heart J.*, Feb., 1955, 49(2): 162-87.
29. McAnulty JH, Rahimtoola SH. Bundle branch block. *Prog. Cardiovasc. Dis.*, Jan./Feb., 1983, 26(4): 333-54.
30. Duke DM. Intraventricular conduction blocks, Part I. *Crit. Care Nurse*, May/Jun., 1982, 2(3): 30-9.
31. Schamroth L. *An Introduction to Electrocardiography*. 6th ed. Oxford: Blackwell Scientific Publications, 1982.
32. Henry EI, Schack JA, Hoffman I. Significance of the relation of QRS and T waves in bundle branch block: a useful electrocardiographic sign. *Am. Heart J.*, Sept., 1957, 54(3): 407-16.
33. Rosenbaum MB, Elizari MV, Kretz A, Taratuto AL. Anatomical basis of AV conduction disturbances. *Geriatrics*, Nov., 1970, 25(11): 132-44.
34. Luck JC, Engel TR. Transient right bundle branch block with "Swan-Ganz" catheterization. *Am. Heart J.*, Aug., 1976, 92(2): 263-4.
35. Gupta PK. The clinical significance of right bundle-branch block. *Pract. Cardiol.*, Sept., 1984, 10(10): 119-27.

36. Rabkin SW, Mathewson FAL, Tate RB. The natural history of right bundle branch block and frontal plane QRS axis in apparently healthy men. *Chest,* Aug., 1981, 80(2): 191-6.
37. Rosenbaum MB. Types of right bundle branch block and their clinical significance. *J. Electrocardiol.,* Feb., 1968, 1(2): 221-32.
38. Massing GK, James TN. Anatomical configuration of the His bundle and bundle branches in the human heart. *Circ.,* Apr., 1976, 53(4): 609-21.
39. Chung EK. ECG interpretations: intraventricular blocks. *Physician Assist.,* May, 1984, 8(5): 95, 98-9, 102-3.
40. Schneider JF, Thomas HE, Sorlie P, Kreger BE, McNamara PM, Kannel WB. Comparative features of newly acquired left and right bundle branch block in the general population: the Framingham study. *Am. J. Cardiol.,* Apr., 1981, 47(4): 931-40.
41. Rabkin SW, Mathewson FAL, Tate RB. Natural history of left bundle-branch block. *Br. Heart J.,* Feb., 1980, 43(3): 164-9.
42. Blackburn T, Dunn M. Evaluating left bundle branch block. *Cardio,* May, 1990, pp 82, 87, 93-4.
43. Rosenbaum MB. Types of left bundle branch block and their clinical significance. *J. Electrocardiol.,* Feb., 1969, 2(2): 197-206.
44. Rosenbaum MB. The hemiblocks: diagnostic criteria and clinical significance. *Mod. Concepts Cardiovasc. Dis.,* Dec., 1970, 39(12): 141-6.
45. Corne RA, Beamish RE, Rollwagen RL. Significance of left anterior hemiblock. *Br. Heart J.,* May, 1978, 40(5): 552-7.
46. Jacobson LB, LaFollette L, Cohn K. An appraisal of initial QRS forces in left anterior fascicular block. *Am. Heart J.,* Oct., 1977, 94(4): 407-13.
47. Duke DM. Intraventricular conduction blocks, Part II. *Crit. Care Nurse,* Jul./Aug., 1982, 2(4): 58-70.
48. Langendorf R. Aberrant ventricular conduction. *Am. Heart J.,* May, 1951, 41(5): 700-7.
49. Sandler IA, Marriott HJL. The differential morphology of anomalous ventricular complexes of RBBB-type in lead V_1. *Circ.,* Apr., 1965, 31(4): 551-6.
50. Bailey JC. The electrocardiographic differential diagnosis of supraventricular tachycardia with aberrancy versus ventricular tachycardia. *Pract. Cardiol.,* May 15, 1980, 6(6): 118-9, 123-6, 129.
51. Cohen SI, Lau SH, Stein E, Young MW, Damato AN. Variations of aberrant ventricular conduction in man: evidence of isolated and combined block within the specialized conduction system. *Circ.,* Nov., 1968, 38(5): 899-916.
52. Sweetwood HM, Boak JG. Aberrant conduction. *Heart & Lung,* Jul./Aug., 1977, 6(4): 673-8.
53. Schwartz AB, Scheinman MM. Ventricular rhythms, aberration, conduction blocks. *Consultant,* May, 1984, 24(5): 238-51.
54. Marriott HJL. Differential diagnosis of supraventricular and ventricular tachycardia. *Geriatrics,* Nov., 1970, 25(11); 91-101.
55. Wellens HJJ, Bär FWHM, Lie KI. The value of the electrocardiogram in the differential diagnosis of a tachycardia with a widened QRS complex. *Am. J. Med.,* Jan., 1978, 64(1): 27-33.
56. Marriott HJL, Sandler IA. Criteria, old and new, for differentiating between ectopic ventricular beats and aberrant ventricular conduction in the presence of atrial fibrillation. *Prog. Cardiovasc. Dis.,* Jul., 1966, 9(1): 18-28.
57. Gulamhusein S, Yee R, Ko PT, Klein GJ. Electrocardiographic criteria for differentiating aberrancy and ventricular extrasystole in chronic atrial fibrillation: Validation by intracardiac recordings. *J. Electrocardiol.,* Jan., 1985, 18(1): 41-50.
58. Gouaux JL, Ashman R. Auricular fibrillation with aberration simulating ventricular paroxysmal tachycardia. *Am. Heart J.,* Sept., 1947, 34(3): 366-73.
59. Schamroth L, Jacobs ML. A study in intracardiac conduction with special reference to the Ashman phenomenon. *Heart & Lung,* Jul./Aug., 1982, 11(4): 381-2.
60. Massumi RA. Bradycardia-dependent bundle branch block: a critique and proposed criteria. *Circ.,* Dec., 1968, 38(12): 1066-73.
61. Giambetta M, Childers RW. Reverse rate related bundle branch block. *J. Electrocardiol.,* Feb., 1973, 6(2): 153-7.
62. Phibbs B. Ventricular ectopy vs. aberrant conduction: the problem, the theory, and some practice. *Ariz. Med.,* Aug., 1981, 38(8): 590-6.
63. Wellens HJJ, Bär FWHM, Vanagt EJDM, Brugada P. Medical treatment of ventricular tachycardia: considerations in the selection of patients for surgical treatment. *Am. J. Cardiol.,* Jan., 1982, 49(1): 186-93.
64. Gozensky C, Thorne D. Rabbit ears: an aid in distinguishing ventricular ectopy from aberration. *Heart & Lung,* Jul./Aug., 1974, 3(4): 634-6.
65. Martell RW, Schamroth L. A study of aberrant ventricular conduction vs. ventricular ectopy. *Heart & Lung,* Sept./Oct., 1981, 10(5): 886-8.
66. Wellens HJJ. The wide QRS tachycardia (editorial). *Ann. Intern Med.,* Jun. 1986, 104:(6) 879.
67. Kindwall KE, Brown J, Josephson ME. Electrocardiographic criteria for ventricular tachycardia in wide complex left bundle branch block morphology tachycardias. *Am. J. Cardiol.,* Jun., 1988, 61: 1279-83.

SELF-ASSESSMENT

MULTIPLE CHOICE
Directions

For each of the questions below, select the correct answer(s) from the choices given. More than one choice may be marked.

Example

Types of AV blocks include:
*a. first degree.
*b. second degree.
*c. third degree.
d. fourth degree.

1. The AV blocks are classified by degrees. Which statement best describes the divisions?
   a. The degrees represent AV conduction. In first degree AV block all P waves are followed by QRS complexes, in second degree AV block some P waves do not conduct QRS complexes, and in third degree AV block there is no AV conduction.
   b. The degrees represent the prognosis. First degree AV block is associated with a good prognosis, whereas second and third degree AV blocks are associated with poorer prognoses.
   c. The degrees categorize the etiology of the block. First degree AV block may occur in normal, healthy individuals, second degree AV block occurs with MI, and third degree AV block is a congenital form of block.
   d. The degrees represent the depth of involvement. First degree AV block is a superficial, temporary block, second degree AV block is a deeper, possibly permanent block, and third degree AV block is a permanent block.

2. First degree AV block is characterized by a PR interval
   a. prolonged with most P waves conducting QRS complexes.
   b. in excess of 0.16 seconds with all P waves conducting QRS complexes.
   c. greater than 0.20 seconds with an occasional dropped QRS complex.
   d. greater than 0.20 seconds with all P waves conducting QRS complexes.

3. Second degree AV block is characterized by
   a. a PR interval greater than 0.20 seconds with all P waves conducting QRS complexes.
   b. some P waves not conducting QRS complexes. This does not include nonconducted APBs.
   c. premature P waves not followed by QRS complexes.
   d. P waves bearing no relation to the QRS complexes.

4. Third degree AV block is characterized by a ventricular rate that is
   a. faster than the atrial rate with AV dissociation.
   b. faster than the atrial rate but both of which are less than 60 bpm.
   c. slower than the atrial rate with AV dissociation.
   d. slower than the atrial rate exhibiting PR intervals that lengthen until a QRS is dropped.

5. Type I second degree AV block differs from Type II in that Type I is
   a. characterized by progressive prolongation of the PR interval until a QRS complex is dropped.
   b. characterized by a consistent prolongation of the PR interval preceding dropped QRS complexes.
   c. usually accompanied by a bundle branch block.
   d. usually not accompanied by a bundle branch block.

6. AV blocks that may occur in healthy individuals include the following:
   a. first degree.
   b. Type I second degree.
   c. Type II second degree.
   d. third degree.

7. The AV blocks which occur in healthy individuals may be due to the following:
   a. decreased vagal tone.
   b. increased vagal tone.
   c. sympathomimetic drugs.
   d. increased sympathetic tone.

8. When 2:1 AV conduction is present, which two ECG signs lend support to the diagnosis of Type II second degree AV block as opposed to Type I?
   a. The presence of a bundle branch block.
   b. A normal QRS complex.
   c. A normal PR interval with conducted beats.
   d. A prolonged PR interval with the conducted beats.

9. Type I second degree AV block is more common with which site of MI?
   a. Anterior.
   b. Anteroseptal.
   c. Lateral.
   d. Inferior.

10. Type II second degree AV block is more commonly associated with which site of MI?
    a. Anterior.
    b. Inferior.
    c. Posterior.
    d. Inferoposterior.

11. Type I second degree AV block is most commonly associated with pathology in which coronary artery?
    a. Left anterior descending.
    b. Left circumflex.
    c. Left main coronary artery.
    d. Right coronary artery.

12. AV dissociation accompanies which of the following arrhythmias?
    a. It is a characteristic of second degree AV block.
    b. It is a characteristic of third degree AV block.
    c. It usually accompanies accelerated idioventricular rhythm.
    d. It is often present with ventricular tachycardia.

13. Intraventricular blocks are classified according to the following:
    a. degrees of involvement.
    b. which fascicle is blocked.
    c. the degree of AV conduction.
    d. the number of impulses reaching the ventricles.

14. The best lead(s) for detecting a bundle branch block is (are)
    a. V_1.
    b. V_3.
    c. I.
    d. II.
    e. aVF.

15. The best lead(s) for detecting a hemiblock is (are)
    a. V_1.
    b. V_6.
    c. I.
    d. II.
    e. aVF.

16. An ECG characteristic of left anterior hemiblock is
    a. left axis deviation.
    b. right axis deviation.
    c. an rSR′ complex in V_1.
    d. a wide QS complex in V_1.

17. An ECG characteristic of left posterior hemiblock is
    a. left axis deviation.
    b. right axis deviation.
    c. an rSR′ complex in V_1.
    d. a wide QS complex in V_1.

18. An ECG characteristic of right bundle branch block is
    a. left axis deviation.
    b. right axis deviation.
    c. an rSR′ complex in V_1.
    d. a wide QS complex in V_1.

19. An ECG characteristic of left bundle branch block is
    a. left axis deviation.
    b. right axis deviation.
    c. an rSR′ complex in V_1.
    d. a QS complex in V_1.

20. A patient with a right bundle branch block and a left anterior hemiblock would be expected to show a predominantly
    a. negative complex on lead II and an rSR′ complex on V_1.
    b. negative complex on lead I with an rSR′ complex on V_1.
    c. positive complex on aVF and a qRs complex on V_6.
    d. positive complex on lead II with a qRs complex on V_6.

21. The most common form of ventricular aberration is
    a. left anterior hemiblock.
    b. left posterior hemiblock.
    c. right bundle branch block.
    d. left bundle branch block.

22. Ventricular ectopy differs from ventricular aberration in that ectopy
    a. is an innocuous arrhythmia.
    b. may be life threatening.
    c. is less common than aberration.
    d. does not require treatment.

MATCHING

Directions

Match each arrhythmia in column A with its correct classification in column B.

Examples

A	B
(B) 1. First degree AV block	A. Intraventricular block
(A) 2. RBBB	B. AV block

A	B
( ) 23. RBBB	A. Monofascicular block
( ) 24. LBBB	B. Bifascicular block
( ) 25. RBBB and LAH	C. Trifascicular block
( ) 26. RBBB and LPH	
( ) 27. LAH	
( ) 28. LPH	
( ) 29. LBBB and RBBB	

A	B
( ) 30. rS on lead II	A. RBBB
( ) 31. Right axis deviation	B. LAH
( ) 32. QRS 0.12 seconds or more	C. LPH
( ) 33. Left axis deviation	D. LBBB
( ) 34. qRs complex in V_6	
( ) 35. QS complex in V_1	
( ) 36. rSR′ complex in V_1	

TRUE/FALSE

Directions

Determine whether each of the following statements is true or false and indicate with a *T* or *F*.

( ) 37. *AV dissociation* and *third degree AV block* are synonymous terms.

( ) 38. Mobitz Type II AV block is also known as *Wenckebach block.*

( ) 39. The etiology most often associated with a left bundle branch block is organic heart disease.

( ) 40. A wide QRS complex with an rSR′ complex in MCL_1 is usually ventricular aberration.

( ) 41. Type I second degree AV block usually requires permanent pacing.

( ) 42. Type I second degree AV block often accompanies inferior wall MI.

( ) 43. The treatment for AV dissociation is permanent pacing.

( ) 44. It is not unusual for third degree AV block to occur in healthy boys during sleep.

( ) 45. The most common form of ventricular aberration is RBBB.

( ) 46. Type I second degree AV block differs from Type II in that Type I is usually transient and requires no treatment.

( ) 47. Ashman's phenomenon is a kind of aberration that occurs during irregular rhythms such as AF.

( ) 48. Axis deviations are best detected on the V leads.

SHORT ANSWER

The following questions require analysis of patient situations and assessment of ECG rhythm strips. Responses required are short answer.

CASE: *Mr. H., a 67-year-old patient in the coronary care unit (CCU), was admitted for evaluation of chest pain. He had a MI 1 year ago. His admitting rhythm strip is shown here:*

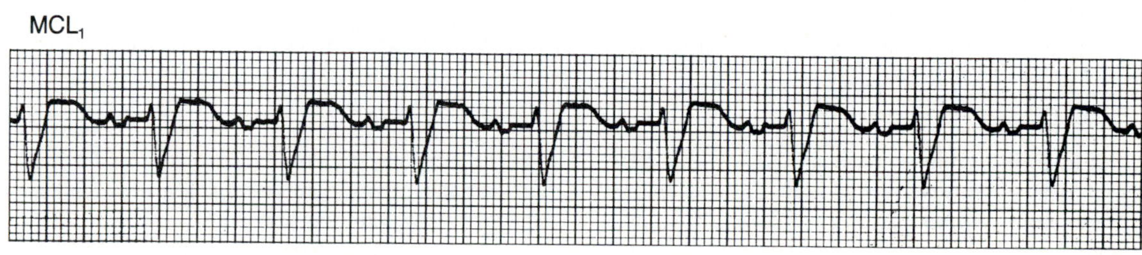

49. Analyze the rhythm.
50. Is the rhythm clinically significant? Why or why not?
51. Mr. H. has a medical diagnosis of acute IWMI. Describe types of AV blocks you would anticipate with an IWMI.

__CASE:__ Ms. A. is an 87-year-old admitted for "palpitations". Her vital signs on admission are temperature (T) 37 degrees C, apical pulse (AP) 155 bpm, respirations (R) 22 per minute, blood pressure (BP) 160/76. Her admitting rhythm strip is shown here:

52. Analyze the rhythm.
53. Describe the ECG features of the series of QRS complexes that are upright. Discuss their morphology and the reason for their appearance.

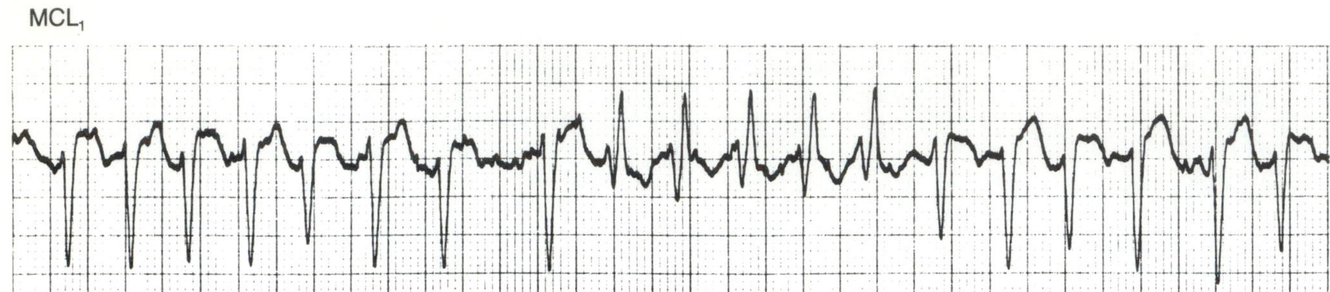

54. Interpret the following rhythm:

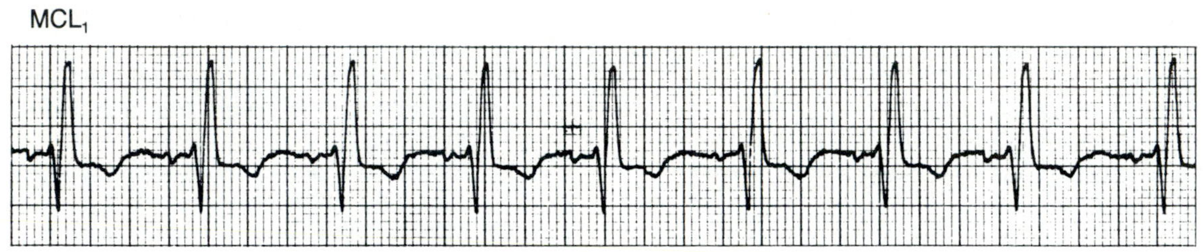

__CASE:__ J.T., 82 years old and active, is admitted to the hospital for evaluation of recent onset fatigue, dependent pitting edema, and shortness of breath with exertion. Her admission vital signs are: B/P 142/90; AP 44 bpm; R 24. She is alert and oriented. Her skin is warm and dry, but her color is slightly pale. The ankles are edematous: 2+ pitting. She admits to mild dyspnea with exertion. Auscultation of her lungs posteriorly reveals fine inspiratory crepitant rales in the bases bilaterally. Her ECG is presented below:

55. Analyze the rhythm.
56. Formulate a nursing diagnosis.
57. Describe nursing interventions.

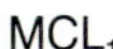

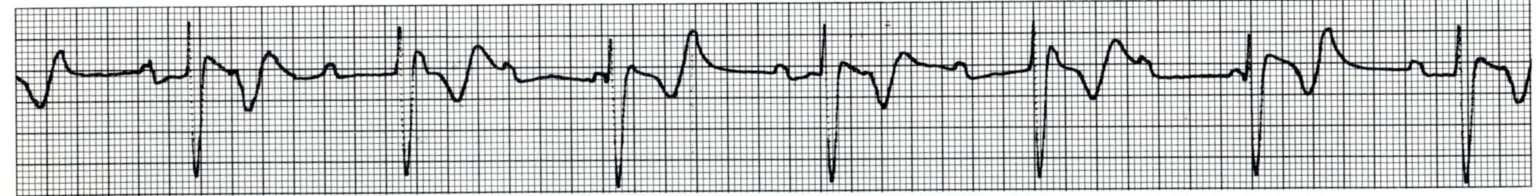

__CASE:__ J.J., a 42-year-old male, was admitted to the CCU with a diagnosis of acute IWMI. On his second day, he developed the arrhythmia in the strip shown here:

58. Analyze the rhythm.
59. What nursing interventions are indicated for treatment of this rhythm disturbance?

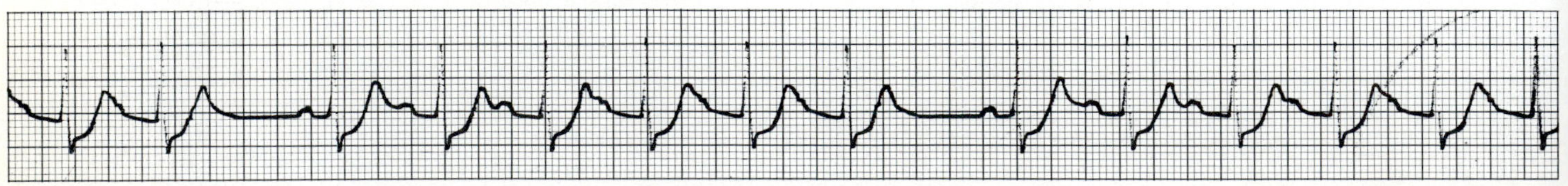

60. Below are the precordial leads of a patient with a wide QRS complex. Determine the bundle branch block. Explain the morphologic characteristics useful in making this differentiation.

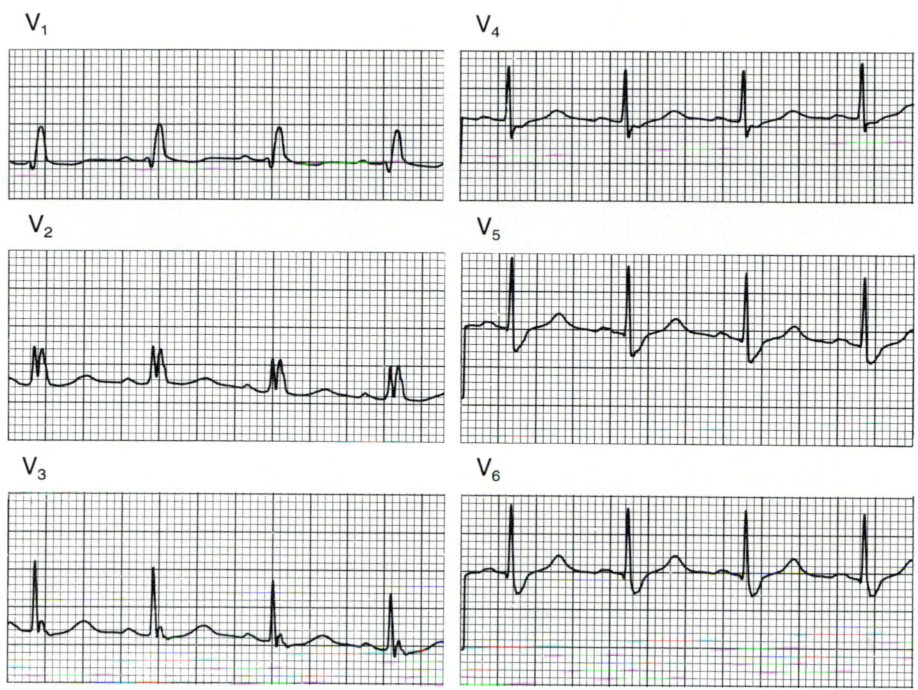

61. Below is a 12-lead ECG. Analyze it and state some considerations that may be made. The patient reports a previous "heart attack."

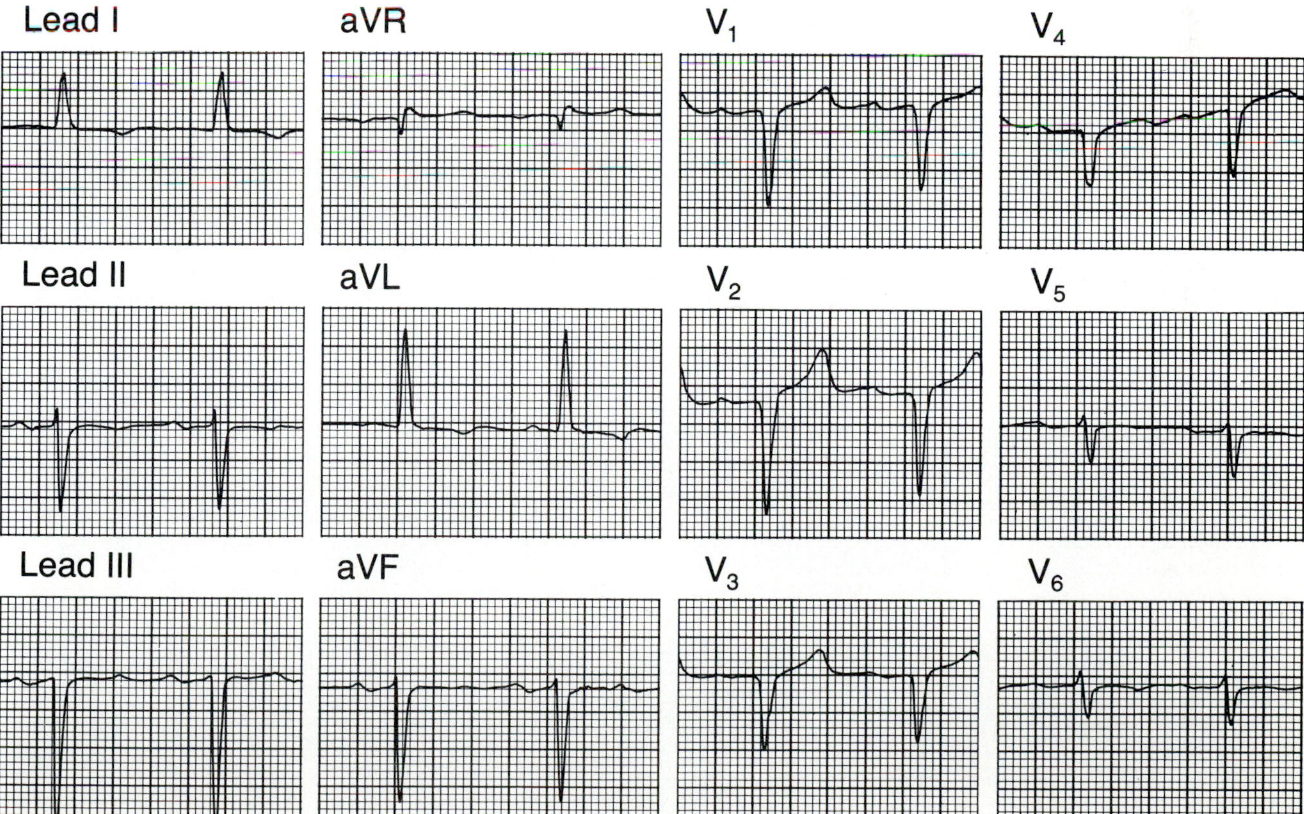

62. Analyze the following rhythm strip.

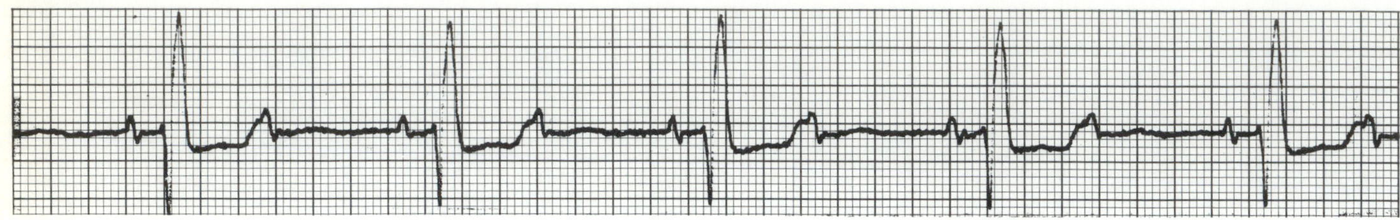

63. The patient with the rhythm strip below was considered for pacemaker therapy. Analyze the rhythm and discuss indications for pacing therapy with this rhythm disturbance.

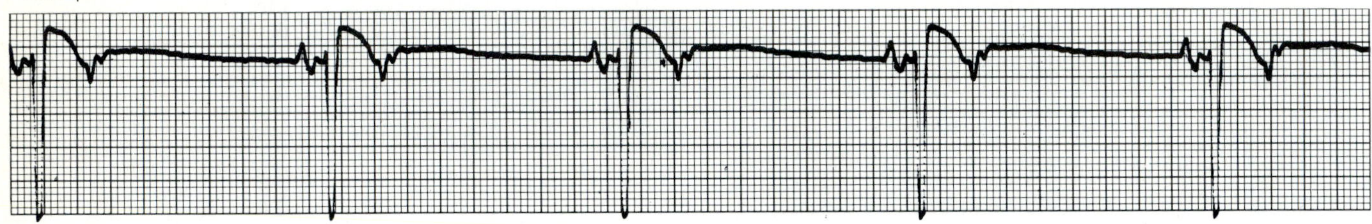

64. Analyze the following 12-lead ECG and determine what kind of intraventricular conduction disturbance is present.

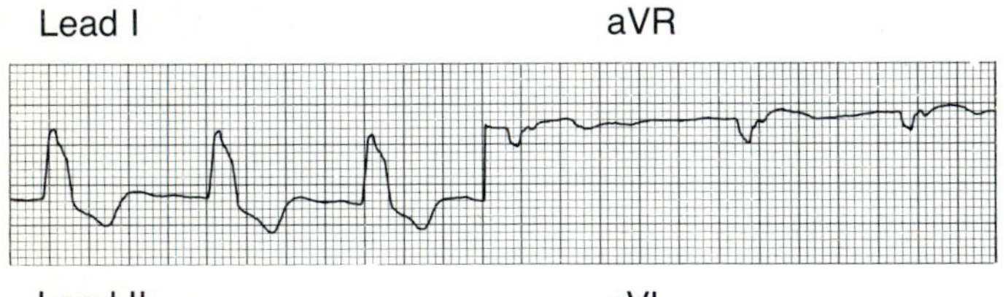

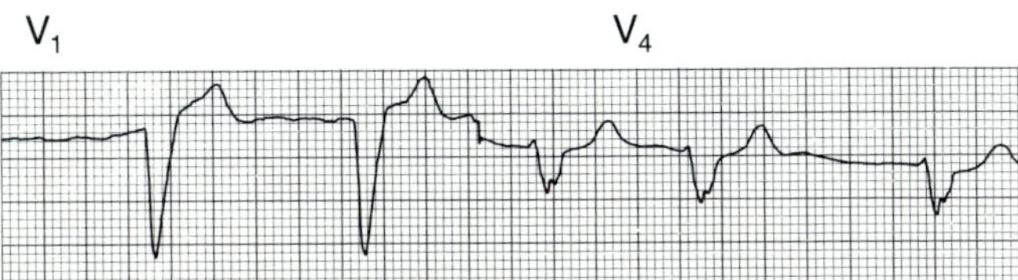

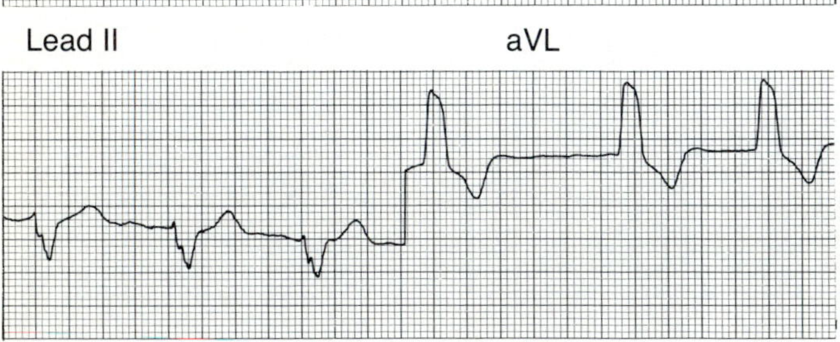

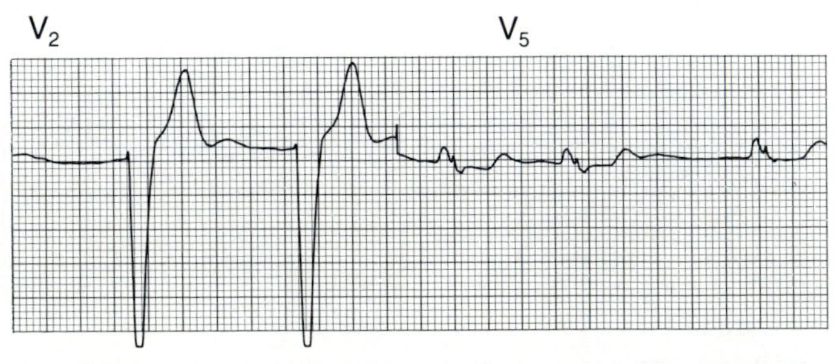

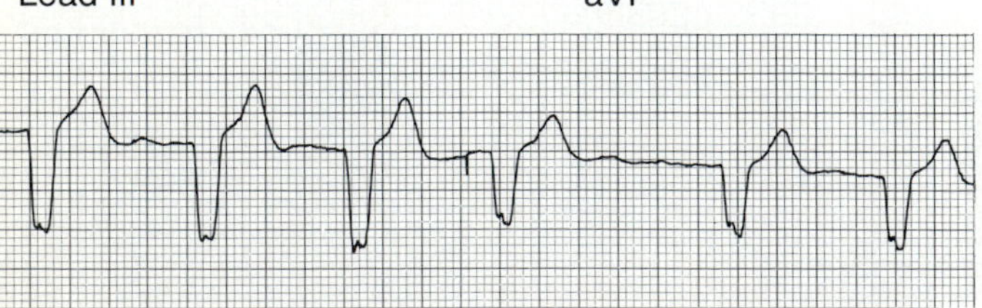

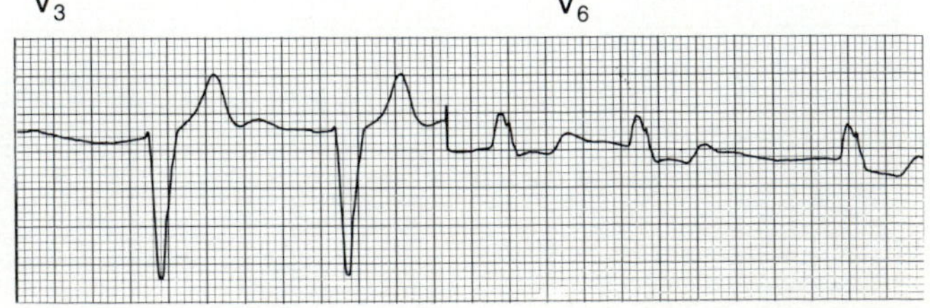

65. Analyze the rhythm strip presented here.

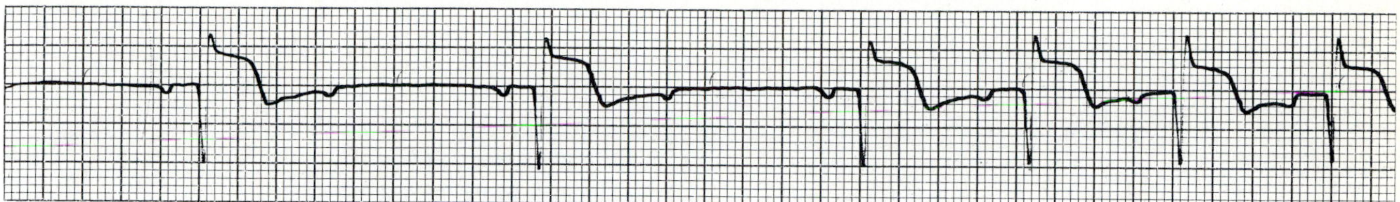

66. Analyze the rhythm strip presented here.

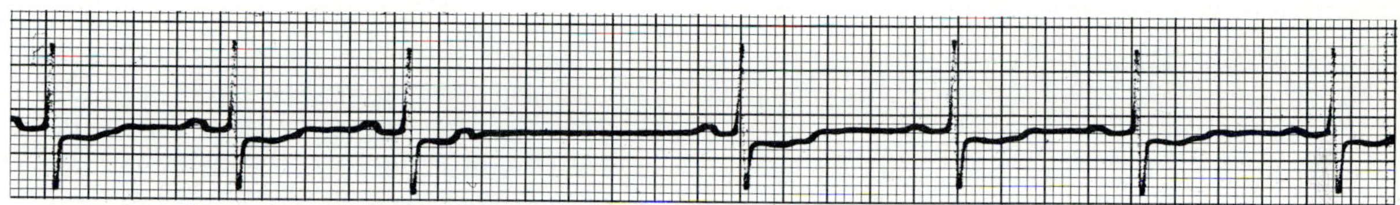

67. The patient with the rhythm strip displayed below has a history of AF for which digoxin 0.25 mg/day is prescribed. Interpret the rhythm, consider a nursing diagnosis, and delineate possible appropriate nursing interventions.

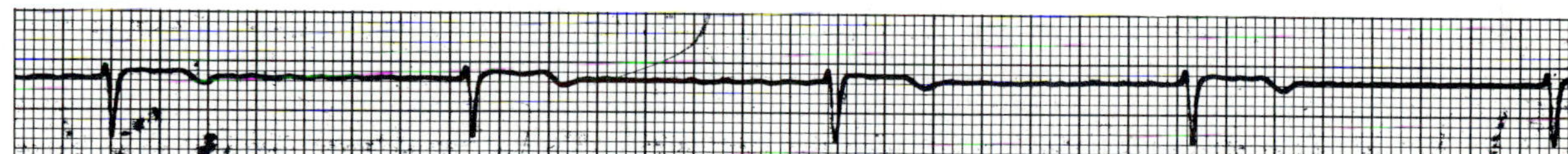

ANSWERS TO SELF-ASSESSMENT

1. a
2. d
3. b
4. c
5. a, d
6. a, b
7. b
8. a, c
9. d
10. a
11. d
12. b, c, d
13. b
14. a
15. c, d, e
16. a
17. b
18. c
19. d
20. a
21. c
22. b

23. A
24. B
25. B
26. B
27. A
28. A
29. C
30. B
31. C
32. A, D
33. B
34. A
35. D
36. A

37. F
38. F
39. T
40. T
41. F
42. T
43. F
44. F
45. T
46. T
47. T
48. F

49. *Rate:* 88 bpm
 Rhythm: Regular
 P wave: 0.12 seconds, prolonged
 PR interval: 0.23 seconds
 QRS complex: 0.16 seconds. The complex is an rS configuration on lead MCL_1. Since the QRS is wide, we can diagnose a BBB. There is no terminal, wide R wave; instead the terminal portion of the QRS is negative so we diagnose LBBB even though more commonly LBBB exhibits a QS configuration.
 Interpretation: Sinus rhythm with first degree AV block, LBBB, and intraatrial block.
50. First degree block is generally discovered by ECG only. If the PR interval had been extremely prolonged, the atrial kick may have been lost, resulting in decreased ventricular ejection.
 Since there is an LBBB present, the only fascicle remaining is the right bundle branch. First degree AV block in the presence of LBBB may be significant in situations where the integrity of the right bundle branch is threatened, such as in anterior infarction or ischemia, since the left anterior descending coronary artery also supplies the right bundle branch.
51. An acute IWMI may cause first degree AV block. Examining previous ECGs may help determine if the block is an acute finding. Mobitz I and third degree AV blocks may also occur in the presence of acute IWMI.
52. *Rate:* 170 bpm
 Rhythm: Irregular
 P wave: None distinguishable
 PR interval: Unable to determine
 QRS complex: 0.10 seconds; 0.12 seconds in the 9th to 13th complexes. These wider, upright complexes exhibit an rSR′ configuration in MCL_1 and therefore resemble RBBB. These beats also occur as the previous long cycle is followed by a relatively short cycle.
 Interpretation: Uncontrolled AF with a rapid ventricular response and a five-beat run of RBBB aberration exhibiting Ashman's phenomenon
53. Ashman's phenomenon is ventricular aberration in the presence of AF and is characterized by ventricular aberration when a long cycle is followed by a relatively short cycle. The aberration is terminated once the R-R interval becomes long enough to permit recovery of both bundle branches. RBBB aberration is the type of aberration displayed in this strip. The rSR′ configuration in MCL_1 or V_1 is characteristic of RBBB aberration.
54. *Rate:* 86 bpm
 Rhythm: Regular
 P wave: Normal
 PR interval: 0.14 seconds
 QRS complex: 0.14 seconds. On lead MCL_1, the QRS morphology is rSR′.
 Interpretation: Sinus rhythm with RBBB
55. *Rate: Atrial:* 98 bpm
 Ventricular: 43 bpm
 Rhythm: Atrial: Regular
 Ventricular: Regular
 P wave: Normal in configuration. More P waves than QRS complexes; Ps do not bear constant relation to QRSs.
 PR interval: Not applicable in presence of AV dissociation
 QRS complex: 0.12 seconds rS configuration, possible idiojunctional rhythm (IJR) with LBBB
 Interpretation: Third degree AV block, IJR with LBBB at rate 43 bpm; atrial rate 98.
56. Decreased cardiac output related to bradycardia and loss of atrial kick.
57. Administer oxygen.
 Start an IV infusion.
 Have external pacemaker at bedside ready for use.
 Have atropine ready.
 Prepare for possible pacemaker insertion.
 Bed rest with head of bed elevated.
 Intake and output with daily weights.
 Administer diuretics as ordered by physician.
 Because the patient is alert with adequate blood pressure, atropine is not indicated at this time in this situation.

58. *Rate: Atrial:* 97 bpm
Ventricular: 80 to 90 bpm
Rhythm: Atrial: Regular
Ventricular: Irregular, grouped beating. R-R interval shortens slightly before a pause. Longest R-R interval is less than twice the shortest.
P wave: Normal; more Ps than QRSs
PR interval: 0.19 to 0.30 seconds gradually increases until a P is not followed by a QRS.
QRS complex: 0.07 to 0.08 seconds, depressed J point and ST segment
Interpretation: 7:6 Type I second degree AV block
59. No treatment is indicated at this time. Continue to monitor.
60. V_1 shows an rsR′ configuration with a wide terminal R′ wave. V_6 shows a qRs with a wide terminal s wave. The bundle branch block is right.
61. *Rate:* 70 to 84 bpm
Rhythm: Unable to determine
P wave: 0.10 to 0.12 seconds, too wide. P precedes each QRS and bears a constant relation to it.
PR interval: 0.24 seconds, prolonged
QRS complex: 0.10 seconds. Left axis deviation with rS pattern in II, III, aVF. No r wave in V_1 and absence of R wave progression in V_2 to V_4 with low amplitude R wave in V_5, V_6.
Interpretation: Sinus rhythm with first degree AV block, possible intraatrial conduction disturbance. Consider left anterior hemiblock; consider anteroseptal MI.
62. *Rate: Atrial:* 82 bpm
Ventricular: 41 bpm
Rhythm: Atrial: Regular
Ventricular: Regular
P wave: Normal for MCL_1; 2 Ps for each QRS. P waves preceding QRS complexes bear constant relations to the QRSs.
PR interval: 0.18 seconds for those Ps preceding QRSs
QRS complex: 0.16 seconds, rSR′ on MCL_1 indicative of RBBB
Interpretation: Type II second degree AV block with 2:1 conduction, RBBB
63. *Rate: Atrial:* 66 bpm
Ventricular: 33 bpm
Rhythm: Atrial: Irregular
Ventricular: Regular
P wave: 0.11 seconds, too wide. More Ps than QRSs. Ps preceding QRSs bear constant relation to them. Every other P wave is early and not followed by a QRS.
PR interval: 0.17 to 0.18 seconds when present
QRS complex: 0.08 seconds, rS configuration, elevated ST segment
Interpretation: Bigeminal nonconducted APBs.
Pacemaker therapy is not indicated for nonconducted APBs. Treatment would be directed toward controlling the APBs.
64. *Rate: Atrial:* Not able to determine
Ventricular: Approximately 70 bpm
Rhythm: Irregular
P wave: Nonidentifiable
PR interval: —
QRS complex: 0.16 seconds with QS in V_1 and notched wide R in V_6 consistent with LBBB; left axis deviation
Interpretation: AF with LBBB
65. *Rate: Atrial:* 74 bpm
Ventricular: Approximately 50 bpm
Rhythm: Atrial: Regular
Ventricular: Irregular
P wave: Normal. More Ps than QRSs. Ps preceding QRSs bear constant relation to them.
PR interval: 0.21 seconds
QRS complex: 0.08 to 0.09 seconds, elevated J point and ST segment
Interpretation: Second degree AV block with 2:1 conduction, probable Type I resulting from absence of BBB
66. *Rate: Atrial:* 60 to 75 bpm
Ventricular: Approximately 60 bpm
Rhythm: Atrial: Irregular
Ventricular: Irregular
P wave: Normal, one precedes each QRS, one APB not followed by QRS
QRS complex: 0.07 seconds
Interpretation: Sinus rhythm with 1 nonconducted APB
67. *Rate: Atrial:* Not discernible
Ventricular: 41 bpm
Rhythm: Ventricular: Regular
P wave: Unidentifiable
QRS complex: 0.08 seconds normal rS morphology for MCL_1
Interpretation: AF with complete AV block and resultant AV dissociation with IJR
After checking the patient's tolerance of the arrhythmia by assessing sensorium, blood pressure, skin color, and so forth, a possible nursing diagnosis to consider would be alteration in cardiac output: decreased related to bradycardia and loss of the atrial contribution to cardiac output.
Nursing interventions would include the following:
- Notify the patient's physician.
- Hold further doses of digoxin as directed by physician.

CHAPTER TEN

Differential Diagnosis of Wide QRS Complexes

▶ GOAL

You will be able to distinguish between ventricular and supraventricular impulses conducted with wide QRS complexes.

▶ OBJECTIVES

After studying this chapter and completing the self-assessment exercises, you should be able to:

1. Differentiate most supraventricular complexes conducted with aberration from ventricular ectopy during atrial fibrillation (AF).
2. List situations in which wide QRS complexes pose dilemmas in differential diagnosis.
3. Recognize Wolff-Parkinson-White (WPW) syndrome with wide QRS complexes in the presence of AF.
4. Identify electrocardiographic (ECG) morphologic clues useful in the differential diagnosis of wide QRS–complex tachycardias.
5. Anticipate which patients are more likely to display ventricular tachycardia (VT).
6. Determine ECG criteria to apply when 12-lead ECG versus bedside or telemetry ECG is available to diagnose wide QRS–complex tachycardia.
7. Describe the value of clinical signs and symptoms in differential diagnosis of wide QRS–complex tachycardias.
8. Describe the consequences of of misdiagnosis and mistreatment of wide-complex tachycardias.
9. List ECG leads most useful in differential diagnosis of wide-complex tachycardias.

To this point, you have learned to identify wide QRS–complex beats (duration of 0.12 seconds or longer) as either ventricular or supraventricular conducted with aberration (temporary bundle branch block). Chapters 6 and 9, discuss under which circumstances supraventricular impulses could be conducted with right bundle branch block (RBBB) and less commonly, left bundle branch block (LBBB) aberration. The wide QRS complexes associated with ventricular ectopy are described in Chapter 8, and it is apparent that differentiating ventricular from supraventricular beats conducted with aberration sometimes poses a dilemma.

Identification of wide QRS complexes is aided by helpful ECG signs such as preceding premature atrial activity, AV dissociation, fixed coupling intervals, typical right and left BBB patterns, and compensatory pauses. However, when the underlying rhythm does not provide helpful signs or when all of the complexes are wide and/or distorted by tachycardia, differentiation can be difficult and sometimes impossible, requiring an electrophysiology (EP) study. EP studies are not always feasible, however, and emergency treatment must be based on an ECG diagnosis. Because any tachycardia is potentially hemodynamically compromising, diagnosis and treatment must be prompt and appropriate. Unfortunately, the pharmacologic treatment for ventricular and supraventricular tachycardias differ, thus a diagnostic mistake not only delays proper treatment but may be fatal if the wrong medication is administered.

HISTORICAL PERSPECTIVE

The primary purpose of the first coronary care units in the 1960s was to provide immediate treatment for lethal ventricular arrhythmias after acute myocardial infarction (AMI). Through the efforts of such pioneers as Henry J.L. Marriott and others, nurses were taught to recognize and treat ventricular tachycardia (VT) and fibrillation (VF) in the CCU setting, resulting in a significant decrease in AMI mortality. With the emphasis on ventricular arrhythmias, it is not surprising that when a wide QRS–complex tachycardia appeared, it was diagnosed as VT without hesitation. The 1960s and early 1970s could be called the *VT decade*.

Shortly after the turn of the century, Sir Thomas Lewis described atrial premature beats (APBs) conducted with aberration. The topic was then quiescent for 60 years. In the mid-1960s, Marriott and Sandler[1,2] described supraventricular impulses conducted with aberration and offered morphologic characteristics for differentiating wide QRS complexes. They sparked clinical concern, research, and debate that continues to this day. To aid in differential diagnosis, Marriott developed and advocated the use of bipolar modified chest leads to enable the bedside ECG to simulate precordial chest leads V_1 and V_6.

Word spread and clinicians learned that wide QRS–complex tachycardias could be supraventricular tachycardia (SVT) with aberration. The pendulum swung too far the other way, however, and by the mid-1970s to mid-1980s, VT was frequently misdiagnosed as SVT with aberration. We had clearly entered what could be called the *SVT-with-aberration decade*.

The pendulum is swinging back again. The mid-1980s to mid-1990s may become known as the *most-is-VT decade*. EP studies have confirmed many of the early differentiating morphologic characteristics and added others so that now in over 90% of cases, an accurate diagnosis can be made by the ECG alone.

BASICS OF WIDE QRS COMPLEXES

The fundamental message has not changed in nearly 30 years: An anomalous beat is either ventricular or supraventricular conducted with aberration.[3] If the beat is aberrant, it is usually either RBBB or LBBB.

Wide QRS complexes that pose the most difficult diagnostic dilemmas fall into two major categories: (1) Anomalous beats in the presence of atrial flutter (AFl) or fibrillation (AF) and (2) wide QRS–complex tachycardias. In discussing wide QRS–complex tachycardias, we are concerned with the two most common types: VT versus SVT with aberration. A third, less-common type, ventricular preexcitation (WPW syndrome) may need to be ruled out. The following discussion of wide QRS complexes addresses these issues. A complete discussion of preexcitation, however, is beyond the scope of this text.

WIDE QRS–COMPLEX BEATS DURING IRREGULAR SUPRAVENTRICULAR RHYTHMS

Data Base: Problem Identification

Definitions, Etiology, and Mechanisms

A review of AF, AFl, ventricular premature beats (VPB), and aberration in Chapters 6, 8, and 9 may be helpful before proceeding. Definitions, etiology, and mechanisms have been discussed previously and thus are not repeated here.

ECG Characteristics

Recall that in the presence of AF and AFl, differential diagnosis of anomalous beats is often difficult because helpful signs (e.g., premature P′ waves, compensatory pauses, and AV dissociation) are not present. In a study of patients in AF, Gulamhusein et al[4] demonstrated that 91% of the anomalous beats were VPBs. Only 9% were supraventricular conducted with BBB aberration and of those, over 93% were conducted with RBBB. Based on this research, chances are greatest that in the presence of AF the following are likely:

- Anomalous beats are most likely VPBs.
- If not, they are most likely RBBB aberration.

Diagnosing RBBB aberration in the presence of AF is not a major problem when the anomalous beat assumes a typical RBBB configuration in V_1 (rSR′)[5] and V_6 (qRs) and measures 0.14 seconds or less. What if the configuration in V_1 is something other than typical? When discussing wide QRS–complex beats, they are categorized as either predominantly negative or predominantly positive in V_1.

Up or down in V_1. Electrophysiologists refer to QRS complexes that are predominantly positive in V_1 as *RBBB morphology* and those that are predominantly negative as *LBBB morphology*. To avoid confusion with true right and left BBBs of supraventricular origin, we refer to this characteristic as either *up* or *down in V_1*.

As stated, most anomalous beats in the presence of AF have been shown to be ventricular.[4] Of those, 63% were predominantly negative (down) in V_1, with most exhibiting an R wave in V_6. Only 37% of the VPBs were predominantly positive (up) in V_1, most of which exhibited either a monophasic R wave or a notched R wave with the left "rabbit ear" taller than the right in V_1, along with a QS or rS complex in V_6.

The most difficult beats to differentiate are anomalous beats that are down in V_1, since LBBB and VPBs very often closely resemble one another. Based on odds alone, the beat that is down in V_1 is most likely a VPB. Going one more step further improves the odds of making a correct diagnosis.

Recall the morphologic characteristics of LBBB described in Chapter 9. Predominantly negative in V_1 and positive in V_6,[6] LBBB writes either an rS or, more commonly, a QS in V_1. When present, the r wave is narrow (< 0.04 seconds). The downstroke of the S or Q wave is slick, reaching its nadir (most negative point) in 0.06 seconds (Fig. 10-1). To summarize, LBBB in V_1 exhibits the following:

- QS (most common) or rS (with r <0.04 seconds).
- Downstroke of Q or S wave slick, reaching nadir within 0.06 seconds.

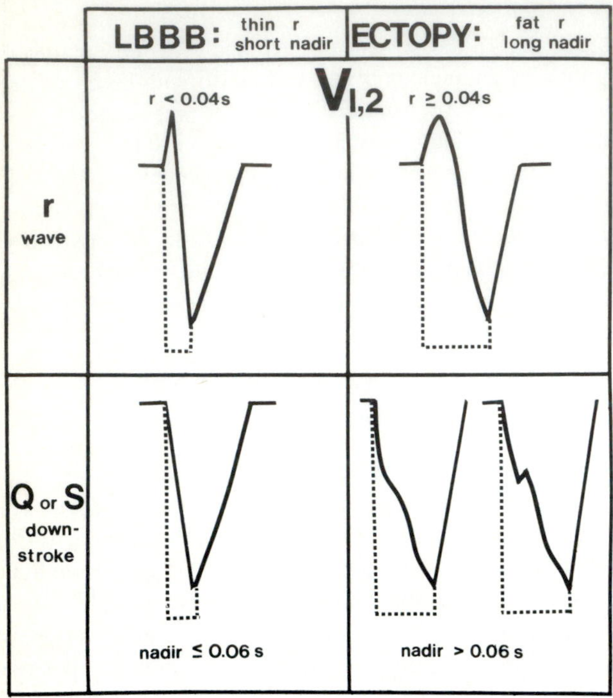

FIGURE 10-1 Comparison of LBBB and ectopy in V_1 and V_2. When present, an r wave in LBBB is often <0.04 seconds. In ventricular ectopy an r wave is often ≥0.04 seconds. The downstroke of the Q or S wave in LBBB is often slick, reaching its nadir in ≤0.06 seconds; in ectopy the downstroke may be slurred or notched with a delayed nadir >0.06 seconds. Note that the presence or absence of a delayed nadir occurs whether or not there is an r wave.

A VPB that is negative in V_1 tends not to exhibit these two features. Rather, if an r wave is present, it often measures 0.04 seconds or wider. The downstroke of the Q wave or S wave will often be slurred or notched, reaching its nadir in excess of 0.06 seconds (see Fig. 10-1). To summarize, a VPB that is negative in V_1 tends to exhibit the following characteristics:

- QS or rS (with r ≥ 0.04 seconds).
- Downstroke of Q or S slurred or notched, reaching nadir in >0.06 seconds.

Axis. The axis of the anomalous beat may also provide diagnostic help in differenting ectopy and aberration. Aberrant QRS complexes usually display a QRS axis in the normal or superior left quadrant. Only 1% of Gulamhusein et al's[4] aberrant QRS complexes were directed to the inferior right quadrant and none was directed to the superior right quadrant. VPBs, on the other hand, display axes in any of the four quadrants. If the axis of an anomalous beat is directed superiorly and to the right, it is highly likely that the beat is ventricular.[6]

Initial vector. For beats that are up in V_1, the initial vector (first 0.02 to 0.04 seconds of QRS) may provide a clue. If the initial vector is the same in both the wide beat on lead MCL_1 or V_1 and the normally conducted beats, chances are good the beat is aberrantly conducted.[6] Chances are enhanced when the initial vector is also the same in leads V_6, I, II, and III[4] (Fig. 10-2). This is also a criterion that can be used for differentiating wide-complex tachycardias that are up in V_1 (Fig. 10-3).

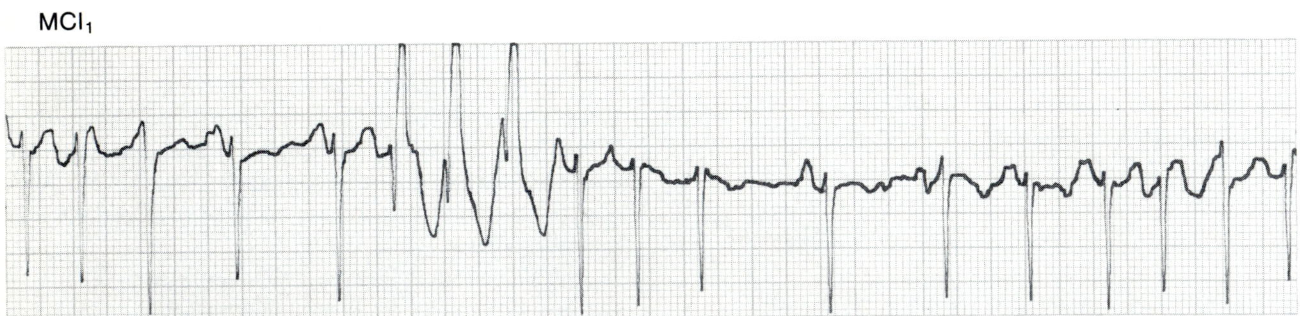

FIGURE 10-2 Paroxysms of AF interrupted by 3-beat run of wide, upright QRS complexes in MCL_1. Note identical initial deflections in wide and narrow beats. Wide beats exhibit triphasic rSR′ pattern, characteristic of RBBB aberration. Note wide complexes end a cycle shorter than the previous R-R interval of 2 narrow complexes, an example of Ashman's phenomenon. Note how rapid rate and superimposition of coarse AF waves distort QRS complexes and T waves of wide beats, and to a lesser extent, narrow beats.

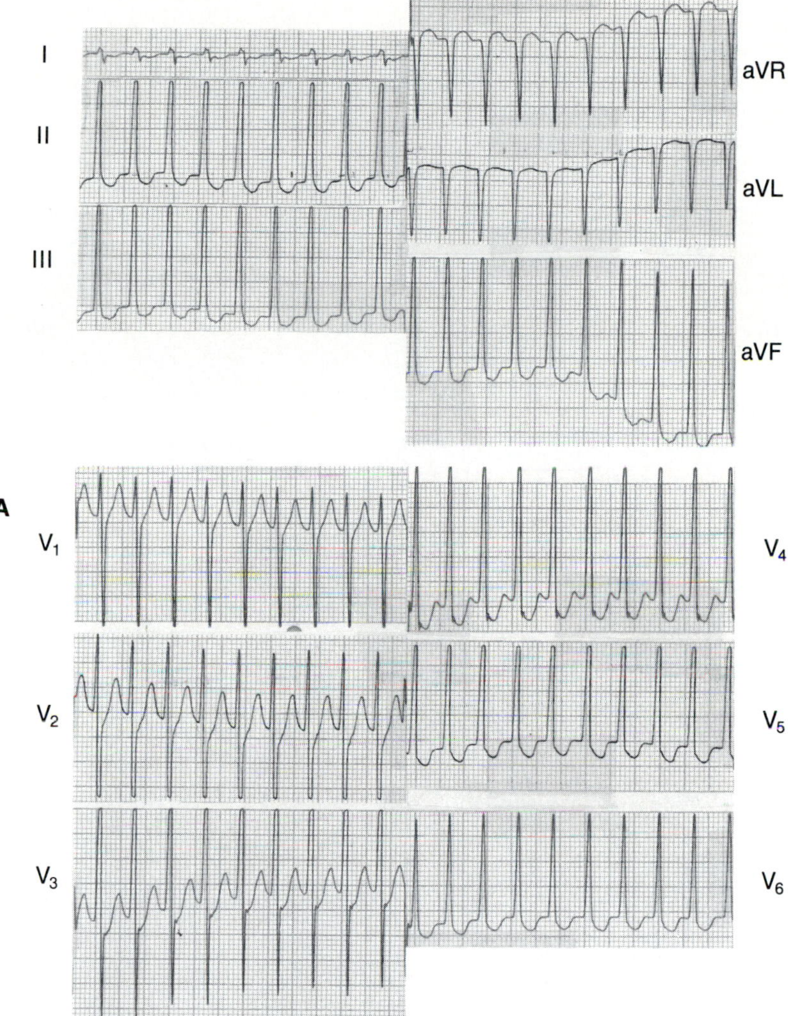

FIGURE 10-3 **A,** SVT with narrow QRS. **B,** Same patient, SVT now with RBBB aberration. One of the few features favoring RBBB aberration in this unusual ECG, that could easily be mistaken for VT, is that the initial deflection is identical in all 12 leads. Note how the rapid rate distorts ST segments and T waves in tracing B.

Continued.

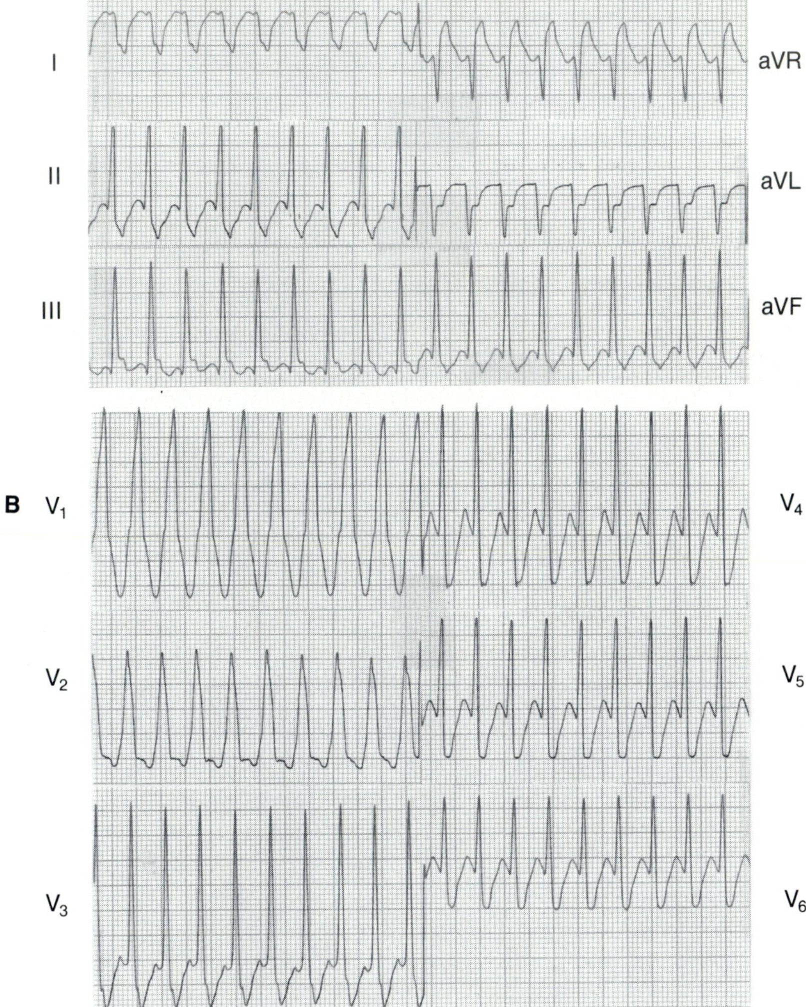

FIGURE 10-3, cont'd. A, SVT with narrow QRS. **B,** Same patient, SVT now with RBBB aberration. One of the few features favoring RBBB aberration in this unusual ECG, that could easily be mistaken for VT, is that the initial deflection is identical in all 12 leads. Note how the rapid rate distorts ST segments and T waves in tracing B.

Fixed coupling interval. Recall from Chapter 8, the coupling interval is the duration from the preceding normal complex to the VPB. In AF, if coupling intervals between the preceding and anomalous beats are within a few hundredths of a second, the diagnosis of ventricular ectopy is favored.[6]

Absence of longer preceding cycle. As you learned in Chapter 9, Ashman's phenomenon[7] is frequently exhibited in AF. Aberration is favored when a shorter cycle follows a longer cycle, but such an arrangement also favors ectopy.[6] Hence, a long-short cycle is not helpful in differentiating the two. What is helpful, though, is absence of a longer preceding cycle, which favors ectopy[6] (Fig 10-4).

For a summary of the ECG criteria supporting both ventricular ectopy and aberration in the presence of AF see the boxes below).

The reader is referred to the references[6] for additional criteria considered beyond the scope of this text.

Applied Nursing Process

See Chapter 6, pp. 150-151 for AF, Chapter 8, pp. 207–209 for VPBs, and Chapter 9, pp. 292–293 for aberration.

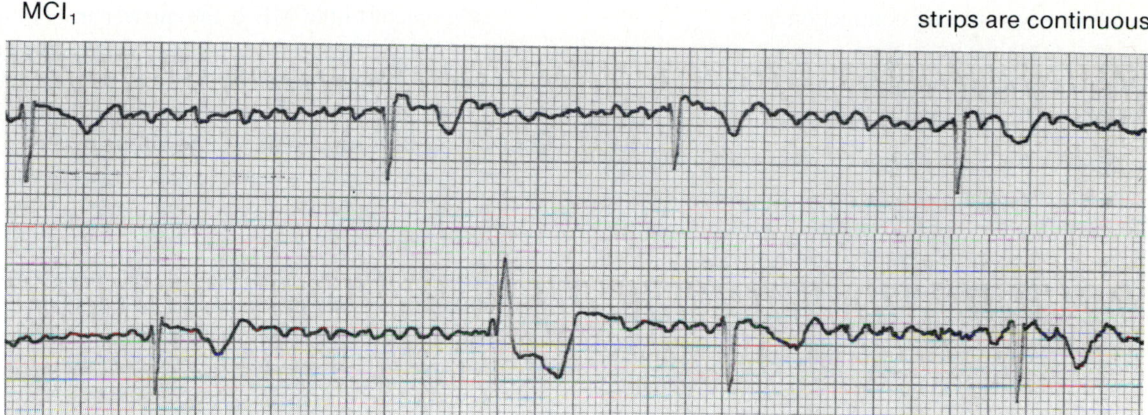

FIGURE 10-4 Atrial fibrillation with anomalous beat (bottom strip), ending a longer cycle, thereby favoring ectopy. The shape of the anomalous beat would lead one to suspect RBBB aberration, but there are no other criteria supporting aberration, such as identical initial vector. Thus the beat is more likely a VPB.

ECG Criteria Supporting Ventricular Ectopy in Presence of Atrial Fibrillation

Odds favor ectopy.
Superior or inferior right axis.
Fixed coupling interval.
Absence longer preceding cycle.
QRSs UP in V_1
- Monophasic R wave in V_1 or
- Taller left rabbit ear in V_1 with
- RS or QS in V_6.

QRSs DOWN in V_1
- Slurred or notched downstroke in V_1.
- Wide r ($\geq$0.04 seconds), if present, in V_1.
- Delayed nadir.

ECG Criteria Supporting Aberrantly Conducted Supraventricular Beats in Presence of Atrial Fibrillation

QRSs UP in V_1
- rSR′ in V_1, qRs in V_6.
- QRS $\leq$0.14 seconds (without preexisting BBB).
- Concordant initial vector in V_1 or more leads.
- Odds favor RBBB if ectopy ruled out.

QRSs DOWN in V_1
- rS or QS in V_1.
- r $\leq$0.03 seconds in V_1.
- Nadir $\leq$0.06 seconds in V_1.

WIDE QRS–COMPLEX TACHYCARDIAS

Data Base: Problem Identification

Definitions, Etiology, and Mechanisms

Uncertainty concerning the differential diagnosis of wide, monomorphic QRS–complex tachycardias has been a topic of clinical concern for many years. Piquing interest have been reports of improper, near-fatal treatment based on diagnostic errors.[8-13] Studies indicate that physicians and nurses misdiagnose VT as SVT with aberration in 39% to 100% of cases.[8-12]

Potential hemodynamic and electrophysiologic consequences of a wide QRS–complex tachycardia include the following[14]:

- Decreased diastolic filling.
- Loss of atrial kick.
- Less-efficient ventricular contraction.
- Functional mitral regurgitation.
- Electrical instability with potential for VF.
- Tachycardia-induced myocardial ischemia.

Although there are many causes of wide QRS–complex tachycardias, the two that pose the most frequent differential diagnostic dilemmas are VT and SVT with either right or left BBB aberration. A third type of wide-complex tachycardia, far less common than the other two, is AF with accessory pathway (AP) conduction to the ventricles, or WPW syndrome (a type of preexcitation). Our discussion focuses on the first two but provides clues to diagnose AF with preexcitation. (It is beyond the scope of this book to provide a complete study of preexcitation.) It would be helpful to review VT, SVT, and BBB in Chapters 6, 8, and 9. Information presented elsewhere is not repeated here.

Rules in differential diagnosis of wide-complex tachycardias (adapted from Marriott)[15]:

- **Play the odds.** VT is more common than SVT with aberration and both are more common than WPW syndrome.[16,17] Based on studies of patients presenting with wide QRS–complex tachycardias,[8,18,19] 81% to 85% can be expected to be diagnosed with VT, 14% to 15% SVT with BBB, and 5% SVT with anterograde conduction over an AP (WPW syndrome). SVT has never been found to be more common in any population of consecutive patients presenting with wide QRS tachycardias,[8,19] yet SVT is diagnosed most frequently, whereas VT is diagnosed correctly in only a minority of cases.[8-10,19]
- **Do not think VT cannot be tolerated.** Hemodynamic collapse and cardiac arrest is a well-known and dreaded complication of VT.[18] Indeed, VT probably accounts for the majority of sudden cardiac deaths. An important factor in the misdiagnosis of wide QRS–complex tachycardias is the pervasive mistaken notion that VT cannot be hemodynamically tolerated. Studies examining misdiagnosis by physicians and nurses confirm this widespread misconception.[9-11] Whether or not a patient tolerates a tachycardia depends more on the rate of the tachycardia and the clinical status of the patient[17] than on the site of the tachycardia. SVTs are certainly capable of causing unconsciousness and deteriorating into VF.[20] VT may persist for hours with a normal blood pressure and level of consciousness, even with rates exceeding 200 bpm.[18] Thus hemodynamic stability is unlikely to provide any clue to the underlying mechanism of wide-complex tachyarrhythmias.
- **Ask the right questions.** If the tachycardiac patient is conscious, and/or if a previous 12-lead ECG is available, determine (1) if the patient has a history of MI and (2) if the spells of rapid heart beating began subsequent to the MI. If the answer to both questions is "Yes," the wide-complex tachycardia is likely VT.[15,18] Approximately 95% of patients with VT have some form of cardiac pathology, and 82% have had a previous MI.[8,21] Of patients presenting with wide-complex tachycardias and a history of MI, 98% are VT.[8] Only 5% to 8% of patients presenting with VT have no cardiac history.[8,21]
- **Do not rely on duration of the tachycardia.** The duration of tachycardia cannot be considered useful in differential diagnosis.[18] Many patients in sustained VT present in a conscious state and report waiting several hours before seeking treatment.[18] It has thus been concluded[18] that **regular wide QRS tachycardia in the conscious adult patient should be considered VT until proved otherwise,** especially when the patient has a history of MI.
- **Do not depend on lead II.** When differentiating wide-complex tachycardias, leads MCL_1 and MCL_6 or V_1 and V_6 are most useful. Determination of axis may be made by frontal plane leads I and aVF. Lead II may be useful when used with other leads to locate P waves to determine if AV dissociation is present.
- **Do not rely on heart rate or rhythm.** It was once thought that differentiation could be based on the rate of the wide tachycardia. This is not the case. Too much overlap exists among three wide QRS–complex tachycardias. The rate of VT ranges from 107 to 270 bpm[8,18]; SVT with aberration ranges from 125 to 273 bpm[8]; and wide-complex tachycardias with preexcitation range from 140 to 300 bpm.[8] Another reason for the misconception is the mistaken belief that hemodynamically tolerated tachycardias with rates exceeding 200 bpm generally imply supraventricular origin.[18] Two thirds of the conscious patients with VT in Steinman et al's[18] study experienced rates of more than 200 bpm, whereas all their patients with SVT had tachycardia rates under 200 bpm.

Rhythm is also not very helpful. Except for WPW

syndrome with AF and AP conduction, which exhibits a very irregular rhythm, frequently with 100% variation in cycle length and RR intervals as short as 0.20 seconds, all paroxysmal tachycardias, regardless of origin, tend to be regular, yet any of them can be irregular.[6] VT is regular in 79% and SVT with aberration in 93% of cases.[22]

ECG Characteristics

VT versus SVT with aberration. Research has identified numerous ECG criteria useful in the differential diagnosis of wide QRS–complex tachycardias. What criteria are used depends largely on whether or not 12-lead ECGs are available before and during the tachycardia. Let us consider the best scenario first (i.e., availability of 12-lead ECGs both before and during the wide QRS–complex tachycardia). Consider the two most common causes of wide-complex tachycardias, VT and SVT with BBB. SVT with BBB should resemble a right or left BBB pattern. Follow the steps below, which are summarized in Figure 10-5:

- **Step 1: Examine previous 12-lead ECG.**
  - If previous ECG shows BBB closely resembling wide QRS–complex tachycardia on all 12 leads, diagnose SVT with BBB.
  - If history of MI and patient reports episodes of rapid heart rate not occurring before MI, diagnose VT.[8]
  - Patients with previous BBB who develop VT will likely exhibit a different QRS during VT[8] (Fig. 10-6).
    - Be aware that VT can sometimes closely resemble patient's sinus rhythm that is conducted with BBB.[23]
    - Of patients presenting with wide-complex tachycardias, 29% of those in SVT with aberration and 12% of those presenting with VT have previous BBB.[8]

Now consider situations in which a 12-lead ECG of the tachycardia is available but not a previous ECG. Brugada et al[24] offer a quick and simple method for initiating differential diagnosis:

- **Step 2: Search for RS complex in all precordial leads (V_1 through V_6).**
  - If **no** RS complex in **any** precordial lead, diagnose VT (Fig. 10-7).
    - Approximately 26% of VTs have no RS.[24]
  - If RS present in any precordial lead, measure from beginning of R wave to nadir (deepest point) of S wave. If duration exceeds 100 msec (0.10 seconds), diagnose VT (Fig. 10-8).
    - In about 50% of those VTs having an RS, the RS exceeds 100 msec.[24]
  - If RS present in any precordial lead but does not exceed 100 msec, procede with additional criteria.

Except for Step 5, the remaining do not require a 12-lead ECG.

- **Step 3: Determine if AV dissociation is present.**
  - If so, diagnose VT (Fig. 10-9).
  - Although very reliable, do not spend a lot of time on this criterion because it is difficult to detect with rapid rates, present in only about half of VTs, and only detectable in a minority (9% to 25%) of cases.[8,15,19,22,24]
  - Three ECG clues[15] that provide evidence of AV dissociation follow. Unfortunately, tachycardias exceeding rates of about 160 bpm are less apt to reveal these signs[15]:
    - Independent P waves.
    - Fusion beats.
    - Capture beats (Fig. 10-10).
  - Physical signs supporting AV dissociation[6,15,20] include the following:
    - Irregular cannon waves noted in jugular pulse.
    - Variation in first heart sound.
    - Variation in Korotkoff sounds of systolic blood pressure.
  - AV dissociation favors VT by ruling out atrial tachycardia but does not rule out the rare occurrence of junctional tachycardia with a BBB and retrograde block.[6,15]
- **Step 4: Determine the QRS axis on the frontal plane.**
  - If −90 to −180 degrees (superior right), diagnose VT.[3-6,19]
    - Between 16% and 24% of VTs meet this criterion.[8,25]
    - This is a good criterion even in patients with preexisting BBB.
- **Step 5: Determine QRS concordance in precordial leads (V_1 through V_6).**
  - If positive concordance (all QRSs upright) and WPW syndrome ruled out, diagnose VT.[6,8,15,22,26]
    - Present in 12% of VTs[8] (Fig 10-11).
    - Although a strong criterion favoring the diagnosis of VT, note one unusual exception in Fig. 10-3, *B*.
  - If negative concordance (all QRSs negative), the diagnosis for VT is supported.[6,15,22,26]
    - Be aware that it can occur in patients with LBBB aberration tachycardia.[6,8]
    - Present in 10% of VTs.[8]
    - Its presence rules out WPW.[15]
- A good criterion even in patients with preexisting BBB.[25]
- **Step 6: Examine morphologic criteria in leads V_1 and V_6.**
  - If **up** in V_1.

    For QRS complexes that are upright in V_1, check for the following three morphologic characteristics typical of RBBB: (1) QRS duration <0.14 seconds, (2) triphasic rSR′ pattern in V_1 with qRs in V_6, and (3) initial vector that is identical to that of the normally conducted beats in V_1 or more leads.[1] If all criteria are met, a diagnosis of RBBB aberration may be made with reasonable certainty.

    Note that the QRS duration criterion has two impor-

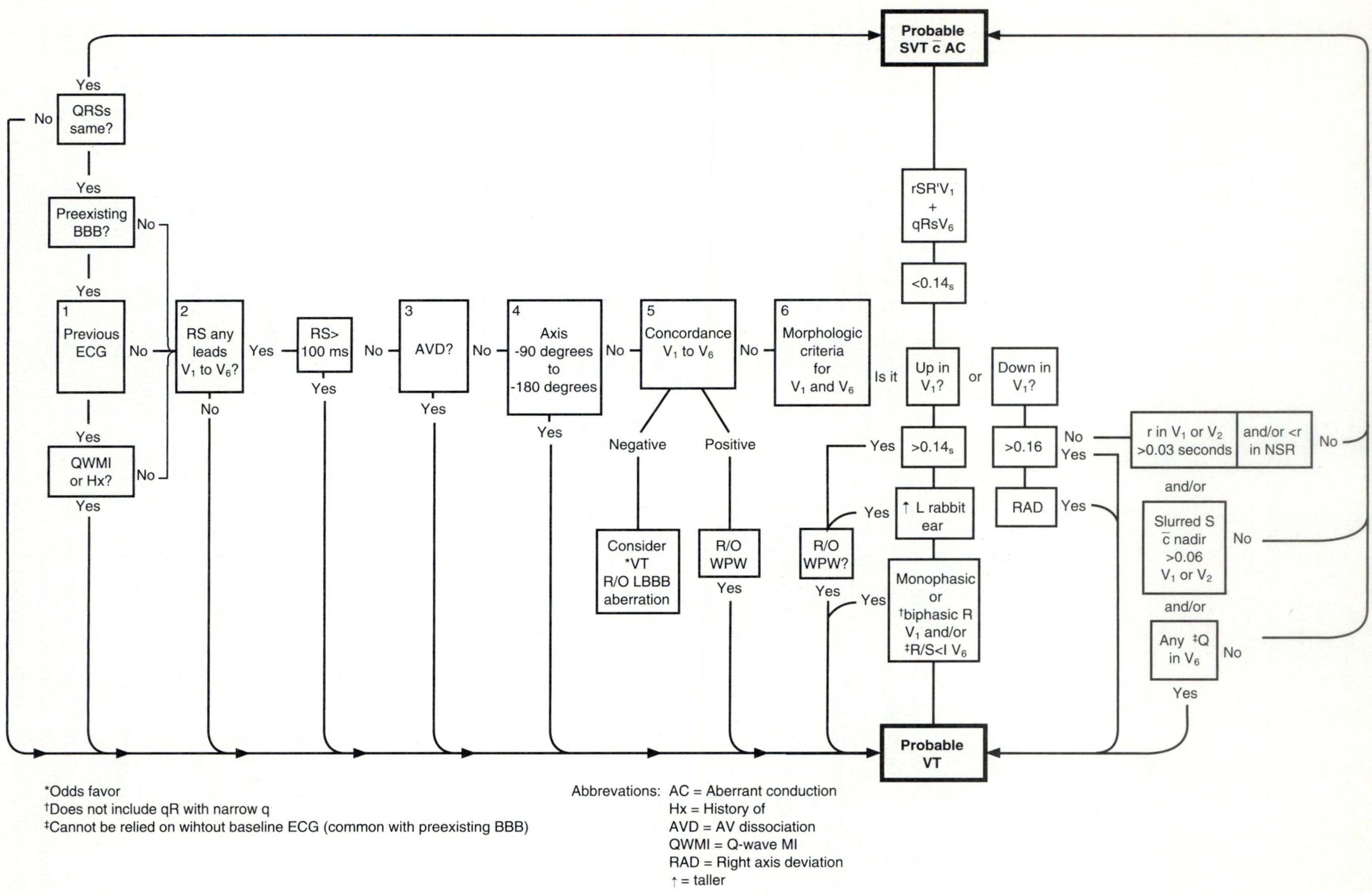

FIGURE 10-5 Wide QRS–complex tachycardia algorithm.

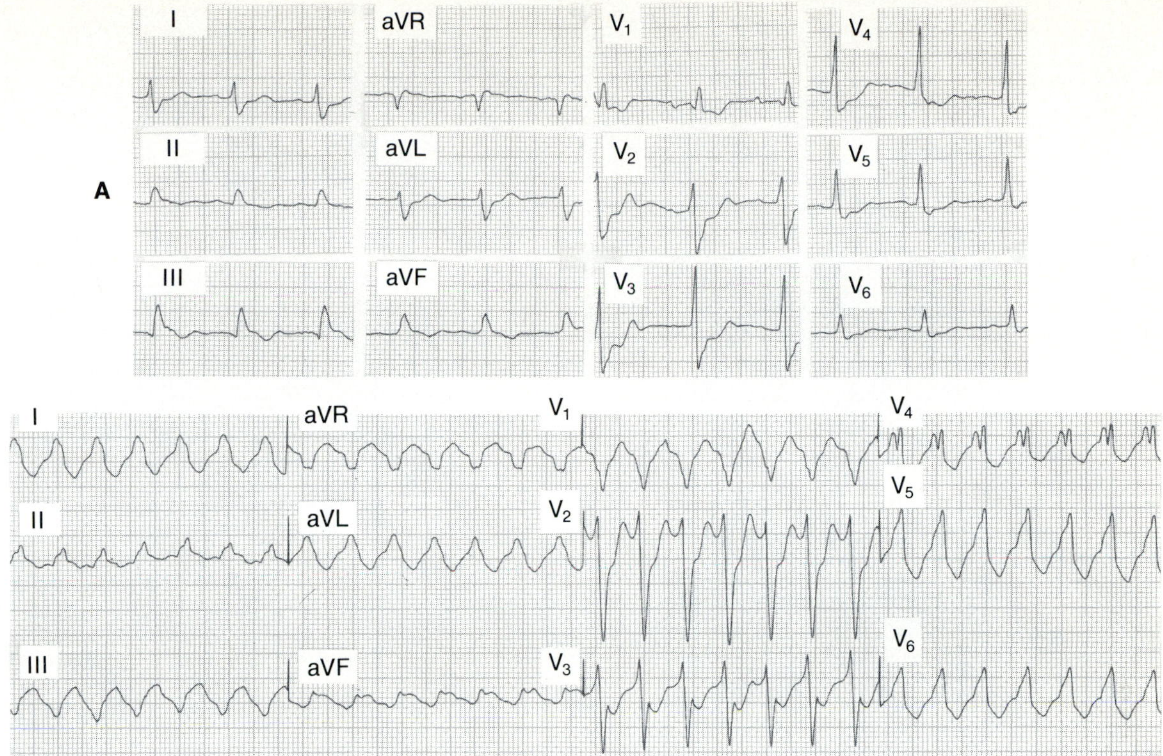

FIGURE 10-6 **A,** ECG of patient with RBBB. **B,** Wide-complex tachycardia with different morphology 1 hour later is diagnosed VT.

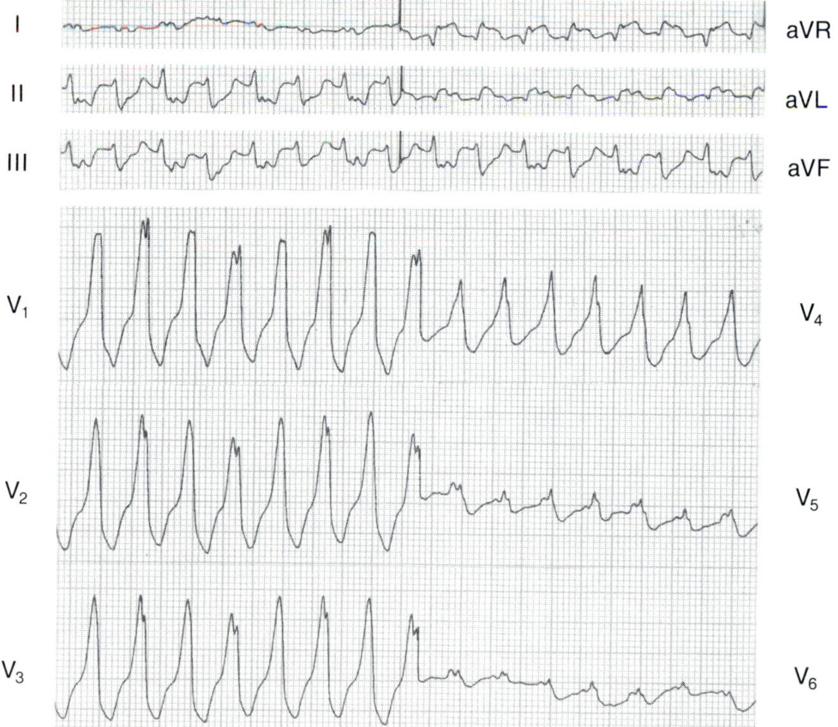

FIGURE 10-7 Ventricular tachycardia. No RS complex on any of the precordial leads is a strong criterion favoring VT. Of interest in this tracing is 2:1 VA conduction from ventricles to atria, producing a negative P′ wave distorting every other QRS complex. Also note positive precordial concordance and monophasic R in V_1, other criteria supporting VT.

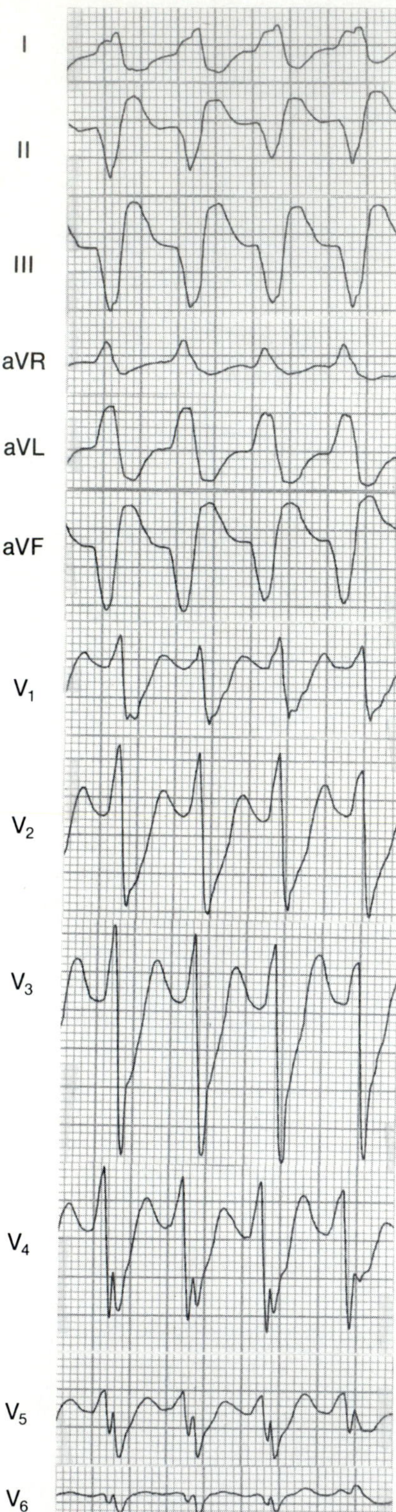

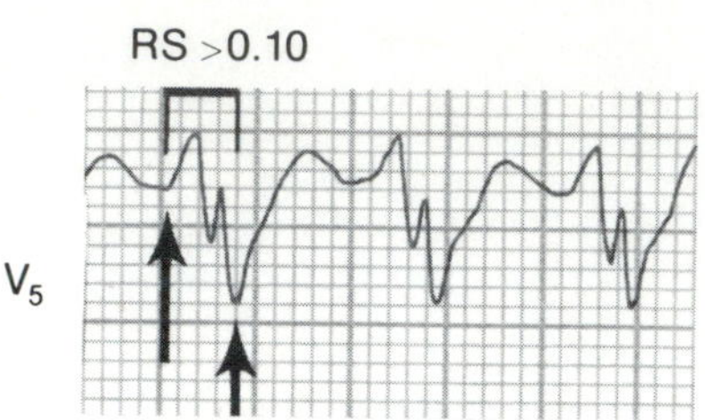

FIGURE 10-8 RS complexes are present in precordial leads V_1 to V_5 and widest in V_2, V_3, and V_5. Measure the widest RS interval from beginning of R wave to sharpest point of S wave. In V_5, RS interval 0.14 to 0.15 seconds, satisfying requirements of exceeding 0.10 seconds as a strong criterion in favor of VT.

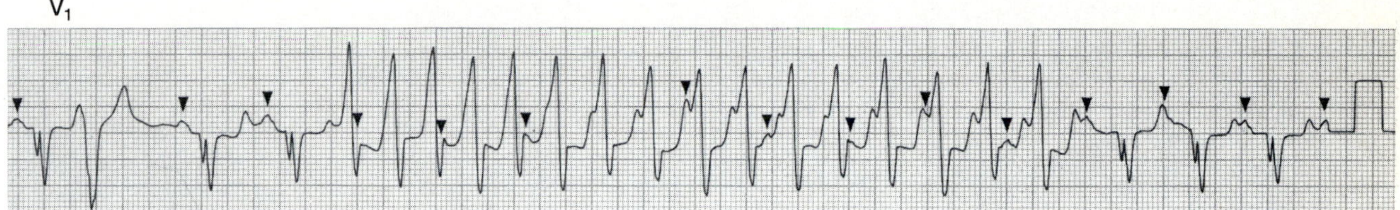

FIGURE 10-9 Nonsustained VT exhibiting AV dissociation (*arrows* mark P waves).

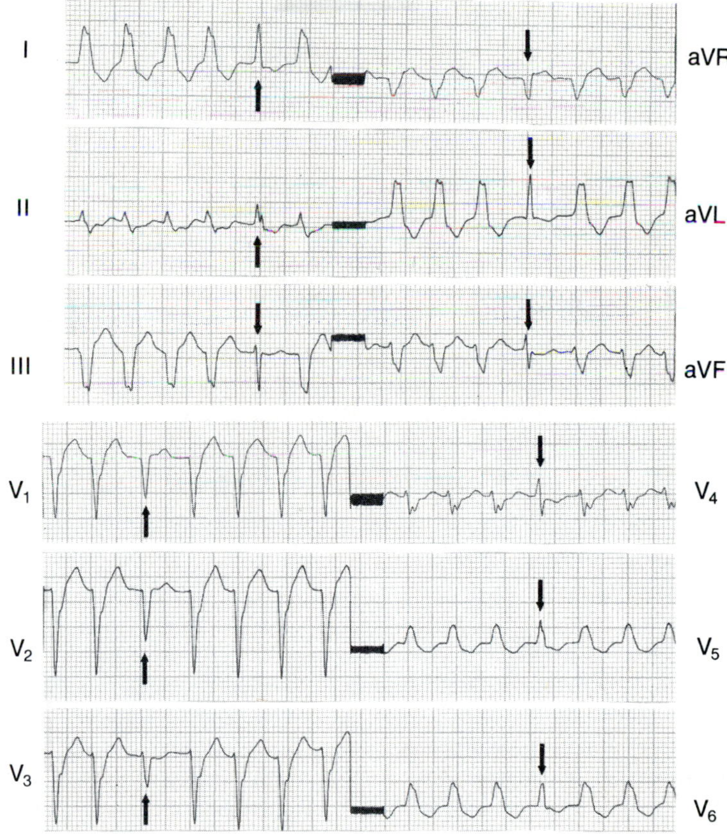

FIGURE 10-10 Capture beats in the midst of VT. Supraventricular beats conducted normally *(arrows)* in VT is a criterion supporting VT.

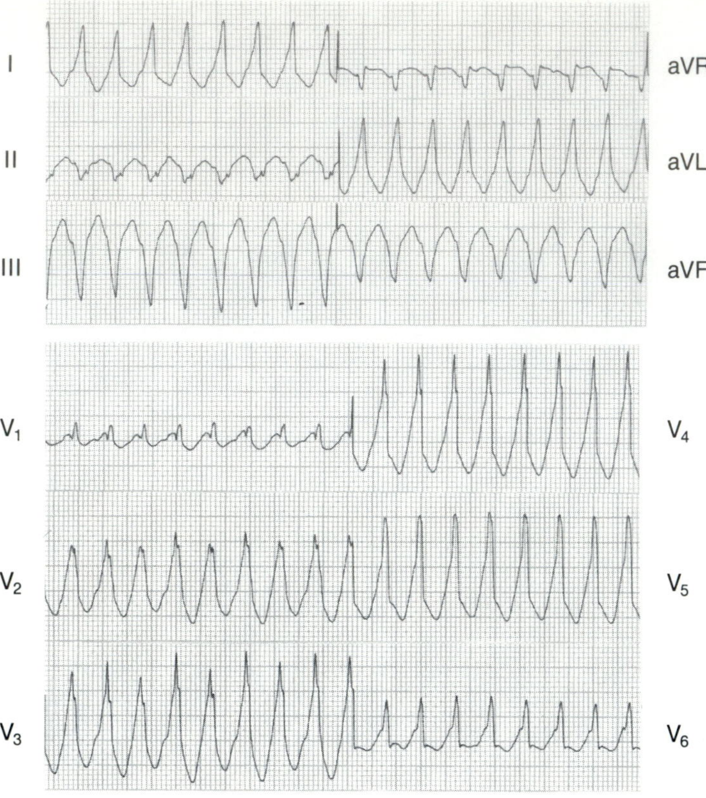

FIGURE 10-11 VT with positive precordial concordance (i.e., all QRSs V_1 to V_6 are positive).

tant features. First, it is applicable only if preexisting BBB has been ruled out.[15,22] In other words, if a patient with a preexisting RBBB develops SVT, the QRS often exceeds 0.14 seconds. Second, be aware that in about 25% of VTs the QRS complexes measure <0.14 sec, and in about 17% of SVTs with aberration the QRS complexes exceed 0.14 seconds.[24]

QRS complexes exceeding 0.14 seconds that are either monophasic R waves [22,25] (including those with a taller left peak)[4,6,22,26,27] or biphasic R waves (RS or QR)[22] in V_1 favor the diagnosis of VT. The monophasic R wave is a good criterion even in patients with preexisting BBB.[25] Indeed, it is seen in about 38% of the VTs that occur in patients with preexisting BBB.[25] A taller left peak points to VT, providing preexcitation has been ruled out.

In looking at V_6 the following two criteria support the diagnosis of VT: (1) a QS or rS complex[4,6,22,26] that is 15 mm or more deep[28] or (2) an R/S ratio <1 (Fig 10-12). The R/S ratio cannot be relied on without a previous ECG because it is common with preexisting RBBB.[25]

- If **down** in V_1.

These tachycardias are much more difficult to differentiate because VTs that are negative in V_1 closely resemble LBBB aberration (see Fig. 10-13). Odds favor the diagnosis of VT by almost 4:1[21] because VT is much more common than LBBB aberration.

If an initial r wave is present in V_1 or V_2 measuring more than 0.03 seconds, diagnose VT. It is important to check both V_1 and V_2 because the initial r wave is sometimes isoelectric in V_1. The *fat little r wave,* as Marriott[6] calls it, is seen in about half of VTs that are negative in V_1. It is a good criterion even in the presence of preexisting BBB and is seen in about 23% of VTs occurring in patients with preexisting BBB,[25] but it is not reliable if the patient is on antiarrhythmic drugs that prolong the QRS.[21,25,29]

If the S wave in V_1 or V_2 is slurred or notched and/or its nadir is delayed beyond 0.06 seconds,[6] diagnose VT. Again, it is important to check both V_1 and V_2.[21] The slurred S and delayed nadir are not reliable criteria in patients on antiarrhythmic drugs that prolong the QRS.[21]

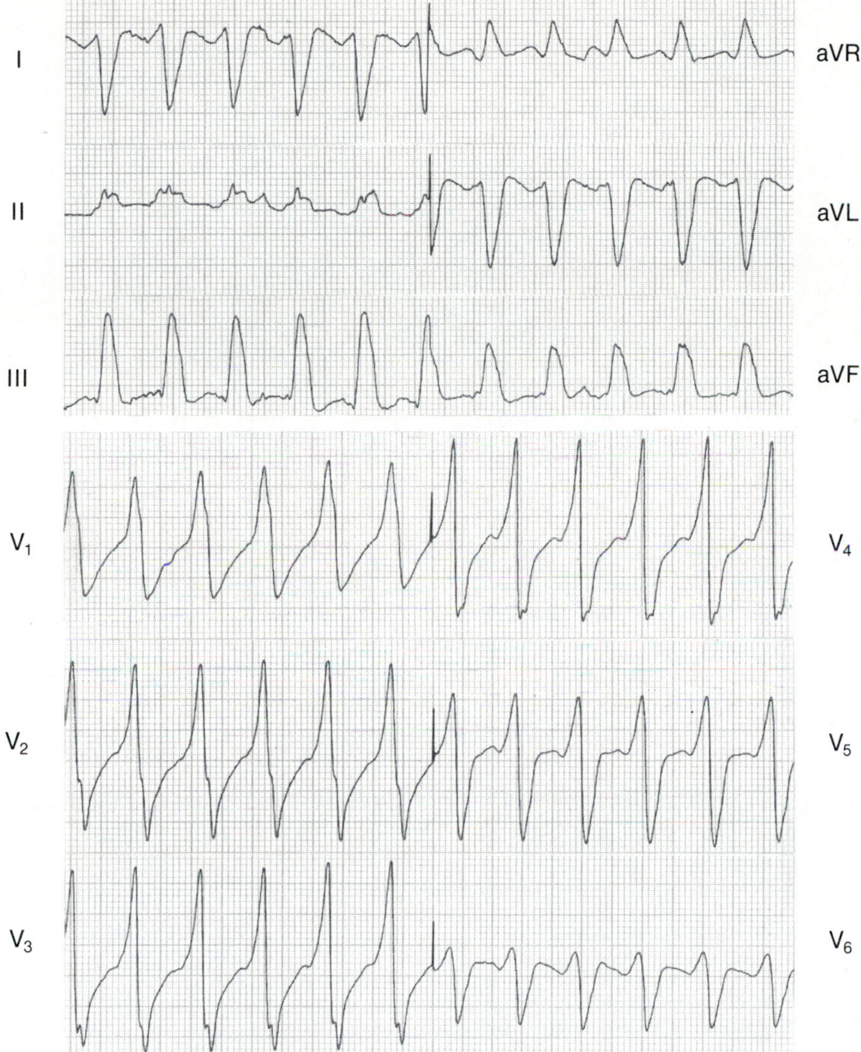

FIGURE 10-12 VT with QRS upright in V_1 with monomophasic R wave, QRS >0.14 seconds, and R/S ratio <1 in V_6. Also note, RS duration in precordial leads V_3 to V_6 exceeds 0.10 seconds.

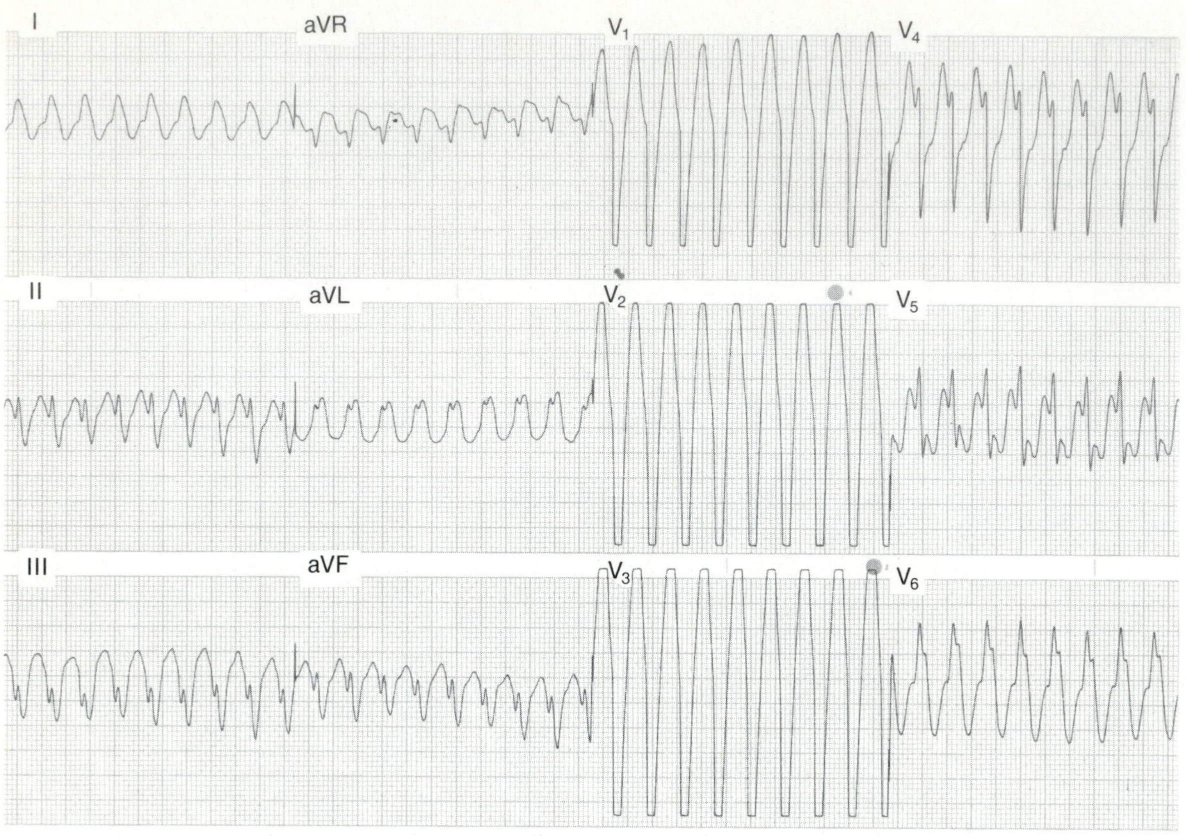

FIGURE 10-13 Wide QRS–complex tachycardia that is negative in V_1. QRS measures 0.12 seconds, axis is superior left. The ECG offers no definitive morphologic clues regarding the origin. The patient, however, is a 46-year-old male with a history of MI. The ECG was confirmed as VT. The patient's history is the strongest criterion supporting the diagnosis.

If the S wave in V_1 shows a slick downstroke, reaching an early nadir (<0.06 seconds), the diagnosis of SVT with LBBB aberration is supported.

QRS complexes measuring >0.16 seconds are likely to be VT. This is not a reliable criterion for patients with preexisting LBBB, for reasons discussed previously.

Check the frontal plane QRS axis. If the axis is directed to the right, diagnose VT. A right axis deviation is present in only about 7% of VTs that are negative in V_1.[8]

Table 10–1 summarizes the morphologic characteristics.

WPW syndrome with AF and preexcitation. WPW syndrome is rare, occurring in only 15 of 10,000 ECGs. However, one of its variations comprises about 5% of patients presenting with wide QRS–complex tachycardias.[19] It is a form of preexcitation in which supraventricular impulses may activate the ventricles via an AP, bypassing portions of the AV junction. There are three ways WPW syndrome can cause wide QRS–complex tachycardias in order of frequency:

Table 10-1 Morphologic Characteristics in Wide QRS–Complex Tachycardias

	Aberration	Ectopy
Up in V_1	<0.14 seconds* rSR′ V_1, qRs V_6 Identical initial vector	>0.14 seconds* Monophasic R or taller left peak‡ RS or QR V_1 R/S <1 V_6 rS or QS V_6 ≥15 mm deep
Down in V_1	Slick S V_1 or V_2† Nadir <0.06 seconds V_1 or V_2† Initial r ≤0.03 seconds V_1 or V_2† QRS <0.16 seconds*	Slurred S V_1 or V_2† Nadir >0.06 seconds V_1 or V_2† Initial r >0.03 seconds V_1 or V_2† QRS >0.16 seconds* Right axis deviation Q in V_6*

*Applicable only if preexisting BBB ruled out.
†Not reliable if patient on antiarrhythmics prolonging QRS.
‡Reliable only if preexcitation ruled out.

1. **Orthodromic reciprocating tachycardia with BBB aberration.** The reciprocating impulse procedes in an anterograde (forward) direction down the AV junction and in a retrograde (backwards) direction up the AP (Fig. 10-14).

   The orthodromic reciprocating SVT with BBB aberration will result in a wide QRS–complex tachycardia fitting the criteria for SVT with BBB aberration as described previously.
2. **Atrial tachycardia (AT), AFl, or AF with anterograde conduction down AP.** When the AV junction is bypassed, the impulse enters the ventricles outside normal conduction pathways. The resultant depolarization procedes much like that of a ventricular ectopic beat (Figs. 10-15 and 10-16).

   Both AT and AFl (AFl is rare in WPW syndrome)[6] with anterograde conduction down the AP produce a wide QRS–complex tachycardia that may be indistinguishable from VT using morophologic criteria.[6]

   AF with anterograde conduction down the AP produces a grossly irregular rhythm, distinguishing it from VT (Fig 10-17). Cycle lengths vary from as short as 0.20 seconds to more than twice the length of the shortest cycles.[6]

   The major determinant of ventricular rate is the length of the refractory period of the accessory pathway. If the refractory period is short, ventricular rates may reach 300 bpm. Thus the danger of WPW Syndrome in the presence of rapid atrial tachyarrhythmias is the possibility of high ventricular rates (up to 300 bpm) causing ventricular fibrillation, either by provoking hypoxia or an impulse arriving during the vulnerable phase of the ventricular cycle.[6]
3. **Antidromic reciprocating tachycardia.** The reciprocating impulse proceeds in an anterograde direction down the accessory pathway and in retrograde direction up the AV junction.

   Antidromic reciprocating tachycardia produces a wide QRS–complex tachycardia that may be indistinguishable from VT using morphologic criteria[6] (Fig. 10-18).

This discussion deals only with those wide-complex tachycardias in which AF is accompanied by anterograde conduction down the AP. ECG characteristics are as follows:

Fast Rate and Irregular Rhythm

- If the rate is rapid (often >250 bpm) with some cycles as short as 0.20 seconds[15] and
- the rhythm is irregular[15] with 100% variation in cycle length, diagnose AF with accessory pathway conduction.

Morphologic Characteristics

- Negative precordial concordance rules out WPW syndrome.[15]
- Positive precordial concordance possible.
- QRS >0.14 seconds in 83%.[19]
- Taller left rabbit ear possible.

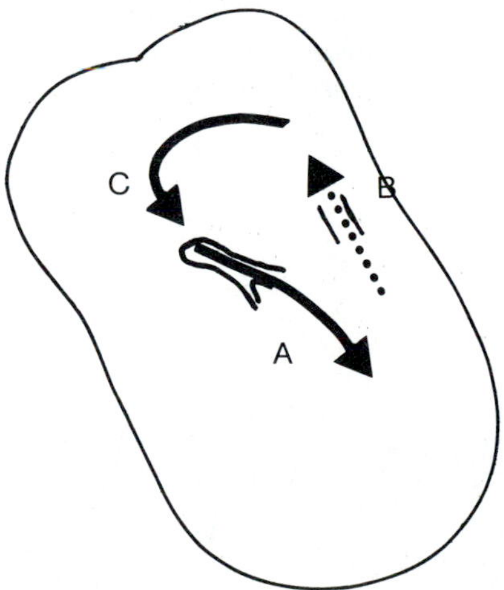

FIGURE 10-14 Orthodromic reciprocating tachycardia with BBB aberration. Impulse enters ventricles via AV junction, activating ventricles *(A)*. Impulse travels retrogradely up accessory pathway *(B)*, activating atria, allowing impulse to again procede down AV junction in a rapid, reciprocating tachycardia *(C)*. The resultant BBB is a result of aberration due to the fast rate.

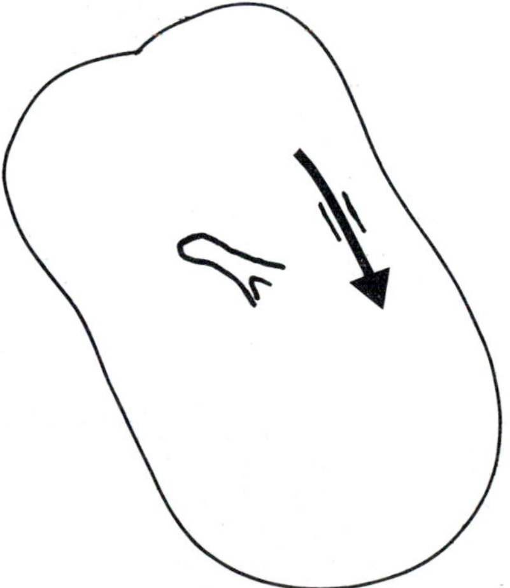

FIGURE 10-15 Supraventricular tachycardia (AT, AFl, or AF) with anterograde conduction down accessory pathway. Impulse enters outside normal conduction pathways, resulting in a wide-complex tachycardia that may be indistinguishable from VT, except when the SVT is AF, in which case, the ventricular rhythm would display typical irregularity that is common with AF.

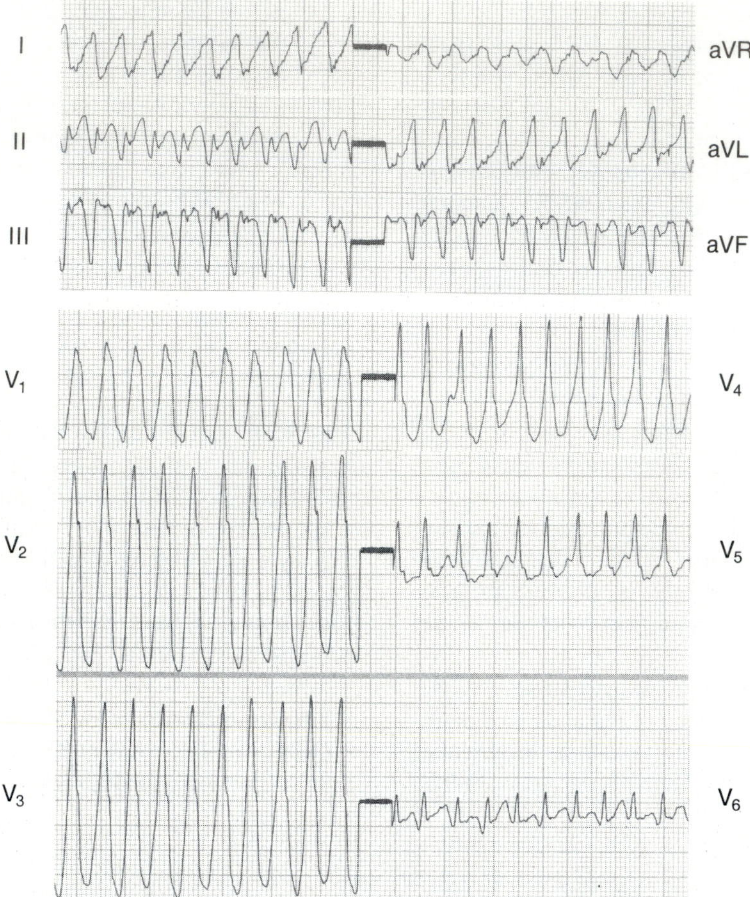

FIGURE 10-16 Fast supraventricular rhythm conducting impulse to ventricles via accessory pathway. The ECG is from a 29-year-old woman with confirmed accessory pathway conduction. Wide-complex tachycardias such as this are often indistinguishable from VT. Note positive precordial concordance and taller left rabbit ear, both criteria support VT, but both are possible with accessory pathway conduction.

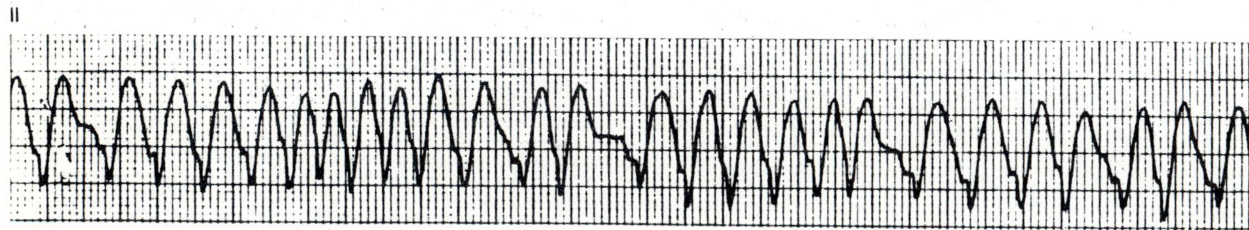

FIGURE 10–17 Atrial fibrillation with conduction over an accessory pathway. From Marriott H, Conover M: *Advanced Concepts in Arrhythmias,* 2nd ed, St. Louis, The CV Mosby Co., 1989.

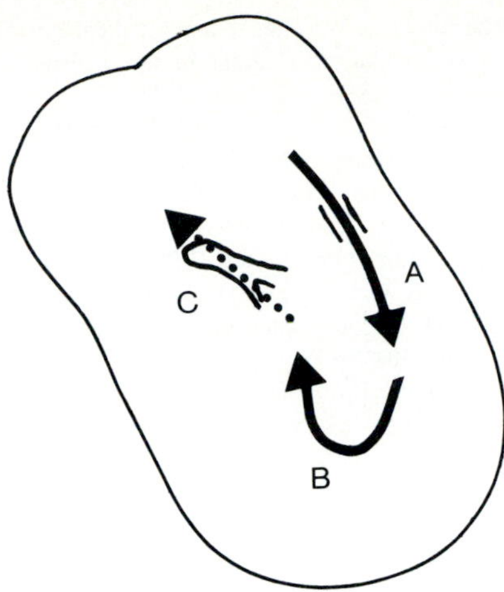

FIGURE 10-18 Antidromic reciprocating tachycardia. The impulse procedes down accessory pathway *(A),* depolarizing the ventricles *(B),* and reenters the atria retrogradely via the AV junction *(C),* resulting in a reciprocating tachycardia that may be indistinguishable from VT.

Applied Nursing Process

Clinical Assessment

The clinical assessment for wide QRS–complex tachycardias is the same as that for VT in Chapter 9 and PSVT in Chapter 6. Presented here are additional points and those that deserve repeating.

- Detect:
  - Rapid, regular pulse (may be thready) or no peripheral pulse and
  - Wide QRS–complex tachycardia on ECG or
  - Rapid, irregular pulse (may or may not be thready) and
  - Irregular, wide QRS–complex tachycardia on ECG.
- Assess patient and ECG.
  - Immediately assess level of consciousness.
  - Check blood pressure.
  - Palpate peripheral pulses.
  - If patient conscious and stable, assess the following:
    Signs and symptoms of myocardial ischemia.
    12-lead ECG.
    Patient's history.
  - Diagnose the arrhythmia. For a wide, regular, monomorphic tachycardia, follow the algorithm in Figure 10-5.

❖ NURSING DIAGNOSIS

(1) Decreased cardiac output related to tachycardia. (2) High risk for decreased tissue perfusion: cardiopulmonary/peripheral/cerebral, related to decreased cardiac output. (3) High risk for knowledge deficit regarding management of tachyarrhythmia at home.

❖ ECG DIAGNOSIS

Wide QRS–complex tachycardia resulting from VT, SVT with aberration, or AF with accessory pathway conduction (specify).

Plan and Implementation

Patient goal. The patient's hemodynamic status will be preserved.
The patient will regain normal sinus rhythm.
Before discharge, the patient will relate appropriate information regarding management of arrhythmia.

Nursing interventions.

- All interventions should be consistent with institutional policy.
- If patient unconscious, consider interventions appropriate for any wide-complex tachycardia:
  - Precordial thump.
  - Electrical cardioversion.
  - CPR.
  - Notify others of cardiac arrest.
  - Notify physician.
- Emergency treatment is directed toward improving hemodynamic status and preventing VF. Pharmacologic therapy is based on ECG diagnosis, not on patient's symptoms. If in doubt, treat as VT.
  - Treating SVT with aberration is often successful with verapamil. However, mistakenly treating VT and WPW syndrome with verapamil often provokes severe hypotension and/or VF in the presence of VT and increases the ventricular rate in WPW syndrome.[11-13,16,30]
- For confirmed **SVT with aberration**:
  - Perform vagal stimulation.
  - Administer verapamil or adenosine.
  - Monitor at least 1 hour after administration of verapamil.[31] Verapamil decreases systemic vascular resistance, heart rate, and cardiac output. Negative inotropic effects are potentiated by beta blockers.[31]
- For **VT**:
  - Administer lidocaine or procainamide.
  - Do not administer verapamil.
- For **WPW syndrome with AP conduction and AF**:
  - Cardioversion (after appropriate anesthesia if conscious).[16]
  - Avoid verapamil, propranolol, or digitalis. These may increase ventricular rate by permitting antegrade conduction over AP unopposed (verapamil, propranolol) or by shortening refractory period of AP (digitalis).[16] By itself, verapamil has no effect on AP conduction but causes peripheral vasodilitation, resulting in reflex catecholamine secretion, which increases conduction velocity over AP.
  - Type IA antiarrhythmics, such as procainamide, quinidine, and lidocaine prolong the refractory period and slow conduction in the AP.

To summarize emergency pharmacologic therapy:

- Never administer verapamil for wide QRS tachycardia unless BBB aberration is confirmed.
- When in doubt, treat wide-complex tachycardia as VT until proved otherwise:
  - Administration of lidocaine (1 to 2 mg/kg) is indicated for VT, it will slow the ventricular rate in WPW syndrome and will not harm patient in SVT with aberration.
  - If necessary, follow with procainamide.

Evaluation

- The patient maintains/regains hemodynamic status during tachycardia as evidenced by maintenance of consciousness and blood pressure.
- The patient regains normal rhythm as evidenced by NSR (or equivalent) on ECG.

Medical Treatment

Confirmed SVT with aberration may be terminated by vagal stimulation or pharmacologic agents such as adenosine or calcium channel blockers, such as verapamil. (See same section, PSVT, Chapter 6.)

VT is treated with lidocaine or procainamide and other antiarrhythmic medications as indicated. (See same section, VT, Chapter 8.)

The treatment for preexcitation may include radiofrequency or surgical ablation of the bypass tract(s).

REFERENCES

1. Sandler JA, Marriott HJL. The differential morphology of anomalous ventricular complexes of RBBB type in lead V_1: Ventricular ectopy versus aberration. *Circ.*, Apr., 1965, 31(4): 551-6.
2. Marriott HJL. Simulation of ectopic ventricular rhythms by aberrant conduction. *JAMA,* May, 1966, 196(9): 107.
3. Marriott HJL. *Workshop in Electrocardiography*. Tampa Tracings, 1972.
4. Gulamhusein S, Yee R, Ko PT, Klein GJ. Electrocardiographic criteria for differentiating aberrancy and ventricular extrasystole in chronic atrial fibrillation: validation by intracardiac recordings. *J. Electrocardiol.*, Jan., 1985, 18(1): 41-50.
5. Vera Z, Cheng TO, Ertem G, Shoaleh-Var M, Wickramasekaran R, Wadhwa K. His bundle electrography for evaluation of critieria in differentiating ventricular ectopy from aberrance in atrial fibrillation. *Circ.,* Oct., 1972, 45(suppl 2): 93550.
6. Marriott HJL. *Practical Electrocardiography*. 8th ed. Baltimore: Williams & Wilkins, 1988.
7. Gouaux JL, Ashman R. Auricular fibrillation with aberration simulating ventricular paroxysmal tachycardia. *Am. Heart J.,* Sept., 1947, 34(3): 366-73.
8. Ahktar M, Shenasa M, Jazayeri M, Caceres J, Tchou PJ. Wide QRS complex tachycardia: Reappraisal of a common clinical problem. *Ann. Intern. Med.,* Dec., 1988, 109(11): 905-12.
9. Cooper J, Marriott HJL. Why are so many critical care nurses unable to recognize ventricular tachycardia in the 12-lead electrocardiogram? *Heart & Lung,* May, 1989, 18(3): 243-7.
10. Morady F, Baerman JM, DiCarlo LA, DeBuitleir M, Krol RB, Wahr DW. A prevalent misconception regarding wide-complex tachycardias. *JAMA,* Nov., 1985, 254(19): 2790-2.
11. Dancy M, Camm AJ, Ward D. Misdiagnosis of chronic recurrent ventricular tachycardia. *Lancet,* Aug., 1985, pp. 320-3.
12. Stewart RB, Bardy GH, Greene HL. Wide complex tachycardia: Misdiagnosis and outcome after emergent therapy. *Ann. Intern. Med.,* Jun., 1986, 104(6): 766-71.
13. Switzer DF, Henthorn RW, Olshansky B. Dire consequences of verapamil administration for wide QRS tachycardia. *Circ.,* 1986, 74(suppl. II):105.
14. Josephson ME. Approach to the patient with wide-complex tachycardia. *Protocols,* 1991, pp. 3-8.
15. Marriott HJL. Differential diagnosis of supraventricular and ventricular tachycardia. *Cardiol.,* 1990, 77: 209-20.
16. Jackman WM, Friday KJ, Naccarelli GV. VT or not VT? An approach to the diagnosis and management of wide QRS complex tachycardia. *Clin. Prog. Pacing Electrophysiol.,* 1983, 1(3): 225-66.
17. Akhtar M. Clinical Spectrum of ventricular tachycardia. *Circ.,* Nov., 1990, 82(5): 1561-73.
18. Steinman RT, Harrera C, Schuger CD, Lehmann MH. Wide QRS tachycardia in the conscious adult. *JAMA,* Feb., 1989, 261(7): 1013-16.
19. Akhtar M. Electrophysiologic bases for wide QRS complex tachycardia. *PACE,* Jan.-Feb., 1983, 6: 81-98.
20. Schwartz AB, Scheinman MM. Ventricular tachycardia: Newer insights. *Clin. Cardiol.,* Jul., 1983, 6: 307-11.
21. Kindwall KE, Brown J, Josephson ME. Electrocardiographic criteria for ventricular tachycardia in wide complex left bundle branch block morphology tachycardias. *Am. J. Cardiol.,* Jun., 1988, 61: 1279-83.
22. Wellens HJJ, Bär FWHM, Lie KI. The value of the electrocardiogram in the differential diagnosis of a tachycardia with a widened QRS complex. *Am. J. Med.,* Jan., 1978, 64: 27-33.
23. Ross DL, Vohra JK, Sloman JG. Similar QRS morphology in sinus rhythm and ventricular tachycardia. *PACE,* 1979, 2: 486-9.
24. Brugada P, Brugada J, Mont L, Smeets J, Andries EW. A new approach to the differential diagnosis of a regular tachycardia with a wide QRS complex. *Circ.,* May, 1991, 83(5): 1649-59.
25. Kremers MS, Black WH, Wells PJ, Solodyna M. Effect of preexisting bundle branch block on the electrocardiographic diagnosis of ventricular tachycardia. *Am. J. Cardiol.,* Dec., 1988, 62: 1208-12.
26. Marriott HJL. Differential diagnosis of supraventricular and ventricular tachycardia. *Geriatrics,* Nov., 1970, pp. 91-101.
27. Gozensky C, Thorne D. Rabbit ears: An aid in distinguishing ventricular ectopy from aberration. *Heart & Lung,* 1975, 3: 634-6.
28. Marriott HJL. Diagnosis of ventricular arrhythmias with thoughts on therapy. *Curr. Concepts Cardiovasc. Disord.,* 1984, 1: 3-12.
29. Rosenbaum MB. Classification of ventricular extrasystoles according to form. *J. Electrocardiol.,* 1969, 2: 289-97.
30. Buxton AE, Marchlinski FE, Doherty JU, Flores BA, Josephson ME. Hazards of intravenous verapamil for sustained ventricular tachycardia. *Am. J. Cardiol.,* May, 1987, 59: 1107-10.
31. Hartshorn JC, Deans K. Cardiovascular pharmacology. *J. Cardiovasc. Nurs.,* Feb., 1988, 2(2): 73-5.

SELF-ASSESSMENT

MULTIPLE CHOICE

Directions

For each of the questions below, select the correct answer(s) from the choices given. If more than one answer is given, mark all that are correct.

Example

Wide QRS-complex beats are caused by
*a. Bundle branch block.
*b. Ventricular ectopy.
c. Atrial ectopy.
*d. Supraventricular beats conducted with aberration.

1. In the presence of atrial fibrillation (AF), anomalous beats are most likely the result of (one answer):
   a. Atrial ectopy.
   b. Junctional ectopy.
   c. Ventricular ectopy.
   d. Supraventricular beats conducted with aberration.

2. Supraventricular beats conducted with aberration in the presence of AF are most likely the result of:
   a. RBBB.
   b. LBBB.
   c. LAH.
   d. LPH.

3. Aberrantly conducted beats that are predominantly negative in V_1 are more likely to exhibit the following characteristics:
   a. Q or S wave that is notched or slurred.
   b. Q or S wave that is slick.
   c. r wave $>$ 0.04 seconds.
   d. r wave $<$0.04 seconds.
   e. nadir reached within 0.06 seconds.
   f. nadir reached after 0.06 seconds.

4. The axis of the QRS complex in ventricular ectopy can be directed to the
   a. superior left.
   b. inferior left.
   c. inferior right.
   d. superior right.

5. In supraventricular tachycardia conducted with aberration, it is rare for the axis to be directed to the
   a. superior left.
   b. inferior left.
   c. inferior right.
   d. superior right.

6. Potential hemodynamic and electrophysiologic consequences of wide QRS–complex tachycardia include:
   a. increased diastolic filling.
   b. loss of atrial kick.
   c. tachycardia-induced myocardial ischemia.
   d. ventricular fibrillation.

7. In differentiating wide QRS–complex tachycardias, the following are good criteria:
   a. duration of the tachycardia.
   b. symptoms.
   c. rate and rhythm.
   d. history of MI.

8. In differentiating wide QRS–complex tachycardias, the following ECG criteria strongly favor ventricular ectopy:
   a. previous 12-lead ECG showing BBB different from wide QRS complex tachycardia.
   b. absence of RS complex in all precordial leads.
   c. AV dissociation.
   d. superior left axis.

9. Morphologic criteria favoring ventricular ectopy include:
   a. wide beats with identical initial vector as patient's normal beats in all leads.
   b. monophasic R wave in V_1.
   c. taller left rabbit ear in lead V_1.
   d. triphasic rSR′ in V_1.

10. Wide-complex tachycardias exhibiting a typical BBB aberration pattern may be caused by
    a. orthodromic reciprocating tachycardia.
    b. antidromic reciprocating tachycardia.
    c. supraventricular tachycardia with anterograde conduction down accessory pathway.
    d. supraventricular tachycardia with BBB aberration.

MATCHING

Directions

Match each arrhythmia in column B with criteria supporting its diagnosis in column A. Choices in column B may be used once, more than once, or not at all.

A

( ) 11. Identical initial vector
( ) 12. Superior right axis
( ) 13. Fixed coupling interval
( ) 14. Absence of longer preceding cycle
( ) 15. Grossly irregular rhythm
( ) 16. 12-lead ECG of wide QRS tachycardia identical to patient's normal ECG
( ) 17. Long-short cycle sequence
( ) 18. AV dissociation
( ) 19. Precordial concordance
( ) 20. Absence of RS complex in all precordial leads
( ) 21. Triphasic rSR′ in V_1
( ) 22. QRS <0.14 seconds
( ) 23. Q or S in V_1 slick downstroke
( ) 24. Delayed nadir in V_1 of >0.06 seconds
( ) 25. Taller left rabbit ear in V_1
( ) 26. R/S ratio <1 in V_6 with positive QRS in V_1

B

A. Supraventricular conducted with aberration.
B. Ventricular ectopy
C. AF with anterograde conduction down accessory pathway

TRUE/FALSE

Directions

Determine whether each of the following statements is true or false and indicate with a *T* or *F*.

Example

(T) Ventricular tachycardia may be a lethal arrhythmia.

( ) 27. Identical initial vector of wide QRSs to patient's normal QRSs is a criterion used in differentiating LBBB aberration from ventricular ectopy.
( ) 28. Long-short cycle sequence exhibited in the presence of AF is strong criterion in favor of aberration.
( ) 29. RBBB aberration is more common than LBBB aberration in the presence of AF.
( ) 30. A "fat little r wave" in V_1 favors ventricular ectopy.
( ) 31. The axis of ventricular ectopic beats may be directed to any quadrant.
( ) 32. The axis of aberrant beats are often directed superiorly and to the right.
( ) 33. SVT with aberration is more common than VT.
( ) 34. VT cannot be tolerated and results in low blood pressure and altered mentation.
( ) 35. The patient presenting with wide-complex tachycardia who has a history of MI is likely to be in VT.
( ) 36. VT is usually of short duration, whereas SVT with aberration may persist for hours.
( ) 37. VT is usually irregular.
( ) 38. RS complex in any precordial lead strongly suggests VT.
( ) 39. Absence of AV dissociation strongly suggests supraventricular tachycardia with aberration.
( ) 40. Anterograde conduction of a SVT down an accessory pathway may be indistinguishable from VT.
( ) 41. Orthodromic reciprocating tachycardia will produce wide QRSs if there is BBB aberration.
( ) 42. Wide QRS–complex tachycardias resulting from BBB aberration usually resemble either a right or a left BBB.
( ) 43. Positive precordial concordance rules out WPW syndrome.
( ) 44. Wide QRS–complex tachycardias are VT until proved otherwise.
( ) 45. Verapamil is the treatment of choice for wide QRS complex tachycardias when the source of the tachycardia is uncertain.

SHORT ANSWER

The remaining questions involve analysis of patient situations and assessment of ECGs.

CASE: *Mr. FK is a 48 year old admitted to the emergency department in a wide-complex tachycardia. It is unknown what, if any, medications he is taking. A previous 12-lead ECG is not available and his previous cardiac history is not known.*

46. Diagnose the tachycardia using the wide QRS tachycardia algorithm.
47. Are any other criteria present to support your diagnosis?

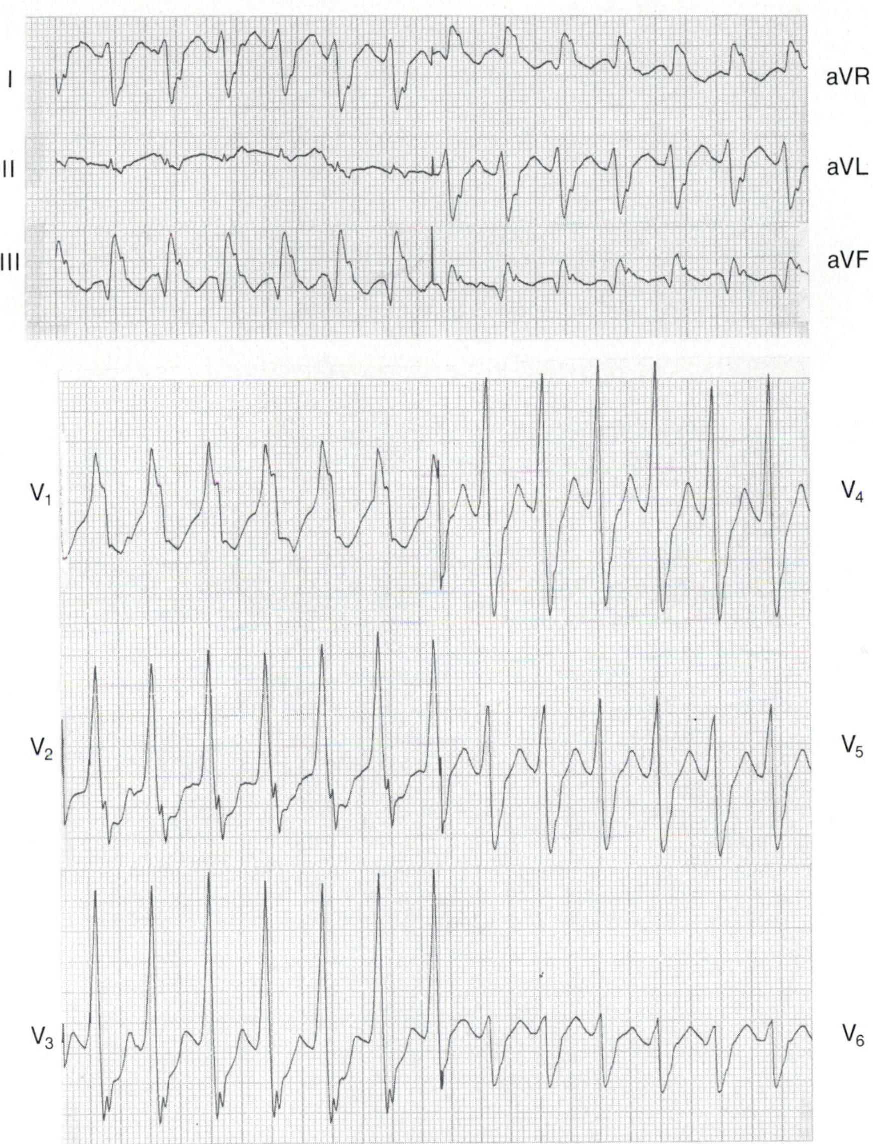

***CASE:** Mr. JH is a 77 year old admitted to the emergency department with a wide-complex tachycardia. The patient is confused and previous records are not available. His vital signs are: HR 136; BP 138/86; R 20.*

48. Diagnose the tachycardia using the wide QRS tachycardia algorithm.

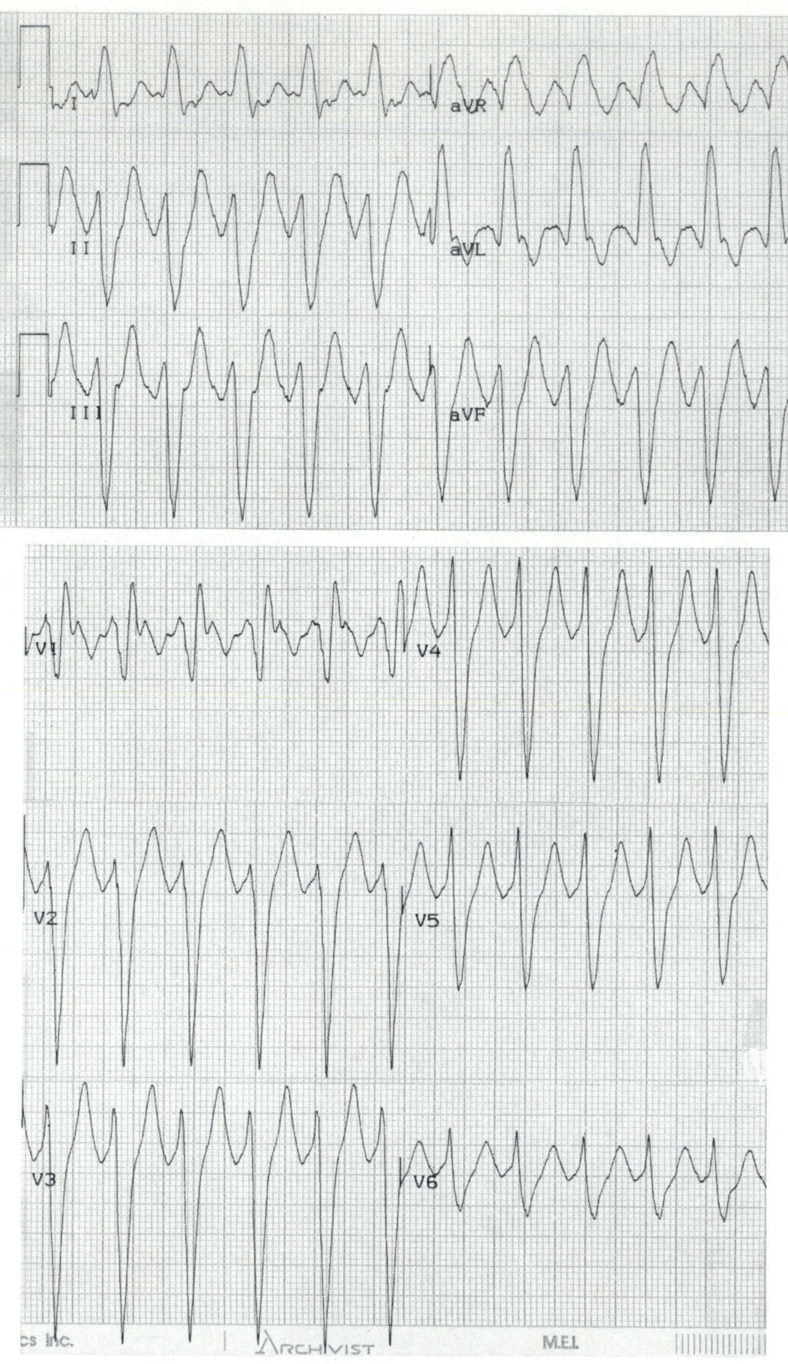

CASE: *Mr. DJ is a 64 year old admitted to the emergency department in a wide-complex tachycardia. He is conscious with a HR of 142 bpm, BP 134/72. He reports having had a myocardial infarction in the past. Previous records are not available. The patient reports having been bothered by occasional "fast heart beats" since his MI, but never lasting as long as the present episode of 5 hours.*

49. Diagnose the tachycardia using the wide QRS tachycardia algorithm.

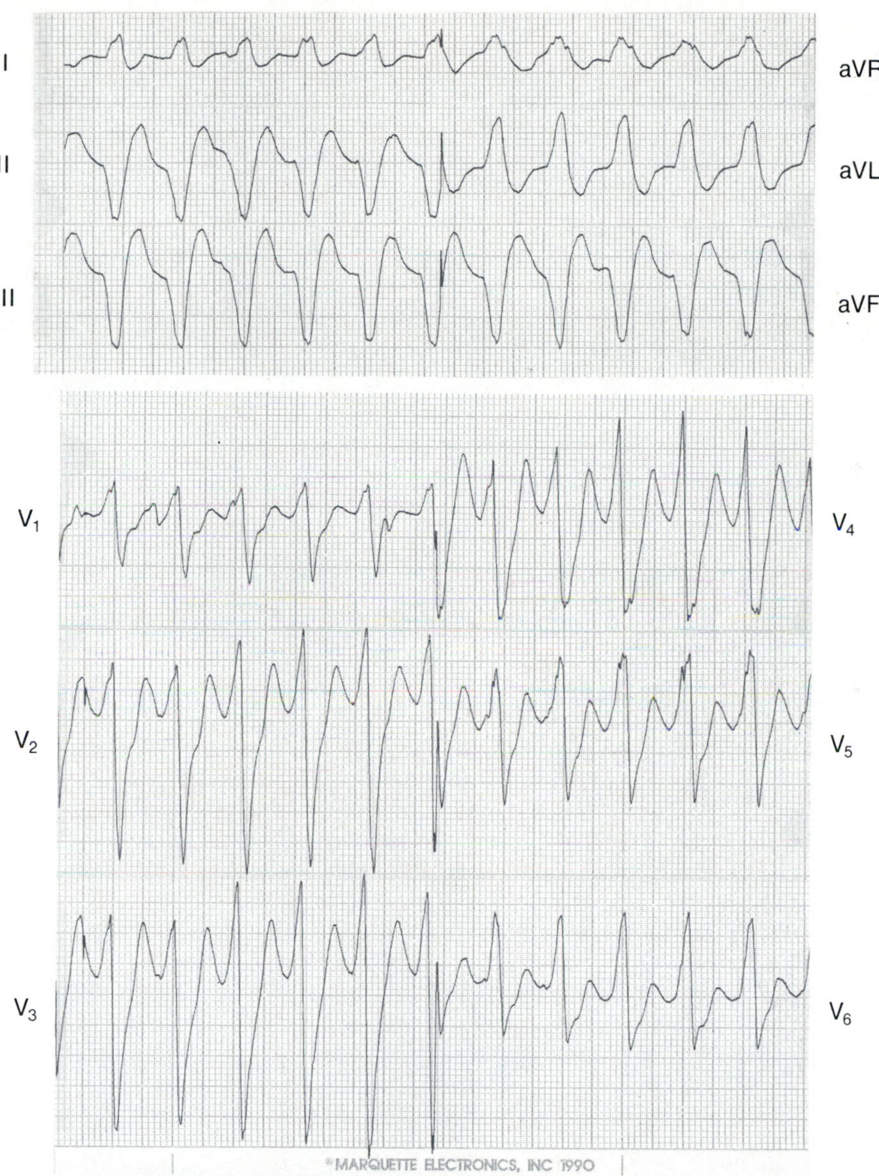

CASE: *Mr. MP is a 60 year old admitted to the telemetry unit to rule out myocardial infarction. He is not taking any medications. He is conscious with a HR of 194 bpm, BP 110/70. He developed the following wide-complex tachycardia shortly after being admitted for evaluation of chest discomfort. Old records are not yet available and the patient reports not having a heart attack in the past. He does report a heavy feeling in his chest with activity during the past few weeks.*

50. Diagnose the tachycardia using the wide QRS tachycardia algorithm.

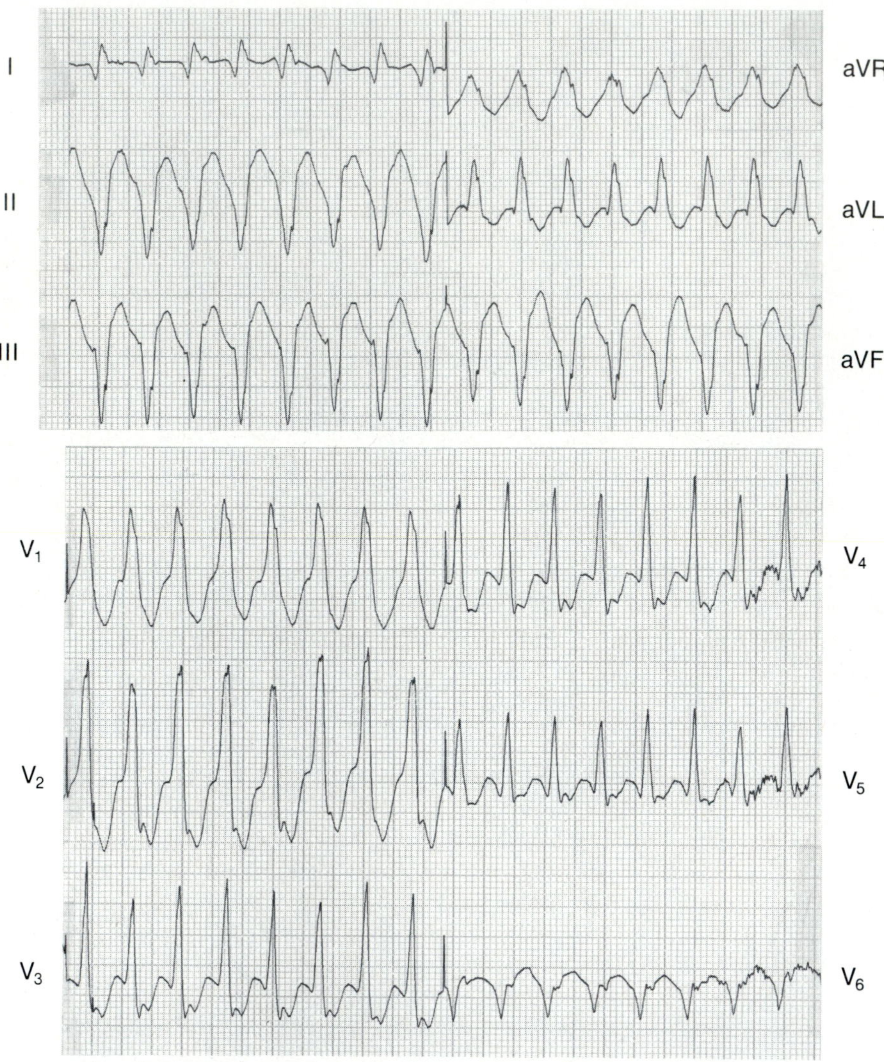

CASE: *Ms. MH is a 73-year-old woman who developed a wide-complex tachycardia* (A) *while hospitalized for evaluation of near-syncopal episodes. Her previous ECG* (B) *is presented for your evaluation and comparison.*

51. Diagnose the tachycardia using the wide QRS tachycardia algorithm.

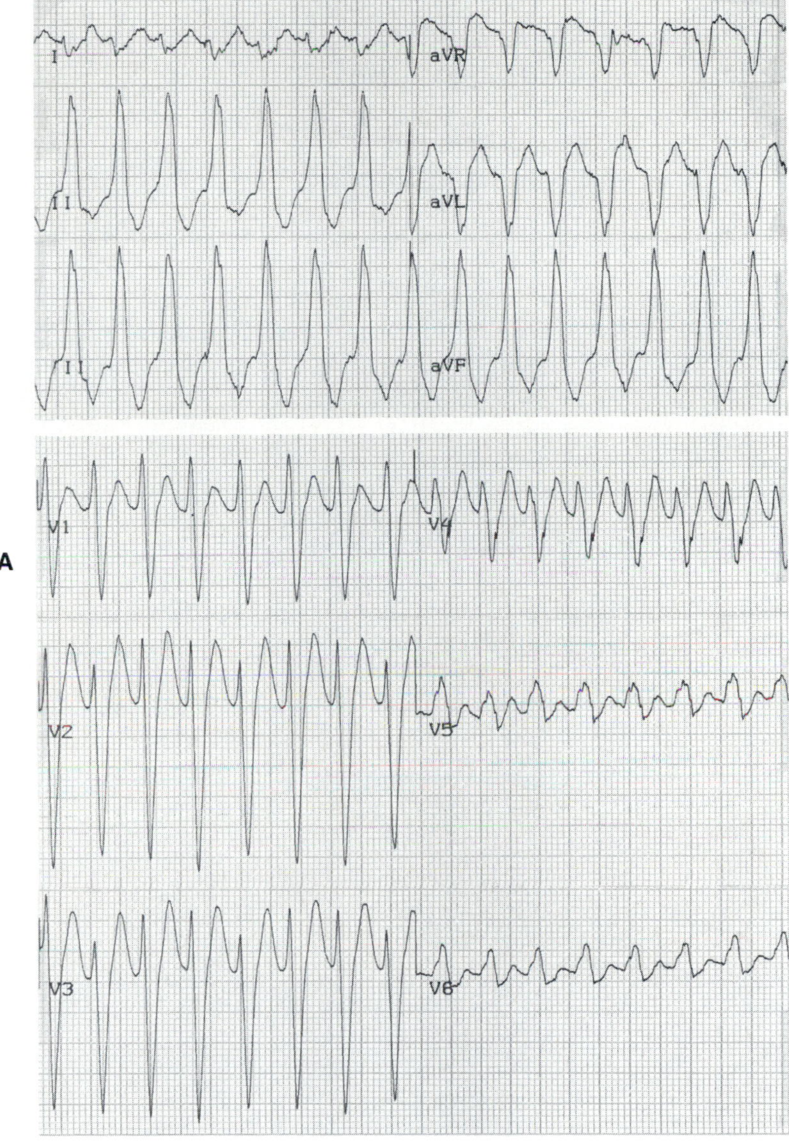

Figure continues.

Figure continued from previous page.

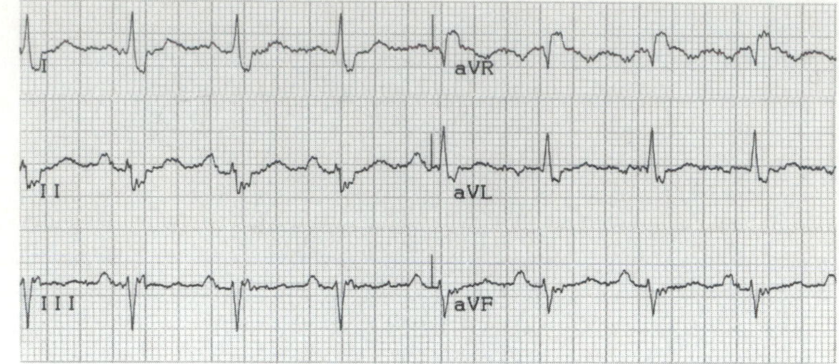

B

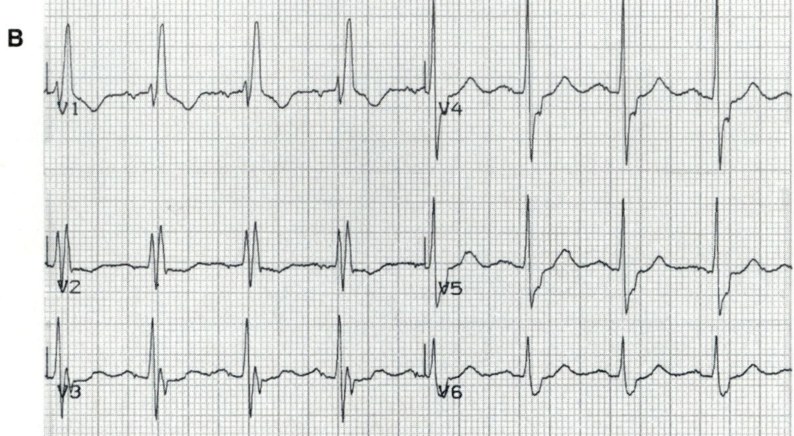

ANSWERS TO SELF-ASSESSMENT

1. C
2. A
3. B, D, E
4. A, B, C, D
5. D
6. B, C, D
7. D
8. A, B, C
9. B, C
10. A, D

11. A
12. B
13. B
14. B
15. C
16. A
17. A
18. B
19. B
20. B
21. A
22. A
23. A
24. B
25. B
26. B

27. F (it can only be used in RBBB aberration vs. ventricular ectopy with upright complex in V_1.)
28. T
29. T
30. T
31. T
32. F
33. F
34. F
35. T
36. F
37. F
38. F
39. F
40. T
41. T
42. T
43. F
44. T
45. F

46. Without a previous ECG, it is necessary to begin with Step 2. There are RS complexes present in the precordial leads V_2 to V_6, the widest of which is found in V_2 where it measures 0.15 to 0.16 seconds, comfortably exceeding 0.10 seconds. The diagnosis is VT.
47. We could stop with Step 2, but other criteria support the diagnosis of VT.

    In proceeding with Step 3, there are hints of independent atrial activity, but they are not definitive. If the clinical situation permits, physical signs of AV dissociation could be sought.

    Step 4: The QRS axis is inferior right (163 degrees), no help.

    Step 5: Precordial concordance is not present.

    Step 6: The QRS is up in V_1 with a monophasic R wave and a taller left peak. Both the monophasic R wave and taller left peak are criteria supporting VT. Additionally, the R/S ratio is <1 in V_6, but we cannot rely on this criterion without ruling out a previous RBBB.

    In summary, Steps 2 and 6 offer criteria supporting the diagnosis of VT.
48. Step 1: Not available.

    Step 2: RS complexes present in V_2 to V_6. In V_1, what at first appears to be an initial r wave, looks suspiciously like AFl waves when we note an identical deflection at the conclusion of the QRS. Indeed, the flutter waves are precisely regular and occur at a rate of 272 bpm. Thus the rhythm is AFl with 2:1 conduction and RBBB aberration. Let's continue with the analysis anyway. In measuring the RS complexes, we know that the initial r wave has an AFl wave superimposed as do the terminal portions of the QRS complex. It is therefore risky to rely on an uncertain RS interval. Even if we were to consider it, the longest RS interval appears to be 0.10 seconds in V_6, not meeting the criterion of exceeding 0.10 seconds.

    Step 3: AV dissociation is not present since flutter waves bear a constant relationship to the QRS complexes.

    Step 4: QRS axis is superior left, no help.

    Step 5: No precordial concordance.

    Step 6: Morphologic criteria are obscured by flutter waves in V_1 and V_6. There is a terminal R wave in V_1 and a terminal S wave in V_6, consistent with RBBB.

    In summary the strongest criterion supporting the diagnosis of supraventricular tachycardia with RBBB aberration is the identification of flutter waves in V_1.
49. Step 1: The patient reports a previous MI and subsequent palpitations so the diagnosis of VT could be made without further investigation. We will proceed with further evaluation to point out additional valuable clues.

    Step 2: RS complexes are present in leads V_1 to V_6 and in all precordial leads appear to measure 0.12 seconds, exceeding the criterion of 0.10 seconds. Again the diagnosis of VT could be made without further investigation, but we will proceed in searching for additional clues to support the diagnosis of VT.

    Step 3: AV dissociation is present and most apparent in lead V_1 with atrial rate of 125 bpm, another strong criterion supporting VT.

    Step 4: QRS axis is superior left, no help.

    Step 5: Precordial concordance not present.

    Step 6: The QRS is biphasic in V_1 with RS configuration, another criterion supporting VT.

    In summary, Steps 1, 2, 3, and to a lesser extent, 6, provide strong evidence supporting VT.

50. Step 1: No previous records are available, but the patient's history is highly suspect of acute MI. In such a situation, we would diagnose VT based on odds alone. However, for instructional purposes, we will proceed with analysis.

    Step 2: RS complexes present in V_3 to V_5 but not sharply demarcated in V_5. In leads V_3 to V_4 the RS measures 0.10 seconds at most, not meeting the criterion, so we will proceed with further analysis.

    Step 3: There is likely atrial activity distoring the pattern, but regular, dissociated P waves are not definitive.

    Step 4: The QRS axis is approximately −85 degrees, no help.

    Step 5: No precordial concordance.

    Step 6: Up in V_1 with a monophasic R wave, a criterion supporting VT.

    In summary, steps 1 and 6 support VT.

51. Step 1: Her previous ECG *(B)* indicates a wide QRS complex resulting from a RBBB. Note rsR′ in V_1 and terminal wide s wave in V_6. Her QRS measures 0.13 seconds. The wide-complex tachycardia does not resemble her RBBB pattern in V_1, since it exhibits a terminal S wave. In examining other leads, the QRS is also markedly different in leads II, III, aVL, aVF and V_2 and does not resemble a typical RBBB pattern. Therefore VT should be diagnosed. For instructional purposes, let's proceed with additional steps.

    Step 2: RS complexes are present in all precordial leads but not sharply demarcated enough in leads V_5 to V_6. In the other leads the RS measures only 0.08 seconds, necessitating further evaluation.

    Step 3: AV dissociation was confirmed by esophageal tracings with an atrial rate of 130 bpm but is not readily discernible on this tracing. Try your luck at identifying the atrial activity at the documented rate of 130 bpm.

    Step 4: The axis is inferior right, of no help at this point.

    Step 5: There is no precordial concordance.

    Step 6: The QRS is predominantly negative in V_1 with the r wave in V_1 approximately 0.06 seconds, exceeding 0.03 seconds, and therefore supporting the diagnosis of VT. The nadir is reached in 0.08 seconds in V_1 and V_2, another point for VT. In the presence of a predominantly negative QRS in V_1 the fact that the QRS axis is right adds support for the diagnosis of VT.

    In summary, Steps 1, 3, 4, and 6 provide clues supporting the diagnosis of VT.

PART THREE

INTERVENTIONS

CHAPTER ELEVEN

Cardioactive Drugs and their Electrocardiographic Effects

▶ GOAL

You will be able to identify and classify the major cardioactive drugs used in the management of cardiac arrhythmias and the primary indications, effects, and nursing responsibilities associated with each classification.

▶ OBJECTIVES

After studying this chapter you should be able to:

1. Classify the antiarrhythmic agents and identify the major drugs of each classification.
2. Describe the general actions of each drug class.
3. Identify the primary indications, electrocardiographic changes, adverse cardiovascular effects, contraindications, and nurse's responsibilities related to the major drugs of each drug class.
4. Identify the dosage administration guidelines for intravenous cardioactive drugs administered in emergency or acute care settings.

▶ CONTENTS

This chapter provides a brief summary and reference to the ECG effects of important cardioactive drugs, as well as the indications and contraindications to their use and the major nursing responsibilities. The purpose is to provide some fundamental guidelines for recognizing significant ECG changes caused by a drug and to supplement information in the text; it is not intended to be a complete reference (see Table 11-1 on p. 336, which describes general actions of the major classifications of antiarrhythmic drugs).

We have presented common or frequently occurring ECG effects only. The text summarizes the drugs listed above. When certain headings are blank, it indicates the effect is not consistently observed. ECG changes (e.g., prolongation of the QT interval) may be therapeutic or a sign of toxicity and are sometimes used as criteria for discontinuing an agent or reducing the dose. It is important to remember that clinical side effects, as well as alterations in the ECG, are frequently dose dependent. Additional precautions are necessary with patients who have renal or hepatic impairment.

Table 11-1 Classification of Antiarrhythmic Agents

Agents	Actions
Class I	
IA Quinidine-like	
Moricizine (IA-IBcombination) Disopyramide Procainamide Quinidine	Suppress sodium channels (block the fast sodium current) Depress depolarization Prolong repolarization and refractoriness ↓ Ectopy ↑ QT interval ↓ Reentry circuits ↑ PR (initially may ↓ PR) ↑ QRS complex Contraindicated in hyperkalemia, IVCD May ↑ left ventricular end-diastolic pressure May ↓ cardiac output *Antidote:* sodium bicarbonate or sodium lactate
IB Lidocaine-like	
Lidocaine Phenytoin Mexiletine Tocainide	Suppress sodium channels (block the fast sodium current) Depress depolarization ↓ Ectopy Shorten repolarization and refractoriness
IC Miscellaneous	
Aprindine Encainide Flecainide Lorcainide Propafenone Indecainide	Suppress sodium channels (block the fast sodium current) Depress depolarization Primarily slow conduction ↑ PR interval ↑ QRS complex ↑ QT interval
Class II Beta-adrenergic blockers	
Metoprolol Atenolol Acebutolol Propranolol Esmolol Timolol	↓ Ectopy ↑ PR interval ↓ Heart rate ↓ Myocardial contractility Bronchial constriction ↓ Myocardial O_2 demand
Class III	
Bretylium Amiodarone Aprindine Sotalol NAPA	Act on repolarization and reentry circuits Prolong repolarization and refractoriness ↓ Intraventricular conduction
Class IV Calcium-channel blockers	
Diltiazem Verapamil	Block the slow calcium channel ↓ Heart rate ↑ PR interval

Dosage considerations, such as pharmacokinetics and combination therapies, have not been addressed. Some of the drugs cited are investigational and conclusive dosage data have not yet been established. Dosage recommendations frequently change as new studies provide us with ever-increasing knowledge about pharmacologic arrhythmia control. Moreover, dosage depends on the patient, the patient's condition and response to a drug, the severity of the arrhythmia, and whether the drug is used in combination with other antiarrhythmic(s). We therefore have limited the inclusion of specific dosage information and intravenous administration guidelines to those drugs that nurses and paramedics administer independently, in emergency situations, according to institutional guidelines.

ACEBUTOLOL (Sectral)

Classification: Class II antiarrhythmic with beta blocker activity (cardioselective).

Route: Oral.

Indications: Hypertension and ventricular arrhythmias.

ECG Effects
- HEART RATE: Decreases.
- PR INTERVAL: Prolongs.
- QRS COMPLEX: No change.
- QT INTERVAL: Shortens.
- T WAVE:
- U WAVE:
- BLOCK: AV Block.

Adverse Cardiovascular Effects: Hypotension and bradycardia.

Contraindications: Severe bradycardia, second and third degree AV blocks, overt congestive heart failure (CHF), and cardiogenic shock.

Nurse's Responsibilities
- As with all patients receiving beta-adrenergic blockers, assess pulmonary status on a regular basis.

- Monitor blood pressure and heart rate.
- Assess for CHF and diminished cardiac output.
- If patient has bronchospastic disease, assess respiratory status.
- Patient teaching: do not interrupt dosage schedule.

Notes: Patient instructions are generally the same as those used for other beta-blocking agents, and the reader should refer to other sources for a full discussion. As with all beta blockers, there should be no abrupt withdrawal of this medication or interruption of its schedule, especially by a patient with coronary artery disease.

Only acebutolol, metoprolol, propranolol, and timolol have been approved to treat arrhythmias or to prevent sudden death after myocardial infarction (MI).

ADENOSINE
Adenocard

Classification: Unclassified. Adenosine is an endogenous nucleoside present throughout the body that has potent electrophysiologic and antiarrhythmic effects.

Route: Parenteral.

Indications: Primary therapy of wide QRS-complex supraventricular tachycardia; paroxysmal supraventricular tachycardia (including PSVT associated with Wolff-Parkinson-White [WPW] syndrome), AV nodal reentrant tachycardia, and circus movement tachycardia.

ECG Effects

- HEART RATE: Biphasic effect: adenosine depresses SA node activity and slows sinus rate. A bolus-induced sinus bradycardia may be followed by sinus tachycardia.
- PR INTERVAL: Prolongs.
- QRS COMPLEX:
- QT INTERVAL:
- T WAVE:
- U WAVE:
- BLOCK: May produce first, second, or third degree heart block after bolus administration.

Adverse Cardiovascular Effects: Adenosine is a potent vasodilator and may reduce systemic blood pressure. It may cause facial flushing and shortness of breath/dyspnea/chest pressure. It may initiate atrial flutter.

Contraindications: Second or third degree AV block and sick sinus syndrome (SSS) (except in patients with functioning artificial pacemaker), atrial flutter/fibrillation, ventricular tachycardia (VT).

Nurse's Responsibilities

- Monitor blood pressure and ECG.
- Adenosine is generally given as a rapid intravenous bolus: the initial adult dose is 6 mg given as a rapid IV bolus over a 1- to 2-second period. A 12-mg dose may be ordered for repeat administration if the first dose does not result in elimination of the arrhythmia. The bolus is generally followed by a saline flush. Termination generally occurs within 30 seconds after drug injection.
- Take precautions in patients taking dipyridamole.

Notes: Fast acting; arrhythmias may recur; side effects are common but transient. The overall efficacy of adenosine is similar to that of verapamil, but its onset of action is more rapid and it has a shorter half-life.

AMIODARONE
Cordarone

Classification: Class III antiarrhythmic.

Route: Oral, parenteral.

Indications: VT, supraventricular tachyarrhythmias including those associated with WPW syndrome, paroxysmal atrial flutter, paroxysmal atrial fibrillation without organic heart disease, AV nodal tachycardia, and circus-movement tachycardia.

ECG Effects

- HEART RATE: Decreases.
- PR INTERVAL: Prolongs.
- QRS COMPLEX: May widen.
- QT INTERVAL: Prolongs.
- T WAVE: Deforms.
- U WAVE: May appear if concurrently taking digoxin.
- BLOCK: May produce bundle branch block. Aggravates intraventricular conduction delay (IVCD). May cause AV block.

Adverse Cardiovascular Effects: In higher doses, it may worsen CHF; sinus bradycardia, polymorphous VT (torsades de pointes). During IV administration, it may cause temporary hypotension, AV block, hot flashes, or complete cardiovascular collapse.

Contraindications: CHF, bradycardia, AV blocks, SSS, and IVCD. IV administration is not advised if cardiomegaly secondary to cardiomyopathy is present.

Nurse's Responsibilities

- Assess for manifestations of CHF.
- Check for improvement in angina, since it has an antianginal effect.
- Measure QT and PR intervals and heart rate often.
- Obtain digoxin level, if indicated.
- Obtain prothrombin time, if on warfarin.
- Neurologic assessment.
- Respiratory assessment.
- Monitor thyroid and hepatic function.
- Administer artificial tears four times daily.
- Patient teaching: Avoid skin exposure to sun; may cause gray-blue discoloration.
- When administering IV, dilute in 20 ml 5% dextrose in water and inject over 10 minutes. Wait 15 minutes be-

fore repeating. May cause tachycardia if injected too quickly.
- Instruct patient that toxic reactions may develop long after hospital discharge.

Notes: Amiodarone has a half-life of 45 days (or longer); side effects are not immediately apparent. Side effects include corneal microdeposits that cause visual halos or blurred vision, nausea, anorexia, vomiting, pulmonary abnormalities including infiltrates and fibrosis, thyroid abnormalities, skin discoloration and photosensitization, hepatic toxicity, and neurologic abnormalities such as sleep disturbances and tremor. It may cause elevated serum digoxin levels. It may potentiate the bradycardic action of beta blockers, digitalis, and some calcium antagonists. It may potentiate the action of warfarin. Amiodarone may also elevate serum total cholesterol and triglyceride levels.

APRINDINE HYDROCHLORIDE

Classification: Class IC antiarrhythmic.

Route: Oral, parenteral.

Indications: Ventricular and supraventricular arrhythmias.

ECG Effects
- HEART RATE:
- PR INTERVAL: May prolong.
- QRS COMPLEX: Widens.
- QT INTERVAL: Prolongs.
- T WAVE:
- U WAVE:
- BLOCK:

Adverse Cardiovascular Effects: Polymorphic VT (torsades de pointes).

Contraindications:

Nurse's Responsibilities
- Neurologic assessment.
- Assess QTc regularly.
- Monitor CBC and bilirubin weekly.

Notes: Aprindine produces a variety of noncardiac side effects, primarily neurologic: tremors, dizziness, ataxia, hallucinations, and seizures, as well as agranulocytosis.

ATENOLOL
Tenormin

Classification: Beta blocker (cardioselective) with antiarrhythmia properties.

Route: Oral.

Indications: Hypertension, angina, and cardiac arrhythmias (SVT and any arrhythmia modulated by the sympathetic nervous system).

ECG Effects
- HEART RATE: Decreases.
- PR INTERVAL: Prolongs.
- QRS COMPLEX:
- QT INTERVAL:
- T WAVE:
- U WAVE:
- BLOCK: AV block possible.

Adverse Cardiovascular Effects: Bradycardia, hypotension, and AV block; may intensify impaired LV function or CHF.

Contraindications: Sinus bradycardia, heart block greater than first degree, cardiogenic shock, overt cardiac failure, asthma, and chronic obstructive pulmonary disease.

Nurse's Responsibilities
- Assess patient for bronchoconstriction.
- Determine whether patient has a history of asthma or wheezing.

Notes: Atenolol is convenient for the patient because it is a once-a-day drug. Atenolol has been shown to be effective in the suppression of paroxysmal VT in children whose tachycardia was precipitated or exacerbated by exercise or catecholamines.

ATROPINE SULFATE

Classification: Parasympatholytic (decreases vagal tone).

Route: Parenteral, endotracheal.

Indications: Symptomatic bradycardias and asystole.

ECG Effects
- HEART RATE: Increases.
- PR INTERVAL: Shortens.
- QRS COMPLEX:
- QT INTERVAL:
- T WAVE:
- U WAVE:
- BLOCK: See "Notes."

Adverse Cardiovascular Effects: May increase heart rate dangerously in the presence of rapid atrial tachyarrhythmias such as atrial fibrillation or flutter. VT and ventricular fibrillation (VF) have been noted after administration in patients with acute MI/acute ischemia.

Contraindications: Rapid atrial tachyarrhythmias. Avoid its use, if possible, in immediate post-MI period (increases myocardial oxygen consumption). Avoid, if possible, in presence of glaucoma (see "Nurse's Responsibilities").

Nurse's Responsibilities
- Assess patient's tolerance of increased heart rate.
- Anticipate complaints of dry mouth and inability to void.
- Administration may precipitate an acute attack of glau-

coma in susceptible individuals. Be certain to administer patient's pilocarpine drops (or similar agent) if atropine is required.
- Since atropine impairs sweat reflex, it is dangerous in hot environments.

Notes: In patients with first degree or Type I second degree AV blocks, atropine may increase the atrial rate to such an extent that the AV junction is not able to conduct as many of the atrial impulses, resulting in what appears to be a worse AV block. This subsides when effects of atropine diminish. Subtherapeutic doses may decrease heart rate. Principal adverse effects are dryness of mouth and skin and pupillary dilatation. Neck-up blush is common. May cause changes in psychologic state.

Dosage
IV

Adults—0.01 to 0.03 mg/kg (this is roughly 0.5 to 1.0 mg). A full vagolytic dose is 2.0 mg in most patients.

Infants and Children—It is important to give a vagolytic dose (minimum dose for infants is 0.1 mg). 0.02 mg/kg every 5 minutes to maximum dose of 1.0 mg in child and 2.0 mg in adolescent.

Endotracheal

Adults—1 to 2 mg diluted in 10 ml sterile water or normal saline.

Infants and Children—Same as IV dose.

Antidote

Physostigmine 0.5 to 2.0 mg IV.

BRETYLIUM TOSYLATE
Bretylol

Classification: Class III antiarrhythmic.

Route: Parenteral, oral.

Indications: Emergency treatment of refractory VT and VF.

ECG Effects
- HEART RATE: Initial increase.
- PR INTERVAL:
- QRS COMPLEX:
- QT INTERVAL:
- T WAVE:
- U WAVE:
- BLOCK:

Adverse Cardiovascular Effects: Postural hypotension after initial hypertension, tachycardia, and an increase in ectopic beats.

Contraindications: None in the presence of VF. Digitalis toxicity contraindicates treatment of ventricular ectopy.

Nurse's Responsibilities
- Monitor blood pressure.
- If the patient is conscious, give IV dose slowly. Nausea and vomiting often accompany rapid administration.
- Since postural hypotension is very common, do not elevate head of bed.

Notes: Bretylium is thought to enhance digitalis toxicity and should be avoided in this situation. Bretylium initially causes release of norepinephrine from nerve terminals, resulting in transient tachycardia and hypertension. However, it ultimately prevents the release of norepinephrine, contributing to orthostatic hypotension and heart rate blunting.

Dosage
IV

Adults—For VF, 5 to 10 mg/kg every 15 to 30 minutes as needed to a total of 30 mg/kg.

For VT, 5 to 10 mg/kg slowly (over 10 minutes). May repeat in 1 to 2 hours, then every 6 to 8 hours. Or may be administered as a continuous infusion at a rate of 2 mg/min.

Children—For VF, 5 mg/kg by rapid IV infusion. Repeat 10 mg/kg.

For VT, 5 mg/kg slowly (over 8 to 10 minutes). May repeat in 20 minutes.

DIGOXIN
Lanoxin

Classification: Cardiac glycoside.

Route: Oral, parenteral.

Indications: CHF. Paroxysmal supraventricular tachycardia, atrial fibrillation, atrial flutter, and AV nodal tachycardia.

ECG Effects
- HEART RATE: Decreases.
- PR INTERVAL: Prolongs.
- QRS COMPLEX:
- QT INTERVAL: Shortens.
- T WAVE: Alters configuration, flattens.
- ST SEGMENT: Sags, depresses.
- U WAVE: Present.
- BLOCK: May cause AV and SA block.

Adverse Cardiovascular Effects: Bradycardia, SA block, sinus arrhythmia, AV block, junctional rhythms, ventricular ectopy, atrial tachycardia (AT) with block, asystole. May accelerate AV conduction in WPW syndrome.

Contraindications: AV block and WPW syndrome.

Nurse's Responsibilities
- Monitor serum potassium and digoxin levels.
- Assess PR interval frequently.
- Detect signs of toxicity: anorexia, nausea, vomiting, diarrhea, abdominal pain, yellow vision, accelerated junctional rhythm, AT with block, ventricular bigeminy, AV block, bradycardia, and SA block.

Notes: Hypokalemia facilitates and hyperkalemia suppresses digitalis-induced arrhythmias. Quinidine enhances the effect of digoxin. Concomitant use with beta blockers may cause severe bradycardia. Generally digoxin is discontinued before elective cardioversion if the patient is clinically digoxin toxic.

DILTIAZEM HYDROCHLORIDE
Cardizem

Classification: Class IV antiarrhythmic, calcium-channel blocker.

Route: Oral.

Indications: Exertional angina, angina because of coronary artery spasm, moderate essential hypertension, atrial flutter, circus-movement tachycardia, SVT, and controlling the ventricular response to atrial fibrillation/flutter.

ECG Effects
- HEART RATE: May decrease.
- PR INTERVAL: Prolongs.
- QRS COMPLEX:
- QT INTERVAL:
- T WAVE:
- U WAVE:
- BLOCK: AV block.

Adverse Cardiovascular Effects: May cause/worsen AV block, bradycardia, and hypotension.

Contraindications: Severe hypotension, SSS, second and third degree AV blocks unless pacemaker in use.

Nurse's Responsibilities
- Monitor blood pressure.
- Assess PR interval frequently.

Notes: Diltiazem favorably affects lipid metabolism with an increase in high density lipoproteins and decrease in triglycerides. Side effects may include dizziness and edema.

DISOPYRAMIDE
Norpace, Norpace-CR

Classification: Class IA antiarrhythmic.

Route: Oral.

Indications: Ventricular arrhythmias, AV nodal tachycardia, and circus-movement tachycardia.

ECG Effects
- HEART RATE: Variable changes.
- PR INTERVAL: Variable changes, AV block.
- QRS COMPLEX: Widens.
- QT INTERVAL: Prolongs.
- T WAVE:
- U WAVE: Present.
- BLOCK: AV block.

Adverse Cardiovascular Effects: Negative inotropic effect may worsen CHF. Hypotension, ventricular tachyarrhythmias including torsades de pointes, and AV block.

Contraindications: Cardiogenic shock, second and third degree AV blocks unless functioning pacemaker in use, uncompensated heart failure, obstructive uropathy, glaucoma, long QT syndrome, hypokalemia, and torsades de pointes.

Nurse's Responsibilities
- Monitor blood pressure.
- Measure QT and PR intervals and QRS complex.
- Assess for CHF.
- Take measures to relieve complaints of persistent dry mouth.
- Instruct patient to prevent constipation by increasing dietary intake of fresh fruits and vegetables. Request dietitian consultation.
- Notify physician to discontinue administration if AV block develops, QRS widens by more than 25%, or QT interval lengthens by more than 25% above baseline.

Notes: Disopyramide causes dry mouth, urinary retention, esophageal reflux, and constipation. Warfarin enhances the drug's effect.

ENCAINIDE
Enkaid

Classification: Class IC antiarrhythmic.

Route: Oral, parenteral.

Indications: Ventricular (malignant ventricular tachyarrhythmias) and supraventricular arrhythmias, AV nodal tachycardia, circus-movement tachycardia, refractory atrial fibrillation/flutter.

ECG Effects
- HEART RATE:
- PR INTERVAL: Prolongs. Also prolongs P wave.
- QRS COMPLEX: Widens.
- QT INTERVAL: May prolong.
- T WAVE:
- U WAVE:
- BLOCK: AV block possible.

Adverse Cardiovascular Effects: Polymorphous ventricular tachycardia; possible atrial proarrhythmic effects.

Contraindications: SSS and conduction block (unless a pacemaker is present).

Nurse's Responsibilities
- Assess for new or modified symptomatic atrial arrhythmias with rapid ventricular response.
- Assess for recurrence of ventricular arrhythmias.

- Measure PR and QT intervals and QRS complex regularly. Expect a 20% to 40% increase in PR interval and QRS complex at therapeutic dosages.
- Good oral hygiene may help alleviate metallic taste.
- Assess the presence of side effects (see "Notes").
- Administer with meals.

Notes: Encainide produces a variety of neurologic side effects including tinnitus, dizziness, diplopia, ataxia, and tremors; metallic taste is common.

The recent Cardiac Arrhythmia Suppression Trial reported that patients with decreased left ventricular function and asymptomatic ventricular arrhythmias after MI experienced increased sudden cardiac death mortality when treated with flecainide or encainide compared with similar placebo-treated patients.

Encainide has been effective in the treatment of some resistant forms of permanent junctional reciprocating tachycardia and AV reciprocating tachycardia in children who are otherwise healthy. However, children with previous proarrhythmic events or severe cardiac dysfunction, and children under 6 months of age, have had a high incidence of adverse effects from the drug.

Based on continuing uncertainty regarding the implications of the recent Cardiac Arrhythmia Suppression Trial (CAST), in addition to the availability of a growing number of alternative therapies, Bristol Laboratories discontinued sales and commercial distribution of Enkaid effective December 16, 1991. However, certain patients with life-threatening, documented ventricular arrhythmias remain on Enkaid therapy through the Enkaid Continuing Patient Access Program sponsored by Bristol Laboratories.*

EPINEPHRINE
Adrenalin Chloride

Classification: Sympathomimetic amine.

Route: Parenteral, endotracheal.

Indications: Asystole, electromechanical dissociation, fine VF, agonal rhythms, IVR, and shock.

ECG Effects
- HEART RATE: Increases.
- PR INTERVAL: Decreases.
- QRS COMPLEX:
- QT INTERVAL:
- T WAVE:
- U WAVE:
- BLOCK:

Adverse Cardiovascular Effects: May cause VT or VF. Increases myocardial oxygen consumption. Hypertension.

Contraindications: Tachycardia.

*Personal correspondance, Bristol Laboratories, 2400 West Lloyd Expressway, Evansville, Indiana 47721-0001, September 30, 1991.

Nurse's Responsibilities

Never mix with alkaline solutions such as sodium bicarbonate. Epinephrine and other related sympathomimetic drugs are inactivated in alkaline solution.

Notes: Epinephrine is used during resuscitation to produce increases in systemic vascular resistance, blood pressure, heart rate, coronary and cerebral blood flow, myocardial contraction, and automaticity; and to make VF more susceptible to DC countershock.

Dosage

IV

Adults—0.5 to 1.0 mg (1:10,000 solution) every 5 minutes or more as needed.

Children—0.1 ml/kg (1:10,000 solution) every 5 minutes as needed.

Endotracheal

Adults—Inject 1.0 mg diluted with 10 ml normal saline or sterile water into endotracheal tube then apply positive pressure ventilation.

Children—0.1 ml/kg (1:10,000 solution) every 5 minutes as needed.

Continuous IV infusion

Adults—1 mg in 250 ml 5% dextrose in water initially at 2 μg/min and titrated to effect.

Children—Formula for infusion: 0.6 × body weight (kg) = mg dose added to make 100 ml. Then 1 ml/hr delivers 0.1 μg/kg/min. Initiate infusion at 0.1 μg/kg/min.

ESMOLOL
Brevibloc

Classification: Class II antiarrhythmic (cardioselective beta blocker).

Route: Parenteral.

Indications: Supraventricular tachyarrhythmias (sinus tachycardia, atrial flutter, atrial fibrillation), perioperative tachycardia, and hypertension.

ECG Effects

- HEART RATE: Decreases.
- PR INTERVAL: May prolong.
- QRS COMPLEX:
- QT INTERVAL: May shorten.
- T WAVE:
- U WAVE:
- BLOCK: AV block possible.

Adverse Cardiovascular Effects: Transient hypotension, AV block, and heart failure. Decreases left ventricular ejection fraction.

Contraindications: Severe renal impairment markedly increases the drug's elimination half-life. Administer with caution to those with left ventricular dysfunction.

Nurse's Responsibilities
- Monitor hemodynamics closely in those patients with left ventricular dysfunction.
- Assess for skin irritation at the IV site. Avoid the use of butterfly needles and administration of esmolol concentrations greater than 10 mg/ml.
- Do not mix IV preparation with sodium bicarbonate or with other drugs before dilution.
- Closely monitor patients with coronary artery disease when esmolol administration is abruptly discontinued.
- Assess pulmonary status on a regular basis.

Notes: Esmolol is an ultrashort-acting beta-adrenergic blocking agent (with a half-life of only 9 minutes) and may be safe in patients with mild valvular heart disease, mild chronic obstructive pulmonary disease, and mild congestive heart failure because of a tachycardia. Side effects include hypotension, nausea, and, rarely, somnolence, confusion, headache, agitation, fatigue, paresthesia, asthenia, depression, abnormal thinking, anxiety, anorexia, light-headedness, bronchospasm, dyspnea, and nasal congestion.

FLECAINIDE ACETATE
Tambocor

Classification: Class IC antiarrhythmic.

Route: Oral.

Indications: Ventricular arrhythmias, AV nodal tachycardia, circus-movement tachycardia, and atrial arrhythmias (including refractory atrial fibrillation/flutter).

ECG Effects
- HEART RATE: May decrease.
- PR INTERVAL: Prolongs.
- QRS COMPLEX: Widens.
- QT INTERVAL: Prolongs (because of widening of QRS).
- T WAVE:
- U WAVE:
- BLOCK: Possible SA, AV, and bundle branch blocks.

Adverse Cardiovascular Effects: Exacerbation of ventricular arrhythmias. May worsen conduction abnormalities in AV and SA nodes. May exacerbate CHF. Possible atrial proarrhythmic effects.

Contraindications: Second and third degree AV blocks (unless pacemaker functioning). Cardiogenic shock. Right bundle branch block (RBBB) with hemiblock (unless pacemaker). Use with extreme caution in SSS.

Nurse's Responsibilities
- Assess for new or modified symptomatic atrial arrhythmias with rapid ventricular response.
- Assess continuous ECG monitor frequently during initial dosing.
- Measure PR and QT intervals and QRS complex at regular intervals. Almost all patients develop first degree AV block. When the PR interval exceeds 0.30 seconds or the QRS increases by 50%, notify physician to decrease or discontinue drug.
- If patient has pacemaker, assess frequently for failure to pace.
- Assess for development of side effects (below).
- Assess for signs and symptoms of CHF.
- Evaluate frequency of ventricular arrhythmias.
- Patient teaching: instruct patient that drug should be taken every 12 hours.

Notes: Flecainide has been reported to produce dizziness, visual disturbances, headache, nausea, dyspnea, chest pain, and tremor. It raises endocardial pacing thresholds and may suppress ventricular escape rhythms. Pacemaker-dependent patients may need reprogramming of their pacemaker.

The recent Cardiac Arrhythmia Suppression Trial (CAST) reported that patients with decreased left ventricular function and asymptomatic ventricular arrhythmias after MI experienced increased sudden cardiac death mortality when treated with flecainide or encainide compared with similar placebo-treated patients.

Flecainide has been found to be effective for the treatment of supraventricular and ventricular arrhythmias in children and young adults.

INDECAINIDE

Classification: Class IC antiarrhythmic.

Route: Oral, parenteral.

Indications: Ventricular arrhythmias.

ECG Effects
- HEART RATE:
- PR INTERVAL: May prolong.
- QRS COMPLEX: May widen.
- QT INTERVAL:
- T WAVE:
- U WAVE:
- BLOCK:

Adverse Cardiovascular Effects: Aggravation of arrhythmia.

Contraindications:

Nurse's Responsibilities
- Assess neurologic system.
- Monitor ECG regularly and frequently.

Notes: Neurologic side effects are common. The potentially serious neurologic and cardiovascular side effects that occur after indecainide administration limit its usefulness.

ISOPROTERENOL HYDROCHLORIDE
Isuprel

Classification: Sympathomimetic amine.

Route: Parenteral, sublingual.

Indications: Immediate and temporary control of hemodynamically significant and atropine-refractory second and third degree AV blocks, bradycardia, and idioventricular rhythm.

ECG Effects
- HEART RATE: Increases.
- PR INTERVAL: Shortens.
- QRS COMPLEX: Increases ectopic activity.
- QT INTERVAL:
- T WAVE:
- U WAVE:
- BLOCK: Decreases AV block.

Adverse Cardiovascular Effects: Ventricular arrhythmias, including VT and VF. Markedly increased myocardial oxygen demand that may induce or exacerbate myocardial ischemia. Decreased systemic arterial resistance (decreased blood pressure). Potent inotropic and chronotropic effects. Lowers coronary perfusion pressure during cardiac arrest.

Contraindications: Tachyarrhythmias resulting from digoxin toxicity or hypokalemia. Ischemic heart disease. Cardiac arrest. Acute MI. Hypertension.

Nurse's Responsibilities
- Monitor for ventricular arrhythmias, VT, and VF.
- Monitor for signs and symptoms of myocardial ischemia.
- Assess blood pressure frequently.
- Gradually increase IV dose only until desired effect achieved, then stabilize dosage.
- Never administer undiluted.
- Use only until artificial pacing can be initiated.

Notes: Isoproterenol should not be administered with epinephrine. Safer agents have replaced isoproterenol in most clinical settings.

Dosage
IV infusion

Adults—1 mg diluted in 500 ml 5% dextrose in water at 2 to 10 μg/min.

Children—Formula for infusion: 0.6 × body weight (kg) = mg dose added to make 100 ml. Then 1 ml/hr delivers 0.1 μg/kg/min. Initiate infusion at 0.1 μg/kg/min.

LIDOCAINE HYDROCHLORIDE
Xylocaine

Classification: Class IB antiarrhythmic.

Route: Parenteral, endotracheal

Indications: Ventricular arrhythmias. Prophylaxis against VF in presence of acute MI.

ECG Effects
- HEART RATE:
- PR INTERVAL:
- QRS COMPLEX: May widen.
- QT INTERVAL:
- T WAVE:
- U WAVE:
- BLOCK: AV block possible.

Adverse Cardiovascular Effects: May accelerate AV conduction initially. Hypotension may occur. Sinus arrest, bradycardia, cardiac standstill, and AV blocks may occur with toxic dosages. May worsen ventricular arrhythmias.

Contraindications: Idioventricular rhythm, Stokes-Adams syndrome, WPW syndrome, and severe heart block.

Nurse's Responsibilities
- Monitor blood pressure.
- Watch for symptoms of lidocaine toxicity (see "Notes.")
- Use with caution in presence of atrial flutter with rapid ventricular response.
- Precede increases in infusion rate with 50 mg bolus.
- 360 mg/hour is considered maximum dosage.
- Elderly patients and those with impaired hepatic blood flow (acute MI, congestive heart failure, or shock) require decreased dosages (half).
- Monitor blood lidocaine level closely after 24 hours of administration.
- Bolus administered at a rate greater than 50 mg/min may cause seizures.

Notes: Lidocaine produces a variety of noncardiac (primarily neurologic) side effects: respiratory depression, light-headedness, apprehension, slurred speech, confusion, dizziness, tinnitus, blurred vision, tremors, convulsions, and coma. See the ACC/AHA Task force report.

Dosage
Cardiac arrest IV

Adults—1 mg/kg initial bolus (not to exceed a total of 100 mg). Repeat 0.5 mg/kg every 8 to 10 minutes to a total of 3 mg/kg as indicated. After restoration of circulation, continuous infusion at 2 to 4 mg/min (1 g diluted in 250 ml 5% dextrose in water = 4 mg/ml).

Children—1 mg/kg. May repeat in 10 to 15 minutes. Continuous infusion of 120 mg in 100 ml 5% dextrose and water at 20 to 50 μg/kg/min (1 to 2.5 ml/kg/hr).

Endotracheal

Children—same dose as IV.

Primary prophylaxis against VF

Adults—1.5 mg/kg (not to exceed a total of 100 mg) followed by continuous infusion of 2 to 4 mg/min. Repeat bolus of 0.5 mg/kg in 10 minutes. Titrate infusion upward if ventricular ectopy present.

LORCAINIDE

Classification: Class IC antiarrhythmic.

Route: Oral, parenteral.

Indications: Ventricular and supraventricular arrhythmias.

ECG Effects
- HEART RATE:
- PR INTERVAL: Prolongs.
- QRS COMPLEX: Widens.
- QT INTERVAL: Prolongs.
- T WAVE:
- U WAVE:
- BLOCK: AV block.

Adverse Cardiovascular Effects: AV block and aggravation of ventricular arrhythmias.

Contraindications:

Nurse's Responsibilities
- Measure PR and QT intervals and QRS complexes.
- Monitor serum sodium, especially with concomitant diuretic therapy.
- Evaluate effectiveness in suppressing arrhythmias.
- Assess for presence of side effects (see "Notes," below).

Notes: Lorcainide may cause neurologic side effects including dizziness, tremors, blurred vision, nightmares, diaphoresis, and insomnia. Nausea is fairly common. Lorcainide often causes hyponatremia.

MAGNESIUM SULFATE

Classification: Unclassified.

Route: Parenteral.

Indications: Ventricular arrhythmias: particularly polymorphous VT associated with a long QT interval and torsades de pointes.

ECG Effects
- HEART RATE: May increase.
- PR INTERVAL:
- QRS COMPLEX:
- QT INTERVAL: May shorten.
- T WAVE:
- U WAVE:
- BLOCK:

Adverse Cardiovascular Effects: Hypotension resulting from vasodilitation.

Contraindications:

Nurse's Responsibilities
- Monitor blood pressure.

Notes: Transient cutaneous flushing may occur.

METOPROLOL
Lopressor

Classification: Class II antiarrhythmic with beta blocker activity (cardioselective).

Route: Oral, parenteral.

Indications: Multifocal atrial tachycardia, hypertension, angina, post-MI to reduce cardiovascular mortality, and atrial and ventricular arrhythmias that are modulated by the sympathetic nervous system.

ECG Effects
- HEART RATE: Decreases.
- PR INTERVAL: Prolongs.
- QRS COMPLEX:
- QT INTERVAL:
- T WAVE:
- U WAVE:
- BLOCK: AV block possible.

Adverse Cardiovascular Effects: Hypotension, AV block, sinus bradycardia; may intensify impaired LV function or CHF.

Contraindications: Second or third degree heart block, bronchospasm, CHF, and hypotension.

Nurse's Responsibilities
- Continuous ECG and hemodynamic monitoring is required for intravenous, short-term therapy.
- Monitor pulmonary status.
- Monitor heart rate and blood pressure.
- Measure PR interval.
- Determine history of asthma, CHF, and COPD.

Notes: Only metoprolol, acebutolol, propranolol, and timolol have been approved to treat arrhythmias or to prevent sudden cardiac death after MI.

MEXILETINE
Mexitil

Classification: Class IB antiarrhythmic.

Route: Oral, parenteral.

Indications: Ventricular arrhythmias.

ECG Effects
- HEART RATE: Variable.
- PR INTERVAL:
- QRS COMPLEX:
- QT INTERVAL: May shorten.
- T WAVE:
- U WAVE:
- BLOCK:

Adverse Cardiovascular Effects: Bradycardia and hypotension after IV administration. Aggravation of preexisting ventricular arrhythmias and exacerbation of VT.

Contraindications: Cardiogenic shock and second or third degree block unless pacemaker in use.

Nurse's Responsibilities
- Assess for neurologic toxicity (see "Notes," below).
- Administer drug with food or antacids to alleviate gastrointestinal (GI) symptoms.
- Use cautiously in presence of congestive heart failure or severe hypotension.
- Use cautiously in presence of sinus node dysfunction.
- Monitor blood pressure, heart rate, and rhythm.
- Evaluate effectiveness in suppressing arrhythmia.
- Assess for development of side effects (see "Notes," below).

Notes: Mexiletine commonly produces a variety of GI and neurologic side effects similar to those of lidocaine. Side effects may or may not be be dose related and include headache, tremor, dizziness, nystagmus, confusion, blurred vision, ataxia, paresthesias, slurred speech, impaired memory, sleep disturbances, nausea, and vomiting. Occasionally this drug is most effective when used in combination with a Class IA antiarrhythmic. The daily dose of mexiletine should not exceed 1200 mg.

MORICIZINE HYDROCHLORIDE
Ethmozine

Classification: Class IA, IB antiarrhythmic. (This drug is not easily classified.)

Route: Oral.

Indications: Malignant ventricular arrhythmias.

ECG Effects
- HEART RATE:
- PR INTERVAL: Prolongs.
- QRS COMPLEX: Widens.
- QT INTERVAL:
- T WAVE:
- U WAVE:
- BLOCK: May cause AV block.

Adverse Cardiovascular Effects: The incidence of exacerbation of CHF is about 2%.

Contraindications: Second or third degree AV block, bifascicular block, cardiogenic shock, and known hypersensitivity to phenothiazines.

Nurse's Responsibilities
- Assess PR interval and QRS complex regularly.
- Assess for AV block.
- Assess patients with CHF or history of CHF for development of, or increase in, symptoms.

Notes: Moricizine enhances metabolism of diltiazem, decreasing its serum level by about 50%. Diltiazem inhibits metabolism of moricizine so that moricizine level increases.

N-ACETYLPROCAINAMIDE (NAPA)

Classification: Class III antiarrhythmic (even though NAPA is the main metabolite of procainamide). NAPA is a metabolic, degradation byproduct of procainamide.

Route: Oral.

Indications: Ventricular arrhythmias, particularly ventricular tachycardia; atrial arrhythmias and supraventricular tachycardia.

ECG Effects
- HEART RATE:
- PR INTERVAL:
- QRS COMPLEX:
- QT INTERVAL: Prolongs.
- T WAVE:
- U WAVE:
- BLOCK:

Adverse Cardiovascular Effects: Marked QT prolongation and torsades de pointes.

Contraindications: History of torsades de pointes.

Nurse's Responsibilities
- Monitor ECG.
- Measure QT interval and calculate QTc.

Notes: Some patients who are unresponsive to NAPA respond to procainamide and vice versa.

NOREPINEPHRINE
Levophed

Classification: Sympathomimetic amine.

Route: Parenteral.

Indications: Temporary management of hemodynamically significant hypotension that is refractory to other sympathomimetic amines.

ECG Effects
- HEART RATE: Increases.
- PR INTERVAL: Shortens.
- QRS COMPLEX: Increases ventricular ectopic activity.
- QT INTERVAL:
- T WAVE:
- U WAVE:
- BLOCK:

Adverse Cardiovascular Effects: Increases systemic vascular resistance. Increases myocardial oxygen demand. May precipitate arrhythmias.

Contraindications: Hypotension resulting from hypovolemia. In presence of myocardial ischemia, its use is a last resort.

Nurse's Responsibilities
- Infuse into a large vein, preferably a central one.

- Watch for IV infiltration. It will cause sloughing of skin and possibly distal necrosis; infiltrate the IV infiltration site with phentolamine 5 to 10 ml diluted in 10 to 15 ml saline.
- Monitor blood pressure closely (every 5 minutes or preferably with intraarterial monitoring).
- Abrupt cessation may lead to acute severe hypotension.
- Avoid bolus effect, which causes severe hypertension.
- Never administer undiluted.

Notes: Causes renal and mesenteric vasoconstriction.

Dosage

IV infusion

Adults—1 ampule (4 ml) diluted in 500 ml 5% dextrose in water or 5% dextrose in normal saline. Titrate to maintain systolic blood pressure >90 mmHg.

Children—Formula for infusion: 0.6 × body weight (kg) = mg dose added to make 100 ml. Then 1 ml/hr delivers 0.1 μg/kg/min. Initiate infusion at 0.1 μg/kg/min.

PHENYTOIN SODIUM
Dilantin

Classification: Class IB antiarrhythmic, anticonvulsant.

Route: Oral, parenteral.

Indications: Digitalis-induced arrhythmias and seizure disorders.

ECG Effects
- HEART RATE: Decreases.
- PR INTERVAL: Variable.
- QRS COMPLEX:
- QT INTERVAL:
- T WAVE:
- U WAVE:
- BLOCK: AV block possible.

Adverse Cardiovascular Effects: Hypotension, bradycardia, AV block, VF, and asystole.

Contraindications: Complete heart block, sinus bradycardia, and Stokes-Adams attacks.

Nurse's Responsibilities
- Monitor blood pressure and ECG.
- Assess for respiratory depression.
- Watch for early signs of toxicity: nystagmus and slurred speech.
- Do not mix with 5% dextrose in water (will crystallize).
- Flush IV tubing with sterile normal saline before and after administering.
- Rapid IV administration (greater than 50 mg/min) may cause cardiovascular collapse, asystole, VF, and AV blocks.
- Use cautiously in presence of congestive heart failure, hepatic or renal dysfunction, hypotension, myocardial insufficiency, and in patients who are elderly or debilitated.
- Administer oral preparations with food or large glass of water.
- Monitor serum blood levels.
- Patient teaching: do not drink alcohol.
- Dental hygiene is very important.
- Take measures to prevent constipation.
- Check compatibility with patient's other medications.

Notes: Phenytoin causes a wide variety of adverse neurologic, gastrointestinal, dermatologic, hematologic, and connective tissue effects, including ataxia, nystagmus, drowsiness, blood dyscrasias, fever, and rash. It also interacts with many drugs.

PIRMENOL HYDROCHLORIDE

Classification: IA (some IB properties).

Route: Oral.

Indications: Ventricular arrhythmias.

ECG Effects
- HEART RATE:
- PR INTERVAL:
- QRS COMPLEX: Widens.
- QT INTERVAL: Prolongs.
- T WAVE:
- U WAVE:
- BLOCK:

Adverse Cardiovascular Effects: Possible proarrhythmic effect.

Contraindications:

Nurse's Responsibilities
- Regular ECG monitoring.

Notes: Clinical studies to date have reported a noncardiac side effect profile that is quite favorable. Pirmenol may produce an odd taste in the mouth. The drug is used in Europe and remains investigational in this country.

PROCAINAMIDE HYDROCHLORIDE
Pronestyl, Procan SR, Pronestyl-SR

Classification: Class IA antiarrhythmic.

Route: Oral, parenteral.

Indications: Ventricular and supraventricular arrhythmias, including AV nodal tachycardia and circus-movement tachycardia. Emergency treatment of life-threatening ventricular arrhythmias if lidocaine is not effective.

ECG Effects
- HEART RATE: Variable.
- PR INTERVAL: Prolongs.

- QRS COMPLEX: Widens; may decrease QRS voltage (height).
- QT INTERVAL: Prolongs.
- T WAVE: May decrease voltage.
- U WAVE:
- BLOCK: AV block and bundle branch block possible.

Adverse Cardiovascular Effects: Worsening of ventricular arrhythmias including VT, VF, and torsades de pointes. Hypotension. May worsen AV block and bundle branch block. Asystole.

Contraindications: Severe or complete heart block, myasthenia gravis, long QT syndrome, hypokalemia, and history of torsades de pointes.

Nurse's Responsibilities
- Monitor blood pressure.
- Measure PR and QT intervals and QRS complex duration regularly.
- Obtain serum procainamide levels.
- Administer IV doses cautiously to patients with acute MI.
- Assess for signs of systemic lupus erythematosus (SLE) and fully inform the patient of the symptoms of SLE, which are reversible on discontinuation of procainamide.
- Monitor serum potassium.
- Discontinue IV dosage if one of the following occurs:
    The arrhythmia is suppressed.
    Hypotension.
    QRS widens by 50%.
    A total of 1 gm has been administered.
- Patients with left ventricular dysfunction and/or renal failure require decreased dosages.
- Take measures to improve the patient's appetite. Offer oral care frequently. Request consultation with a dietitian.

Notes: When used for the treatment of atrial flutter/atrial fibrillation, the ventricular rate may increase as the atrial rate decreases. Procainamide may also cause SLE-like syndrome and agranulocytosis. Hyperkalemia enhances procainamide toxicity. Anorexia, nausea, and bitter taste commonly occur. A high percentage of patients must discontinue procainamide therapy in the first 6 months because of adverse effects.

Dosage

IV

Adults—50 mg every 5 minutes to maximum dose of 1 gm or discontinuation criterion met (see "Nurse's Responsibilities"). For urgent situations: 100 mg every 5 minutes as needed to maximum of 10 doses (1 gm), no faster than 20 mg/min.

IV infusion

1 to 4 mg/min.

PROPAFENONE HYDROCHLORIDE
Rythmol

Classification: Class IC antiarrhythmic.

Route: Oral, parenteral.

Indications: Ventricular (sustained VT) and supraventricular arrhythmias, paroxysmal atrial fibrillation without organic heart disease (catecholamine sensitive), AV nodal tachycardia, circus-movement tachycardia, and atrial flutter.

ECG Effects
- HEART RATE: Slight decrease at high doses.
- PR INTERVAL: Prolongs.
- QRS COMPLEX: Widens.
- QT INTERVAL:
- T WAVE:
- U WAVE:
- BLOCK: SA, AV, and bundle branch block possible.

Adverse Cardiovascular Effects: Exacerbation of CHF, AV block, sinus arrest, intraventricular conduction delay, new bundle branch block, aggravation of ventricular arrhythmias, and atrial flutter in patients treated for atrial fibrillation.

Contraindications: Uncontrolled CHF, cardiogenic shock, SSS, AV block, bradycardia, marked hypotension, bronchospastic disorders, and electrolyte imbalance.

Nurse's Responsibilities
- Assess PR interval and QRS complex regularly.
- Assess CHF patients for increase in symptoms.
- Evaluate suppression of arrhythmias.
- Assess for development of side effects (see "Notes").
- If alteration in taste is present, alert patient to avoid use of excessive salt in seasoning foods. Obtain dietitian consultation.
- Assess prothrombin time in patients taking warfarin (may be increased in prothrombin time by 25%).

Notes: Gastrointestinal side effects commonly reported include nausea, vomiting, constipation, and alteration in taste or smell. Dizziness and fatigue may also occur. Propafenone also has beta-blocking properties.

On the basis of the Cardiac Arrhythmia Suppression Trial findings, the Food and Drug Administration relabeled encainide and flecainide as being indicated only in patients with documented life-threatening ventricular arrhythmias. Propafenone has FDA approval with the same labeling. Therefore the other indications listed are unapproved uses under FDA standards.

PROPRANOLOL
Inderal, Inderal LA, Inderide

Classification: Class II antiarrhythmic (nonselective beta blocker).

Route: Oral, Parenteral.

Indications: Hypertension, angina, hypertrophic cardiomyopathy, supraventricular and ventricular arrhythmias, postmyocardial infarction, atrial flutter, and AV nodal tachycardia.

ECG Effects

- HEART RATE: Decreases.
- PR INTERVAL: Prolongs.
- QRS COMPLEX:
- QT INTERVAL: May shorten.
- T WAVE:
- U WAVE:
- BLOCK: May worsen existing AV block.

Adverse Cardiovascular Effects: Bradycardia, sinus arrest, AV block, hypotension, may worsen CHF or existing AV block.

Contraindications: Sinus bradycardia, second or third degree AV blocks, cardiogenic shock, severe CHF, cardiogenic shock, and bronchial asthma.

Nurse's Responsibilities
- Assess pulmonary status on a regular basis.
- Monitor blood pressure and ECG continually during IV administration.
- Administer IV dose slowly (no faster than 1 mg/5 min).
- Assess for signs and symptoms of CHF.
- Patient teaching: Avoid abrupt cessation of drug.
- Administer before meals and at bedtime. (Inderal LA is a long-acting, once-a-day preparation.)

Notes: Produces a variety of noncardiac side effects: pulmonary (bronchospasm), neurologic (insomnia, nightmares, fatigue, depression), renal, hepatic, and metabolic (altered glucose and lipid metabolism). Abrupt withdrawal or interruption of the drug schedule can be dangerous, especially in the presence of coronary artery disease.

Only propranolol, acebutolol, metoprolol, and timolol have been approved to treat arrhythmias or to prevent sudden death after MI.

QUINIDINE
Cardioquin, (quinidine polygalacturonate), Quinidex (quinidine sulfate), Quinaglute, and Duraquin (quinidine gluconate)

Classification: Class IA antiarrhythmic.

Route: Oral, parenteral.

Indications: Ventricular and supraventricular arrhythmias, including circus-movement tachycardia.

ECG Effects
- HEART RATE: Variable changes.
- PR INTERVAL: Early toxic sign is prolonged PR interval.
- QRS COMPLEX: Widens (development of bundle branch block [BBB] is sign of toxicity).
- QT INTERVAL: Prolongs.
- T WAVE:
- U WAVE:
- BLOCK: May cause SA block; AV block is sign of toxicity as is tall, notched P waves; may cause BBB.

Adverse Cardiovascular Effects: May worsen AV block. Ventricular arrhythmias, including VT and polymorphic VT (torsades de pointes), quinidine syncope, and hypotension. Can create reentry circuits, causing reentrant tachyarrhythmias.

Contraindications: Arrhythmias resulting from digitalis toxicity, complete heart block, BBB, myasthenia gravis, congenital long QT syndrome, history of torsades de pointes, and hypokalemia.

Nurse's Responsibilities
- Monitor serum digoxin and quinidine levels.
- Monitor serum potassium level.
- Ensure patient is digitalized before receiving quinidine for treatment of atrial flutter. (Quinidine decreases atrial rate and improves AV conduction early in treatment.)
- Monitor for quinidine cardiotoxicity: progressive prolongation of PR interval, QRS complex, QT interval; tall, notched P waves.
- Administer with food.
- Assess for development of side effects (see "Notes").

Notes: Enhances digitalis effect; digoxin toxicity occurs in a significant percentage of patients receiving quinidine and digoxin concurrently. The quinidine effect is enhanced by potassium and reduced in hypokalemia. Causes a variety of neurologic (tinnitus, blurred vision, dizziness, headache, light-headedness, and tremor) and gastrointestinal (nausea, vomiting, and diarrhea) side effects. Diarrhea may be persistent.

SOTALOL

Classification: Class III antiarrhythmic with beta blocker activity (nonselective) (also possesses Class II properties).

Route: Oral, parenteral.

Indications: Ventricular (serious) and supraventricular arrhythmias; paroxysmal atrial flutter, AV nodal tachycardia, and circus-movement tachycardia.

ECG Effects
- HEART RATE: Decreases.
- PR INTERVAL: Prolongs.
- QRS COMPLEX:
- QT INTERVAL: Prolongs; lengthens QTc.
- T WAVE:
- U WAVE:
- BLOCK: AV block possible.

Adverse Cardiovascular Effects: Ventricular tachycardia and torsades de pointes. Reduces systolic blood pressure.

Contraindications: Uncontrolled CHF, disorders of impulse generation and/or conduction, bradycardia, and marked hypotension.

Nurse's Responsibilities
- Calculate PR interval and QTc regularly.
- Evaluate suppression of arrhythmias.
- Monitor ECG and blood pressure regularly and frequently.

TIMOLOL
Blocadren

Classification: Class II antiarrhythmic with beta blocker activity (nonselective).

Route: Oral.

Indications: Hypertension, post-MI to reduce cardiovascular mortality and the risk of reinfarction, atrial and ventricular arrhythmias modulated by the sympathetic nervous system, and SVT.

ECG Effects
- HEART RATE: Decreases.
- PR INTERVAL: Prolongs.
- QRS COMPLEX:
- QT INTERVAL:
- T WAVE:
- U WAVE:
- BLOCK: AV block possible.

Adverse Cardiovascular Effects: Sinus bradycardia, AV block, and hypotension. May intensify diminished LV function or CHF.

Contraindications: Bronchial asthma, severe chronic obstructive pulmonary disease, sinus bradycardia, second and third degree AV block, and cardiac failure.

Nurse's Responsibilities
- Determine history of asthma or chronic obstructive pulmonary disease.
- Monitor heart rate and blood pressure.
- Measure PR interval regularly.
- Assess patient for manifestations of CHF.

Notes: Only timolol, acebutolol, metoprolol, and propranolol have been approved to treat arrhythmias or to prevent sudden death after MI.

TOCAINIDE HYDROCHLORIDE
Tonocard

Classification: Class IB antiarrhythmic.

Route: Oral.

Indications: Ventricular arrhythmias.

ECG Effects
- HEART RATE: May decrease.
- PR INTERVAL: Variable.
- QRS COMPLEX: May widen.
- QT INTERVAL: Variable effect.
- T WAVE:
- U WAVE:
- BLOCK: AV block possible.

Adverse Cardiovascular Effects: Bradycardia, sinus arrest, conduction disturbances, VF, and hypotension. May accelerate ventricular rate in atrial fibrillation/atrial flutter. May worsen ventricular arrhythmias. Potentially aggravates heart failure.

Contraindications: Second and third degree AV blocks without functioning artificial pacemaker.

Nurse's Responsibilities
- Monitor heart rate, rhythm, and blood pressure regularly.
- Assess for neurotoxicity.
- Assess for presence of side effects (see "Notes") and note if side effects are reversible with dosage reduction.
- Administer with food or antacid to reduce nausea, vomiting, and abdominal pain.
- Evaluate suppression of arrhythmias.

Notes: Tocainide is an oral analog of lidocaine and has similar electrophysiologic, antiarrhythmic, and hemodynamic properties. Approximately 30% of patients receiving tocainide develop intolerable side effects (pulmonary fibrosis and agranulocytosis are rare but severe reactions). More commonly, it produces a variety of noncardiac (gastrointestinal and neurologic) adverse side effects, similar to those resulting from lidocaine: tremor, nausea, vomiting, and paresthesia. Side effects may or may not be dosage related. Occasionally this drug is most effective when used in combination with a Class IA antiarrhythmic.

VERAPAMIL
Calan, Isoptin

Classification: Class IV antiarrhythmic, calcium-channel blocker, antihypertensive.

Route: Oral, parenteral.

Indications: Chronic stable angina, supraventricular tachyarrhythmias (particularly AV nodal reentrant tachycardias), atrial flutter, circus-movement tachycardia, control of ventricular response to atrial fibrillation, selected cases of exercise-induced VT, cardiomyopathy, and hypertension.

ECG Effects
- HEART RATE: Decreases but may increase as a reflex

tachycardia. Can dangerously increase rate in patients with WPW syndrome.
- PR INTERVAL: Prolongs.
- QRS COMPLEX:
- QT INTERVAL:
- T WAVE:
- U WAVE:
- BLOCK: SA and AV block possible.

Adverse Cardiovascular Effects: AV nodal block. Worsens intraventricular conduction delay and SSS. Sinus bradycardia and sinus arrest. Has negative inotropic effect; may cause or worsen CHF. Hypotension. In patients with WPW syndrome, it may dangerously accelerate ventricular rate and lead to cardiac arrest.

Contraindications: VT, SSS, second or third degree AV blocks without artificial pacemaker, and WPW syndrome. Concomitant use of IV beta blockers. Avoid administering to patients with severely compromised left ventricular function, cardiogenic shock, and severe hypotension.

Nurse's Responsibilities
- Monitor blood pressure and ECG constantly during IV administration and have defibrillator/cardioverter present.
- Assess for hypotension.
- Obtain serum digoxin levels if indicated.
- Assess for signs and symptoms of CHF.
- Headache and constipation occur with verapamil therapy and can be treated.
- Use caution when administering IV. In patients over age 55, administer dose over 3 minutes.
- Use caution when administering IV to patients on oral beta blockers.

Notes: Verapamil interacts with other cardiac drugs such as beta blockers (worsens SA and AV nodal disease, potentiates AV block, and decreases left ventricular function); digoxin (increases serum digoxin levels and may potentiate heart block); and disopyramide (decreases myocardial function).

Dosage
IV

0.075 to 0.15 mg/kg (maximum 10 mg) over 1 to 2 min, 3 minutes if 55 or older. May repeat 0.15 mg/kg (maximum 10 mg) in 30 minutes, not to exceed 15 mg.

Age 8 to 15 years: 0.1 to 0.3 mg/kg (maximum 2 to 5 mg). May repeat 0.1 to 0.2 mg/kg (maximum 2 to 5 mg) in 30 minutes.

BIBLIOGRAPHY

ACC/AHA Task force report. Guidelines for the early management of patients with acute myocardial infarction. *J. Am. Coll. Cardiol.*, Aug., 1990, 16(2): 249-292.

American Heart Association. *Textbook of Advanced Cardiac Life Support*. Dallas: American Heart Association, 1987.

Alboni P, Paparella N, Cappato R, Candini GC. Direct and autonomically mediated effects of oral flecainide. *Am. J. Cardiol.*, Apr. 1, 1988, 61: 759-63.

Anastasiou-Nana MI, Gilbert EM, Miller RH, Singh S, Freedman RA, Keefe DL, Saksena S, MacNeil DJ, Anderson JL. Usefulness of d, l sotalol for suppression of chronic ventricular arrhythmias. *Am. J. Cardiol.*, Mar. 1, 1991, 67: 511-16.

Anderson JL, Stewart JR, Perry BA, Van Hamersveld DD, Johnson TA, Conard GJ, Chang SF, Kvam DC, Pitt B. Oral flecainide acetate for the treatment of ventricular arrhythmias. *N. Engl. J. Med.*, Aug. 27, 1981, 305(9): 473-7.

Antman EM. *Supraventricular Arrhythmias*. Upper Montclair, NJ: HealthScan, 1981.

Barbey JT, Thompson KA, Echt DS, Woosley RL, Roden DM. Tocainide plus quinidine for treatment of ventricular arrhythmias. *Am. J. Cardiol.*, Mar. 1, 1988, 61: 570-3.

Benning CA, Burke PA. Tocainide in the cardiac ICU. *Crit. Care Nurse*, Feb., 1989, 9(2): 45-6, 48-9, 53.

Berns E, Rinkenberger RL, Jeang MK, Dougherty AH, Jenkins M, Naccarelli GV. Efficacy and safety of flecainide acetate for atrial tachycardia or fibrillation. *Am. J. Cardiol.*, Jun. 1, 1987, 59: 1337-1341.

Bigger JT (ed). Symposium on flecainide acetate. *Am. J. Cardiol.*, Feb. 27, 1984, 53(5).

Bigger JT, Coromilas J, Rolnitzky LM, Fleiss JL, Kleiger RE. Effect of diltiazem on cardiac rate and rhythm after myocardial infarction. *Am. J. Cardiol.*, Mar. 1, 1990, 65: 539-46.

Braunwald E (ed). *Heart disease: A Textbook of Cardiovascular Medicine*. 3rd ed. Philadelphia: WB Saunders, 1988.

Buckley MM, Grant SM, Goa KL, McTavish D, Sorkin EM. Diltiazem. A reappraisal of its pharmacological properties and therapeutic use. *Drugs*, May, 1990, 39(5): 757-806.

Byrd RC, Sung RJ, Marks J, Parmley WW. Safety and efficacy of esmolol (ASL-8052: an ultrashort-acting beta-adrenergic blocking agent) for control of ventricular rate in supraventricular tachycardias. *J. Am. Coll. Cardiol.*, Feb., 1984, 3(2): 394-9.

Cardiac arrhythmia pilot study investigators. Effects of encainide, flecainide, imipramine and moricizine on ventricular arrhythmias during the year after acute myocardial infarction: the CAPS. *Am. J. Cardiol.*, Mar. 1, 1988, 61: 501-509.

Cardiac arrhythmia suppression trial. Preliminary report: Effect of encainide and flecainide on mortality in a randomized trial of arrhythmia suppression after myocardial infarction. *N. Engl. J. Med.*, 1989, 321: 406-412.

Catalano JT. Antiarrhythmic medications classified by their autonomic properties. *Crit. Care Nurse*, May-Jun., 1986, 6(3): 44-9.

Cetnarowski AB, Rihn TL. A review of adverse reactions to mexiletine and tocainide. *Cardiovasc. News Rep.*, Dec., 1985, (12): 1335-42.

Chouty F, Coumel P. Oral flecainide for prophylaxis of paroxysmal atrial fibrillation. *Am. J. Cardiol.*, Aug. 25, 1988, 62: 35-37.

Crijns HJ, Gelder IC, Lie KI. Supraventricular tachycardia mimicking ventricular tachycardia during flecainide treatment. *Am. J. Cardiol.*, Dec. 1, 1988, 62: 1303-6.

Dance D, Yates M. Nursing assessment and care of children with complications of congenital heart disease. *Heart & Lung*, May, 1985, 14(3): 209-14.

Dimarco JP. Electrophysiology of adenosine. *J. Cardiovasc Electrophysiology*, Aug., 1990, 1(4): 340-48.

Dimarco JP, Miles W, Akhtar M, Milstein S, Sharma AD, Platia E, McGovern B, Scheinman MM, Govier WC. Adenosine for paroxysmal supraventricular tachycardia: dose ranging and comparison with verapamil. Assessment in placebo-controlled, multicenter trials. *Ann. Intern. Med.*, Jul., 15, 1990, 113(2): 104-10.

Dimarco JP, Sellers TD, Lerman BB, Greemberg ML, Bern RM, Belardinelli L. Diagnostic and therapeutic use of adenosine in patients with supraventricular tachyarrhythmias. *J. Am. Coll. Cardiol.*, Aug., 1985, 6(2): 417-25.

Doherty JV, Waxman HL, Kienzle MG, Cassidy DM, Marchlinski FE, Buxton AE, Josephson ME. Limited role of intravenous propafenone hydrochloride in the treatment of sustained ventricular tachycardia: electrophysiologic effects and results of programmed ventricular stimulation. *J. Am. Coll. Cardiol.*, Aug., 1984, 4(2): 378-81.

Douglas JH 3d, Ross JD, Burce DL. Delayed awakening due to lidocaine overdose. *J. Clin. Anesth.*, Mar.-Apr., 1990, 2(2): 126-8.

Encainide-Ventricular Tachycardia Study Group. Treatment of life-threatening ventricular tachycardia with encainide hydrochloride in patients with left ventricular dysfunction. *Am. J. Cardiol.*, Sept., 1988, 62: 571-75.

Frei J. Amiodarone: therapeutics and guidelines. *Prog. Cardiovasc. Nurs.*, Oct.-Dec., 1989, 4(4): 113-8.

Flecainide Ventricular Tachycardia Study Group. Treatment of resistant ventricular tachycardia with flecainide acetate. *Am. J. Cardiol.*, Jun. 1, 1986, 57(15): 1299-1304.

Funck-Brentano C, Kroemer HK, Lee JT, Roden DM. Propafenone. *N. Engl. J. Med.*, Feb. 22, 1990, 322(8): 518-22.

Garson A. Dosing the newer antiarrhythmic drugs in children: considerations in pediatric pharmacology. *Am. J. Cardiol.*, Jun. 1, 1986, 67: 1405-7.

Gillette PC. Supraventricular arrhythmias in children. *J. Am. Coll. Cardiol.*, Jun., 1985, 5(6): 122B-9B.

Goodman SL, Gliderman JM, Bernstein IJ. Prophylactic lidocaine in suspected acute myocardial infarction. *J. Am. Coll. Emerg. Phys.*, Jun., 1979, 8(6): 221-4.

Heger JJ, Prystowsky EN, Zipes DP. New drugs for treatment of ventricular arrhythmias. *Heart & Lung*, May: Jun., 1981, 10(3): 475-83.

Hoff PI, Tronstad A, Oie B, Ohm OJ. Electrophysiologic and clinical effects of flecainide for recurrent paroxysmal supraventricular tachycardia. *Am. J. Cardiol.*, Sept. 15, 1988, 62: 585-89.

Hoshino PK, Blaustein AS, Gaasch WH. Effect of propranolol on the left ventricular response to the Valsalva maneuver in normal subjects. *Am. J. Cardiol.*, Feb. 1, 1988, 61: 400-4.

Howland-Gradman J. Flecainide acetate. *Crit. Care Nurse*, Mar.-Apr., 1987, 7(2): 28-9.

Hurst JW (ed). *The Heart, Arteries, and Veins*. 7th ed. New York: McGraw-Hill, 1990.

Jordaens L, Gorgels A, Stroobandt R, Temmerman J. Efficacy and safety of intravenous sotalol for termination of paroxysmal supraventricular tachycardia. *Am. J. Cardiol.*, Jul. 1, 1991, 68: 35-40.

Kennedy GT. Slow channel calcium blockers in the treatment of chronic stable angina. *Cardiovasc. Nurs.*, Jan.-Feb., 1984, 20(1): 1-5.

Kerr CR, Klein GJ, Axelson JE, Cooper JC. Propafenone for prevention of recurrent atrial fibrillation. *Am. J. Cardiol.*, Apr. 15, 1988, 61: 914-16.

Kienzle MG, Martins JB, Wendt DJ, Constantin L, Hopson R, McCue ML. Enhanced efficacy of oral sotalol for sustained ventricular tachycardia refractory to type I antiarrhythmic drugs. *Am. J. Cardiol.*, May 1, 1988, 61: 1013-17.

Kim SS, Smith P, Ruffy R. Treatment of atrial tachyarrhythmias and preexcitation syndrome with flecainide acetate. *Am. J. Cardiol.*, Aug. 25, 1988, 62: 29-34.

Kolar JA, Dracup K. Psychosocial adjustment of patients with ventricular dysrhythmias. *J. Cardiovasc. Nurs.*, Feb., 1990, 4(2): 44-55.

Kopelman HA, Woosley RL, Lee JT, Roden DM, Echt DS. Electrophysiologic effects of intravenous and oral sotalol for sustained ventricular tachycardia secondary to coronary artery disease. *Am. J. Cardiol.*, May 1, 1988, 61: 1006-11.

Krapf R, Gertsch M. Torsade de pointes induced by sotalol despite therapeutic plasma sotalol concentrations. *Br. Med. J.*, Jun. 15, 1985, 290(6484): 1784-5.

Kuck KH, Kunze KP, Schluter M, Duckeck W. Encainide versus flecainide for chronic atrial and junctional ectopic tachycardia. *Am. J. Cardiol.*, Dec. 20, 1988, 62: 37-44.

Kus T, Costi P, Dubuc M, Shenasa M. Prolongation of ventricular refractoriness by class Ia antiarrhythmic drugs in the prevention of ventricular tachycardia induction. *Am. Heart. J.*, Oct., 1990, 120(4): 855-63.

Lerman B, Belardinelli L. Cardiac electrophysiology of adenosine. *Circ.*, May, 1991, 83(5): 1499-1509.

Lui HK, Lee G, Dhurandhar R, Hungate EJ, Laddu A, Dietrich P, Mason DT. Reduction of ventricular ectopic beats with oral acebutolol: a double blind randomized crossover study. *Am. Heart J.*, May, 1983, 105(5): 722-6.

Mäkynen PJ, Koskinen PJ, Saaristo TE, Liisanantti RK. Comparison of encainide and quinidine for supraventricular tachyarrhythmias. *Am. J. Cardiol.*, Dec., 1988, 62: 55-59.

Manolis AS, Deering TF, Cameron J, Estes NAM 3d. Mexiletine: pharmacology and therapeutic use. *Clin. Cardiol.*, May, 1990, 13: 349-59.

Marden SF, Chuley M. Esmolol HCl. *Crit. Care Nurse.*, Nov.-Dec., 1989, 9(10): 12-4.

Marriott HJL, Bieza CF. Alarming ventricular acceleration after lidocaine administration. *Chest*, Jun., 1972, 61(7): 682-3.

McGovern B, Garan H, Ruskin JN. Precipitation of cardiac arrest by verapamil in patient with Wolff-Parkinson-White syndrome. *Ann. Intern. Med.*, Jun., 1986, 104(6): 791-4.

Miles WM, Zipes DP, Rinkenberger RL, Markel ML, Prystowsky EN, Dougherty AH, Heger JJ, Naccarelli GV. Encainide for treatment of atrioventricular reciprocating tachycardia in the Wolff-Parkinson-White Syndrome. *Am. J. Cardiol.*, Dec. 20, 1988, 62: 20-25.

Monk JP, Brogden RN. Mexiletine. A review of its pharmacodynamic and pharmacokinetic properties, and therapeutic use in the treatment of arrhythmias. *Drugs*, Sept., 1990, 40(3): 374-411.

Moosvi AR, Goldstein S, VanderBrug Medendorp S, Landis JR, Wolfe RA, Leighton R, Ritter G, Vasu CM, Acheson A. Effect of empiric antiarrhythmic therapy in resuscitated out-of-hospital cardiac arrest victims with coronary artery disease. *Am. J. Cardiol.*, May 15, 1990, 65: 1192-7.

Morganroth J for the Mexiletine-Quinidine Research Group. Comparative efficacy and safety of oral mexiletine and quinidine in benign or potentially lethal ventricular arrhythmias. *Am. J. Cardiol.*, Dec. 1, 1987, 60(16): 1276-81.

Murdock CJ, Kyles AE, Yeung-Lai-Wah JA, Qi A, Vorderbrugge S, Kerr CR. Atrial flutter in patients treated for atrial fibrillation with propafenone. *Am. J. Cardiol.*, Sept. 15, 1990, 66: 755-7.

Musto B, D'Onofrio A, Cavallaro C, Musto A, Greco R. Electrophysiological effects and clinical efficacy of flecainide in children with recurrent paroxysmal supraventricular tachycardia. *Am. J. Cardiol.*, Aug. 1, 1988, 62: 229-233.

Naccarelli GV, Jackman WM, Akhtar M, Rinkenberger RL, Friday KJ, Dougherty AH, Tchou P, Yeung-Lai-Wah JA. Efficacy and electrophysiologic effects of encainide of atrioventricular nodal reentrant tachycardia. *Am. J. Cardiol.*, Dec. 20, 1988, 62: 31-36.

Neuss H, Schlepper M. Long term efficacy and safety of flecainide for supraventricular tachycardia. *Am. J. Cardiol.*, Aug. 25, 1988, 62: 56-61.

New drugs, drug news. *Drug Therapy*, Feb., 1987, 17(2): 11-12.

Nicholson WJ, Martin CE, Gracey JG, Knoch HR. Disopyramide induced ventricular fibrillation. *Am. J. Cardiol.*, May, 1979, 43: 1053-6.

Personal correspondence, Bristol Laboratories, 2400 West Lloyd Expressway, Evansville, Indiana 47721-0001, September 30, 1991.

Pelleg A, Porter RS. The pharmacology of adenosine. *Pharmacotherapy*, 1990, 10(3): 157-74.

Pietersen AH, Hellemann H. Usefulness of flecainide for prevention of paroxysmal atrial fibrillation and flutter. *Am. J. Cardiol.*, Apr. 1, 1991, 67: 713-17.

Podrid PJ, Lown B. Mexiletine for ventricular arrhythmias. *Am. J. Cardiol.*, Apr. 1981, 47: 895-902.

Podrid PJ, Lown B. Tocainide for refractory symptomatic ventricular arrhythmias. *Am. J. Cardiol.*, Apr. 1, 1982, 49: 1279-84.

Pollak PT, Sharma AD, Carruthers SG. Elevation of serum total cholesterol and triglyceride levels during amiodarone therapy. *Am. J. Cardiol.*, Sept. 15, 1988, 62: 562-5.

Pool PE, Seagren SC, Salel AF. Effects of diltiazem on serum lipids, exercise performance and blood pressure: Randomized, double-blind, placebo-controlled evaluation for systematic hypertension. *Am. J. Cardiol.*, Dec. 6, 1985, 56: 86H-91H.

Pottage A. Clinical profiles of newer class I antiarrhythmic agents—tocainide, mexiletine, encainide, flecainide and lorcainide. *In* Harrison DC (ed). Symposium on Perspectives on the Treatment of Ventricular Arrhythmias. *Am. J. Cardiol.*, Sept. 22, 1983, 52(6): 24C-31C.

Rae AP. Supraventricular tachyarrhythmias: atrial flutter and atrial fibrillation. Horowitz L (series ed). Interpreting an ECG. *Geriatrics*, Mar., 1985, 40(3): 93-108.

Ramoska EA, Spiller HA, Myers A. Calcium channel blocker toxicity. *Ann. Emerg. Med.*, Jun., 1990, 19(6): 649-53.

Robinson KC, McKenna WJ, Krikler DM. Amiodarone: current perspectives from Europe. *Heart & Lung*, Nov., 1987, 16(6): 636-9.

Rowland TW. Augmented ventricular rate following verapamil treatment for atrial fibrillation with Wolff-Parkinson-White syndrome. *Pediatrics*, Aug., 1983, 72: 245-6.

Ryan C. Calcium-channel blockers and the elderly. *Compr. Ther.*, Jun., 1990, 16(6): 51-4.

Scagliotti D, Strasberg B, Hai HA, Kehoe R, Rosen K. Aprindine-induced polymorphous ventricular tachycardia. *Am. J. Cardiol.*, Apr., 1982, 49: 1297-1301.

Scher DL, Arsura EL. Effectiveness of metoprolol versus verapamil therapy for multifocal atrial tachycardia. *Cardiol. Bd. Rev.*, Jan., 1990, 7(1): 110-22.

Scherer P. New drugs of 1985 in theory and in practice. *Am. J. Nurs.*, Apr., 1986, 86(4): 406-15.

Scherer P. New drugs. *Am. J. Nurs.*, May, 1987, 87(5): 645-9.

Sharma A, Klein G. Comparative quantitative electrophysiological effects of adenosine triphosphate on the sinus node and atrioventricular node. *Am. J. Cardiol.*, Feb., 1988, 61: 330-35.

Sheldon RS, Mitchell LB, Duff HJ, Wyse DG, Manyari DE, Reynolds K. Right and left ventricular function during chronic amiodarone therapy. *Am. J. Cardiol.*, Oct. 1, 1988, 62: 736-40.

Shenasa M, Kus T, Fromer M, LeBlanc RA, Dubuc M, Nadeau R. Effect of intravenous and oral calcium antagonists (diltiazem and verapamil) on sustenance of atrial fibrillation. *Am. J. Cardiol.*, Sept. 1, 1988, 62: 403-7.

Singh JB, Rasul AM, Shah A, Adams E, Flessas A, Kocot SL. Efficacy of mexiletine in chronic ventricular arrhythmias compared with quinidine: a single-blind, randomized trial. *Am. J. Cardiol.*, Jan., 1984, 53: 84-7.

Singh SN, Cohen A, Chen Y, Wish M, Thoben-O'Grady L, Peralba J, Gottdiener J, Fletcher RD. Sotalol for refractory sustained ventricular tachycardia and nonfatal cardiac arrest. *Am. J. Cardiol.*, Sept. 1, 1988, 62: 399-402.

Singh S, Klein R, Eisenberg B, Hughes E, Shand M, Doherty P. Long-term effect of mexiletine on left ventricular function and relation to suppression of ventricular arrhythmia. *Am. J. Cardiol.*, Nov. 15, 1990, 66: 1222-7.

Smith A. Amiodarone; clinical considerations. *Focus Crit. Care*, Oct., 1984, 11(5): 30-7.

Soyka LF. Safety consideration and dosing guidelines for encainide in supraventricular arrhythmias. *Am. J. Cardiol.*, Dec., 1988, 62: 63L-68L.

Strasberg B, Prechel D, Bauman J, Cielho A, Swiryn S, Bauernfeind R, Rosen KM. Long-term follow-up of patients receiving aprindine. *Arch. Intern. Med.*, Nov., 1983, 143(11): 2131-3.

Strasburger JF, Smith RT, Moak JP, Gothing C, Garson A. Encainide for resistant supraventricular tachycardia in children: follow-up report. *Am. J. Cardiol.*, Dec. 20, 1988, 62: 50-54.

Sung R. Beta blockade in the treatment of arrhythmias. *Cardio.*, Sept., 1985: 37-9.

Tiovonen LK, Neiminen MS, Maanninen V, Frick H. Pirmenol in the termination of paroxysmal supraventricular tachycardia. *Am. J. Cardiol.*, Jun. 15, 1987, 59: 35H-38H.

Vigorito C, Giodano A, Ferraro P, Acanfor D, DeCaprio L, Naddeo C, Rengo F. Hemodynamic effects of magnesiun sulfate on the normal human heart. *Am. J. Cardiol.*, Jun. 15, 1991, 67: 1435-7.

Vinsant MO, Spence MI. *Commonsense Approach to Coronary Care*. 5th ed. St. Louis: The CV Mosby Co., 1988.

Vukmir RB, Stein KL. Torsade de pointes therapy with phenytoin. *Ann. Emerg. Med.*, Feb., 1991, 20(2): 198-200.

Weintraub AR, Manolis AS, Estes NA. Electrophysiologic and electrocardiographic effects, efficacy and safety of encainide in malignant ventricular arrhythmias associated with coronary artery disease. *Am. J. Cardiol.*, Oct., 1990, 66(12): 947-53.

Wilkerson RD (ed). *Cardiac Pharmacology*. New York: Academic Press, 1981.

Woelfel A, Foster JR, McAllister RG, Simpson RJ, Gettes LS. Efficacy of verapamil in exercise-induced ventricular tachycardia. *Am. J. Cardiol.*, Aug. 1, 1985, 56: 292-7.

Zeigler V, Gillette PC, Hammill B, Ross BA, Ewing L. Flecainide for supraventricular tachycardia in children. *Am. J. Cardiol.*, Aug. 25, 1988, 62: 41-43.

Zeigler V, Gillette PC, Ross BA, Ewing L. Flecainide for supraventricular arrhythmias in children and young adults. *Am. J. Cardiol.*, Oct. 1, 1988, 62: 818-20.

CHAPTER TWELVE

Countershock

The Nurse's Role

▶ **GOAL**

You will be able to identify the types of countershock therapy and describe the indications for their use.

▶ **OBJECTIVES**

After studying this chapter you should be able to do the following:

1. Define defibrillation and identify the procedural steps in defibrillating adults and children.
2. Identify the energy dose used in adult and pediatric defibrillation.
3. Define cardioversion.
4. Describe preparatory procedures for elective cardioversion.
5. Identify the procedural steps and primary nursing responsibilities in cardioverting a patient.
6. Describe the nurse's role in assisting patients with internal automatic defibrillation or cardioversion-defibrillation devices.

Electrical intervention in the form of countershock is a common method of bringing tachyarrhythmias under control. When a countershock is delivered to the myocardium, it causes all the cells to depolarize at once, thus terminating a chaotic rhythm or a rhythm that is too fast to allow optimal cardiac output. The sinus node is allowed to resume control of the rhythm. If the sinus node is not functioning properly, a subsidiary, or lower, pacemaker should take control.

There are two types of countershock therapy, defibrillation and cardioversion. Defibrillation, the emergency treatment of choice for ventricular fibrillation (VF), consists of delivery of a direct current (DC) charge to the external chest or directly onto the myocardial surface (internal defibrillation). Cardioversion is delivery of a synchronized charge to the external chest for treatment of ventricular or supraventricular tachycardias. The delivery of the charge is synchronized with the ECG so that it will not occur during the T wave, possibly causing VF. The current that is delivered to the paddles in either type of countershock is several thousand volts and lasts 4 to 12 milliseconds (msec). This current is expressed as energy and measured as joules (j) or watt-seconds (w-s).

DEFIBRILLATION

Defibrillation is performed as soon as possible after VF is recognized. The sooner defibrillation takes place, the more likely it will be successful. (Sometimes VF can be converted immediately after onset with a precordial thump causing enough mechanical stimulation (0.4 j) to depolarize the myocardium. Precordial thumps are not administered to children.) Factors other than time play a role in the likelihood of successful defibrillation. Conditions such as hypoxemia, acidosis, hypothermia, electrolyte imbalance, and drug toxicity can contribute to failure to correct VF.

Precautions

- Make certain you are standing on dry floor.
- Make certain neither you nor anyone else is touching the bed or the patient.

- Disconnect all ungrounded equipment as defibrillation may damage it.

Procedure
Preparation

Use correct *paddle size.*

Adults:	10 to 13 cm circular diameter
Children:	8 cm circular diameter
Infants:	4.5 cm circular diameter

Cover paddle surface with conductive medium. Saline pads or special conductive pads may be used. These will reduce skin resistance to current flow, decrease burning, and prevent the likelihood of arcing. When using a conductive gel or cream or saline-soaked pads, avoid using too much. The current, taking the path of least resistance, will traverse the excessive cream, gel, or saline, resulting in burns and ineffective shock. Never use alcohol, since it will burst into flames when the current is released.

For internal defibrillation, sterile saline moistened gauze pads may be placed between the myocardium and the internal defibrillation paddles.

Initial Energy Dose

- Adults: 200 j.
- Infants and Children: 1j/lb (or 2j/kg).
- Infant on digitalis: Begin at lowest machine setting.
- Internal: 5 to 50j.

Paddle Placement.

- Standard placement:
  - One paddle below the right clavicle, just to the right of the upper sternum.
  - One paddle to the left of the apex (to the left and below the left nipple in the midaxillary line) (Fig. 12-1).
  - Make certain paddles are at least 2 inches apart and that they are flat on the skin. If these two precautions

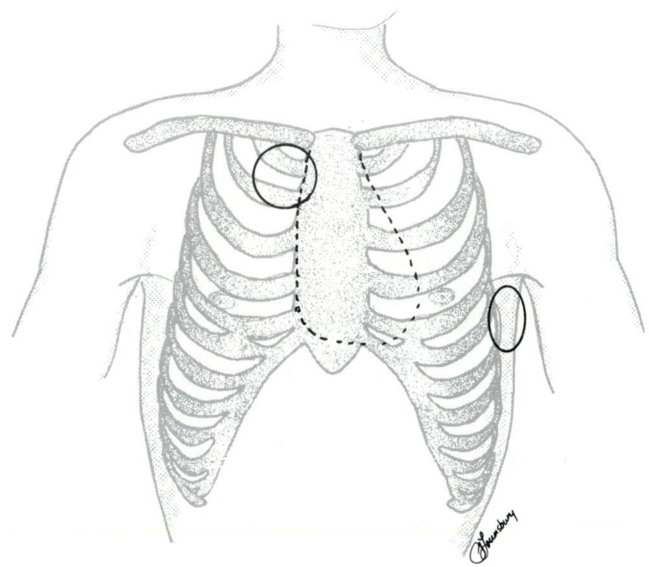

FIGURE 12-1 Standard paddle placement.

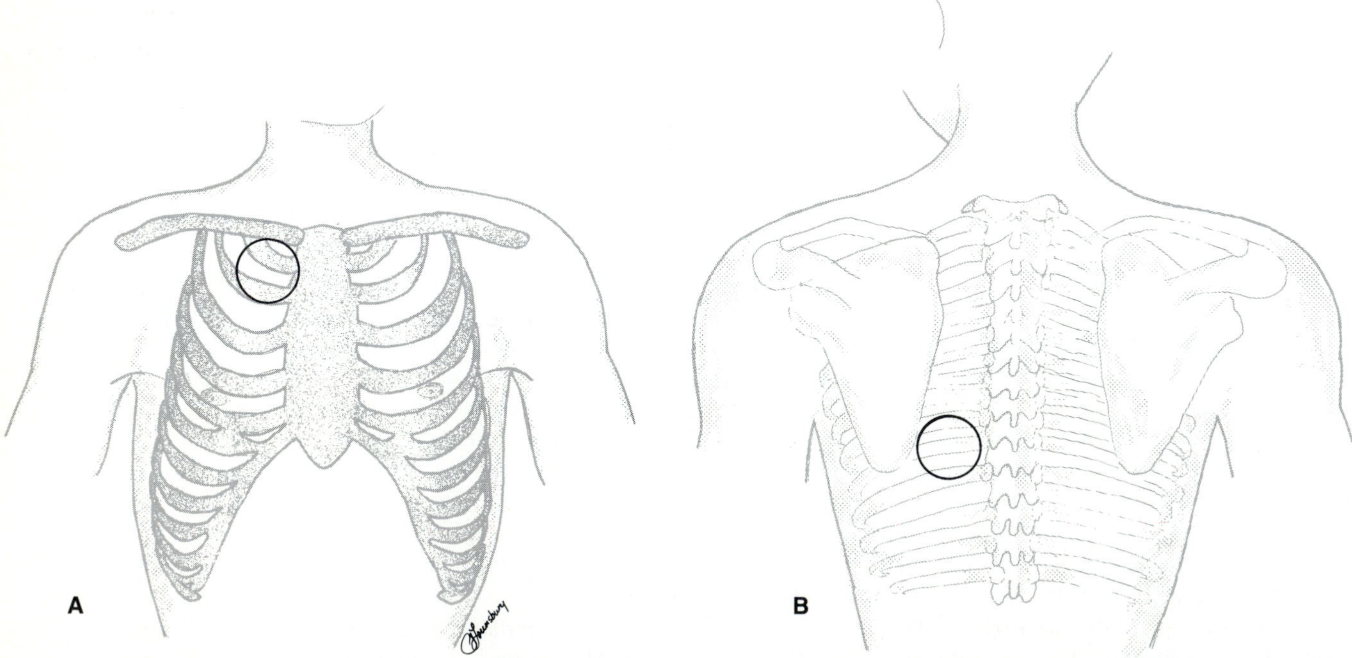

FIGURE 12-2 Anteroposterior paddle placement. **A,** Anterior paddle: right parasternal area or left precordium. **B,** Posterior paddle: left infrascapular region.

are not taken, dangerous arcing can occur.

- Anteroposterior placement:
  - Anterior paddle over the left precordium or right parasternal area.
  - Posterior paddle in the left infrascapular region (Fig. 12-2).
- For internal defibrillation during surgery:
  - One paddle over the right atrium.
  - One paddle at the apex.
- For defibrillation with a pulse generator (permanent pacemaker):
  - Do not place paddles over the pulse generator or the electrodes. Place paddles at least 5 inches from the pulse generator.

Steps in Performing Emergency Defibrillation.

1. Identify VF on the ECG.
2. Establish unresponsiveness. (Make certain rhythm is not artifact.)
3. Prepare paddles with conduction medium.
4. Place paddles.
5. Charge machine.
6. Press firmly, using 25 to 30 pounds of pressure, for external defibrillation.
7. Stand clear, state "all clear," visually verify.
8. Check rhythm again.
9. Depress both buttons simultaneously until machine discharges.
10. Check rhythm.
11. Continue CPR if not successful and repeat procedure with increased energy dosage.
12. If successful, assess patient, support ventilations as needed.
13. Insert IV if not already in.
14. Administer bolus of lidocaine if returning rhythm is not idioventricular rhythm (IVR) or asystole. Initiate a lidocaine infusion at 2 to 4 mg/min.
15. Monitor blood pressure and ECG continuously.
16. Assess mental status, respiratory status, and skin temperature.
17. Obtain arterial blood gases.
18. Obtain 12-lead ECG.
19. Inspect skin surface for burns.
20. Make certain all events have been recorded.
21. Offer emotional support to the patient and significant other(s).

CARDIOVERSION

Cardioversion is defined as delivery of a synchronized direct current charge to the myocardium. It is used in emergency and elective treatment of tachyarrhythmias. The shock is synchronized with the patient's QRS complexes so that accidental delivery of shock during the vulnerable period, which is during repolarization (in the vicinity of the T wave on the ECG), is avoided, thus preventing VF. Like defibrillation, the shock causes all the cells to depolarize simultaneously, allowing the sinoatrial (SA) node to resume control of the rhythm. Cardioversion may be indicated in paroxysmal supraventricular tachycardia (PSVT), atrial flutter (AFl), atrial fibrillation (AF), and ventricular tachycardia (VT). For VT, the procedure is often performed as emergency treatment if the patient is symptomatic.

Precautions

To prepare the patient for elective cardioversion, precautions are taken to diminish the likelihood of complications.

Digitalis Toxicity

If the patient is clinically digitalis toxic, cardioversion is postponed until the toxicity subsides (2 or more days) because cardioversion in this situation may result in VF. If cardioversion cannot be delayed start with the lowest energy and increase until effective. Check serum digoxin level.

Atrial Fibrillation

For patients in atrial fibrillation, the left atrial appendage is a notorious site for thrombus formation, therefore presenting a risk of thromboembolism after conversion. For these patients, it is recommended they be anticoagulated for 3 weeks before cardioversion. If AF is of recent onset, anticoagulation may not be necessary. After cardioversion, the patient is often maintained on warfarin for several days.

Postconversion Arrhythmias

Since there is always a period of electrical instability after countershock therapy, which may lead to arrhythmias, it is prudent to eliminate factors that may enhance electrical instability before treatment, if possible. These arrhythmogenic factors include hypokalemia, hypoxia, and acidosis or alkalosis.

- Check serum potassium.
- Assess arterial blood gases.
- Obtain 12-lead ECG for postconversion comparison.
- Assess vital signs, peripheral pulses, and mentation for postconversion comparison.

Procedure

Preparation

Explain the procedure to the patient and family in terms that will not frighten. Try to avoid terms like *electric shock*. Explain the procedure will send a signal to the heart causing the heart to beat more regularly or more slowly. Assure the patient that medication will be given so no pain will be experienced. Have the patient sign a consent form.

Since the patient will be lightly anesthetized (the physician usually chooses a short-acting barbiturate, midazolam hydrochloride, or diazepam), implement the following:

- Nothing by mouth for 6 to 12 hours before the procedure.
- Have emergency resuscitation equipment available.
- Start IV infusion.
- Monitor patient on ECG.
- Remove patient's dentures.
- Administer oxygen before the procedure.
- Discontinue oxygen during procedure (in the presence of electrical arcing, oxygen may support combustion).
- Maintain patient in supine position with patent airway.
- Assist ventilations as needed.

Set the machine to "synchronize" and attach the patient to the ECG that is synchronized with the cardioverter. The machine senses the patient's QRS complexes, so make sure a lead has been chosen that displays them well. Adjust amplitude so other waves, such as T waves, are not triggering the rate sensor. (The cardioverter will give some indication it is sensing the QRS complexes; machines vary.)

Apply conduction medium to the paddles to decrease skin resistance to the flow of current. This decreases skin burning and the possibility of arcing. Use appropriate paddle size (see "Defibrillation," pp. 353–355). Sometimes self-adhesive electrodes are used instead of paddles. Their advantages include safety (the patient is not touched by the nurse to administer the shock) and a good ECG signal.

Energy

The larger the chest, the greater the transthoracic impedance. Therefore large-chested, emphysematous patients may require a higher dosage. Usual initial dosages are as follows:

AFl: 25 j
AF and PSVT: 75 to 100 j
VT: 50 j

Paddle Placement

Use 25 to 30 pounds of pressure to the same paddle sites as for defibrillation.

Steps in Performing Cardioversion

1. Connect patient's monitor cable to oscilloscope synchronized with cardioverter.
2. Make certain QRS complexes are triggering synchronizer.
3. Select energy dosage.
4. Place paddles with firm pressure.
5. Discontinue oxygen.
6. Check ECG rhythm.
7. State "all clear" and visually check that no one is touching patient or bed.
8. Depress buttons on paddles and wait for the shock to be delivered.
9. Assess ECG rhythm.
10. Assess respirations, administer oxygen.
11. Repeat cardioversion, if necessary, at higher dose as ordered. Failure to cardiovert may be because of hypoxia, acidosis, or alkalosis.
12. After successful cardioversion, assess the patient's level of consciousness and respiratory status.
13. Continually monitor ECG. Ectopic beats are common but rarely require antiarrhythmic therapy.
14. Obtain 12-lead ECG.
15. Inspect patient's skin for presence of burns.

INTERNAL AUTOMATIC DEFIBRILLATORS AND INTERNAL AUTOMATIC CARDIOVERSION DEFIBRILLATION

Recently developed, internal cardioversion or defibrillation treats patients who are at high risk of sudden cardiac death resulting from VT and VF. For patients who continue to experience life-threatening ventricular arrhythmias, despite antiarrhythmic medications or surgical or nonsurgical ablation, such a device (the internal cardioverter defibrillator [ICD] and the Automatic Internal Cardioverter Defibrillator [AICD]) may be the only life-saving alternative. The device has reduced the death rate resulting from recurring arrhythmia in patients refractory to antiarrhythmic drug therapy.

A generator is placed subcutaneously with lead wires inserted in and over the heart. The generator automatically and continuously monitors the heart rhythm. It is programmed to respond once a specific rate threshold is reached and delivers an electrical current of 25 j to the heart within 10 to 35 seconds of sensing VT or VF. It repeats the shock if the arrhythmia persists. External defibrillation can be applied using standard paddle placement without harming the ICD.

In selected patients with sustained VT, automatic cardioverter defibrillators have been implanted along with antitachycardia pacemakers to provide back-up in the event of tachycardia accelerated by the pacemaker.

Patient Teaching

Patient teaching is an important aspect of nursing the patient with an AICD or ICD. Before beginning, assess the patient's and significant other's emotional adaptation to the treatment. Some time and counseling may be necessary before proceeding with the details of home management.

Consult with the physician and the manufacturer for specific information on the instructions to give the patient. You will want to include the following main topics in your patient teaching plan:

- Purpose of device, how it works, other means of

treating arrhythmias, such as antiarrhythmic medications.

- Work, driving, and activity (including lifting) restrictions.
- Cough CPR. Instruct the patient to cough every 2 seconds for 30 seconds when palpitations or other prodromal symptoms are noted.
- What patient will feel when the device fires and actions to be taken by others. The patient should be told to keep a record of how often the device fires to inform the physician.
- Electrical and magnetic concerns.
- Medical identification and an ICD identification card are mandatory.
- The need to inform the physician if beeping tones from the generator are heard.
- The importance of follow-up appointments with the physician.
- Exercise regimen.

In addition, include the following in teaching the family:

- CPR.
- Actions to take if ICD malfunctions.
- Actions to take when ICD fires.
- Touching the patient when ICD fires will not result in injury, only mild muscular contraction.
- EMT service and emergency rooms in the area.

Magnetic and Electrical Concerns

Normal household appliances and small electric motors will not interfere with the ICD. However, contact with strong magnetic fields may cause the device to fire or malfunction. The patient should not touch the antenna of a ham or citizen's band radio or the spark plug or distributor wire of a running car or lawn mower. The patient should also stay clear of radio or television transmitting towers and avoid using diathermy or electrocautery. The ICD will trigger airport weapon detectors but will not be affected by them.

Support Groups

The clinical population with this implanted device has unique psychological and social needs. Support groups for AICD recipients and their families are useful in assisting nurses to meet those needs.

BIBLIOGRAPHY

American Heart Association. Standards and guidelines for cardiopulmonary resuscitation and emergency cardiac care. *JAMA,* Jun. 6, 1986, 255 (21): 2841.

American Heart Association. *Textbook of Advanced Cardiac Life Support.* Dallas: American Heart Association, 1987.

Cooper DK, Valladares BK, Futterman LG. Care of the patient with the automatic implantable cardioverter defibrillator: a guide for nurses. *Heart & Lung,* Nov., 1987, 16(6, part 1): 640-8.

Crocetti SS, DeBorde R, Falsetti J, Pardoe P. AICD: Some lifesaving advice. *Am. J. Nurs.,* Sept., 1986, 86(9): 1006-8.

Dance D, Yates M. Nursing assessment and care of children with complications of congenital heart disease. *Heart & Lung,* May, 1985, 14(3): 209-14.

De Borde R, Aarons D, Biggs M. The automated implantable cardioverter. *AACN Clin. Issues Crit. Care Nurse,* Feb., 1991, 2(1): 170-7.

DeSilva RA, Graboys TB, Podrid PJ, Lown B. Cardioversion and defibrillation. *Am. Heart J.,* Dec., 1980, 100(6): 881-95.

Dibianco R, Esses M III, Horowitz LN. Nondrug treatment for arrhythmias. *Patient Care,* Feb. 15, 1991, 25(3): 24-8, 37-42, 45.

Fisher JD, Kim SG, Mercando AD. Electrical devices for treatment of arrhythmias. *Am. J. Cardiol.,* Jan. 15, 1991, 61: 45A-57A.

Guzzetta CE. The person requiring cardiopulmonary resuscitation. *In* Guzzetta CE, Dossey BM (eds). *Critical Care Nursing: Bodymind Tapestry.* St. Louis: The CV Mosby Co., 1984.

Higgins CA. The AICD: a teaching plan for patients and families. *Crit. Care Nurse,* Jun. 1990, 10(6): 69-74.

Horowitz LN. The implantable cardioverter defibrillator. *Pract. Cardiol.,* Apr., 1991, 17(4): 61-2.

Hurst JW (ed-in-chief). *The Heart, Arteries, and Veins.* 7th ed. New York: McGraw-Hill, 1990.

Kay GN, Plumb VJ, Dailey SM, Epstein AE. Current role of the automatic implantable cardioverter-defibrillator in the treatment of life-threatening ventricular arrhythmias. *Am. J. Med.,* Jan., 1990, 88(1N): 25N-34N.

Kerber RE. When and how to perform cardioversion. *Hosp. Ther.,* Mar., 1985, pp. 44-53.

Keren R, Aarons D, Veltri EP. Anxiety and depression in patients with life-threatening ventricular arrhythmias: Impact of the implantable cardioverter-defibrillator. *PACE,* Feb., 1991, 14(2 Pt. 1): 181-7.

Koler JA, Dracup K. Psychosocial adjustment of patients with ventricular dysrhythmias. *J. Cardiovasc. Nurs.,* Feb., 1990, 4(2): 44-55.

Lehmann MH, Steinman RT, Schuger CD, Jackson K. The automatic implantable cardioverter defibrillator as antiarrhythmic treatment modality of choice for survivors of cardiac arrest unrelated to acute myocardial infarction. *Am. J. Cardiol.,* Oct. 1, 1988, 62: 803-5.

Mann DL, Maisel AS, Atwood JE, Engler RL, LeWinter MM. Absence of cardioversion-induced ventricular arrhythmias in patients with therapeutic digoxin levels. *J. Am. Coll. Cardiol.,* Apr., 1985, 5(4): 882-90.

Noel DK, Burkke LJ, Martinez B, Petrie K, Stack T, Cudworth KL. Challenging concerns for patients with automatic implantable cardioverter defibrillators. *Focus Crit. Care,* Dec., 1986, 13(6): 50-8.

Saksena S, Mehta D, Krol RB, Tullo NG, Saxena A, Kaushik R, Noglia J. Experience with a third generation implantable cardioverter-defibrillator. *Am. J. Cardiol.,* Jun. 15, 1991, 67: 1375-84.

Singer I, Kupersmith J. AICD Therapy: drug/pacemaker interactions and future directions. *Prim. Cardiol.,* Jul., 1990, 16(7): 67-73.

Singer I, Kupersmith J. AICD Therapy: implantation techniques and clinical results. *Prim. Cardiol.,* June, 1990, 16(6): 37-49.

Spence MI. Cardioversion. *In* Millar S, Sampson L, Soukup M. *AACN Procedure Manual for Critical Care.* Philadelphia: WB Saunders, 1985.

Spence MI. Defibrillation. *In* Millar S, Sampson L, Soukup M. *AACN Procedure Manual for Critical Care.* Philadelphia: WB Saunders, 1985.

Thomson JE, Olash J. Antitachycardia pacing with cardioverter-defibrillator backup for malignant ventricular dysrhythmias. *J. Cardiovasc. Nurs.,* Feb., 1990, 4(2): 33-43.

Veseth-Rogers J. A practical approach to teaching the automatic implantable cardioverter-defibrillator patient. *J. Cardiovasc. Nurs.,* Feb., 1990, 4(2): 7-19.

Vinsant MO, Spence MI. *Commonsense Approach to Coronary Care.* 5th ed. St. Louis: The CV Mosby Co., 1988.

Wilson L, Miller PG. The automatic implantable cardioverter defibrillator: A lifesaving device. *Am. J. Nurs.,* Sept., 1986, 86(9): 1004-7.

CHAPTER THIRTEEN

Pacemakers

▶ **GOAL**

You will be able to identify and describe the various pacing theories and modes, and the primary indication of temporary and permanent cardiac pacing.

▶ **OBJECTIVES**

After studying this chapter you should be able to do the following:

1. Describe the major pacing modes.
2. Identify the cardiac chamber(s) stimulated.
3. Define pacing codes.
4. Describe primary nursing responsibilities in temporary transvenous endocardial pacing.
5. Describe primary nursing responsibilities in permanent transvenous endocardial pacing.
6. Describe primary nursing responsibilities in temporary epicardial and temporary external (transcutaneous) pacing.
7. Identify components of the teaching plan for patients with permanent pacemakers.
8. Identify common pacemaker electrocardiographic rhythms.

Once used only for the patient with intractable bradycardia, pacemaker therapy is now used in a variety of clinical settings to treat tachy- and bradyarrhythmias. Regardless of the arrhythmia being treated, various pacemaker therapies have certain features in common. A catheter composed of a wire with one or more electrodes is placed in contact with the myocardium, either passed intravenously into the right atrium and/or the right ventricle to make endocardial contact or sewn directly onto the epicardium during a thoracotomy. The catheter is connected to a pulse generator that emits electrical impulses to stimulate depolarization. Emergency pacemakers, allowing faster pacing capabilities, use a transthoracic approach where the pacing catheter is inserted through a needle entering the thorax, or the pacing stimulus is delivered directly to the thorax through electrodes placed on the chest and back for an emergency noninvasive approach.

The purpose of this chapter is to define briefly the various transvenous pacing techniques used for arrhythmia control and to acquaint you with some of the characteristic electrocardiographic patterns pacemakers produce. It does not provide a full discussion of pacemaker electrocardiography and therapy; that is a study of its own.

Transvenous pacemakers may be temporary or permanent. The temporary pacemaker is an external device used for short-term treatment. Permanent pacemakers are internal and used for long-term use with the pulse generator inserted subcutaneously.

MODE

Most pulse generators are of the *demand* type. This means that they are able to sense the heart's own (intrinsic) electrical activity and fire only when the heart does not. Demand pacemakers are either *synchronous triggered* or *synchronous inhibited*.

In contrast the *fixed rate* type is *asynchronous* and does not sense the patient's own ventricular beats. Consequently, if the patient generates her own heart beats, the pacemaker is not inhibited and dual rhythms exist.

CHAMBER

The chamber of the heart that is stimulated may be the atrium, the ventricle, or both in sequence. *Atrial pacing* is achieved by placing the pacing catheter into the right atrium. It is indicated for use in patients who have normal atrioventricular (AV) conduction but require atrial stimulation because of sinus node dysfunction. The atrial stimulation produces a spike or pacing artifact on the ECG followed by a P wave and normal conduction to the ventricles.

Ventricular pacing is achieved with the pacing catheter inserted into the right ventricle. The ventricle is stimulated and results in a complex, preceded by a spike, that looks like a ventricular ectopic beat on the ECG.

The *A-V sequential* pacing mode enables the atria to contract before the ventricles, mimicking more closely the

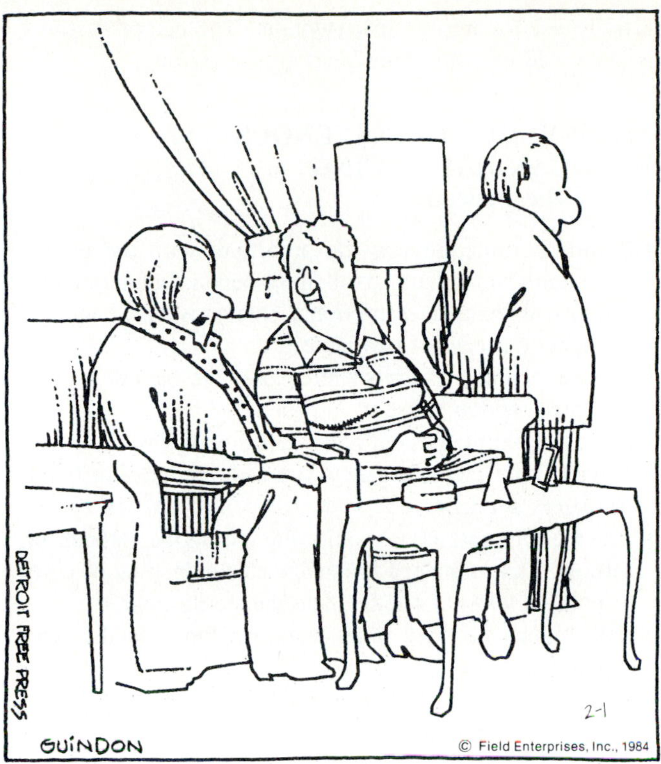

"Now that Jesse has a pacemaker, he's become as accurate, up to 15 seconds a year, as a quartz watch."

normal conditions. The advantage to this mode over the ventricular mode is that the atrial kick is not lost. The pattern on the ECG consists of a spike preceding a P wave and a spike preceding the QRS complex. The PR interval is set to accomodate a wide range of AV intervals.

PACEMAKER CODES

Many pacing combinations and modes are available. A coding system has been developed so the type of pacemaker can be communicated using three or four letters.

The first letter represents the chamber that is paced.

A = Atrium.
V = Ventricle.
D = Dual, or both.

The second letter denotes the chamber that is sensed.

A = Atrium.
V = Ventricle.
D = Dual, or both.
O = Neither is sensed—the pacemaker's rate is fixed rather than demand.

The third letter represents the manner in which the pacemaker operates.

T = Triggered (e.g., triggered by a sensed beat).
I = Inhibited (e.g., inhibited by a sensed beat).
D = Both inhibited and triggered.
O = Neither triggered nor inhibited.

The fourth letter denotes a special function such as rate responsive pacing or antitachycardia pacing.

Combinations encountered in clinical pacing include:

VVI Ventricular Synchronous Demand. The ventricle is paced, the ventricle is sensed, and the pacemaker operates by being inhibited when the patient has his/her own QRS complex (so it is demand). The pacemaker fires when the patient's ventricular rate falls below a certain preset level. This is a very common type of pacemaker.

DVI Atrioventricular Sequential Pacemaker. Both the atrium and ventricle are paced but only the ventricle is sensed, and the pacemaker operates by being inhibited when there is ventricular depolarization. So if the patient generates a spontaneous QRS complex, the pacemaker will not fire because it has been inhibited. When the patient does not generate ventricular depolarization, the pacemaker senses this and discharges both atrial and ventricular stimuli in sequence. The interval between these two stimuli, the A-V interval, is a programmable feature. The A-V interval is analogous to the PR interval. During the A-V interval, the sensing may or may not be continuous. If sensing is continuous the mode of operation is known as *noncommitted*. If sensing does not occur during the A-V interval, the mode of operation is called *committed*. Committed pacing systems put out a ventricular stimulus whenever an atrial stimulus is emitted, regardless of whether or not normal conduction proceeds to the ventricles and results in spontaneous ventricular depolarization.

VOO Ventricular Asynchronous Fixed Rate. The ventricle is paced; there is no sensing mechanism. There is neither inhibition nor triggering because the pacemaker fires at a fixed rate regardless of the patient's own intrinsic rhythm. It is easy to see how potentially problematic this type of pacemaker could become if the patient developed a rhythm of his/her own. This type of pacemaker is not used frequently.

VAT Atrial Synchronous Triggered. The ventricles are paced, the atria are sensed, and the pacemaker fires when triggered. In other words, the pacemaker is able to sense atrial depolarization and responds with a ventricular paced beat after a preset time interval. This mode is rarely used.

VDD Atrial Synchronous Pacemakers. The ventricles are paced, both the atria and the ventricles are sensed, and the pacemaker works by both triggering and inhibition. The pacemaker senses atrial depolarization and triggers a ventricular paced beat. If the patient has his/her own QRS complex, though, the pacemaker will not fire. This pacemaker can function in either the VAT or VVI modes.

VVT Ventricular Synchronous Triggered. The ventricles are paced, the ventricles are sensed, and the pacemaker functions by being triggered. When ventricular depolarization is begun, the pacemaker triggers a stimulus and a spike is seen at the start of the QRS complex. If an intrinsic ventricular depolarization does not occur, the pacemaker stimulates a ventricular beat. The VVT pacemaker mode is not in common use.

AAI Atrial Synchronous Demand. The atria are paced, the atria are sensed, and the pacemaker functions by inhibition. If the patient's own SA node fails, this pacemaker stimulates the atria to depolarize. Normal conduction proceeds through the AV node and ventricles. This mode may only be applied to patients with intact AV conduction.

DDD Pacemakers. Both atria and ventricles are paced, both are sensed, and the pacemaker functions by both inhibition and being triggered. This pacemaker mode functions by triggering atrial depolarization when there is no intrinsic atrial depolarization and triggers a ventricular depolarization when there is no QRS after a P wave.

VVIR Ventricular Rate Responsive (Adaptive). The ventricles are paced. The ventricles are sensed. The pacemaker is inhibited by ventricular sensed events, and the pacing rate is determined by the activity of a sensor-circuitry system designed to increase or decrease heart rate depending on cardiovascular requirements.

DDDR Dual Chamber Rate Responsive (Adaptive). This pacemaker has the same properties and capabilities of a DDD pacemaker, coupled with the same sensor circuitry of the VVIR. It is the ideal pacemaker for the patient with AV block and sinus node dysfunction.

PACEMAKER THERAPY FOR TACHYARRHYTHMIA CONTROL

Pacemakers used in the treatment of tachyarrhythmias consist of implantable and temporary types. Certain implantable pacemakers are programmed to sense a tachycardia and respond with the pacemaker firing stimuli at a normal fixed rate range, delivering stimuli at different times during the tachycardia, and eventually interrupting the tachycardia circuit. This is known as *underdrive pacing*.

Another mode responds to the tachycardia with strategically timed stimuli during the tachycardia, eventually interrupting the tachycardia. This type is known as a *scanning pacemaker*.

Still another type responds to a tachyarrhythmia with rapid, fixed-rate pacing at a rate faster than the tachycardia. This is known as a *burst pacemaker,* a type of overdrive pacing. Overdrive pacing is also used when ectopic activity occurs during slow rhythms. The ectopic activity is depressed by pacing the heart at a faster rate.

TEMPORARY TRANSVENOUS ENDOCARDIAL PACING

Before the Procedure

- If time permits, review the procedure with the patient and significant others, explaining benefits of temporary pacing, movement restrictions, safety aspects, and the therapeutic aspect of treatment.
- After explaining the procedure, have the patient sign an informed written consent.
- Make certain the patient has a functioning IV.
- Make certain the emergency cart with defibrillator is immediately available.
- Provide for continuous monitoring during the catheter insertion. You may need to change electrode sites so wires or patches will not contaminate the sterile field.
- Have lidocaine and other antiarrhythmic medications available.
- Familiarize yourself with the basic functioning of the external pulse generator.
  - On/off switch.
  - Indicator light or needle for pacing and sensing.
  - Stimulus output dial: know the proper setting for the pacing output required for the patient.
  - Sensitivity dial: know the proper setting for your patient.
  - Rate control or stimulus frequency control: know the proper rate for your patient.
  - AV interval control: for dual chamber models, know the correct interval to ensure proper AV synchrony.

During the Procedure

- Reassure the patient, administer analgesia as ordered, and assist as required.
- Maintain patent airway and assist ventilations as needed.
- Monitor the patient's heart rhythm continuously.
- When the catheter reaches the right ventricle, frequent VPBs and short runs of VT are often noted.
- Record in nurse's progress notes the following:
  - Location of electrode catheter.
  - Pacing mode.
  - Rate.
  - Milliamperes.

After the Procedure

- Maintain patent airway.
- Assess for signs and symptoms of the following:
  - Myocardial perforation.
  - Cardiac tamponade.
  - Pneumothorax.

  - Hemothorax.
  - Pulmonary embolization.
- Observe insertion site for hematoma, swelling, and drainage.
- Obtain 12-lead ECG.
- Continue cardiac monitoring. Watch for ventricular ectopy, which is common, and proper pacemaker capture and sensing.
  - Identify the features of the paced rhythm for the particular pacing mode (e.g., DVI).
  - Locate the stimulus artifact and differentiate it from the QRS complex.
  - Differentiate the paced P waves and QRS complexes from spontaneous beats.
  - Measure the A-V interval (for A-V sequential pacemakers) from the atrial pacing artifact to the ventricular pacing artifact.
  - Determine the QRS axis of the paced beats and observe for changes in the axis.
  - Determine the paced rate.
  - Analyze the paced rhythm for consistency of capture and notify the physician of loss of capture (when the pacing artifact does not produce a ventricular depolarization).
  - Analyze the rhythm for evidence of proper sensing. For example, when there is a spontaneous depolarization, the pacemaker should not fire again until the interval between the spontaneous beat and subsequent paced beat is the same as the interval between two paced beats.
  - Observe for competitive rhythms, such as runs of atrial, junctional, or ventricular tachycardia or accelerated rhythms, and other arrhythmias.
  - Observe for changes in the electrical axis of the pacing spike.
  - Note increases or decreases in amplitude of the pacing spike and QRS complex.
- Obtain chest x ray to check for catheter position.
- Assess vital signs every 15 minutes until stable.
- Assess for signs and symptoms suggestive of thrombophlebitis, catheter-induced arrhythmias, and infection.
- Assess level of discomfort and administer analgesics as needed.
- Inspect and clean site daily using sterile technique.
- Keep pacing wires stabilized by restricting the patient's movement as necessary.
- Cover the dials of the pacemaker with transparent tape to prevent accidental malfunctions.
- Obtain chest x rays and 12-lead ECGs as clinically indicated.
- Note pacing parameters every shift.

Pacing Therapy Discontinuation

When temporary transvenous pacing is no longer required, the lead wires are removed.

  - Explain what you are about to do to the patient, assuring that the procedure will not be painful.
  - Turn unit off.
  - Remove dressings.
  - Remove any sutures holding the pacing wire in place.
  - Watch the monitor for ectopic beats during removal.
  - Remove the wire, checking that it is intact.
  - Dress the site with sterile bandage.
  - Observe the site periodically for bleeding.

Preventing Pacemaker Malfunction

Electrical hazards. With a temporary transvenous pacemaker, your patient has an electrical connection from the outside of his body to the inside of his heart. Small electrical currents that normally would not be harmful may now initiate ventricular fibrillation! Protecting your patient from stray current is a nursing responsibility. Make certain that all equipment in the patient's environment is grounded, including the bed, intravenous infusion pump, cardiac monitor, any pressure monitoring devices, electric shaver, heating pad, bedside light, and anything else that comes in contact with the patient. Static electricity must also be eliminated.

Accidental malfunction. Protect the pulse generator from accidental adjustments with clear tape over the dials. A child or confused patient may require additional safety measures including restraints.

Electrical countershock. If your patient requires countershock, either defibrillation or cardioversion, make certain the paddles stay clear of the pacing wires and pulse generator.

PERMANENT TRANSVENOUS ENDOCARDIAL PACING

Preoperatively

- Explain the procedure to the patient. Include the following:
  - Where the procedure will be performed.
  - The patient will receive medications to facilitate relaxation during the procedure.
  - The patient will be asked to lie very still during a portion of the procedure.
  - Approximately how long it will take.
- Obtain informed written consent.
- Check the patient's allergies and post on front of chart.
- Document the arrhythmia for which the pacemaker is being used.
- Obtain a 12-lead ECG.
- Order a coagulation profile (according to hospital policy).
- Insert IV in left arm with an extension (surgeon usually works from the patient's right side).

- Place electrodes off chest and away from insertion site, making certain that lead wires will not cross the sterile field or impede fluoroscopic visualization.
- Prepare the site according to hospital procedure.
- Administer preoperative medication as ordered by physician.

Postoperatively

- Assess for the following complications of lead displacement.
  - Pacemaker failure to capture.
  - Failure of pacemaker to sense.
  - Myocardial perforation with cardiac tamponade.
  - Perforation of interventricular septum.
- Take blood pressure and pulse according to standard postoperative policy.
- Assess the peripheral pulses and determine if pulse deficit exists.
- Obtain a chest x ray.
- Assess for the patient's perception of palpitations, chest pain, shortness of breath, dizziness, light-headedness, and discomfort during pacing, such as hiccoughs or a thumping feeling.
- Bed rest first 24 hours, gentle range-of-motion exercises.
- Assess for signs and symptoms of local and systemic infection.
- Check dressings, perform wound care with sterile technique.
- Administer short-term antibiotics as ordered by physician.
- Obtain 12-lead ECG.
- Analyze the ECG.
  - Identify the features of the paced rhythm for the particular pacing mode (e.g., DVI).
  - Locate the stimulus artifact and differentiate it from the QRS complex.
  - Differentiate the paced P waves and QRS complexes from spontaneous beats.
  - Measure the A-V interval (for AV sequential pacemakers) from the atrial pacing artifact to the ventricular pacing spike.
  - Determine the QRS axis.
  - Determine the paced rate.
  - Analyze the paced rhythm for consistency of capture and notify physician if loss of capture (pacing artifact is not followed by a ventricular depolarization) occurs.
  - Analyze the rhythm for proper sensing (e.g., when there is a spontaneous depolarization, the pacemaker should not fire again until the interval between the spontaneous beat and subsequent paced beat is the same as the interval between two paced beats.)
  - Observe for competitive rhythms, such as runs of atrial, junctional, or ventricular tachycardia or accelerated rhythms and other arrhythmias.
  - Observe for changes in the electrical axis of the paced beats.
  - Note increases or decreases in amplitude of the pacing spike and QRS complex.

Electrical Countershock

If a patient requires countershock, either defibrillation or cardioversion, it is necessary to protect the pacemaker from electrical current damage. If anterior paddle placement is used, place the paddles at least 4 to 5 inches from the pulse generator and leads. Anteroposterior placement would lessen the likelihood of pacemaker damage, since current would then flow at right angles to the pacemaker and lead system. Although newer models of pacemakers are built to resist damage from countershock, paddles should never be placed directly over the pulse generator or lead. After countershock is completed, check the monitor for proper functioning of the pacemaker.

Teaching Plan for the Patient with a Permanent Pacemaker

Patients who have had permanent pacemakers implanted require comprehensive patient teaching to ensure continued therapeutic benefit. Presented here is a teaching plan in outline form. The plan should be supplemented with specific information from the manufacturer's literature and individualized to fit your patient's situation.

I. Anatomy and physiology of the heart.
   A. Circulation through the heart.
      You will need to determine the appropriate level of instruction for your patient. It is not necessary to include any more than the following. You will often elect to delete some of this information.
      1. Right atrium.
      2. Right ventricle.
      3. Pulmonary circulation.
      4. Left atrium.
      5. Left ventricle.
      6. Systemic circulation
   B. Normal electrical activation of the heart.
      1. Depolarization of the atria.
      2. The AV junction.
      3. Depolarization of the ventricles.
II. The patient's rhythm disturbance.
   A. Compare the patient's rhythm disturbance to normal electrical functioning.
   B. The pacemaker and how it will help the patient's rhythm disturbance.
   C. Symptoms of low cardiac output.
      1. Light-headedness.
      2. Syncope or near-syncope.

3. Fatigue.
4. Symptoms of congestive heart failure.
   a. Shortness of breath.
   b. Cough.

III. Pacemaker.

A. The pulse generator.
   1. Location of generator under skin.
   2. Diagram where the electrodes are located in the heart.
   3. How pacemaker causes chambers to depolarize.
   4. Provide the name of the manufacturer, the model, expected term of battery life, and in understandable terms, the mode. Fill out the identification card with the model and serial numbers.
   5. Arrange for the patient to obtain a "Medic Alert" bracelet or necklace.

B. Proper functioning of the pacemaker.
   1. Rate at which pacemaker has been set.
      a. Demand pacemakers will be activated when the patient's rate falls below a certain value.
         (1) Patient must know how to take his/her own pulse.
         (2) At least one significant other should know how to assess the pulse rate.
      b. Some pacemakers respond to increased activity with increased rate.
         (1) If your patient has this type of pacemaker, find out what the maximum preset rate is for the patient and inform the patient.
      c. Write the rate parameters on an information sheet for the patient.

C. Antitachycardia pacemakers.
   1. Patient-activated pacemakers.
      a. Patient must be able to recognize the onset and termination of the tachycardia.
      b. Teach the patient how to activate this mode by one of the following means:
         (1) A magnet is held over the implantation site to induce slow competitive or underdrive pacing.
            (a) Instruct the patient on the length of time magnet is applied.
         (2) Radiofrequency unit that has programmable rates for underdrive or overdrive pacing.
            (a) Apply unit to the chest over the implanted receiver.
            (b) Press button to activate. Depress button for 1 to 3 seconds (consult manufacturer's literature).
            (c) Number of bursts necessary to achieve desired outcome (usually one or two).
            (d) Teach the patient how and when to change the batteries.
      c. Make certain the patient knows what emergency room or physician to contact if reprogramming or disabling the pacemaker is necessary.

D. Maintenance of the pacemaker.
   1. Transtelephonic checking of function.
      a. Teach the patient how to use this service and the recommended times for its use.
      b. Technique.
         (1) Patient places electrodes on both wrists (electrodes are connected to a transmitter box).
         (2) Place telephone receiver on the transmitter and a recording is taken over the telephone.
   2. Instruct the patient to take his or her pulse on a regular basis and whenever symptoms of low cardiac output are present. Instruct patient to notify physician if pulse is slower than the preset rate.
   3. Inform when the patient needs to have a new battery pack inserted. (Lithium iodide batteries last 6 to 12 years.)
   4. Clinical examinations.
      a. Inform the patient that above measures do not take the place of regular clinical examinations.
      b. List dates and times for clinic visits on the patient's information sheet.
   5. Inform the patient of extrinsic sources of radiofrequency and electromagnetic interference.
      a. Devices that do affect pacemaker function.
         (1) Therapeutic electrocautery.
         (2) Diathermy.
         (3) Electrosurgical units.
      b. Devices that may affect pacemaker function (depending on model, proximity to device, and duration of exposure).
         (1) Microwave ovens.
         (2) High-energy electromagnetic fields.
            (a) Industrial arc-welding units (resistance welding).
            (b) Smelting inducting furnaces.
            (c) High-energy radar, television, and radio transmitters; CB radios with high-powered amplifiers.
            (d) Radiofrequency-activated fuses for explosives.
         (3) Electric razors.

(4) Ultrasonic dental instrument cleaners.
(5) Car, tractor, and boat engines (if working on the motor).

c. Devices that do not affect pacemaker function.
(1) Household appliances.
(2) Household tools.
(3) Theft-prevention equipment (pacemaker may activate the alarm).
(4) Magnetometer weapon detectors (pacemaker may activate the alarm).
(5) Garage door openers.

TEMPORARY EPICARDIAL PACING AFTER OPEN-HEART SURGERY

The purpose of temporary epicardial pacing postoperatively is to provide access for diagnostic recordings and therapeutic electrical stimulation of the myocardium. Pacing wires are attached during surgery to the right atrium and the right ventricle. The pacemaker is then available to pace the heart during periods of bradycardia or to terminate a tachyarrhythmia. Arrhythmias that commonly occur in the postoperative cardiothoracic patient include sinus bradycardia, junctional and atrial arrhythmias, and AV block. The epicardial wires are removed after the time when arrhythmias are most frequent, usually 5 days.

The nurse must guard against and observe for the following epicardial pacemaker wire-related complications that may be encountered during the postoperative period.

- Dislodgement and misidentification of wires.
  - If wires are not to be connected to an external pulse generator, coil them loosely, wrap in a gauze pad, and tape to the dressing. Make certain the ends of the wires are visible and readily accessible by covering them with transparent nonconductive, water-resistant tape.
  - Identify the atrial and ventricular wires.
    Atrial wires are usually shorter and on the patient's right side.
    Ventricular wires are usually longer and on the patient's left side.
- Local and systemic infection.
  - Cleanse area around insertion site daily with iodine or 70% isopropyl alcohol.
  - Apply antibiotic ointment.
  - Cover with sterile gauze pad and tape securely.
- Myocardial irritation causing arrhythmias.
- Cardiac tamponade.
- Microshocks that may initiate ventricular fibrillation.
  - The source may be any stray current.
  - The patient's environment must therefore be electrically insulated.

After removal of the wires the nurse must take the following steps:

- Examine wires to make sure they are intact.
- Apply elastic bandage to site.
- Check the patient's blood pressure and heart rate every 15 minutes for 1 hour and then at least every 4 hours.
- Observe closely for signs of hemorrhage, hemopericardium, and cardiac tamponade: hypotension, distended neck veins, elevated central venous pressure, distant heart sounds, pulsus paradoxus.

TEMPORARY EXTERNAL PACING

Temporary external (transcutaneous) pacing is a method of pacing the heart externally and noninvasively. A method used on a temporary basis, the external pacemaker does not pose risks to the patient that an invasive pacemaker would. There is no risk of infection, hemopericardium, or endocardial irritation.

Indications for its use are the same as for transvenous pacing: bradyarrhythmias or overdriving tachyarrhythmias. The electrodes can be applied with the machine turned off for prophylactic use in a patient who is at risk for developing a bradyarrhythmia. Or the electrodes can be applied quickly for emergency use.

The electrical currents pass through the thorax, anterior to posterior, causing depolarization of the myocardium. As the current passes, the muscles of the thorax also contract, often causing the patient some discomfort.

Follow these guidelines in initiating external pacemaker therapy:

- If time permits and the patient is conscious, explain the therapy to the patient. Prepare the patient for the probability of muscle discomfort during pacing but offer assurance that the lowest amount of energy required will be used and that the physician will order medication to facilitate rest.
- Wash entire chest and left side of the back with soap and water. Rinse and dry well.
- Do not apply any flammable liquids such as alcohol or benzoin.
- Place ECG electrodes on the patient's chest and choose a lead that displays a strong signal.
- Apply the pacing electrodes. They are usually labeled front and back.
  - Back electrode (applied first): Place between the spine and left scapula at the level of the heart (Fig. 13-1, *A*).
  - Front electrode: Place on anterior chest in the V_2, V_3, or V_5 lead position (Fig. 13-1, *B*). The best location is determined by the stimulation threshold, the minimum amount of energy (milliampere) required to stimulate the myocardium. The V_3 position offers the advantage of minimizing pectoral and trapezius muscle stimulation. If possible, use a position that will not interfere with placement of defibrillation paddles.
- Determination of stimulation threshold by the physician.
  - The front electrode is placed at various locations, and

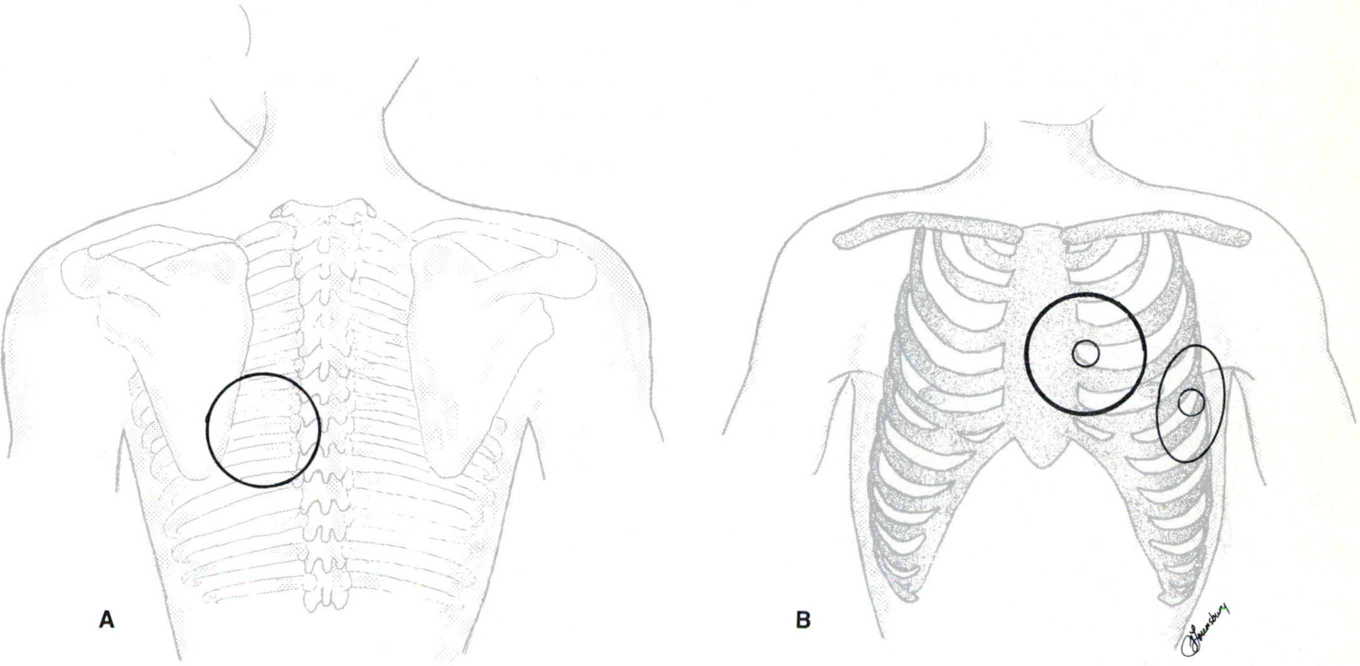

FIGURE 13-1 Electrode sites for transcutaneous pacing. **A,** Site for back electrode. **B,** Sites for front electrode.

increasing milliamperes (mA) are administered until ventricular depolarization occurs.
  - When the desirable location has been established, remove the adhesive pads and attach the electrode.
- After the electrodes are in place, the mA is increased 2 to 3 above threshold. Average threshold is approximately 55 mA; large individuals require higher mA.
- Assess the patient's level of discomfort. Administer medications to promote comfort and rest as ordered.
- Check pacemaker function.
  - Note wide pacing spikes followed by QRS complexes on the ECG.
  - Each QRS should be accompanied by a palpable radial pulse.
  - Changes in the patient's physiologic homeostasis, such as electrolyte imbalance, hypoxia, drug therapy, myocardial ischemia, and congestive heart failure may affect mA required to pace.
- Check vital signs frequently.
  - Take blood pressures in the right arm as falsely elevated blood pressures have been reported in the left arm with external pacing.
- Record in nurse's notes the following:
  - The amount of time the pacemaker is functioning.
  - The mA setting on the pacemaker.
  - How well the patient is tolerating the procedure.
- Check the pacing electrodes every 2 to 4 hours to make certain they are securely attached. Change pacing electrodes as needed, usually every 24 to 48 hours. If the patient is diaphoretic, electrodes may need to be changed more frequently. When changing the electrodes, turn the power switch to "monitor" position.
- Assess threshold daily or with changes in the patient's condition.

COMMON PACEMAKER ECG RHYTHMS

The following rhythm strips present the main features of various types of paced rhythms, both normal and abnormal. These examples are not intended to provide sufficient instruction for proficiency with pacemakers and their ECG characteristics but to familiarize you with some of the most common forms. (Figs 13-2 to 13-16).

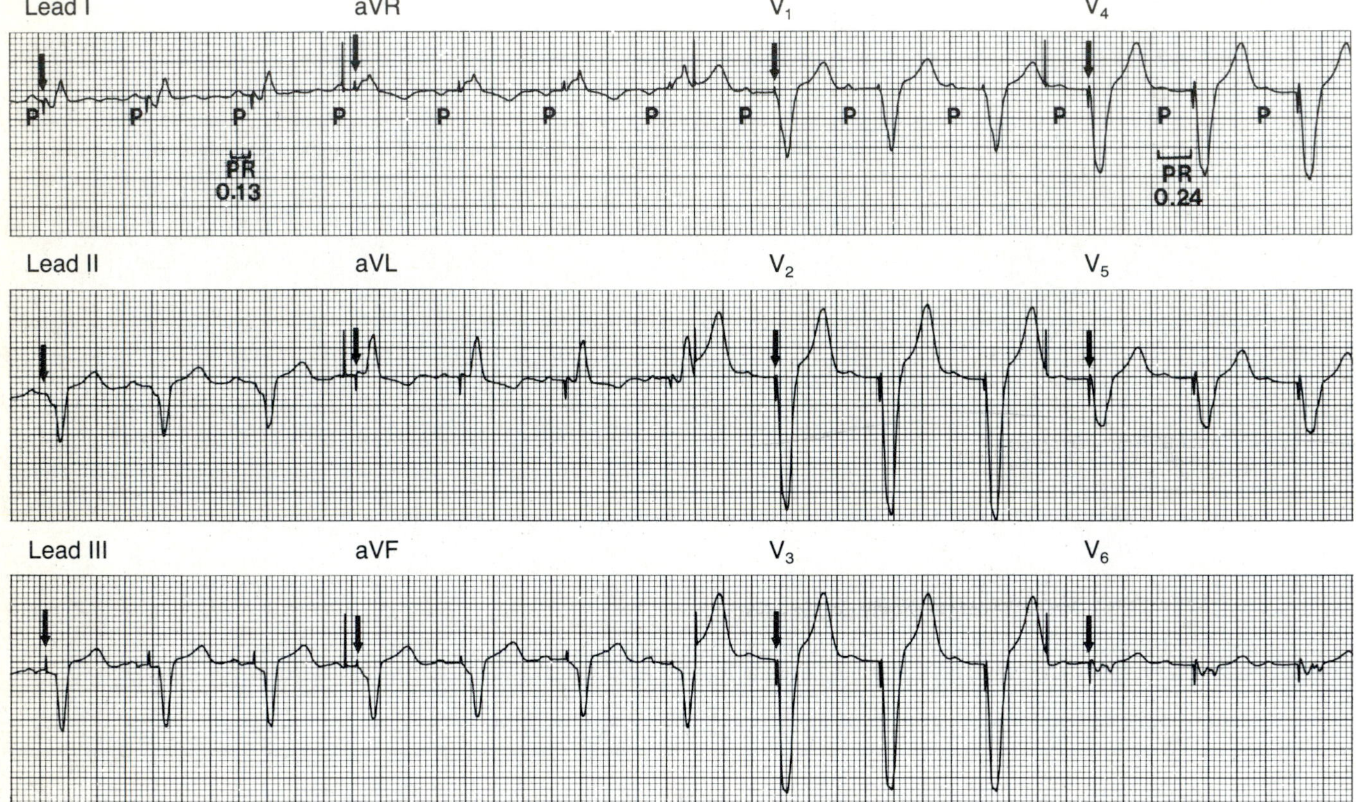

FIGURE 13-2 VVI pacemaker, also known as a *ventricular demand pacemaker.* This pacing style is a standard mode that was one of the first pacing methods used. The pacing catheter in the ventricle senses and paces only the ventricles. The atria beat independently, resulting in AV dissociation. Pacing spikes *(arrows)* precede ventricular complexes. P waves are coincidentally preceding QRS complexes, but note that they do not bear a constant relationship to the QRS complexes. The atrial rate is 85 bpm and regular throughout and the paced ventricular rate is 82 bpm and regular. Note in leads II and V_1 the pacing spike is not visible. Discuss the reasons for this and possible clinical implications. The QRS complex is 0.18 seconds in duration and has an axis of −76 degrees.

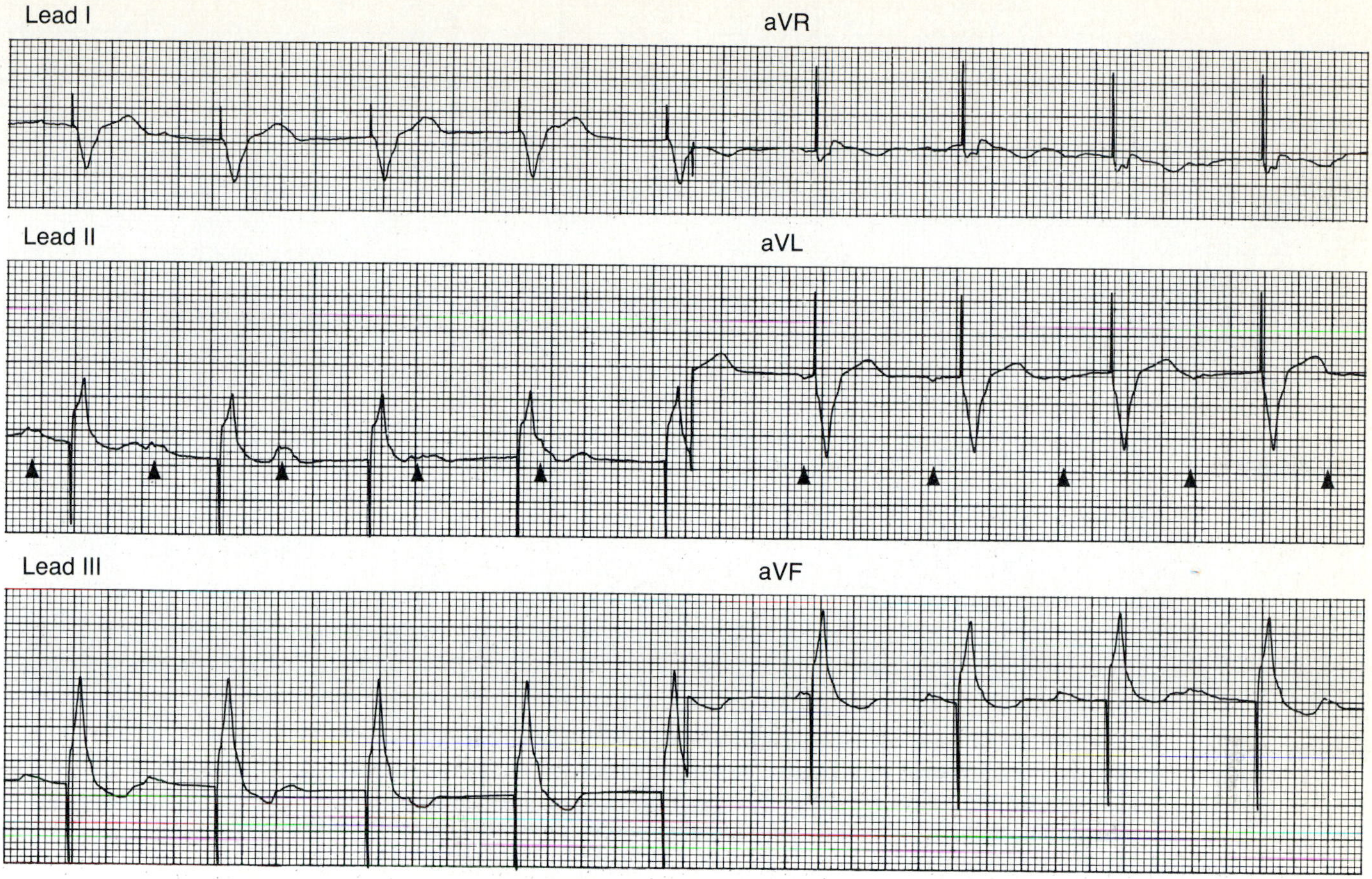

Lead I

aVR

Lead II

aVL

Lead III

aVF

FIGURE 13-3 VVI pacemaker with unipolar epicardial lead. Again note AV dissociation. The atria *(arrows)* and ventricles are beating independently. Also note the QRS axis. It is right and inferior. This is because the epicardial lead is attached at the upper anterior septum.

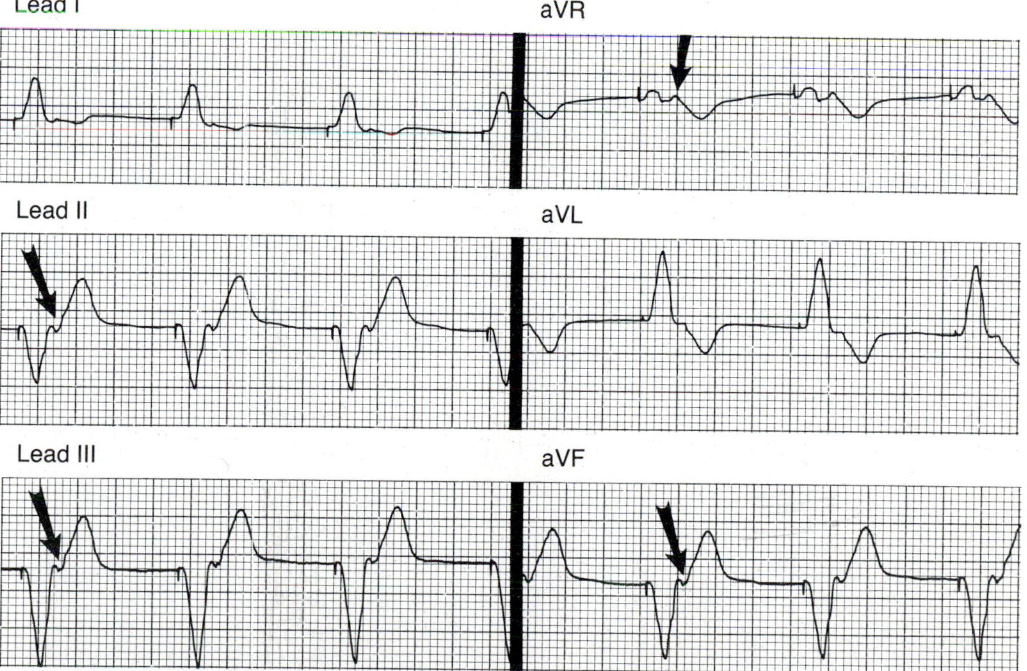

FIGURE 13-4 VVI pacemaker with 1:1 V-A (ventricular-to-atrial) conduction. In this tracing the VVI pacemaker causes ventricular depolarization after the spike. The ventricular depolarization in turn causes retrograde atrial depolarization, best seen on the inferior leads II, III, and aVF with inverted P waves *(arrows)*, and on aVR with upright P waves.

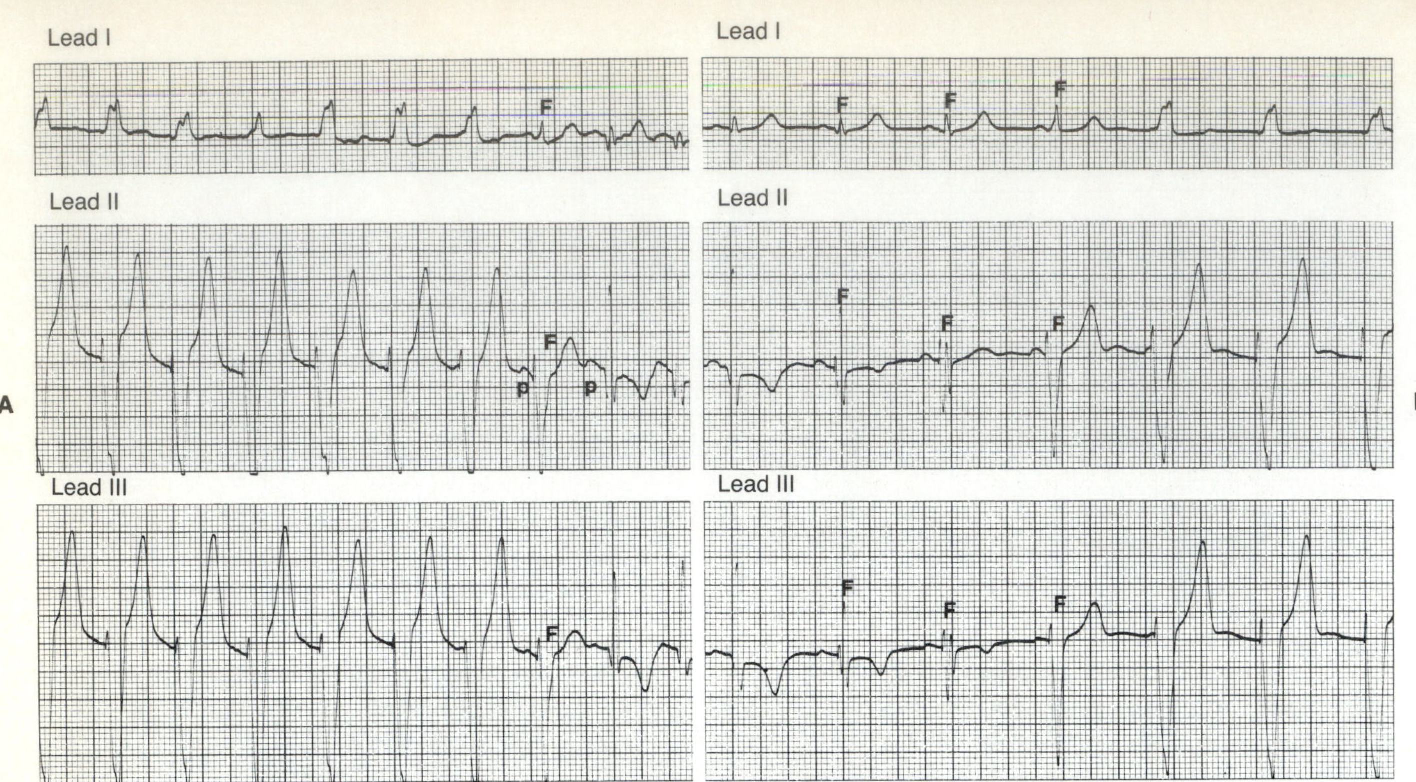

FIGURE 13-5 Activity sensing rate responsive ventricular pacemaker. This ECG was obtained from a 20-year-old male with sinus node disease. **A,** His pacemaker senses activity and increases the ventricular rate. **B,** With activity, the pacemaker rate increases to 120 bpm and with rest, the rate decreases to 78 bpm. Note fusion beats produced when a sinus-conducted QRS and ventricular paced beat occur simultaneously (F). Sinus P waves capture the rhythm in the last three beats in **A** and the first four beats in **B.** AV dissociation then ensues when the paced ventricular rhythm usurps in the last three beats in **B.**

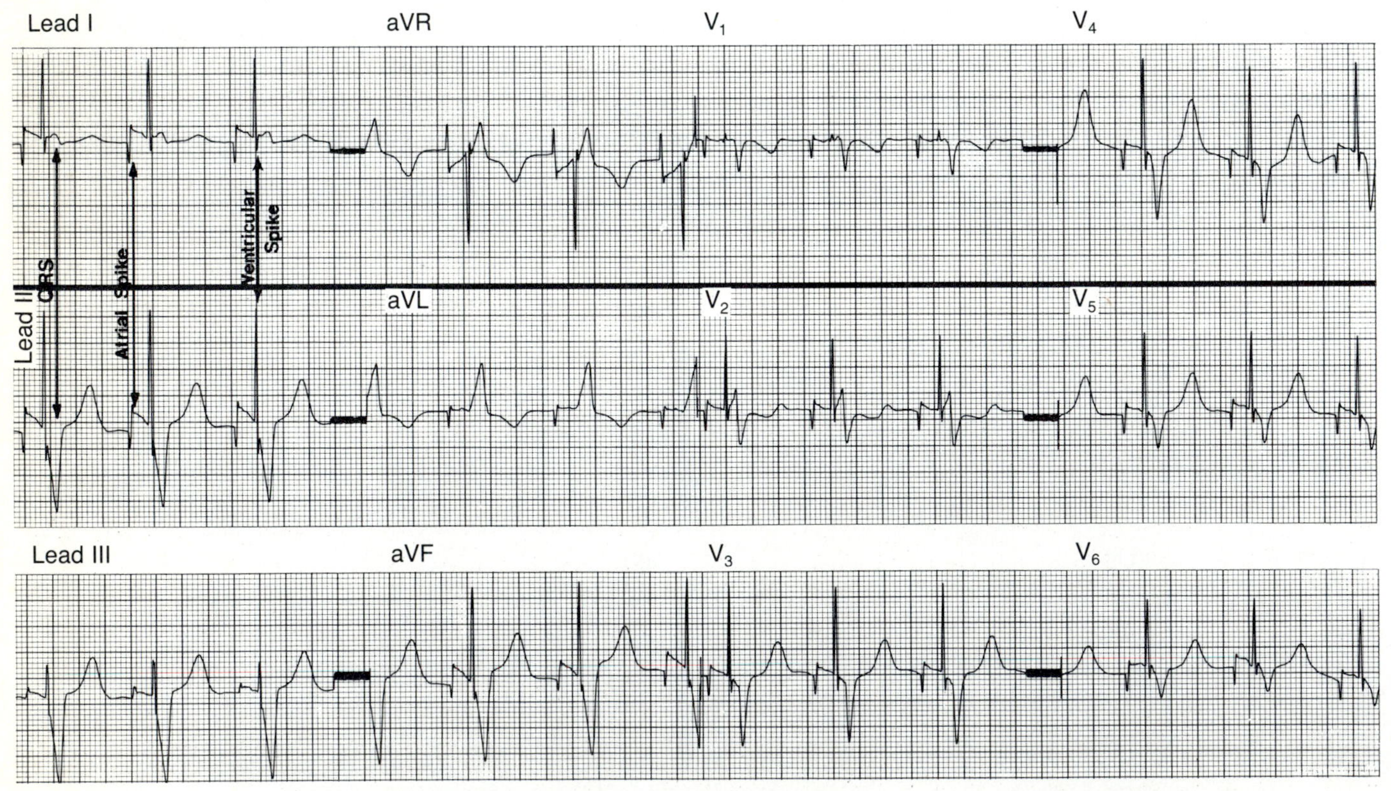

FIGURE 13-6 DVI pacemaker, also known as *AV sequential pacemaker.* Note pacing spikes *(arrows)* that precede both P waves and QRS complexes. The atrial spike precedes the ventricular spike by 0.16 seconds. Why do ventricular pacing spikes not show on lead aVL? When you have difficulty locating the beginning and end of a particular ECG component, such as the QRS complex in lead I, find a QRS that is displayed well simultaneously. In this case the QRS is displayed well in leads II and III. Locate the QRS in the exact location on lead I.

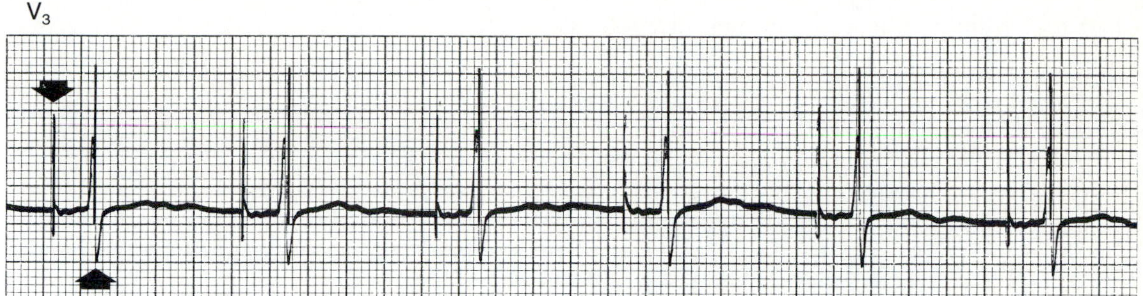

FIGURE 13-7 Committed DVI pacemaker. The term *committed* pertains to sensing during the interval from the atrial to ventricular spikes, the *A-V interval.* If the pacemaker's mode of operation is committed, then sensing does not occur during the A-V interval. So if an atrial spike producing a P wave conducts normally to the ventricles, resulting in spontaneous ventricular depolarization, and therefore a normal QRS complex, the pacemaker has not sensed this activity and a ventricular spike is emitted. Once the atrial stimulus has been emitted, the pacemaker is *committed* to produce a ventricular stimulus. This often results in fusion beats and so-called pseudo-fusion beats. In this example atrial pacing spikes appear regularly (*arrow* above tracing) followed by normal conduction to the ventricles. In each QRS, however, is a pacing spike (*arrow* below tracing). This is because the pacemaker fired simultaneously with ventricular depolarization. This is considered a normal finding with this type of pacemaker.

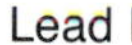

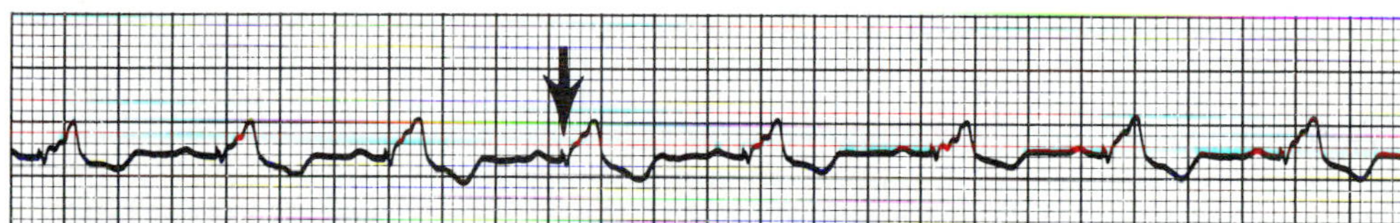

Lead II

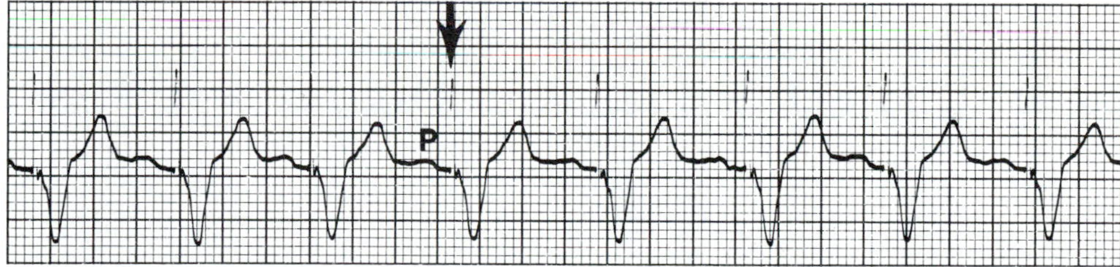

Lead III

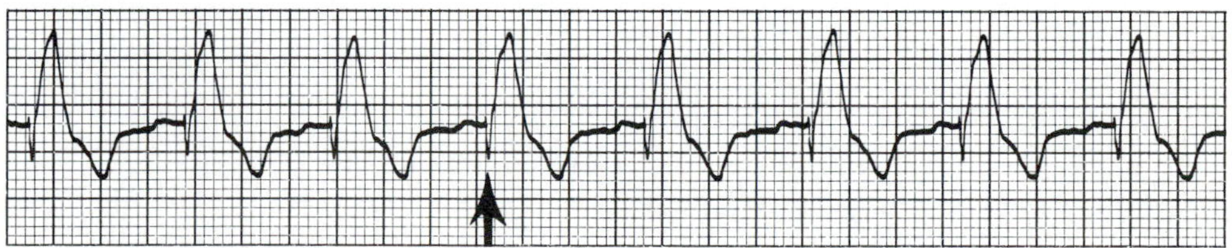

FIGURE 13-8 DDD pacemaker. In this example the atrial rate is adequate and therefore inhibits the atrial pacing component. Each of the patient's P waves *(P)* is followed within 0.16 seconds by a pacing spike *(arrow)* and subsequent paced ventricular complex.

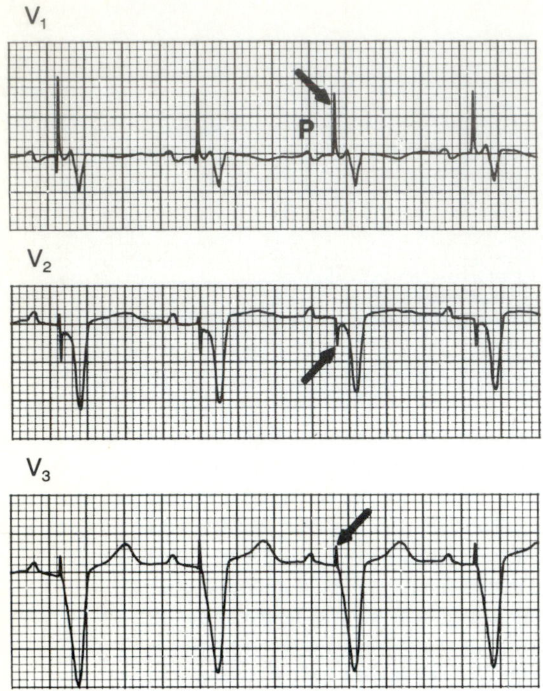

FIGURE 13-9 VDD pacemaker. In this example, normal P waves *(P)* are followed within 0.16 seconds by pacing spikes *(arrows)* producing ventricular complexes.

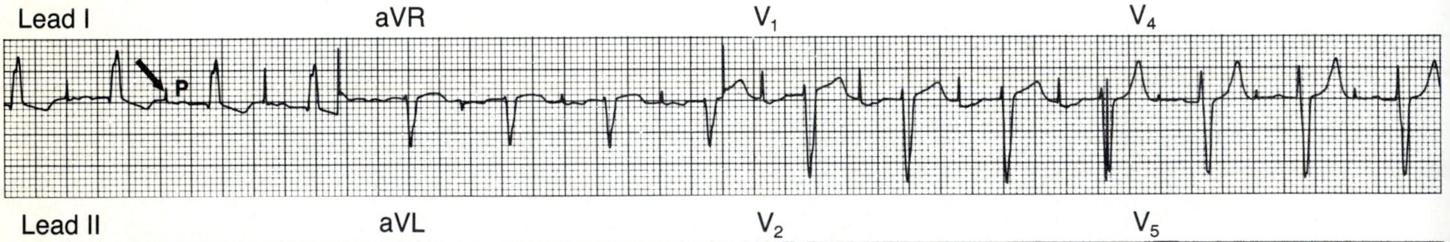

FIGURE 13-10 Atrial pacemaker. Atrial pacing spikes *(arrows)* result in P waves *(P)*. Normally conducted QRS complexes follow the P waves.

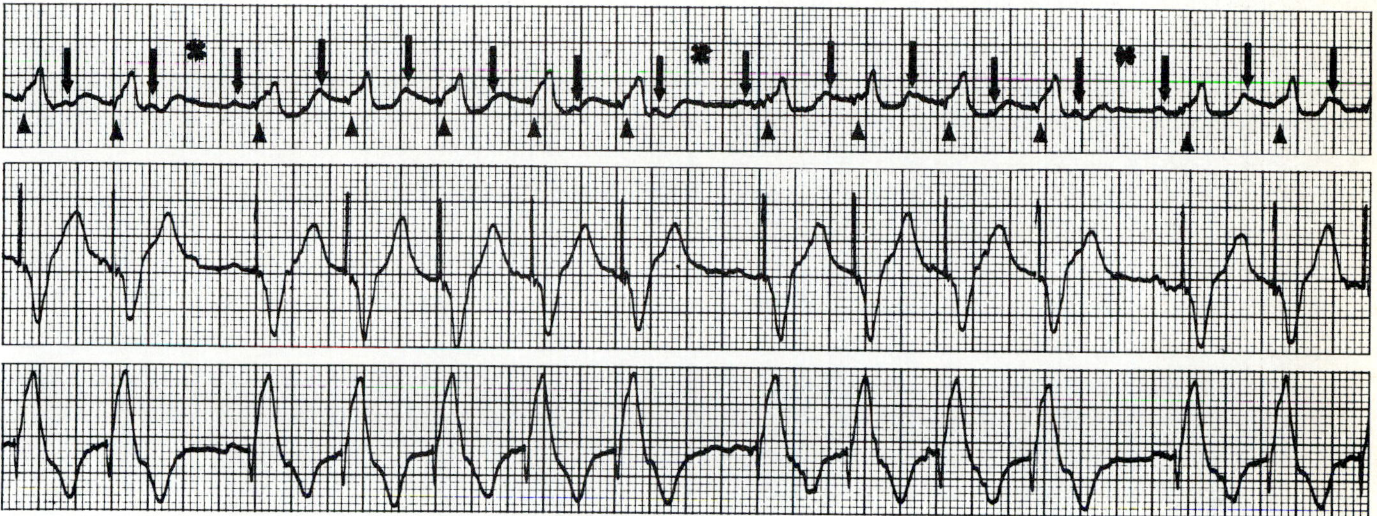

FIGURE 13-11 DDD pacemaker Wenckebach block, a normal function. As the atrial rate exceeds the programmed upper rate limit of the pacemaker, a Wenckebach pattern of ventricular pacing is produced. These three tracings are simultaneous recordings. Note regular occurring atrial activity (*arrows* above trace). Pacing spikes (*arrow* below trace) following the P waves occur with increasing distance until a pacing spike and QRS complex do not occur at all *(asterisk)*.

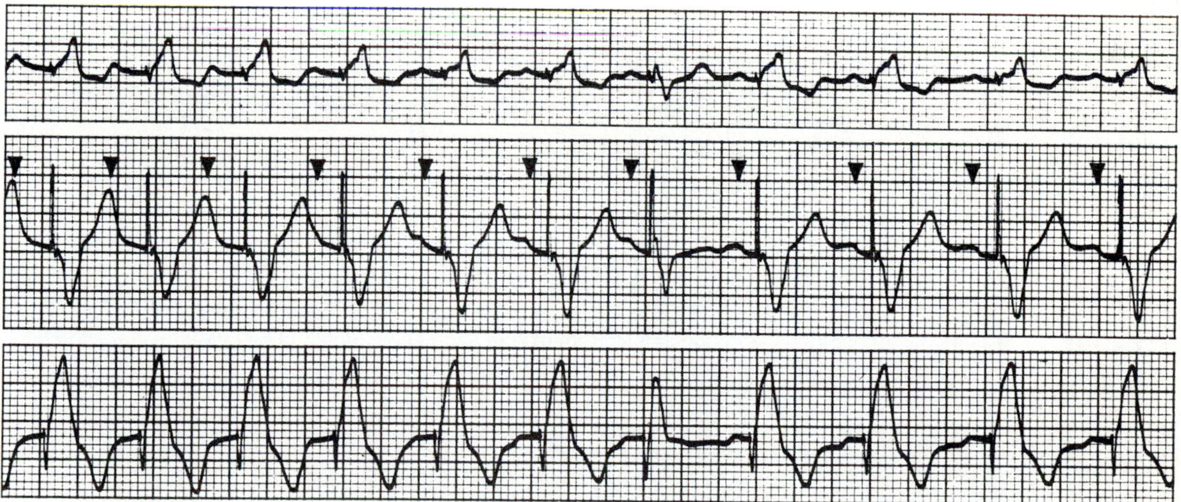

FIGURE 13-12 DDD pacemaker with atrial tracking during deceleration of heart rate. In these three simultaneous tracings, note as the atrial rate *(arrow)* declines, the atrial lead senses this and emits ventricular pacing spikes at a correspondingly slower rate.

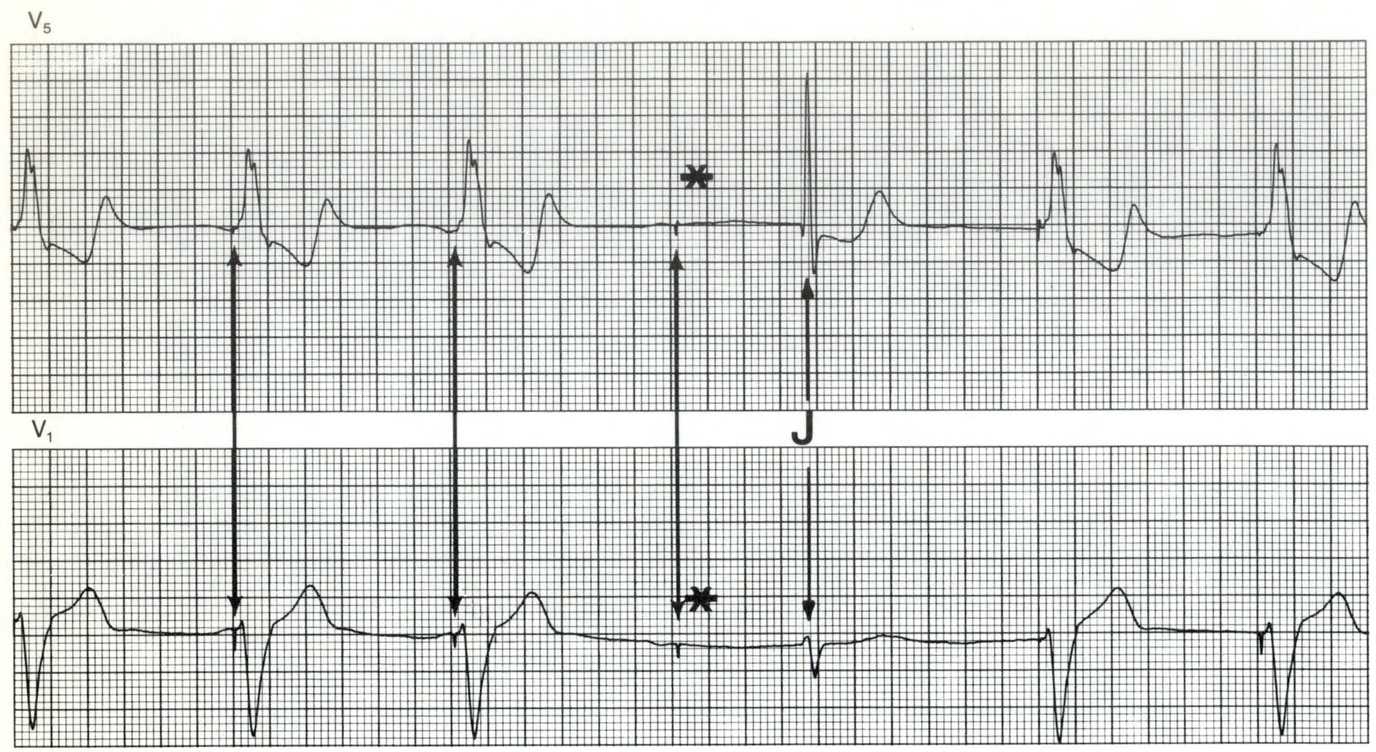

FIGURE 13-13 Failure to capture. Ventricular pacing spike *(arrow)* fails to produce a ventricular beat *(asterisk)*. The resultant pause in ventricular activity is interrupted by a junctional escape beat *(J)*.

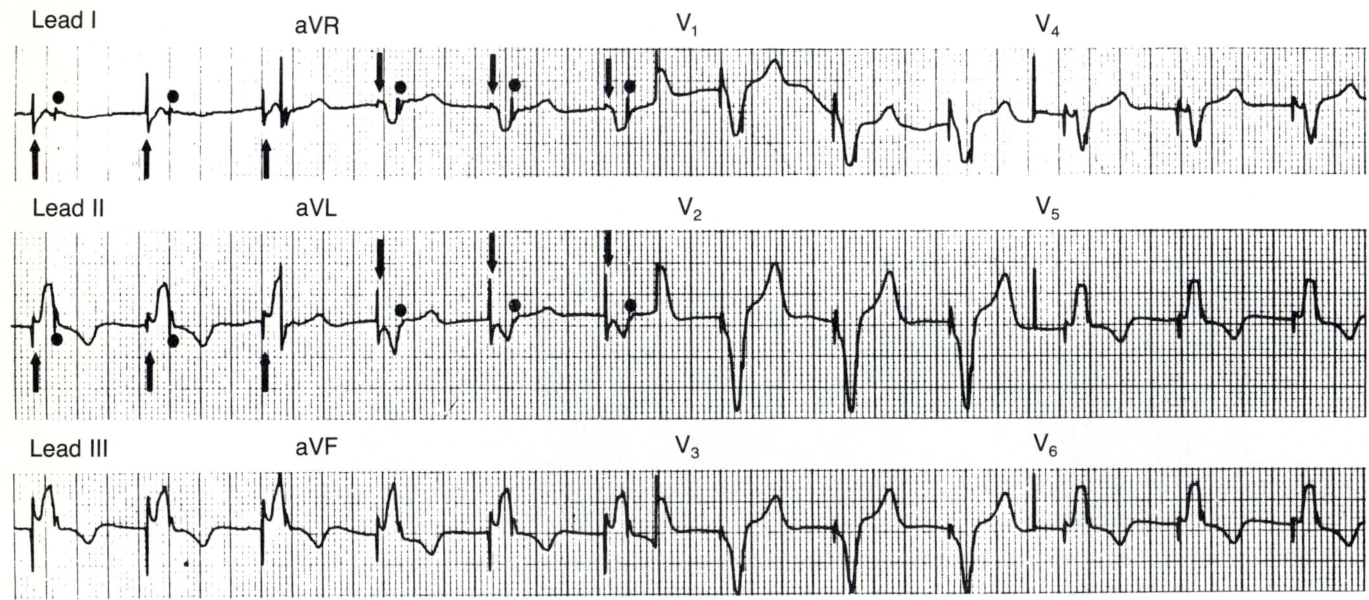

FIGURE 13-14 Pacemaker malfunction? Post-open-heart surgery with external dual chamber pacemaker. The atrial and ventricular epicardial wire leads are reversed, resulting in ventricular pacing from the atrial output *(arrows)*. Atrial capture does not appear to occur. The wire lead attached to the atrium results in only a pacing spike *(dot)*.

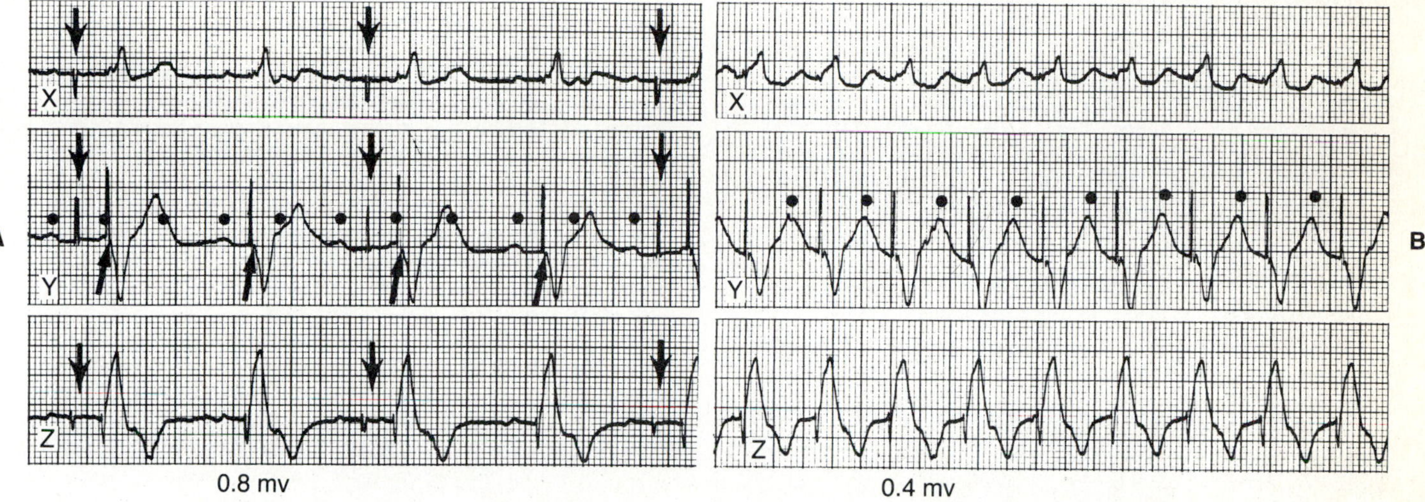

FIGURE 13-15 DDD pacemaker with atrial sensing malfunction. **A,** With sensitivity set at 0.8 mV, P waves *(dots)* are not all sensed so atrial pacing spikes appear (*arrows* above tracing) at times. Ventricular pacing occurs regularly (*arrows* below tracing). **B,** After reprogramming the sensitivity in the atrium to 0.4 mV, left atrial sensing is adequate to track atrial activity even during exercise as shown. Note there are no atrial pacing spikes. Each P wave is followed by a ventricular pacing spike with resultant ventricular paced beat. With the rate at 120 bpm, the P waves are all perched on top of the T waves.

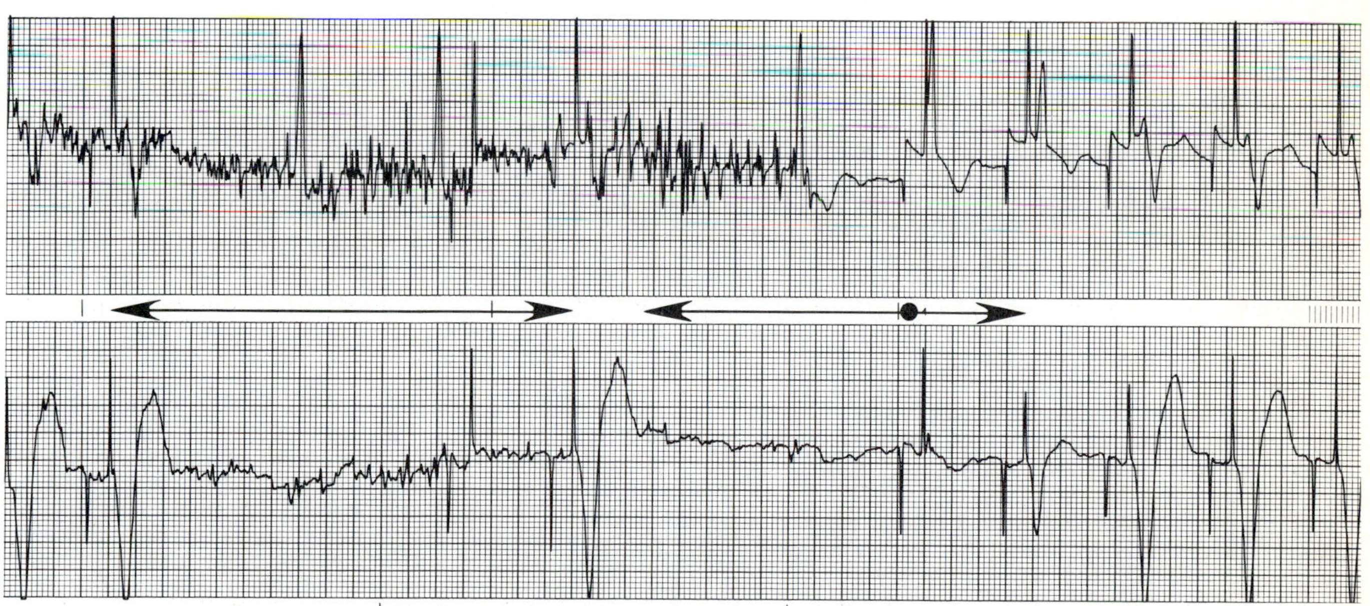

FIGURE 13-16 Myopotential inhibition of DVI pacemaker. The sensing circuit of the pacemaker detects electrical activity from forceful skeletal muscle contraction in the vicinity of the pulse generator resulting in output inhibition. Note the long asystolic pauses *(arrows)* in these two simultaneous recordings.

BIBLIOGRAPHY

Barredo J. What really interferes with pacemakers? *Am. J. Nur*, Dec., 1990, 90(12): 24-5.

Braunwald E. (ed). *Heart Disease: A Textbook of Cardiovascular Medicine*. 3rd ed. Philadelphia: WB Saunders, 1988.

Dibianco R. Estes M III, Horowitz LN. Nondrug treatment for arrhythmias. *Patient Care,* Feb. 15, 1991, 25(3): 24-8, 37-42, 45.

Fisher JD, Kim SG, Mercando AD. Electrical devices for treatment of arrhythmias. *Am. J. Cardiol.,* Jan. 15, 1991, 61: 45A-57A.

Frye SJ, Yacone LA. Cardiac pacing: A nursing perspective. *In* Hakki A-H (ed). *Ideal Cardiac Pacing* (Vol. 31 in the Series *Major Problems in Clinical Surgery*). Philadelphia: WB Saunders, 1984.

Hurst JW (ed). *The Heart, Arteries, and Veins*. 7th ed. New York: McGraw-Hill, 1990.

Kesten KS, Norton CK. *Pacemakers: Patient Care, Troubleshooting, Rhythm Analysis*. Baltimore: Resource Applications, 1985.

Mickus D, Monehan KJ, Brown C. Exciting external pacemakers. *Am. J. Nurs.,* Apr., 1986, 86(4): 403-5.

Persons CB. Transcutaneous pacing: Meeting the challenge. *Focus Crit. Care,* Feb., 1987, 14(1): 13-9.

Porterfield L, Porterfield JG. What you need to know about today's pacemakers. *RN,* Mar., 1987, pp. 44-9.

Roman-Smith P. Pacing for tachydysrhythmias. *AACN Clin. Issues Crit. Care Nurs.,* Feb., 1991, 2(1): 132-9.

Singer I, Kupersmith J. AICD Therapy: drug/pacemaker interactions and future directions. *Prim. Cardiol.,* July, 1990, 16(7): 67-73.

Spielman, SR. New advances in cardiac pacemaking. *In* Hakki A-H (ed). *Ideal Cardiac Pacing* (Vol. 31 in the Series *Major Problems In Clinical Surgery*). Philadelphia: WB Saunders, 1984.

Thomson JE, Olash J. Antitachycardia pacing with cardioverter-defibrillator backup for malignant ventricular dysrhythmias. *J. Cardiovasc. Nurs.,* Feb., 1990, 4(2): 33-43.

Vinsant MO, Spence MI. *Commonsense Approach to Coronary Care*. 5th ed. St. Louis: The CV Mosby Co., 1988.

Witherell CL. Permanent pacemakers. Questions nurses ask. *Am. J. Nurs.,* Dec., 1990, 90(12): 20-8.

Index

Page numbers in italics indicate illustrations; t indicates tables.

Q

R